HANDBOOK OF DIABETES

Hana Smalley

ALLIED
HEALTH
PRESS

Handbook of Diabetes

Author: **Hana Smalley**

Allied Health Press
4164 Lakeshore Road
Burlington ON L7L 1A4
Canada
www.alliedhealthpress.com
Email: orders@arclereducation.com

ISBN: 978-1-77956-863-2

ABOUT THE AUTHOR

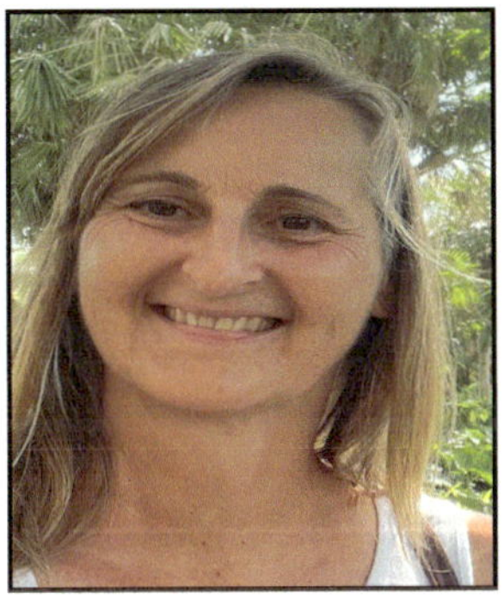

Hana Smalley is a pharmacist with a passion for optimizing medications for her patients and educating her audiences in the field of pharmacology. Hana has a diverse background in hospital care, long term care, geriatric and palliative care, pain management, and education. With her expertise in pharmacology, she has been working with multi-disciplinary care teams along with patients and care-givers to adjust medications, including collaborating with prescribers to select medications, identify and prevent adverse reactions, and educate medical staff and patients about the risks and benefits of medications. She also creates and teaches pharmacology courses for beginner and advanced levels. Hana's academic journey includes earning her pharmacy degree from the "Université de Montréal". She further obtained a doctorate of pharmacy (Pharm.D) at the Medical University of South Carolina in Charleston, USA. Hana has vast experience as a clinician, a manager and pharmacology instructor. Her knowledge of pharmacology and passion for health makes her an asset to a care team and a key educator for health care students.

Brief Table of Contents

Detailed Table of Contents

CHAPTER 5

Other Types of Diabetes 121

CHAPTER 6

Diabetes Control and Its Measurement 147

CHAPTER 7

Management of Type 1 Diabetes 177

LIST OF FIGURES

PREFACE

The understanding of metabolic control has undergone profound shifts in the past century. Advances in science have progressively elucidated the biological mechanisms of nutrient intake, energy storage, and hormonal signals, revealing an exquisite balance maintained in the human body. Among the most crucial control mechanisms is the glucose homeostasis mechanism, which is based on finely regulated cell-to-cell communication and organ system interactions. When this balance is upset, the effects are widespread, impacting various physiological systems and necessitating complex therapeutic interventions. Clinical experience and laboratory findings have increasingly clarified these mechanisms, providing a foundation for effective treatment and diagnostic approaches.

Throughout the decades, rising morbidity and mortality trends with associated metabolic disturbances have prompted the global medical community to examine causes and effects at both the population and individual levels. This has spurred the creation of clinical specialties and public health agendas founded on disorders that interfere with the body's ability to regulate glucose. Different genetic susceptibility, environmental challenges, immune responsiveness, and lifestyle combined come together to influence the incidence and progression of illness. As knowledge grows and treatment options expand, the need for a handy and encyclopedic guide is increasingly greater, especially for individuals whose profession is at the boundary of both the scientific and clinical treatment of care.

This need is filled by the Handbook of Diabetes, a small and accessible guide to healthcare professionals, students, and researchers in endocrinology, internal medicine, primary care, and allied disciplines. Written as much as possible for both introductory and clinical use, the text finds a middle ground between scientific rigor and clinical relevance. It distills recent evidence-based information into chapters organized to reflect both biological principles and the spectrum of clinical presentations. With close attention to relevance, coherence, and clarity, this volume conveys information required for correct diagnosis, successful management, and ongoing patient care.

Chapter 1 is a conceptual introduction that features definitions and classifications needed for the initial understanding of the condition in all its accepted forms. It establishes the terminological accuracy and diagnostic format on which the later chapters build. Chapter 2 covers the physiological regulation of insulin, outlining mechanisms of secretion and action and the incretin effect on which postprandial glucose regulation hinges. An appreciation of this physiological standard is necessary for a proper analysis of pathological states and their therapeutic implications.

Chapter 3 reviews the epidemiological pattern and etiologic foundation of type 1 diabetes, emphasizing genetic susceptibility, autoimmune processes, and environmental triggers of the disease. Chapter 4 has its twin in the overview of type 2 diabetes against the background of lifestyle, genes, and patterns of insulin resistance. Both chapters synthesize current trends, global statistics, and risk stratification models to contextualize prevalence and incidence rates. Chapter 5 covers less common types like monogenic diabetes, secondary diabetes due to other diseases, and gestational diabetes, with observations on the diagnostic challenges and management nuances. Chapter 6 outlines the recommendations for glycemic control and outlines the methods presently used for determining glucose and glycemic trends in the long term. It includes laboratory tests, point-of-care testing, and the use of continuous glucose monitoring. Chapter 7 addresses type 1 diabetes care and includes a discussion on insulin regimens, delivery systems, education plans, and technical aids such as insulin pumps and CGM systems. The strategy combines pharmacological and behavioral treatments necessary for long-term success.

Chapter 8 proceeds with type 2 diabetes management with a focus on broad therapy from lifestyle modification to pharmacotherapy with newer drug classes that have cardiovascular and renal effects. Individualized treatment planning and algorithms are also shown in this chapter. Chapter 9 presents a comprehensive overview of acute metabolic emergencies like diabetic ketoacidosis, hyperglycemic hyperosmolar state, and lactic acidosis. Etiology, clinical presentation, diagnosis criteria, and treatment regimens are arranged systematically for easy use in the clinic. Hypoglycemia, a common life-threatening complication, is discussed in Chapter 10. It explains physiological cut-offs, risk factors, symptomatology, and protective and therapeutic approaches. Chapter 11 discusses diabetic eye disease in the form of retinopathy. The chapter addresses staging systems, screening guidelines, and intervention options such as laser and intravitreal injection.

Chapter 12 deals with diabetic neuropathy, categorizing its various types, sensory, motor, autonomic, and offering tips on symptom identification and treatment control. Chapter 13 continues the theme of complication management by dealing with diabetic nephropathy. The chapter discusses early indicators such as albuminuria, progression stages, and renal protective strategies in the form of blood pressure and glycemic control targets. Chapter 14 discusses blood lipid abnormalities, which are also quite frequent in diabetic patients, their contribution to cardiovascular risk, and their management with lifestyle and drug therapy. Chapter 15 proceeds to hypertension in diabetes, a serious comorbidity that contributes significantly to vascular disease. It gives recommendations for screening, diagnostic criteria, treatment objectives, and drug selection, focusing especially on interactions with glucose metabolism and renal function.

This book is intended for a broad readership within the health sciences. Medical students and house officers will find it a useful primer structured to facilitate rapid comprehension of essential facts and clinical judgment. Clinicians in practice, generalists, internists, endocrinologists, nurse practitioners, and diabetes educators, will appreciate its no-nonsense, straightforward format and ease of access to clinically relevant information. Researchers will also find useful summaries provided, offering current references for key concepts and points of information. Although not exhaustive in describing all controversies or new theories, the book strikes a balance between clarity and trustworthiness, making it suitable for both initial learning and quick reference during patient care. Handbook of Diabetes is designed to advise, inform, and assist. As global health systems respond to the rising workload of chronic metabolic disease, ready access to intelligible, contemporary, clinically oriented information is essential. This book is part of a joint effort, equipping its audience with the knowledge to cope with both everyday problems and innovative developments in the field.

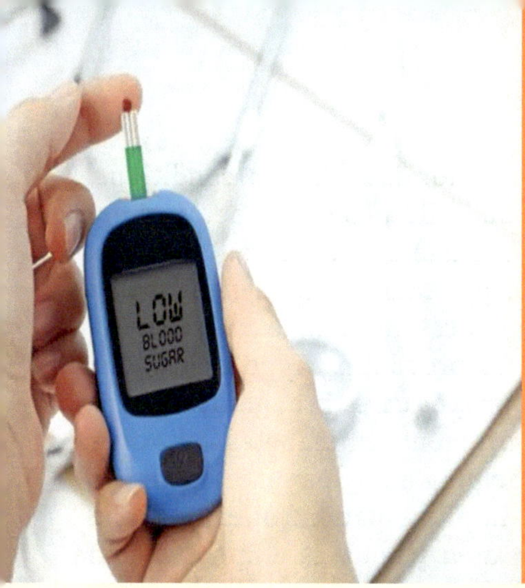

Chapter 1

OVERVIEW OF DIABETES

Contents

Introduction

Diabetes is a chronic metabolic disorder characterized by elevated levels of glucose in the bloodstream, commonly referred to as hyperglycemia. Either the pancreas does not produce enough insulin or the body does not make use of the insulin it produces. Insulin is important because it helps manage blood sugar and lets glucose enter cells to be used for energy. There are mainly two types of diabetes: Type 1, where the body's immune system attacks insulin-producing cells and causes little or no insulin, and Type 2, which is linked to insulin resistance and is often associated with being overweight and not exercising. To come up with good prevention and treatment approaches, it is important to understand these types because each one requires a different way of managing and caring for them. All over the world, diabetes is now considered a serious public health problem. The study reveals that the number of diabetes-related cases has gone up as people are living longer and the population ages.

As a result of more diabetes cases, more people are suffering from non-fatal health conditions, showing that chronic diseases are now a main concern in health globally. Because of diabetes, many people suffer from cardiovascular problems, kidney failure, and nerve damage, which all put extra pressure on the healthcare system and reduce the quality of life for patients and their families. To handle diabetes properly, people should adopt healthy habits, take medications, and learn about the disease. Promoting healthy eating and exercise is very important for preventing Type 2 diabetes, especially among people who are at risk. Also, early detection and proper care through healthcare services help reduce the problems that come with diabetes. Improvements in diabetes care over the past years include new technologies and medicines, which are helping many patients. However, the challenge remains great, as ongoing research is necessary to improve patient outcomes and reduce the overall burden of diabetes on individuals and society as a whole, as emphasized in literature that focuses on comprehensive diabetes management strategies (Livingston et al., 2020) and the overarching impact of non-fatal health losses attributable to the condition (James et al., 2018) (Figure 1.1).

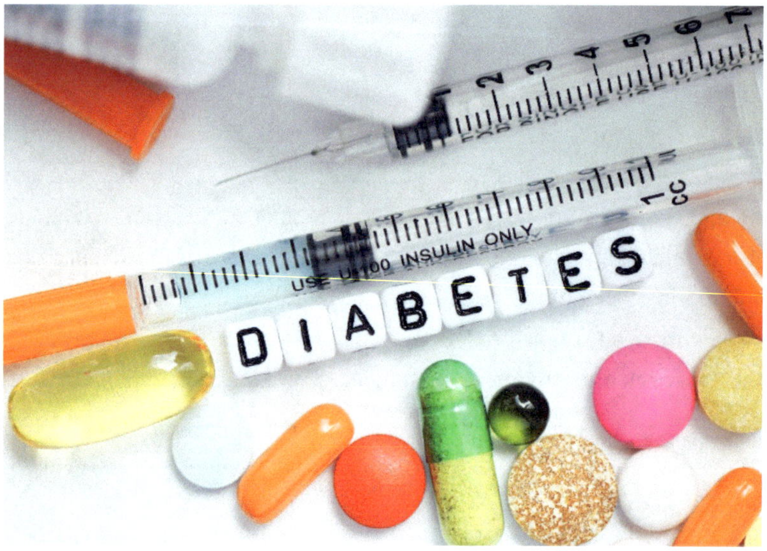

Figure 1.1. Diabetes.

Source: https://intrustcare.co.uk/wp-content/uploads/2020/06/diabetes-symptoms.jpg

1.1. Causes and Risk Factors

Some of the causes and risk factors for diabetes relate to genetics, while others are connected to how a person lives. Obesity is a major factor, since it is closely connected to the development of type 2 diabetes. Too much body fat, mainly visceral fat, may cause insulin resistance, which stops the body's cells from responding to insulin and leads to high blood glucose. Sedentary behavior also makes the problem worse, because being inactive can cause extra weight gain and disturbances in metabolism. Staying active regularly can make it easier for insulin to work and help you manage your weight, so your chances of getting diabetes are reduced. It is clear from this relationship that living a healthier life can help fight the increasing number of diabetes cases. The risk of diabetes also depends on a person's age. As people get older, their chances of getting type 2 diabetes rise a lot. The extra risk is usually linked to less exercise, different body changes, and an increase in insulin resistance. Also, older people are often diagnosed with hypertension and dyslipidemia, which can make diabetes more likely. It is very important to screen for early signs of prediabetes and diabetes among people in this group. As evidenced by research where 27.0% of participants showed undiscovered alterations in clinical parameters, early intervention can lead to effective management and the prevention of diabetes-related complications, thereby improving outcomes for aging populations (Cuffari et al., 2022).

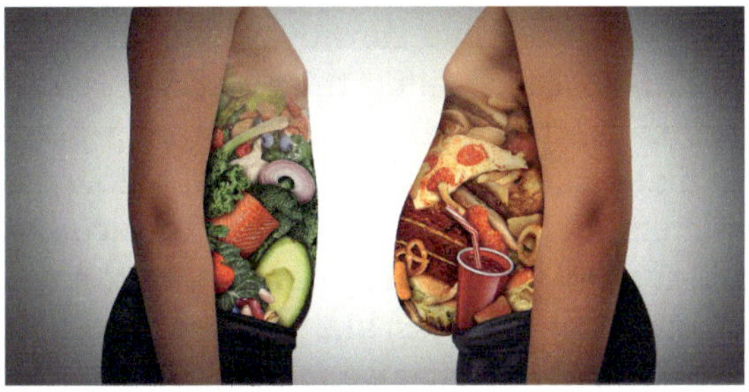

Figure 1.2. Excess body fat, particularly visceral fat, can lead to insulin resistance, a condition where the body's cells do not respond effectively to insulin, resulting in elevated blood glucose levels.

Source: https://lowcarbdownunder.com.au/wp-content/uploads/2015/04/AdobeStock_261656106-1024x510.jpeg

Family history and genes are very important when determining the risk of diabetes. If diabetes runs in the family, a person is much more likely to develop the condition, which shows that genetics plays a big role. It has been found through research that some genetic markers can affect insulin resistance and the work of beta cells, both of which are important in diabetes. In addition, environmental factors that go along with genetic background, for example, diet and economic status, can make diabetes more likely. It is necessary to consider these factors when making prevention strategies. It is important to recognize that effective intervention must address both the behavioral aspects and the genetic predispositions to create a comprehensive approach to diabetes prevention, highlighting the need for personalized healthcare strategies and community support initiatives in tackling this global health concern (Apullan et al., 2012) (Figure 1.2).

1.1.1. Genetic Predisposition and Family History

It is very important to know how family history and genetic factors can affect someone's risk of Type 2 diabetes. It has been found that those with a family background of diabetes, like relatives with the condition, are much more likely to develop it themselves. Genetics is known to play a role in diabetes, since several genes together with environmental factors can cause insulin resistance. For instance, specific studies have evidenced that even in normoglycemic adults with no clinical overt diabetes, those with a familial background may exhibit early signs of impaired glucose metabolism, suggesting that genetic susceptibility can manifest in varying degrees, underpinning the importance of family medical histories in diabetes-related assessments (Shore et al., 2001). Moreover, the way genetics affects a person's health becomes especially important when looking at obstetric factors and their lasting effects on metabolism. A comprehensive study highlighted that maternal and sibling histories of diabetes correlate strongly with the incidence of gestational diabetes Mellitus (GDM), which later progresses to Type 2 diabetes in some individuals (Chircop et al., 2003). Because of this, it is important for doctors to be more aware, as family patterns may reflect biological factors at work. Especially, while the influences of mothers are stronger, the family history of fathers does not seem as reliable in predicting diabetes risk, which points to the specific effects of genes and environment. In addition, we need to consider both the effects of genes and the way we live to understand genetic predisposition. Even though family history is important, it's also necessary to remember that diet, exercise, and lifestyle have a big impact on getting diabetes. A person's genetic makeup and the way they live can either increase or decrease the chances of getting diabetes. For this reason, people with a family background of diabetes should be advised to change their lifestyle to protect themselves from diabetes. The way genetics and environment interact in diabetes demonstrates that each individual's healthcare needs should be considered when dealing with this disease (Figure 1.3).

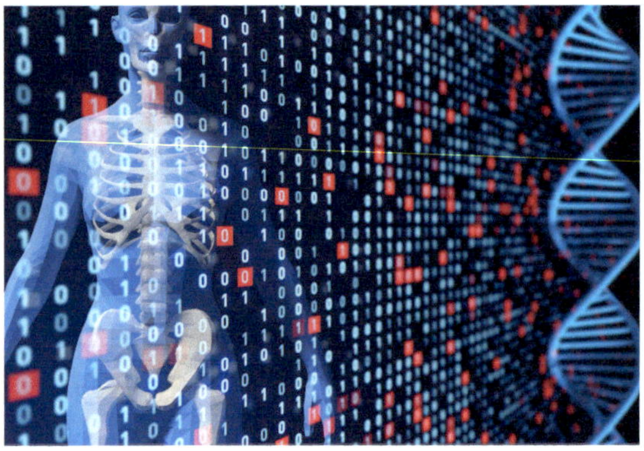

Figure 1.3. Understanding the role of genetic predisposition and family history is vital in the context of diabetes, particularly Type 2 diabetes.

Source: https://cdn.prod.website-files.com/5cdafe18a28089d0b3d79559/6802d3ec65ab0af8102e1dbe_67a5b40cfe6504fbac1524ae_1.png

1.1.2. Lifestyle Factors: Diet, Exercise, and Obesity

How much people eat, how active they are, and their weight can have a major impact on diabetes. What we eat is very important for metabolic health, so it's best to include foods rich in vitamins, minerals, and fiber in our diet. Studies have shown that a lot of sugar and processed foods can make individuals gain weight and develop insulin resistance. Because obesity is on the rise in many groups, it is obvious that people with excess weight are more likely to develop diabetes. Those who are obese have a higher chance of developing type 2 diabetes, so it is important for them to be careful with their diet and learn more about it. Ongoing dietary interventions are needed to avoid serious problems linked to diabetes. Being physically active is also very important in the discussion of lifestyle and diabetes. Regular exercise helps with weight management and improves the function of insulin thus lowering blood glucose. Both aerobic and resistance exercises have been shown to improve glycemic control and improve cardiovascular health. In addition, research finds that exercise reduces stress and lifts mood, which may help people with diabetes stick to their diet and follow their treatment plans. Yet, it is still hard to encourage individuals to exercise regularly, since there are so many social barriers, like people sitting much of the day and not having enough time. Programs that encourage fitness as a fun and reachable goal are very important for fighting against the growing number of obesity cases and diabetes. The detrimental impact of obesity on metabolic health is also associated with conditions such as polycystic ovary syndrome (PCOS), which highlights the complex relationship between weight, hormonal balance, and diabetes risk. PCOS is frequently accompanied by insulin resistance, which may result in extra weight and a higher risk of developing type 2 diabetes. Dietary changes and exercise have been proven to be useful in dealing with obesity and also for handling the symptoms and complications of PCOS. This way of looking at things demonstrates that adding lifestyle changes to diabetes care can lead to better overall management. Ultimately, public health strategies that promote awareness of the interconnectedness of diet, exercise, and obesity will be vital in forging a path forward in diabetes prevention and management, as outlined in recent studies that draw attention to these critical lifestyle components (Bernier et al., 2012; Karami et al., 2017) (Figure 1.4).

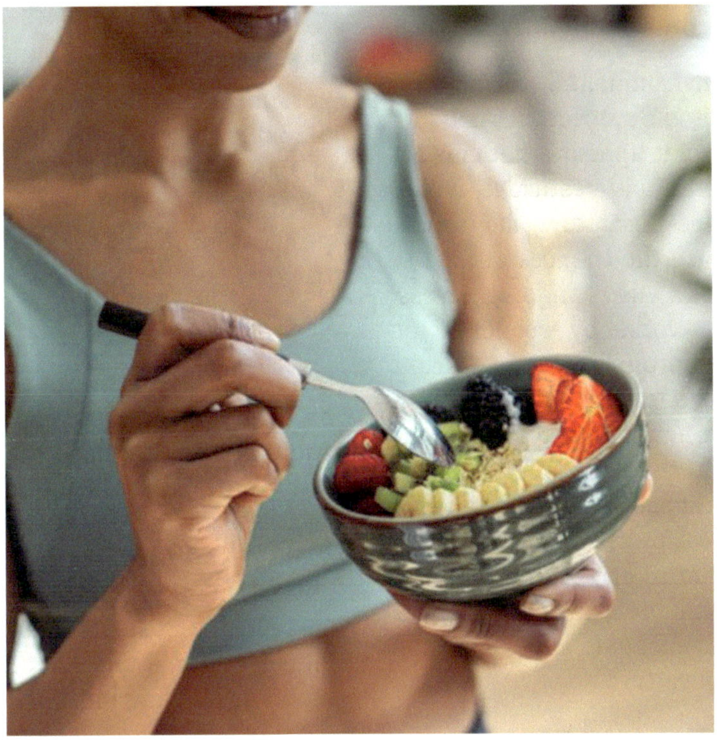

Figure 1.4. Diet plays a crucial role in determining metabolic health, with an emphasis on balanced macronutrient intake that includes whole foods rich in vitamins, minerals, and fiber.

Source: https://www.qntsport.com/img/cms/blog/what-is-healthy-eating.jpg

1.1.3. Environmental Influences and Their Impact on Diabetes Onset

Both the environment and a person's genes play a major role in the development of diabetes. Because of sedentary life, diet changes, and other lifestyle habits, diabetes is now seen more often, which proves how important it is to understand the relationship between health and the environment. Having a diet full of processed foods with lots of sugar and fat, and leading a sedentary lifestyle, can increase a person's chances of getting type 2 diabetes. In addition, a person's socioeconomic status is important since those in lower-income groups may not be able to find healthy food or get the necessary healthcare. Consequently, diabetes is found more often in some places than others, showing that social and environmental differences affect people's health. The combination of these factors makes it clear that diabetes is affected by more than just the body's functions. In addition, the cultural setting plays a major role in shaping what people eat and how they live. In general, people in communities that exercise and eat homemade meals have lower chances of diabetes than those who mostly rely on fast food and do not exercise. Also, having access to unhealthy food and its frequent marketing mostly impacts vulnerable people, resulting in more people eating high-calorie diets and becoming obese, which increases their risk of diabetes. Such influences can also be seen in how people act socially, as friends may encourage unhealthy eating and less physical exercise.

For this reason, knowing about these factors is crucial to creating public health plans that encourage healthy habits and lower diabetes risk among people in the community.

The link between environmental toxins and pollutants and diabetes is a subject that is being studied more and more. It appears that contact with chemicals in plastics and pesticides, which are known as endocrine disruptors, may upset metabolism and increase the chances of insulin resistance and diabetes. Also, ongoing stress, which is often made worse by economic or safety issues in the environment, may disrupt hormones and cause people to eat more than usual. The many environmental factors involved in diabetes reveal the need for public health interventions that look at people's habits and also the environment where they live and work. Using what we learn from studies on the environment and its effects on health, we can better explain the factors that lead to diabetes and search for effective solutions (Figure 1.5).

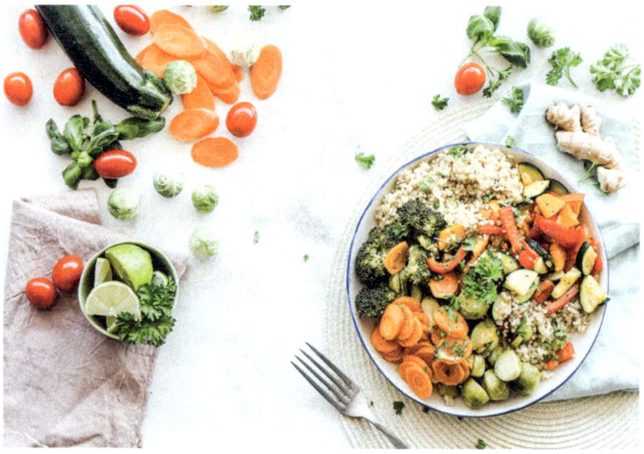

Figure 1.5. Urbanization, altered dietary patterns, and lifestyle changes have shifted the incidence of diabetes, highlighting the importance of understanding the interplay between environment and health.

Source: https://www.cabidigitallibrary.org/cms/asset/7ecae18a-d7b5-40a6-8b7b-c863f595c1aa/igr01.jpg

1.2. Symptoms and Diagnosis

The signs of diabetes may differ widely from one person to another and depend on the type of diabetes they have. Some of the first symptoms are frequent urination, increased thirst, and a lot of weight loss. Because insulin does not work properly in the body, blood glucose levels rise. In people with Type 1 diabetes, the symptoms may show up very quickly, usually in children and young adults. On the other hand, symptoms for Type 2 diabetes can appear slowly and may not be noticed until something serious happens. Some people can have the disease without any symptoms, so it is important to check them regularly, mainly in groups at higher risk. Since the symptoms can be tricky to notice, it is important to understand them well to make a correct diagnosis, proving that early action is vital for managing diabetes. Most of the time, blood tests that measure glucose are used to diagnose diabetes. The most frequently used tests are the fasting plasma glucose test, the oral glucose tolerance test, and the A1C test, as each one is meant for a different use. The A1C test gives a good overview of blood glucose levels over the past two to three months and is very helpful for long-term care. Based on current guide,ines, the diagnosis of diabetes is made when the fasting blood glucose is greater than 125 mg/dL, and the A1C level is higher than 6.5%. When diabetes is diagnosed early and correctly, treatment can start right away and the risk of complications, such as nerve and heart problems, is lowered, so it is important to follow strict diagnostic procedures. The process of diagnosing diabetes shows that the disease affects different populations differently, mainly because of socioeconomic factors. It is believed that people from low-income families usually have more health problems, but may not receive the proper care and treatment for diabetes. The link between money and health makes us think about how fairly healthcare is provided to everyone. Many poor people may experience a lot of diabetes-related problems, but they are not diagnosed as often as their reports would suggest, according to research. This disconnection necessitates a more integrated approach to healthcare that not only aims to improve diagnostic accuracy but also addresses the social determinants of health, ensuring that all individuals, regardless of their socioeconomic status, receive timely and adequate diabetes care (Bachmann et al., 2014) (Figure 1.6).

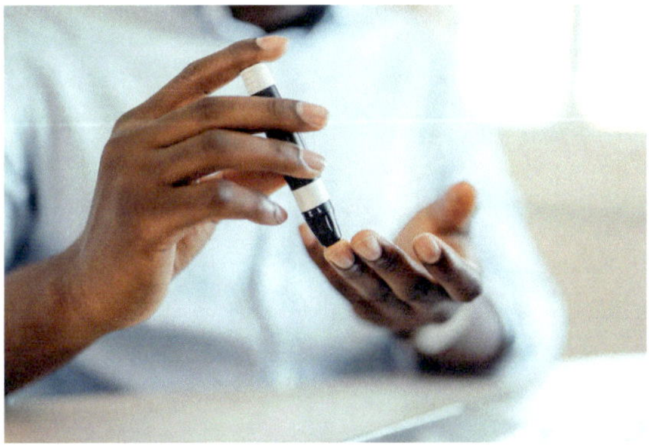

Figure 1.6. Diagnosis of diabetes is predominantly determined through a combination of blood tests that measure glucose levels.

Source: https://img.lb.wbmdstatic.com/vim/live/webmd/consumer_assets/site_images/articles/health_tools/why_your_feet_are_always_cold_and_what_to_do_about_it_slideshow/1800ss_getty_rf_diabetes_blood_glucose_test.jpg

1.2.1. Common Symptoms of Diabetes

The symptoms of diabetes mellitus may seriously influence a person's daily routine. In most cases, people with diabetes feel the need to urinate more, drink more water, and eat more, which are known as polydipsia and polyphagia. Because the body does not use insulin well, blood glucose levels become too high. The process of the kidneys removing excess glucose from the body results in more frequent urination, which then causes dehydration and makes people feel very thirsty. The cycle may lead to tiredness and pain for the patients.

Although elevated blood glucose levels are high in both type 1 and type 2 diabetes, type 1diabetes is asoociated with a lack of insulin production by pancreatic beta cells, whereas type 2 diabetes is associated with insulin resistance at the cellular level where insulin usually triggers the passage of glucose out of the circulation and into cells where it is used for storage or energy. Type 1 diabetes is often accompanied by significant weight loss despite adequate food intake. Due to the lack of insulin, the use of glucose as energy is compromised. The body adapts by using fat and muscle rather than glucose for energy, resulting in weight loss, fatigue and, in more severe situations, a condition called ketoacidosis.

Conversely, type 2 diabetes is accompanied by increased weight.

In the long term, elevated blood glucose due to poorly managed type 1 or 2 diabetes causes damage to neuron, resulting in peripheral neuropathy, vision loss, cardiovascular disease, and renal disease. Rarely, type 1 diabetes can be accompanied by extreme liver enlargement due to deposition of glycogen in the liver, regardless of glycemic control. This is called Mauriac syndrome and children and adolescents affected by this syndrome have problems with growth, delayed puberty, and features similar to Cushing's disease. Even though modern insulin treatments have cut down on Mauriac syndrome, it still highlights the serious results of not controlling diabetes well. Additionally, conditions like maternally inherited diabetes and deafness (MIDD) highlight the complex nature of diabetes symptoms as they relate to genetic factors Hearing loss in both ears and digestive problems are symptoms of MIDD, showing that diabetes can damage various body organs. Understanding these variations in symptoms emphasizes the need for comprehensive diabetes education and individualized patient care strategies to manage the disease effectively in diverse populations (Jainta et al., 2017) (Figure 1.7).

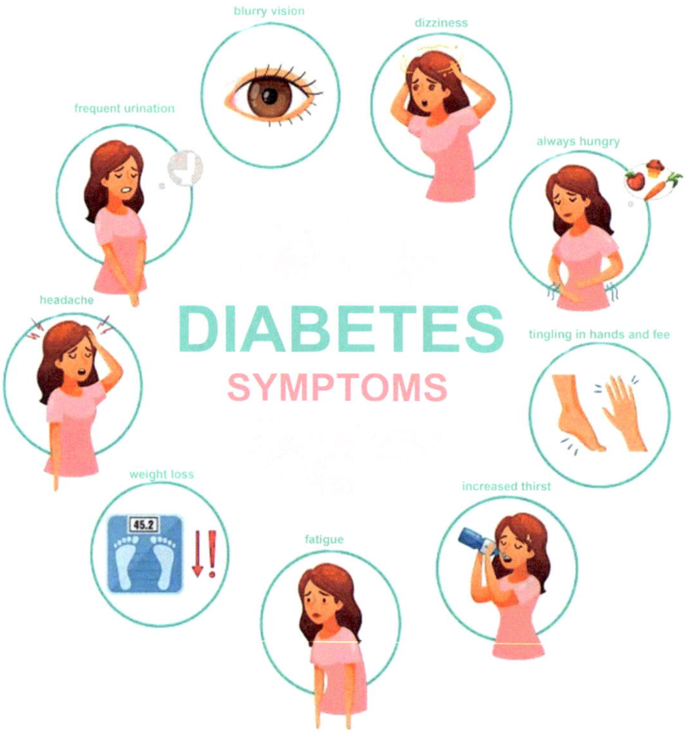

Figure 1.7. The symptoms of diabetes are multifaceted and can vary significantly depending on the type of diabetes and the individual.

Source: https://longlivelives.com/wp-content/uploads/2020/08/1907.i203.006.diabetes-cartoon.jpg

1.2.2. Diagnostic Criteria and Tests for Diabetes

The process of diagnosing diabetes has changed a lot, and now includes several useful criteria used by healthcare professionals. The National Institute for Health and Care Excellence (NICE) and the American Diabetes Association (ADA) both recommend key tests for diagnosing diabetes, which include fasting plasma glucose (FPG) tests, oral glucose tolerance tests (OGTT), and hemoglobin A1c assays. Having an FPG level of 126 mg/dL or more, an A1c level of 6.5% or higher, or a two-hour OGTT result of 200 mg/dL shows that diabetes is present. These guidelines along with the clinical presentation, help identify type 1, type 2 and gestational diabetes, which has its own set of issues and affects both the mother and the baby.

The screening process for gestational diabetes mellitus (GDM) serves as a crucial component of prenatal care. It is primarily performed between the 24th and 28th weeks of pregnancy, utilizing the glucose challenge test (GCT). When the GCT is positive, a 100-gram OGTT is done to make sure the diagnosis is accurate. The study of 1276 pregnant women in northern Iran showed that 15.8% of the women had GCT and 4.9% were diagnosed with GDM according to Carpenter and

Coustan's criteria. The identification of independent risk factors such as maternal age, BMI, and a history of obesity underscores the need for targeted screening practices tailored to women at risk, thereby optimizing the management of GDM and enhancing maternal and neonatal outcomes (Eshghinia et al., 2015).

Although there are many diagnostic tests available, their use must be balanced with the clinical presentation. Frequent testing can be costly and should be used with effective interventions including diet, lifestyle and medications to improve health outcomes. (Buhagiar et al., 2005). When research advances, new tests that give special insight into diabetes management should be given priority to improve how diabetes is diagnosed. It is necessary to use this approach for managing patients, as well as for making sure health resources are used wisely and that testing helps achieve better health results in diabetes (Figure 1.8).

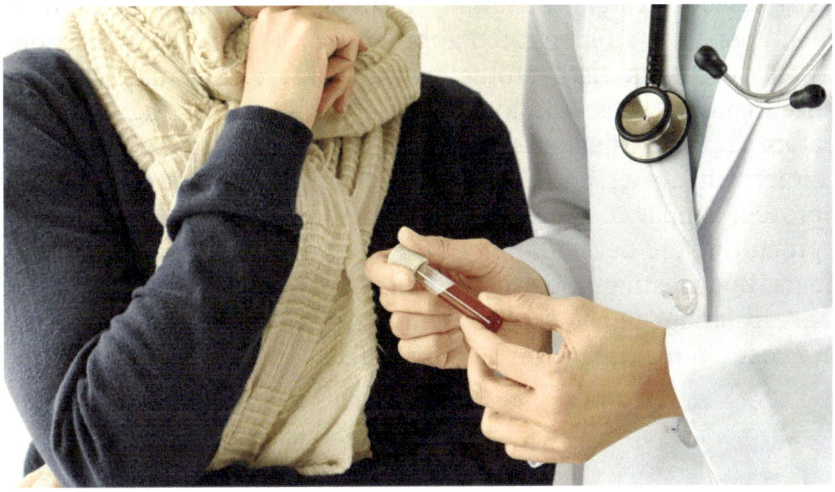

Figure 1.8. Oral glucose tolerance tests (OGTT).

Source: https://www.thomsonmedical.com/_next/image?url=https%3A%2F%2Fimages.contentstack.io%2Fv3%2Fassets%2Fblt5f400315f9e4f0b3%2Fblt5fc1a33c4c061a9d%2F66a793c6bc6ec2db64f983ae%2FOral_Glucose_Tolerance_Test_(OGTT)_%CE%93%C3%87%C3%B4_What_do_you_need_to_know_1440x810.png%3Fbranch%3Dprod&w=3840&q=75

1.2.3. Importance of Early Detection and Screening

The significance of early detection and screening in the context of diabetes cannot be overstated, as timely identification of the disease can dramatically influence outcomes. The asymptomatic nature of Type 2 diabetes often leads to late diagnoses, which can result in severe complications such as cardiovascular disease, kidney failure, and nerve damage. Screening efforts, particularly in at-risk populations, are crucial in identifying individuals who may have undiagnosed diabetes. Public health initiatives focusing on awareness and education can empower communities to engage in regular screenings, promoting early intervention strategies that could mitigate the long-term health burdens associated with the disease. The urgency for such measures is underscored by studies demonstrating that early management can significantly reduce the onset of complications and enhance patients' overall quality of life, emphasizing the need for systemic changes to incorporate regular glucose screening in healthcare practices. Furthermore, the association between diabetes and other comorbid conditions, such as hypertension and cognitive decline, underscores the necessity for comprehensive screening approaches. For instance, individuals with diabetes are at an increased risk of developing dementia, particularly as they age. The barriers to early detection, including stigma, lack of awareness, and insufficient healthcare infrastructure, must be addressed to facilitate more effective screening and intervention strategies. As observed in demographic studies, such as those examining the rising prevalence of dementia in India, key risk factors, including diabetes and age, highlight the interconnectedness of chronic diseases and the importance of systematic screening. Public health strategies that promote awareness and understanding of these interrelated conditions will not only improve early detection rates but also enhance the overall management of diabetic patients, thereby reducing the strain on healthcare systems. Lastly, implementing a robust screening program for diabetes necessitates collaboration among various sectors, including healthcare providers, community organizations, and public health entities. Such an integrated approach can ensure that detection and subsequent treatment are not only early but also equitable across different populations. This is particularly vital for marginalized communities who may face barriers in accessing healthcare resources. As noted in the literature regarding dementia and diabetes, enhancing healthcare infrastructure and fostering public awareness are essential components of an effective early detection strategy. A multi-sectoral approach, similar to those recommended for dementia care, should be tailored to diabetes as well, promoting the development of targeted interventions that can lead to significant health improvements. By investing in early screening and education, society can take a proactive stance against the escalating diabetes crisis, ultimately leading to healthier communities and reduced healthcare costs in the long term (Figure 1.9).

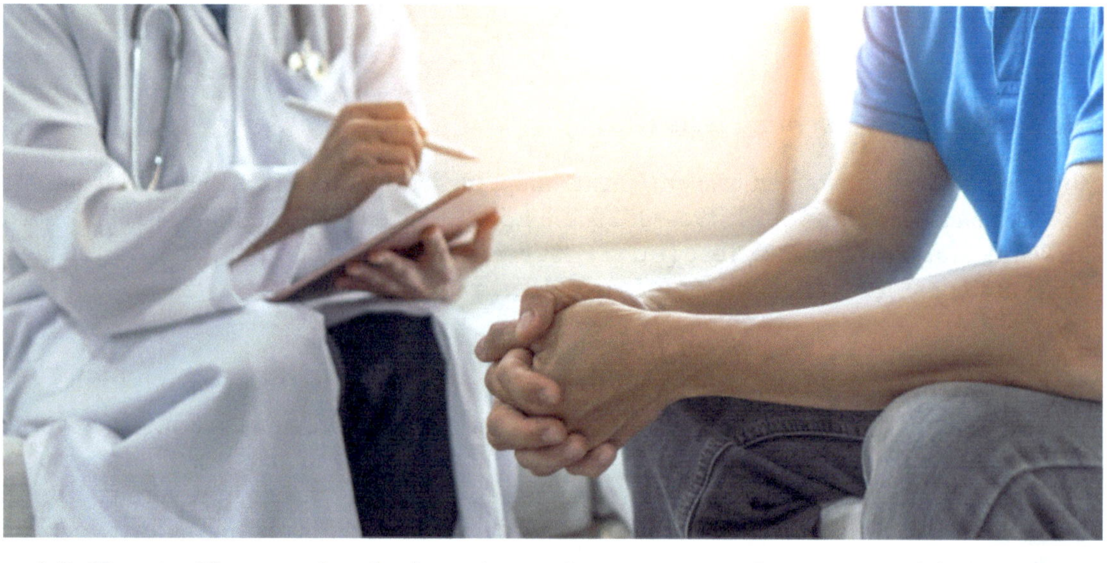

Figure 1.9. The significance of early detection and screening in the context of diabetes cannot be overstated, as timely identification of the disease can dramatically influence outcomes.

Source: https://images.apollo247.in/pd-cms/cms/2023-10/Shutterstock_1489440323.jpg

1.3. Complications of Diabetes

The complications of diabetes are multifaceted, impacting various organ systems and significantly diminishing the quality of life for affected individuals. Chronic hyperglycemia can lead to microvascular complications, such as diabetic retinopathy, nephropathy, and neuropathy, fundamentally altering the physiological landscape of the body. Diabetic retinopathy, an eye condition caused by damage to the blood vessels in the retina, can result in vision loss if not managed appropriately. Similarly, diabetic nephropathy affects the kidneys, often leading to end-stage renal disease requiring dialysis or transplantation. The rising prevalence of these complications highlights the importance of effective diabetes management and patient education, essential components in mitigating risks associated with these conditions, as underscored by the significant role of structured health education programs aimed at increasing patient awareness and self-care practices (Hua et al., 2024). Additionally, macrovascular complications such as cardiovascular disease, which includes coronary artery disease and stroke, pose severe health risks for individuals living with diabetes. The presence of diabetes accelerates the atherosclerotic process due to chronic inflammation and endothelial dysfunction triggered by prolonged hyperglycemia.

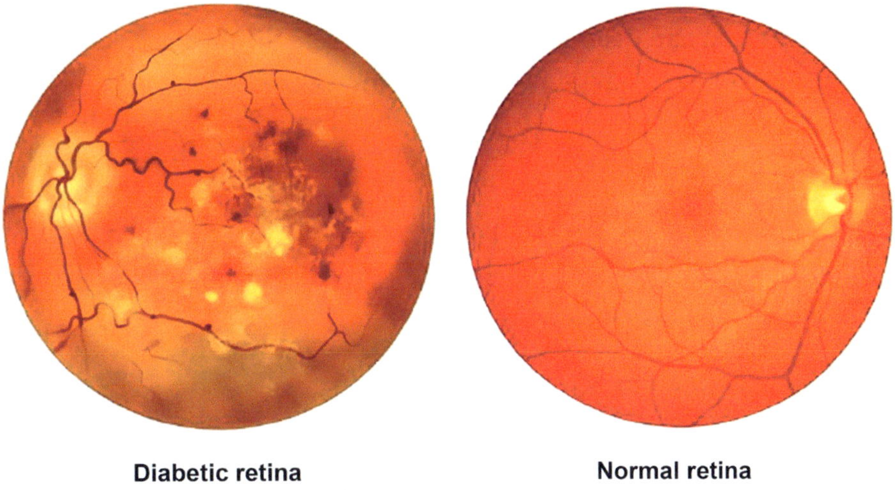

Figure 1.10. Diabetic retinopathy, an eye condition caused by damage to the blood vessels in the retina, can result in vision loss if not managed appropriately.

Source: https://dreyeins.com/wp-content/uploads/2024/06/diabatics.png

These factors contribute to a higher incidence of heart attacks and strokes among diabetic patients compared to their non-diabetic counterparts. The integration of technology in diabetes management has emerged as an important strategy to combat these complications, facilitating better monitoring and more personalized treatment plans. By evaluating the uses and outcomes of technology-enabled programs, it becomes clear that innovative approaches can significantly improve patients' overall health and reduce the incidence of associated complications (Middleton et al., 2007). Ultimately, understanding the complications associated with diabetes is crucial for both healthcare professionals and patients. Empowering diabetic individuals through education and effective management strategies can substantially reduce the risk of microvascular and macrovascular complications. In this context, nurses and allied health professionals play a pivotal role in patient education, demonstrating the need for ongoing research and development of structured educational programs focused on diabetes care. Such programs not only foster a deeper understanding of the disease but also inspire proactive self-management strategies. As the population ages and the prevalence of diabetes increases, the integration of comprehensive education and advanced management technologies is vital. This dual approach will undoubtedly enhance the quality of care and the overall health outcomes for those living with diabetes, paving the way for a future where complications are minimized and quality of life is maximized (Hua et al., 2024) (Figure 1.10).

1.3.1. Short-Term Complications: Hypoglycemia and Hyperglycemia

If blood glucose levels are not controlled in diabetes, people may experience short-term problems such as hypoglycemia and hyperglycemia. Hypoglycemia happens when the body's blood sugar drops too low because insulin or antidiabetic drugs are taken in higher amounts than the glucose can be produced or eaten. Symptoms of hypoglycemia include sweating, confusion, palpitations. If severe it can lead to loss of consciousness, seizures and death.. .

On the other hand, elevated blood glucose levels, or hyperglycemia, occur when the production or effectiveness of insulin are inadequate. Hyperglycemia tends to highten in settings of physiologic stress such as after surgeries or with severe infections. Symptoms of hyperglycemia include frequent urination, fatigue,, increased thirst and blurred vision. Severe hyperglycemia may result in hyperglycemic hyperosmolar syndrome, which involves extreme dehydration and changes in a person's mental state. Studies have shown that surgical patients with diabetes are particularly susceptible to intraoperative hyperglycemia, which is linked to prolonged hospital stays and increased morbidity (Knaak et al., 2019). It is important for people with diabetes to recognize the symptoms of hypoglycemia and hyperglycemia, so they can manage these conditions on time. Also, healthcare providers need to create personalized care plans that take into account a person's way of life, other health conditions, and the possible effects of medications. Strong awareness and active management can greatly decrease the chances and effects of these sudden complications, which helps improve diabetic patients' health in the short and long term. As research advances, diabetes programs should change to include findings that guide the best ways to support people who have unstable blood sugar (Figure 1.11).

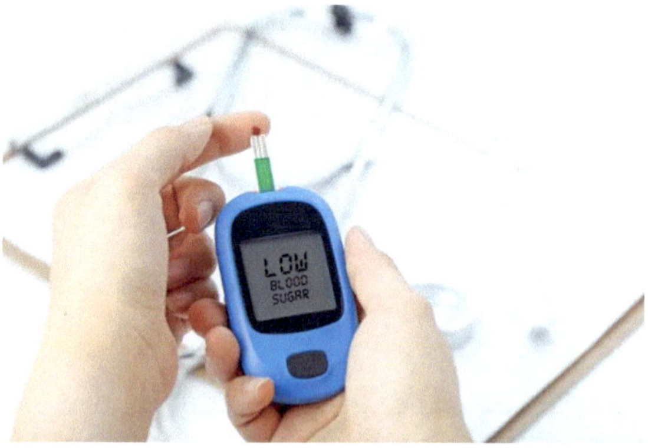

Figure 1.11. Hypoglycemia, characterized by abnormally low blood sugar levels, often manifests when insulin or antidiabetic medications outpace glucose production or intake.

Source: https://www.metropolisindia.com/upgrade/blog/upload/24/02/Hypoglycemia1707207906.webp

1.3.2. Long-Term Complications: Cardiovascular Disease and Neuropathy

Among the long-term problems that diabetes brings are several serious conditions, and cardiovascular disease and neuropathy are the most important. Many diabetics still suffer from serious health problems and death due to cardiovascular disease, mainly because of the long-term high blood sugar in the condition. Maintaining high blood glucose levels for a long time can result in atherosclerosis and raise the chances of heart attacks and strokes. Besides, the link between blood sugar control and heart health proves that it is important for diabetics to maintain their HbA1c in the target range. Even fluctuations in glucose levels may exacerbate cardiovascular issues, as evidenced by recent studies indicating a potential link between glycemic variability and cardiovascular autonomic dysfunction in type 1 diabetes mellitus (Helleputte et al., 2020). Therefore, new strategies for managing blood sugar are needed to help avoid serious cardiovascular problems. In addition, diabetic neuropathy is a long-term problem that can seriously impact a patient's daily life. It appears in many ways, but peripheral neuropathy is most common and usually results in pain, numbness, and a loss of feeling in the extremities. Both metabolic and vascular changes take place, since long-term high blood sugar can damage nerves and reduce blood supply to them. As a result, neuropathy may cause problems such as ulcers on the feet and infections.

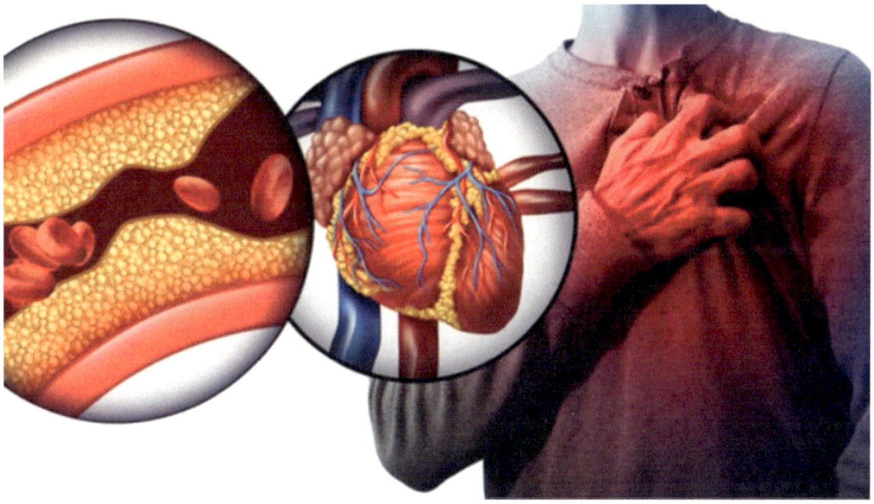

Figure 1.12. Cardiovascular disease remains a leading cause of morbidity and mortality in individuals with diabetes, largely related to the chronic hyperglycemia that characterizes the condition.

Source: https://cardiovascularbusiness.com/sites/default/files/styles/top_stories/public/2021-05/iStock-1141130339.jpg.webp?itok=tv2qWaDz

Research has also highlighted the intricate relationship between neuropathy and cardiovascular health, especially as autonomic neuropathy may complicate the management of cardiovascular disease in diabetic patients (Defeudis et al., 2015). For this reason, it is necessary to notice the symptoms of neuropathy and take care of its management to avoid further health problems, such as cardiovascular events. Cardiovascular disease and neuropathy together show how diabetes has many aspects as a long-term illness. Managing diabetes well involves focusing on blood sugar control as well as preventing its complications. With new treatments appearing, including those that help with nerve and heart problems, it is still very important to keep an eye on patients. Learning about obesity, hypertension, and unhealthy habits is necessary to develop ways to prevent heart disease. Besides, taking part in education and regular health checks allows diabetic patients to handle their health better, which can lead to a lower risk of cardiovascular disease and neuropathy. Thus, managing diabetes well requires a team effort that looks after blood sugar levels and also prevents or manages future problems (Figure 1.12).

1.3.3. Impact on Quality of Life and Daily Functioning

Diabetes has a major effect on how well people live and function each day, including their physical and mental well-being. Many people with diabetes encounter several issues that make it harder for them to take part in daily activities. If blood sugar levels change, it can cause tiredness and difficulties with thinking, which can make work, social life, and entertainment hard. Besides, checking blood sugar levels and following a special diet can be stressful and reduce people's happiness. Dealing with diabetes for a long period can cause emotional stress that often leads to anxiety and depression, affecting the quality of life. In general, the way people with diabetes live each day depends closely on how they handle their condition and the mental effects of having a chronic illness.

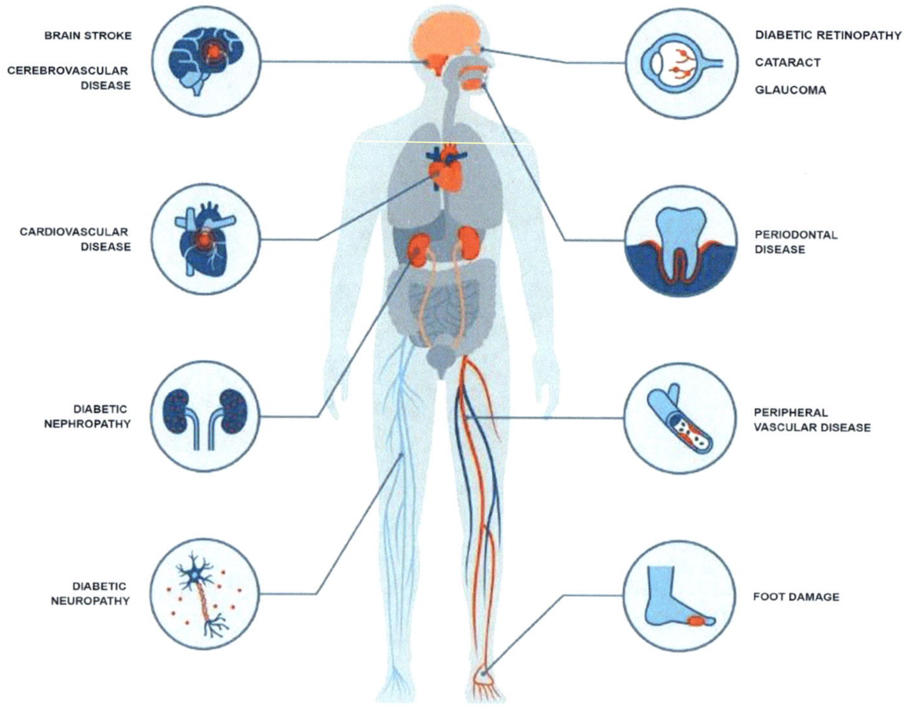

Figure 1.13. Individuals with diabetes experience a myriad of complications that can hinder their ability to engage in everyday activities.

Source: https://www.endocrine.org/-/media/endocrine/images/patient-engagement-webpage/condition-page-images/diabetes-and-glucose-metabolism/diabetes_complications_pe_1796x943.jpg

Research emphasizes the extent to which diabetes influences health-related quality of life (HRQOL) across various domains, especially when considering its complications. A study examining children with inborn errors of metabolism (IEM) highlighted that those with co-existing movement disorders exhibited significantly lower HRQOL compared to other chronic conditions, such as diabetes mellitus. It is clear from this finding that the severity of related diseases, just like diabetes, can have a major effect on HRQOL. Moreover, people with autism usually find it hard to do daily tasks, making it difficult for them to lead an ordinary life. Similar challenges may occur in diabetes when complications affect a person's ability to move, think clearly, or look after themselves daily. So, dealing with the effects of diabetes and adjusting to them points out the importance of finding good management strategies to help people live better. Managing diabetes better is linked to a better quality of life for people. A study exploring diabetes self-management programs found that reductions in glycosylated hemoglobin (HbA1c) levels were correlated with better diabetes-specific quality of life. It means that patients who use self-management strategies do better in their health and also enjoy greater satisfaction in different areas of life. Certain aspects of quality of life revealed that diabetes management aids in controlling blood sugar and improves sexual function, showing that diabetes management affects many areas. For this reason, when patients are empowered and able to manage their health well, their general health and quality of life can improve. This emphasizes the importance of addressing both clinical and patient-centered outcomes in diabetes care, as achieving clinical targets can profoundly influence daily functioning and overall well-being (Khanna et al., 2018) (Figure 1.13).

1.4. Role of Healthcare Professionals

Since diabetes is a difficult condition to manage, healthcare professionals are essential in helping patients. Physicians, nurses, dietitians, and other professionals in health care join forces to plan treatments that suit the needs of people with diabetes. For example, primary care physicians help diagnose diabetes, watch its progress, and give the right treatments. Since nurses often interact with patients, they need to explain self-care, check that patients take their medications as instructed, and help deal with multiple health issues. When everyone collaborates, patients are more involved and responsible, which leads to better health results for those with diabetes. In addition, good diabetes management depends on clear communication between healthcare workers and patients. It has been found that patients' views on healthcare may not match those of healthcare providers, which means it is important to communicate clearly. Initiatives such as the Advancing Care Coordination & Telehealth Deployment (ACT) Programme have underscored the importance of coordinated efforts in chronic disease management. They indicate that when healthcare providers are involved with their patients, it helps patients stick to their treatment plans and encourages them to take part in their own health. Better communication with patients by healthcare professionals can greatly help people with diabetes follow their treatment plans. More and more, community healthcare nurses are being appreciated for their efforts in helping manage diabetes in a community setting. Through qualitative studies, experts have found out what skills and knowledge nurses should have to manage cases well and teach patients. Practice tools and taking part in diabetes initiatives help community nurses decide on strategies that are useful for patients. Also, these specialists manage child welfare and long-term care, demonstrating a complete awareness of what patients require. The collaborative nature of community nursing, which bridges generalist and specialist practice, illustrates the multifaceted role of healthcare professionals and their commitment to enhancing the quality of care for diabetic patients, as highlighted in various community health initiatives (Baroni et al., 2015; Gray et al., 2010) (Figure 1.14).

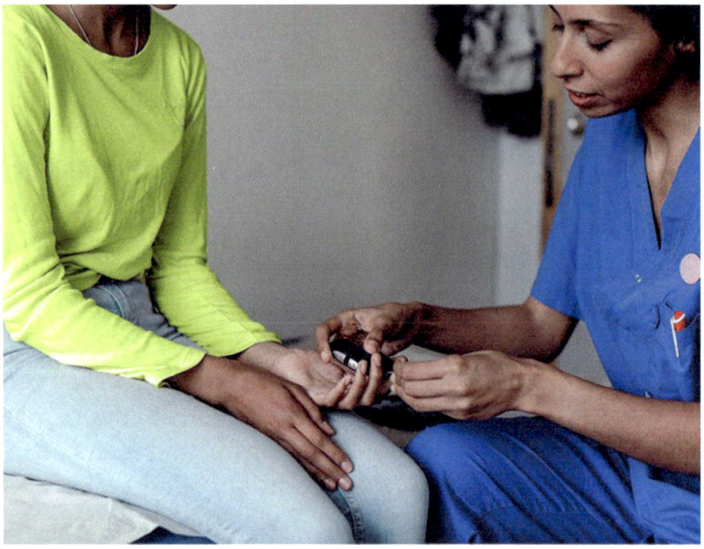

Figure 1.14. Physicians, nurses, dietitians, and other allied health practitioners collaborate to create a comprehensive care plan designed to address the unique needs of diabetic patients.

Source: https://media.post.rvohealth.io/wp-content/uploads/sites/3/2022/04/health_professionals_type1_diabetes_732x549_thumb-732x549.jpg

1.4.1. Importance of a Multidisciplinary Approach

Since diabetes involves many aspects, it is necessary to use a team approach in its management. Diabetes not only involves blood sugar; it usually leads to problems such as nerve damage, vision loss, and foot infections, which can make it difficult for patients to stick to their treatment routines. Recent research shows that managing diabetes well depends on a strategy that brings together several healthcare professionals. For example, occupational therapy is recognized as an important part of diabetes care, showing how several disciplines can unite to help patients. By integrating professionals like dietitians, endocrinologists, nurses, and occupational therapists, patients benefit from a holistic approach that addresses both the medical and psychosocial aspects of their condition, ultimately leading to improved health management and quality of life (Lacey et al. 2025). Besides, the challenges of managing diabetes increase due to issues such as a person's social background, access to medical care, and the availability of educational resources. When the COVID-19 lockdown happened, it was found that people with diabetes faced many problems, making it obvious that a team approach was required. This means that failing to manage self-care often results in not following health advice, so only one doctor is not enough to look after all a person's health needs. In the Caribbean, the recognition of these barriers has prompted calls for a multidisciplinary framework that caters to individual patient needs, thereby fostering an environment of support and education (Smith et al., 2023). Cooperating with patients increases their knowledge and ability to handle changes in health care during emergencies. In addition, uniting different healthcare professions helps create an environment where each patient's needs are addressed individually. Using a team approach from various disciplines, healthcare workers can identify the many needs of people with diabetes and design suitable treatment plans. This teamwork is meant to care for patients' health and also to help them by providing education and support that matches their personal needs. When team members communicate well, all the needs of diabetes management, such as diet and emotional care, are handled properly. This synergy is vital in promoting sustained self-management and enhancing the overall quality of care, thus reinforcing the importance of a multidisciplinary approach in diabetes management (Smith et al., 2023; Lacey et al. 2025) (Figure 1.15).

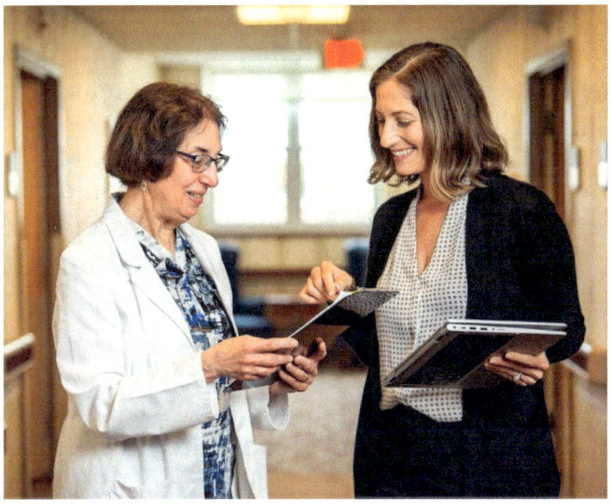

Figure 1.15. By integrating professionals like dietitians, endocrinologists, nurses, and occupational therapists, patients benefit from a holistic approach that addresses both the medical and psychosocial aspects of their condition, ultimately leading to improved health management and quality of life

Source: https://www.hcsgcorp.com/wp-content/uploads/2024/06/Blog-Hero-Images-29.jpg

1.4.2. Education and Support from Healthcare Providers

Good education and continuous help from medical staff are important for managing diabetes. Because of this knowledge, patients can make wise decisions about their health, which helps them manage their own health and improves the results of their treatment. Those who have diabetes benefit a lot from the educational programs that doctors, nurses, and diabetes educators design to meet their needs. The main subjects these efforts address are changing what you eat, checking your blood sugar, and exercising regularly. Moreover, the integration of technology-enabled diabetes management programs has been shown to facilitate these educational efforts, providing accessible and timely information that encourages patient engagement and adherence to treatment protocols (Middleton et al., 2007). Therefore, helping patients learn new things about diabetes enables them to manage it well. The move from pediatric to adult healthcare is often tough for young people with diabetes, which shows why they need special educational support at this time. Such models highlight that adolescents and young adults have specific needs, so they should be given education on self-management during their developmental years. The most successful transition programs are characterized by multidisciplinary collaboration, the involvement of family, and the establishment of designated transition clinics (Bagnall et al., 2013). They help young patients by dealing with issues such as not knowing about their condition and receiving enough support. If these points are included in healthcare, providers can help young people with diabetes adjust better, improve their blood sugar control, and live a better life. Healthcare providers must not be forgotten for the emotional and psychological support they give. Dealing with diabetes often leads to mental health problems like anxiety and depression, which may lessen a patient's desire to take care of their condition. It is important for healthcare providers to pay attention to these feelings and decide when more mental health support is required. When healthcare professionals encourage patients to talk about their feelings, it helps the patients to ask for help and strengthens their ability to manage their health on their own. Also, being part of support groups and community resources can add support and understanding, which can help improve diabetes education. Taking care of both the medical and emotional aspects of diabetes care through education helps patients lead healthier and happier lives (Figure 1.16).

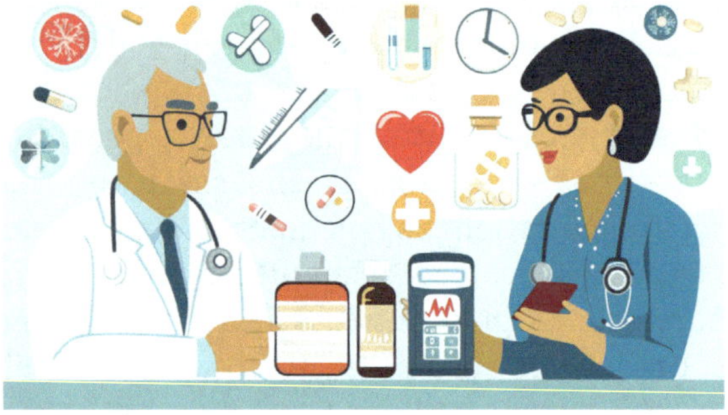

Figure 1.16. Effective education and ongoing support from healthcare providers are vital components in the management of diabetes.

Source: https://coreprescribingsolutions.co.uk/wp-content/uploads/2024/11/Managing-Diabetes-in-Primary-Care-Featured-Image.png

1.4.3. Role of Diabetes Educators and Nutritionists

It is important to use a multidisciplinary strategy for diabetes, and diabetes educators and nutritionists play key roles. They give helpful advice to patients on how to handle diabetes. Since type 2 diabetes is becoming more common, patients should make sure to follow a plan that combines their diet, exercise, and medicine use. Diabetes educators, through patient diabetes education (PDE) programs, strive to enhance patients' understanding of their condition, instilling essential self-care skills necessary for effective glycemic control. However, it is important to recognize that many of these educational frameworks lack consistency and are not firmly rooted in proven behavioral principles, which can limit their overall efficacy in fostering sustainable lifestyle changes (Cilia et al., 2007).

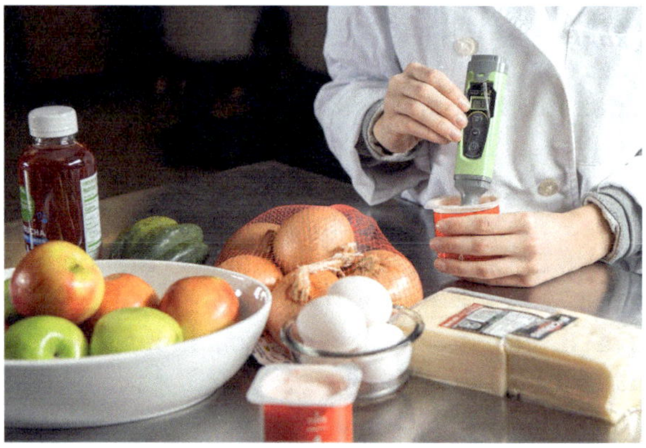

Figure 1.17. Nutritionists play a complementary role by providing a detailed understanding of the dietary requirements essential for managing diabetes.

Source: https://news.ohio.edu/sites/ohio.edu.news/files/2024-04/How%20dieticians%20are%20shaping%20the%20future%20of%20healthcare.jpg

Nutritionists help by giving a clear explanation of what people with diabetes should eat. They evaluate the nutritional status of their patients and design special meal plans for each person. With the help of the Food and Nutrition Guidelines, practitioners can give their patients accurate nutrition information. Since dietary advice keeps changing, it is necessary for nutritionists to follow the latest recommendations. The 2011 review of the Food and Nutrition Guidelines confirms their usefulness in healthcare and stresses that following them helps health practitioners give safe advice on nutrition. By aligning, it becomes easier to handle diabetes and boosts both patient education and health improvements. To summarize, diabetes educators and nutritionists demonstrate that a complete approach is necessary for diabetes care. With the assistance of educators, patients understand their condition, and nutritionists help them manage their diets well. Interventions should help organize the educational material and also make sure patients receive continuous help. It is difficult to connect the ideas from studies with how they are put into practice, so patients stick to their recommended treatments. Cooperating with healthcare professionals, diabetes educators and nutritionists can help patients live better and control their blood sugar, thus reducing the number of diabetes cases (Figure 1.17).

1.5. Current Research and Advances

Today's diabetes studies focus on pharmacogenetics, which examines how our genes impact how certain drugs work in us. It is hoped that this area will enable doctors to manage diabetes in a way that matches each person's unique genetic traits. It has been proven that pharmacogenetics is already being used to treat monogenic diabetes,which is a group of uncommon forms of diabetes caused by variations in a simgle gene. These include maturity-onset diabetes of the young (MODY), and neonatal diabetes. Even so, it is hard to use these findings to enhance treatment for the most common type 2 diabetes. At the moment, researchers are using genome-wide association studies and other genetic approaches to discover links that could affect diabetes treatment. Despite these advancements, numerous barriers persist that hinder the integration of pharmacogenetic discoveries into routine clinical care, necessitating ongoing research to overcome these hurdles and optimize therapeutic outcomes for patients with diabetes (Florez et al., 2013). Apart from pharmacogenetics, technology is greatly helping to enhance diabetes care. In particular, telemedicine makes it possible for people with type 2 diabetes to get medical advice and follow-up care remotely. Studies carried out recently have shown that telemedicine helps patients manage their diabetes and improves their blood sugar levels. Such technologies can give patients instant help, education, and advice, which encourages them to follow their treatment plans. Still, there are some problems with the growth of telemedicine; various studies point out that more research is needed to check the lasting effectiveness and affordability of these programs.

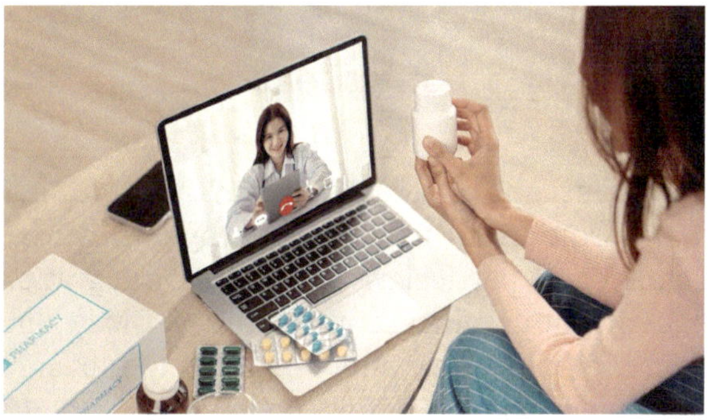

Figure 1.18. Telemedicine has emerged as a vital tool that facilitates remote medical consultations and follow-up care, particularly for individuals with type 2 diabetes.

Source: https://d33xmv9j3wn8v0.cloudfront.net/uploads/2025/02/telehealth-takeover-the-new-era-of-virtual-care.jpg

As healthcare systems continue to adapt to technological innovations, the potential of telemedicine to transform diabetes care is significant, warranting further investigation and investment (Ness et al., 2018). To summarize, diabetes management is being influenced by recent developments in pharmacogenetics and telemedicine. Although pharmacogenetics can provide customized medicine based on a person's genes, telemedicine offers new ways for patients to be involved and supported.

Even though both fields are important in developing new diabetes treatments, there are still problems with using and evaluating them. The combination of genetics and technology creates a special opportunity to help people living with diabetes. It will be very important to overcome the challenges that limit the use of these innovations, so they can help diabetes patients achieve better health and a more efficient healthcare system. As such, continued investment in research and development within these domains is essential for fostering advancements in diabetes treatments (Florez et al., 2013; Ness et al., 2018) (Figure 1.18).

1.5.1. Innovations in Diabetes Technology: Continuous Glucose Monitors and Insulin Pumps

The landscape of diabetes management has been profoundly transformed by innovative technologies, particularly through the integration of continuous glucose monitors (CGMs) and insulin pumps. They allow patients to measure their glucose levels and give insulin with much more accuracy than before. Now that CGMs are available, patients can see their blood sugar levels in real time and find out how their diet or exercise affects them. As a result, users are able to make changes to their diabetes care whenever needed. CGMs also help patients avoid hypoglycemic emergencies by notifying them when their blood sugar goes below the set limit. All these technologies work together to ease the worries and uncertainties that people with diabetes usually experience. Insulin pumps are an important step forward in diabetes technology since they provide a convenient and flexible method of administering insulin. Unlike traditional methods of injection, insulin pumps allow for continuous subcutaneous insulin infusion (CSII), which can be tailored to individual needs, providing both basal and bolus doses of insulin as needed. Because of this, managing patients is easier and they can enjoy more freedom in their daily lives. Moreover, studies have shown a correlation between the use of insulin pumps and improved glycemic control, decreasing average hemoglobin A1c levels significantly over time (Laptev et al., 2024). Improvements are most noticeable in children and adolescents, as both CGMs and insulin pumps have been found to play a big role in helping them manage their diabetes and stay healthy. Using CGMs and insulin pumps has made it possible for diabetes care to become even more thorough and effective. When these devices are linked, users can get better therapy since insulin is delivered based on their glucose readings. When these two devices are combined, innovative systems help patients avoid both high and low blood sugar levels. As highlighted in recent studies, advanced diabetes technologies not only aid in managing blood glucose levels but significantly enhance the quality of life for those with diabetes (Patrycja Łazicka et al., 2024). As a result of these innovations, diabetes care is now more focused on patients and helps them make positive changes in their lives (Figure 1.19).

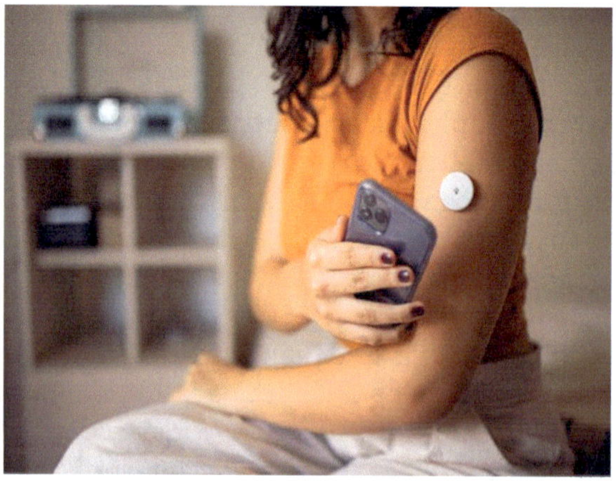

Figure 1.19. Continuous glucose monitors (CGMs).

Source: https://content.health.harvard.edu/wp-content/uploads/2024/06/dea79a4b-bb86-41ff-a53e-31a2f3690d55.jpg

1.5.2. Emerging Treatments and Therapies

The field of diabetes care is always progressing because of new findings and technologies that introduce better ways to treat the condition. Newer treatments are created to handle blood sugar problems and also reduce the risk of hypoglycemia. Hybrid closed-loop insulin delivery systems that use continuous glucose monitoring and automatic insulin delivery are being seen as very promising for managing blood glucose levels. They adjust insulin delivery according to the current glucose level, which helps prevent overreactions and uses a more natural way to give insulin. As a result, using these technologies helps patients become more involved in their diabetes care, pointing to diabetes therapies that are designed to fit each person's needs. Besides new technology, pharmaceutical progress is changing diabetes care by focusing on different aspects that lead to the disease. Recent studies highlight novel compounds such as glucagon-like peptide-1 (GLP-1) receptor agonists and sodium-glucose cotransporter 2 (SGLT2) inhibitors, which have emerged as effective treatments for Type 2 diabetes. They assist in regulating blood sugar and also give added protection to the heart and kidneys, helping with the many problems linked to diabetes. Using these therapies in clinical settings highlights a new approach that looks after metabolic health, which may help decrease the health problems linked to diabetes. When more evidence becomes available, clinicians are advised to review these new treatments for each patient's care plan. The use of personalized medicine in diabetes treatment shows how treatment methods are advancing. Scientists are now acknowledging that genetic, environmental, and lifestyle factors play a big role in the development of diabetes. Because of this, doctors can now use therapies that are designed for each patient's needs, making it easier to manage diabetes. If biomarkers and genetic traits are studied all the time, treatments can be selected that match each patient's unique features. Emerging interventions, as detailed by recent perspectives, are not only focused on glycemic control but also aim to reduce the risk of hypoglycemia without compromising efficacy, particularly in Type 1 diabetes management (Heller et al., 2008). These advancements signify an important step towards a future where diabetes treatment is both more effective and personalized (Briggs et al., 2013) (Figure 1.20).

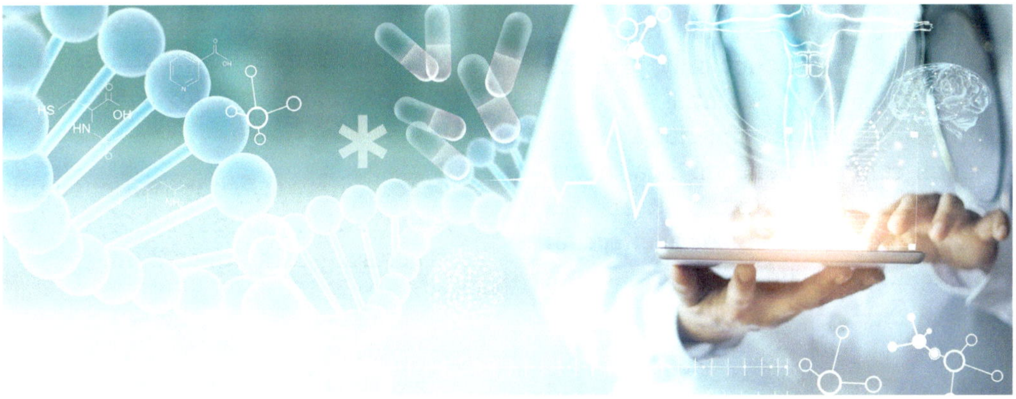

Figure 1.20. The exploration of personalized medicine in the context of diabetes treatment further underscores the progression of therapeutic strategies.

Source: https://images.admiralcloud.com/v5/deliverEmbed/0a5aab94-992c-40f5-8eb8-b90252f7c6fa/image_webp/autocrop/1920/740/1?poc=true

1.5.3. Future Directions in Diabetes Research

Since diabetes is becoming more common around the world, it is important to find new solutions through further research. Using genetics and the environment together in personalized medicine can help doctors choose the best treatment for each patient. If researchers understand the reason for diabetic neuropathy, they may be able to find new ways to spot and treat it. Improved genomic knowledge will guide the development of personalized interventions, enabling better clinical outcomes for diabetes patients (Tavakoli et al., 2023). The move towards personalized care may help save money in healthcare and improve the lives of people with diabetes, since the disease has many aspects. Experts should also concentrate on how technology can be used to handle diabetes. Advances in digital health tools, such as continuous glucose monitoring (CGM) systems and mobile health applications, are transforming how patients manage their condition. Understanding these technologies may help patients keep their blood sugar under control and become more active. Furthermore, the integration of artificial intelligence (AI) and machine learning algorithms to analyze data from these devices may enable proactive management of blood glucose levels. These technological advancements not only promise better outcomes but have the potential to reduce complications associated with diabetes, thereby alleviating significant burdens on healthcare systems (Anger et al., 2019). In the future, it is necessary to focus on the psychosocial effects of diabetes. Investigating the link between mental health and diabetes management may uncover important connections between a person's mental state and their health. Stress reduction, depression management, and anxiety therapy may help patients stick to their medication and self-care plans. So, research should use methods from endocrinology, psychology, and social sciences to design complete care models. This integrated perspective will not only enhance patient care but also ensure that diabetes research remains relevant in addressing the complex challenges faced by individuals living with the disease (Tavakoli et al., 2023) (Figure 1.21).

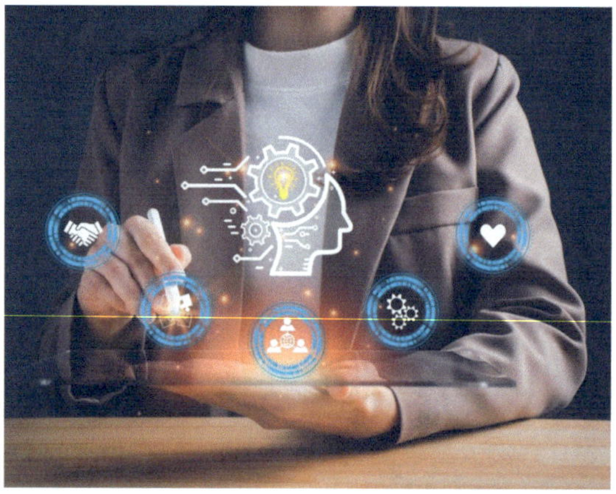

Figure 1.21. Interventions that target stress reduction, depression, and anxiety management may provide holistic treatment frameworks boosting adherence to medication and self-care routines.

Source: https://bayareacbtcenter.com/wp-content/uploads/2024/09/cognitive-restructuring-techniques-3.png

A CLOSER LOOK

BLOOD SUGAR LEVELS

The term blood sugar levels means how much glucose is in the blood. The main source of energy in our bodies is glucose, which comes mostly from the carbs we eat. A person's fasting blood sugar should be between 70 and 99 mg/dL, and it can go as high as 140 mg/dL after a meal. The body controls these levels using insulin, a hormone that comes from the pancreas. Maintaining balanced blood sugar is essential for overall health, as both high (hyperglycemia) and low (hypoglycemia) levels can lead to serious health issues, especially in individuals with diabetes.

Summary

It is clear from studying diabetes that this condition is not only about glucose levels and requires a complete understanding of its effects on health and way of life. Because it is a long-lasting disease with major risks, diabetes is a big challenge for both people who have it and global healthcare systems. Since diabetes is strongly linked to many chronic illnesses and is common today, it is necessary to focus on the social and economic reasons behind its occurrence and treatment. A wider view is necessary to create a setting that helps with effective education and strategies to address the effects of diabetes. A careful study of diabetes management shows that focusing on the patient is essential for better results. When interventions are created to fit a person's needs and worries, it helps them stick to their treatment and live healthier. As highlighted in the literature, a significant proportion of individuals with diabetes experience vaccine hesitancy, underscoring the need for targeted education that addresses specific disease-related fears and beliefs (Day et al., 2022). Also, healthcare providers need to adjust to handle the challenges of diabetes and its related conditions, providing care that covers patients' physical, emotional, and social health. In the end, the effort to fight diabetes is connected to public health programs that help people with diabetes become stronger and enjoy a better quality of life. Implementing integrated healthcare models, as shown through the developments in the Basque healthcare system, can substantially improve care delivery and patient outcomes (Beñat Zubeltzu et al., 2018). They highlight the need for healthcare providers to be united, to use technology, and to manage situations in advance. Going ahead, we should focus on new approaches and teamwork in diabetes care, so that the rising number of diabetes cases is addressed by compassionate and inclusive healthcare.

References

1. Akiyama, H., Alharbi, F., Armitage, R., Armitage, J., Armitage, M., Balin, B., Barbieri, A., et al. (2016). Apolipoprotein E related co-morbidities and Alzheimer's disease. https://core.ac.uk/download/42137999.pdf (accessed on 11th June 2025).
2. Ameer, B., & Weintraub, M. A. (2018). Pediatric Obesity: Influence on Drug Dosing and Therapeutics. *Journal of clinical pharmacology, 58 Suppl 10*, S94–S107. https://doi.org/10.1002/jcph.1092 (accessed on 11th June 2025).
3. Andrada, D., Balalau, C., Manea, M. E., Micu, M., et al. (2019). Alcoholic liver cirrhosis, more than a simple hepatic disease–A brief review of the risk factors associated with alcohol abuse. https://core.ac.uk/download/232440321.pdf (accessed on 11th June 2025).
4. Anger, J. T., Lee, U., Ackerman, A. L., Chou, R., Chughtai, B., Clemens, J. Q., Hickling, D., et al. (2019). Recurrent uncomplicated urinary tract infections in women: AUA/CUA/SUFU guideline. *The Journal of Urology, 202*, 282–289. https://doi.org/10.1097/ju.0000000000000296 (accessed on 11th June 2025).
5. Apullan, M. A., Clark, A., Dorn, J., Stamatakis, E., Franco, O. H., Goldhammer, I., Hamer, M., et al. (2012). Physical activity and cardiovascular mortality risk: Possible protective mechanisms? https://core.ac.uk/download/151162719.pdf (accessed on 11th June 2025).
6. Bachmann, M. O., Campbell, J., Clark, A., Hardcastle, A., et al. (2014). Economic inequalities in burden of illness, diagnosis and treatment of five long-term conditions in England: Panel study. https://core.ac.uk/download/29110729.pdf (accessed on 11th June 2025).
7. Badiu, D. C., Burcea-Dragomiroiu, G. T. A., Gherghiceanu, F., Hainarosie, R., et al. (2019). Management options in the sudden hearing loss of a diabetic patient. https://core.ac.uk/download/216811037.pdf (accessed on 11th June 2025).
8. Bagnall, A., Day, R., & Kime, N. H. (2013). *Systematic Review of Transition Models for Young People with Long-Term Conditions: A Report for NHS Diabetes*. https://core.ac.uk/download/29018738.pdf (accessed on 11th June 2025).
9. Baroni, I., Barrett, D., Bescos, C., Buskens, E., et al. (2015). What does it take to make integrated care work? A 'cookbook' for large-scale deployment of coordinated care and telehealth. https://core.ac.uk/download/155776181.pdf (accessed on 11th June 2025).
10. Bernier, D. (2012). *Polycystic Ovary Syndrome: Pathogenesis, Health Consequences, And Treatment of PCOS in Relation to Insulin Resistance*. https://core.ac.uk/download/72048051.pdf (accessed on 11th June 2025).
11. Boyle, F. M., Brooker, K. S., Mutch, A. J., Young, D., et al. (2015). Incorporating patient preferences in the management of multiple long-term conditions: Is this a role for clinical practice guidelines? https://core.ac.uk/download/pdf/30317024.pdf (accessed on 11th June 2025).
12. Briggs, A., Frank, B., Unal, B., Murray, C. J., Ford, E. S., Ben Romdhane, H., Ghozzi, H., et al. (2013). Analyzing recent coronary heart disease mortality trends in Tunisia between 1997 and 2009. https://core.ac.uk/download/17298046.pdf (accessed on 11th June 2025).
13. Buhagiar, G. (2005). Rationalization of the biochemistry laboratory: Which way forwards? https://core.ac.uk/download/46602008.pdf (accessed on 11th June 2025).

14. Helleputte, S., De Backer, T., Lapauw, B., Shadid, S., Celie, B., Van Eetvelde, B., Vanden Wyngaert, K., & Calders, P. (2020). The relationship between glycaemic variability and cardiovascular autonomic dysfunction in patients with type 1 diabetes: A systematic review. *Diabetes/ metabolism research and reviews, 36*(5), e3301. https://doi.org/10.1002/dmrr.3301(accessed on 11th June 2025).
15. Cherukuri, L., Smith, M. S., & Tayek, J. A. (2018). The durability of oral diabetic medications: Time to A1c baseline and a review of common oral medications used by the primary care provider. https://core.ac.uk/download/323082829.pdf (accessed on 11th June 2025).
16. Chircop, M., Savona-Ventura, C., & Schranz, A. G. (2003). Family history in the etiology of gestational diabetes mellitus and type 2 diabetes. https://core.ac.uk/download/46601850.pdf (accessed on 11th June 2025).
17. Cilia, S. (2007). Educational programmed for patients with type 2 diabetes at community health centers: What is the evidence? https://core.ac.uk/download/46602122.pdf (accessed on 11th June 2025).
18. Collins, S., & Reynolds, F. (2008). How do adults with cystic fibrosis cope following a diagnosis of diabetes? https://core.ac.uk/download/337114.pdf (accessed on 11th June 2025).
19. Cosentino, F., Grant, P. J., Aboyans, V., Bailey, C. J., Ceriello, A., Delgado, V., Federici, M., et al. (2019). 2019 ESC Guidelines on diabetes, pre-diabetes, and cardiovascular diseases developed in collaboration with the EASD. *European Heart Journal, 41*, 255–323. https://doi.org/10.1093/eurheartj/ehz486 (accessed on 11th June 2025).
20. Cuffari, R., D'Andrea, G., Di Pietro, A., Facciolà, A., et al. (2022). Prevention of cardiovascular diseases and diabetes: Importance of a screening program for the early detection of risk conditions in a target population. https://core.ac.uk/download/539311408.pdf (accessed on 11th June 2025).
21. Cuschieri, S. (2020). The diabetes epidemic in Malta. https://core.ac.uk/download/288638679.pdf (accessed on 11th June 2025).
22. Czerska, M. A., Furtak, K., Kamińska-Omasta, K., Krupa, M., et al. (2025). Effective treatment strategies for adults with type 2 diabetes. https://core.ac.uk/download/646079936.pdf (accessed on 11th June 2025).
23. Davies, M. J., D'Alessio, D. A., Fradkin, J., Kernan, W. N., Mathieu, C., Mingrone, G., Rossing, P., et al. (2018). Management of hyperglycemia in type 2 diabetes, 2018. A consensus report by the American Diabetes Association (ADA) and the European Association for the Study of Diabetes (EASD). *Diabetes Care, 41*, 2669–2701. https://doi.org/10.2337/dci18-0033 (accessed on 11th June 2025).
24. Day, D., Grech, L., Nguyen, M., Bain, N., Kwok, A., Harris, S., Chau, H., et al. (2022). Serious underlying medical conditions and COVID-19 vaccine hesitancy: A large cross-sectional analysis from Australia. *Vaccines, 10*. https://www.semanticscholar.org/paper/b38dbfc205625946df10ab8717867fcf95784c80 (accessed on 11th June 2025).
25. Defeudis, G., Di Emidio, C., Gianfrilli, D., Lenzi, A., et al. (2015). Erectile dysfunction and its management in patients with diabetes mellitus. https://core.ac.uk/download/54528262.pdf (accessed on 11th June 2025).
26. DeGaetano, A., Ferrara, A., Gaetano De, A., Hayes, A., Topp, B., Athukorala, C., Knight-Agarwal, C.

R., et al. (2019). Multi-scale simulation modeling for prevention and public health management of diabetes in pregnancy and sequelae. http://arxiv.org/abs/1905.02552 (accessed on 11th June 2025).

27. Dickinson, F. M., Kalk, J., Payne, K., Soltani, H., et al. (2007). Breast feeding practices and views among diabetic women: A retrospective cohort study. https://core.ac.uk/download/99945.pdf (accessed on 11th June 2025).

28. Eshghinia, S., Mohammadzadeh, F., & Vakili, M. A. (2015). The prevalence of gestational diabetes mellitus and its related risk factors in Gorgan, north of Iran. Selective or universal screening test is cost-effective? https://core.ac.uk/download/52205664.pdf (accessed on 11th June 2025).

29. Florez, J. C., & Huang, C. (2013). Pharmacogenetics in type 2 diabetes: Potential implications for clinical practice. https://core.ac.uk/download/28942477.pdf (accessed on 11th June 2025).

30. Gowda, R. J., Mehta, A., & Jayanna, K. (2025). Dementia: A public health challenge in India. https://core.ac.uk/download/640070567.pdf (accessed on 11th June 2025).

31. Gowda, R., Jeevitha, Jayanna, Krishnamurthy, & Mehta, A. (2025). Dementia: A public health challenge in India. https://core.ac.uk/download/640070552.pdf (accessed on 11th June 2025).

32. Gray, C. M., James, B., Lauder, W., McCulloch, J., et al. (2010). Developing community nursing practice: Promoting case management and skill enhancement to support shifting the balance of care. https://core.ac.uk/download/110605.pdf (accessed on 11th June 2025).

33. Heller, S. (2008). Minimizing hypoglycemia while maintaining glycemic control in diabetes. https://core.ac.uk/download/50935.pdf (accessed on 11th June 2025).

34. Hua, K. K., Kumaravelu, P., & Wah, Y. C. (2024). The impact of diabetes mellitus structured health education program on knowledge, attitude and practice of diabetes care and management among nursing students. https://core.ac.uk/download/640070116.pdf (accessed on 11th June 2025).

35. Jainta, N., & Otto-Buczkowska, E. (2017). Mauriac syndrome–Is already a history? https://core.ac.uk/download/268454797.pdf (accessed on 11th June 2025).

36. James, S. L., Abate, D., Abate, K. H., Abay, S. M., Abbafati, C., Abbasi, N., Abbastabar, H., et al. (2018). Global, regional, and national incidence, prevalence, and years lived with disability for 354 diseases and injuries for 195 countries and territories, 1990–2017: A systematic analysis for the Global Burden of Disease Study 2017. *The Lancet, 392*, 1789–1858. https://doi.org/10.1016/s0140-6736(18)32279-7 (accessed on 11th June 2025).

37. Karami, A., & Shaw, G. (2017). Computational content analysis of negative tweets for obesity, diet, diabetes, and exercise. http://arxiv.org/abs/1709.07915 (accessed on 11th June 2025).

38. Khanna, A. (2018). Hemoglobin A1C improvements and better diabetes-specific quality of life among participants completing diabetes self-management programs: A nested cohort study. https://core.ac.uk/download/212897283.pdf (accessed on 11th June 2025).

39. Knaak, C., Kuenz, S., Kurpanik, M., Lachmann, B., et al. (2019). Risk factors of intraoperative dysglycemia in elderly surgical patients. https://core.ac.uk/download/225124691.pdf (accessed on 11th June 2025).

40. Lacey, A. (2025). Exploring occupational therapy's role in diabetes: An experiential internship. https://core.ac.uk/download/pdf/86427529.pdf (accessed on 11th June 2025).

41. Laptev, D., Knyazeva, T. T., & Bezlepkina, O. (2024). The introduction of new technologies for insulin therapy and glycemic control in clinical practice in the period 2016–2023, and their impact on achieving treatment targets in children with type 1 diabetes mellitus. *Diabetes Mellitus*. https://www.semanticscholar.org/paper/c6b143697a6813db94063cdb73b0d22fde201262 (accessed on 11th June 2025).

42. Łazicka, P., Tarnowska, J., & Jakubowska, E. (2024). The use of insulin pumps as an innovative approach of diabetes therapy to improve glycemic control, patients' comfort of life and daily activity. *Journal of Education, Health and Sport*. https://www.semanticscholar.org/paper/41adbbc8f1a09cefb5311561495f868a2993f950 (accessed on 11th June 2025).

43. Livingston, G., Huntley, J., Sommerlad, A., Ames, D., Ballard, C., Banerjee, S., Brayne, C., et al. (2020). Dementia prevention, intervention, and care: 2020 report of the Lancet Commission. *The Lancet, 396*, 413–446. https://doi.org/10.1016/s0140-6736(20)30367-6 (accessed on 11th June 2025).

44. Marchetti, A. L. (2019). Building prediction models for dementia: The need to account for interval censoring and the competing risk of death. https://scholarworks.indianapolis.iu.edu/items/9ce8f985-808b-48ac-9307-15f0392a90a4 (accessed on 11th June 2025).

45. Middleton, B., Cusack, C. M., Kendrick, D., Bates, D. W., Bu, D., Johnston, D., Pan, E., et al. (2007). The value of information technology-enabled diabetes management. https://core.ac.uk/download/71355637.pdf (accessed on 11th June 2025).

46. Moats, A. (2019). Hypoglycemia in mitochondrial disorders. https://core.ac.uk/download/228022820.pdf (accessed on 11th June 2025).

47. Muhali, S. S., Muhali, F. S., Mfinanga, S., Sadiq, A. M., Marandu, A. A., Kyala, N. J., Said, F. H., et al. (2024). Impact of self-monitoring blood glucose on glycemic control among insulin-treated patients with diabetes mellitus in northeastern Tanzania: A randomized controlled trial. *Journal of Diabetes Research, 2024*. https://www.semanticscholar.org/paper/a168b90b8cd130422aadbe105aa15031c4e89d64 (accessed on 11th June 2025).

48. Mustafa, M. (2025). Self-care management practices among patients with diabetes mellitus in a tertiary care hospital in Karachi, Pakistan: An analytical cross-sectional study. *Social Science Review Archives*. https://www.semanticscholar.org/paper/99efe7619a629da770bdf879515e4341c4fb9ed8 (accessed on 11th June 2025).

49. Ness, E. (2018). Telemedicine and type 2 diabetes. https://core.ac.uk/download/217656868.pdf (accessed on 11th June 2025).

50. Peall, K. (2014). Rare inborn errors of metabolism with movement disorders: A case study to evaluate the impact upon quality of life and adaptive functioning. https://core.ac.uk/download/42532112.pdf (accessed on 11th June 2025).

51. Preston, S., & Stokes, A. (2017). Deaths attributable to diabetes in the United States: Comparison of data sources and estimation approaches. https://open.bu.edu/bitstream/2144/31144/1/stokes_deaths.pdf (accessed on 11th June 2025).

52. Shore, A. C., Rumley, A., Hattersley, A. T., Lee, B. C., Balletshofer, B., Caballero, A. E., Lowe, G. D., et al. (2001). Skin microvascular vasodilatory capacity in offspring of two parents with type 2 diabetes. https://core.ac.uk/download/9349833.pdf (accessed on 11th June 2025).

53. Smith, P. (2023). Barriers to diabetes self-management in Grenada during the COVID-19

pandemic: A qualitative study. https://core.ac.uk/download/595875465.pdf (accessed on 11th June 2025).

54. Zubeltzu, B., Mitxelena, A., Alberdi, A., Elola, M., Errasti, U., Berroeta, A., Vaquero, M., et al. (2018). Multipronged management strategy for patients with complex needs using an integrated organizational model. *International Journal of Integrated Care*. https://www.semanticscholar.org/paper/3ead3d2de57f5bc8d6427f3a1903d7e5e63e5567 (accessed on 11th June 2025).

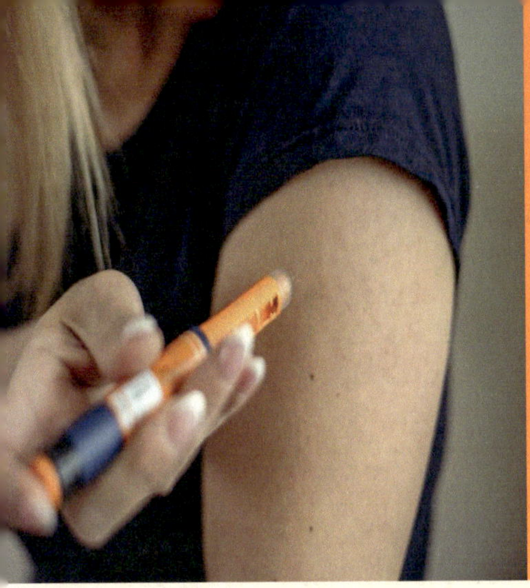

Chapter 2

NORMAL PHYSIOLOGY OF INSULIN SECRETION AND ACTION, AND THE INCRETIN EFFECT

Contents

Introduction

Research on how insulin is secreted and how it works is important for learning about the body's regulation of glucose. The pancreas's beta cells make insulin, which is necessary for tissues to absorb glucose and keep energy balance and metabolism steady. Insulin is important in normal physiology as it helps use glucose and also affects how energy is stored and released in the body, depending on the body's needs. The complex regulation of insulin secretion involves a variety of signals, including blood glucose levels, neuronal inputs, and other hormones, emphasizing the dynamic nature of this regulatory system that can become dysfunctional in conditions such as type 2 diabetes and metabolic syndrome (Farrugia et al., 2014). Besides the effects of insulin, the incretin effect is also very important for regulating glucose. Incretin hormones, such as glucagon-like peptide-1 (GLP-1) and gastric inhibitory polypeptide (GIP), are released from the gut in response to food intake and enhance insulin secretion from the pancreas. Thanks to these hormones, insulin is released when blood sugar goes up, even when it is not a steady increase. In addition to insulin resistance, the incretin effect is greatly reduced in people with type 2 diabetes, which is why it is important to know what stops these hormones from working properly. Research has revealed intricate interactions between incretin hormones and insulin secretion dynamics, shedding light on complications associated with obesity and glucose intolerance (Lee et al., 2019).

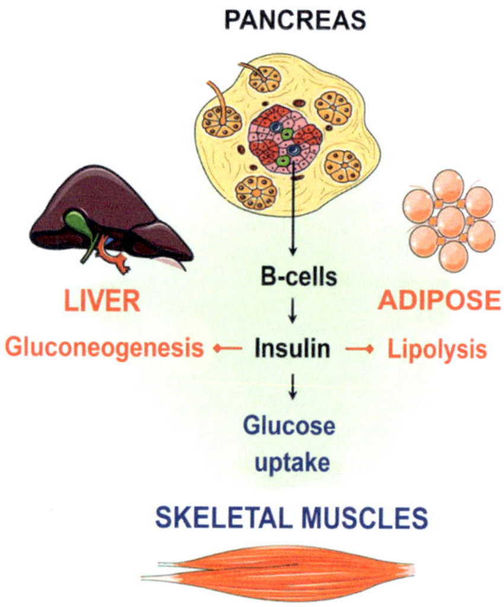

Figure 2.1. Insulin, a crucial hormone produced by the beta cells of the pancreas, plays a vital role in mediating glucose uptake by tissues, thereby maintaining energy balance and metabolism.

Source: Rahman MS, Hossain KS, Das S, Kundu S, Adegoke EO, Rahman MA, Hannan MA, Uddin MJ, Pang M-G. Role of Insulin in Health and Disease: An Update. *International Journal of Molecular Sciences*. 2021; 22(12):6403. https://doi.org/10.3390/ijms22126403

Having knowledge of insulin's normal secretion and its effects, as well as the incretin effect, is necessary for designing good treatments for metabolic problems. Looking at β-cell function helps explain the reasons behind prediabetes and diabetes, which improves how these conditions are handled. New mathematical approaches and evaluations of the Disposition Index, which measures insulin sensitivity, have shown that checking β-cell function is necessary for understanding the details of glucose homeostasis. Still, future studies should examine if factors such as incretin hormone interaction and β-cell aging have an impact on the whole process of insulin regulation. By linking these concepts, a more comprehensive understanding of insulin physiology could contribute significantly to the prevention and treatment of type 2 diabetes (Farrugia et al., 2014) (Figure 2.1).

2.1. Anatomy of the Pancreas

The pancreas, a vital organ located in the abdominal cavity behind the stomach, plays a crucial role in both the endocrine and exocrine systems. Its unique anatomical structure allows for the dual functionality necessary for proper metabolic regulation and digestion. The pancreas is divided into four regions: the head, body, tail, and uncinate process. The head is nestled in the curve of the duodenum, while the tail extends towards the spleen, providing a relevant anatomical context for understanding its intricate relationships with surrounding organs. This strategic positioning facilitates the pancreas's vital functions, especially regarding insulin secretion. Moreover, the relationship between the pancreas and the digestive system underscores its importance in the regulation of glucose metabolism, thereby linking its anatomical structure to its physiological roles in the body. The endocrine component of the pancreas is primarily composed of the islets of Langerhans, which contain various cell types responsible for hormone secretion. Among these, beta cells are particularly significant due to their role in producing insulin, a hormone crucial for glucose homeostasis. The architecture of the islets allows for the precise regulation of insulin release into the bloodstream, influenced by multiple factors including blood glucose levels and neural signals. This information directly ties into the incretin effect, wherein hormones like glucagon-like peptide-1 (GLP-1) amplify insulin secretion following food intake. Understanding the anatomical organization of the islets provides insight into how these cells efficiently communicate with one another and with the rest of the body, ultimately influencing metabolic processes and maintaining energy balance, a core aspect of the normal physiology of insulin action.

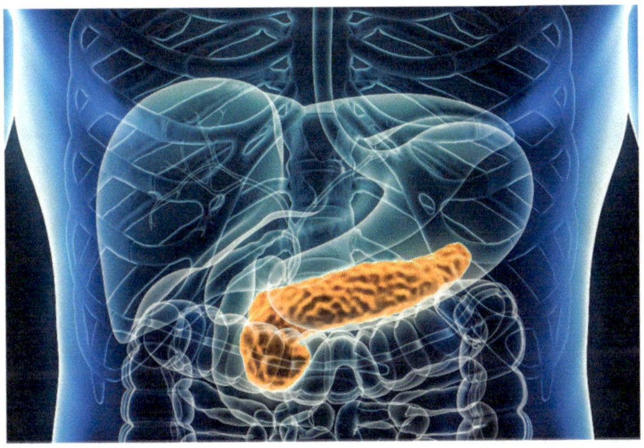

Figure 2.2. Pancreas.

Source: https://gastrofl.com/wp-content/uploads/2024/03/Inflamed-Pancreas-scaled.jpg

Moreover, the interactions between the pancreatic endocrine cells and incretin hormones highlight the intricate relationships that govern insulin secretion and action. The secretion of insulin occurs in response to both direct glucose levels and the incretin hormones released from the gut, such as GLP-1 and glucose-dependent insulinotropic polypeptide (GIP). Notably, the effects of Dipeptidyl peptidase 4 (DPP4) on these incretin hormones further complicate this dynamic. DPP4 is an enzyme responsible for the cleavage of certain peptides, including GLP-1, which can alter their receptor selectivity and bioactivity, thus impacting insulin secretion (Elmansi et al., 2019). This raises essential questions about the regulatory mechanisms at play and underscores the importance of ongoing research into pancreatic functions and incretin endocrine profiles, as advancements in this field could have significant clinical implications for diabetes treatment and management (Gunton & Girgis, 2012) (Figure 2.2).

2.1.1. Structure and Function of Pancreatic Islets

The endocrine pancreas relies on the islets of Langerhans to manage the levels of glucose in the body. The islets are made up of beta, alpha, and delta cells, and all of them work together to keep blood glucose levels in a narrow range. Cells in the islets react to many things besides the amount of glucose in the blood. There are various hormones, chemical messengers, and nerve signals that impact their release of hormones. A comprehensive understanding of the interplay between these diverse inputs is essential to appreciate how the pancreatic islets adapt to physiological changes, particularly in the context of metabolic disorders such as diabetes, where dysregulation can lead to significant health consequences (Huising et al., 2019). The way pancreatic islets function is greatly affected by the incretin effect, which means insulin is released more strongly after eating than after receiving nutrients through an IV. Key incretin hormones, such as glucagon-like peptide-1 (GLP-1) and gastric inhibitory polypeptide (GIP), play pivotal roles in this enhanced response. They mostly affect beta cells, causing them to release insulin when blood glucose is high, so hyperglycemia is prevented. Besides acting outside the pancreas, GLP-1 and GIP also work inside the islets, which greatly influence the structure and function of the pancreas. For instance, recent studies reveal that the co-expression of GLP-1 and GIP with other hormones in alpha cells demonstrates a complex interplay that underlies islet adaptation during metabolic stress, such as insulin resistance induced by prolonged glucocorticoid exposure (Flatt et al., 2014). The way pancreatic islets are organized supports good communication among their cells, which helps them all react efficiently to changes in metabolism. Every islet has an extensive network of blood vessels that speed up the delivery of hormones into the blood. The precise organization of the islets highlights the role of signals within the islets, making sure the endocrine cells cooperate well. Also, the ability of the islets to grow and change allows them to manage increased insulin resistance and maintain proper glucose levels. The intricate feedback mechanisms, shaped by both local signaling and systemic conditions, emphasize the significance of understanding the structure-function relationship in pancreatic islets, particularly for developing potential therapeutic strategies aimed at improving diabetes management (Huising et al., 2019) (Figure 2.3).

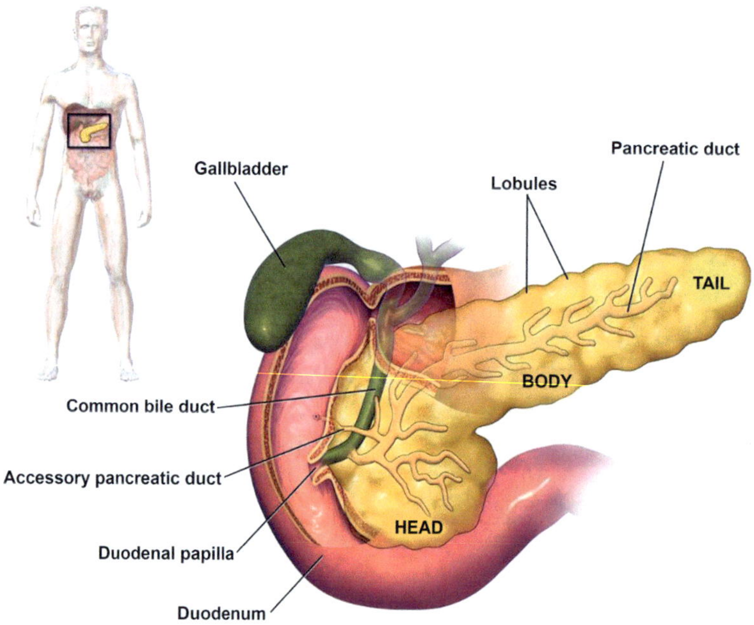

Figure 2.3. The pancreatic islets, also known as the islets of Langerhans, serve as critical components of the endocrine pancreas, orchestrating the regulation of glucose homeostasis.

Source: https://upload.wikimedia.org/wikipedia/commons/thumb/7/7e/Blausen_0699_PancreasAnatomy2.png/1200px-Blausen_0699_PancreasAnatomy2.png

2.1.2. Types of Cells in the Islets of Langerhans

The pancreas has islets of Langerhans, which house different types of endocrine cells needed to keep blood glucose levels stable. Among them are beta cells that release insulin, and these account for 60-80% of the total islet cells. They mainly react to changes in blood glucose, and this leads them to release insulin that allows glucose to enter peripheral tissues. Additionally, beta cells are influenced by the incretin hormones such as GLP-1 and GIP, which enhance glucose-induced insulin secretion through mechanisms involving cyclic AMP (cAMP) signaling pathways. These pathways not only amplify insulin release but also play pivotal roles in the differentiation and survival of beta cells, highlighting their central importance in the physiological processes governing insulin secretion and action (Furman et al., 2010). About 15-20% of the islet cells are alpha cells that secrete glucagon, which helps raise blood glucose levels when a person is not eating. Glucagon is released only when glucose levels are low and when there are other signals from neighboring cells in the islet. When the pancreas receives different nutrients, alpha cells react to messages from beta cells, demonstrating their interconnections. As a result, balanced amounts of insulin and glucagon help maintain the right level of glucose in the body. Furthermore, somatostatin-secreting delta cells, which inhibit both insulin and glucagon release, add another layer of regulatory control, ensuring that these hormones are released in appropriate proportions based on physiological needs (Huising et al., 2019). The islet also houses PP (pancreatic polypeptide) cells and epsilon cells, although they are less abundant. Pancreatic polypeptide, mainly produced by PP cells, controls the pancreas' exocrine work and also affects appetite. Epsilon cells, which make ghrelin, help regulate hunger and the amount of food people eat. All these cell types in the islets of Langerhans regulate insulin and glucagon secretion and also sense signals coming from the body's general environment. This coordination is vital for achieving glucose homeostasis and responds to various metabolic states, indicating that the islet functions as a key player in overall metabolic regulation (Huising et al., 2019) (Figure 2.4).

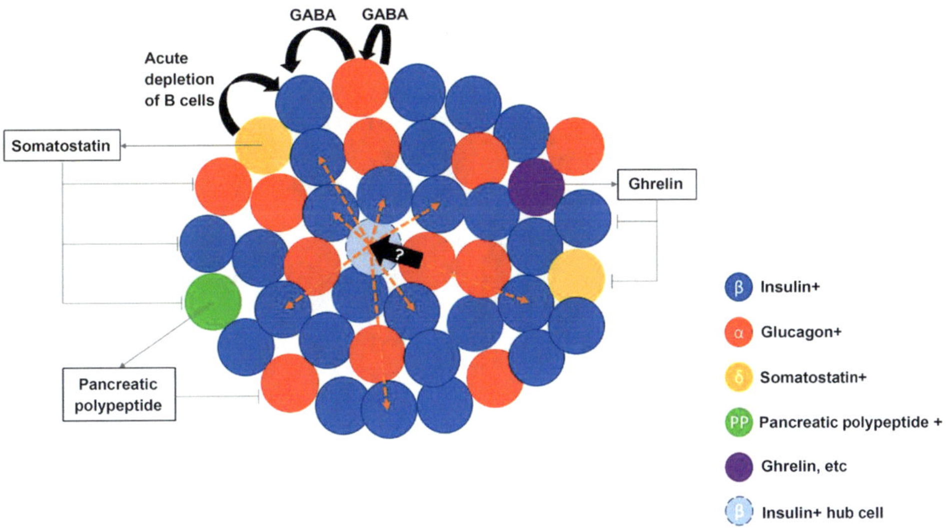

Figure 2.4. The cells of the islets of Langerhans.

Source: Da Silva Xavier G. The Cells of the Islets of Langerhans. *Journal of Clinical Medicine*. 2018; 7(3):54. https://doi.org/10.3390/jcm7030054

2.1.3. Blood Supply and Innervation of the Pancreas

The pancreas is mainly supplied by the celiac trunk and the superior mesenteric artery to ensure it gets the nutrients and oxygen it needs. To be specific, the splenic artery from the celiac trunk feeds the body and tail of the pancreas, and the gastroduodenal artery, also from the celiac trunk, supplies the head and neck of the pancreas. In addition, the pancreas has a wide network of pancreatic blood vessels that help with its metabolism and also control the release of insulin. Blood supply to the pancreas is designed in a way that hormones are delivered to the liver through the portal vein, underlining the organ's importance in glucose control and the action of hormones, mainly the incretin effect. The pancreas is innervated by both the sympathetic and parasympathetic parts of the autonomic nervous system. The sympathetic fibers are mainly connected to the celiac plexus, and they release norepinephrine to stop insulin secretion and increase glucagon secretion during stressful periods. Alternatively, the parasympathetic system, mainly through the vagus nerve, increases the secretion of insulin and helps move food through the digestive tract, which is necessary after a meal. This demonstrates that the central nervous system and the pancreas communicate to manage the pancreas's secretions according to various body conditions. Importantly, recent evidence points to the fact that the integrity of autonomic signaling is key for the incretin effect, which is needed for a strong insulin response after eating. Also, the connection between the nerves of the pancreas and the incretin effect is very important for understanding type 2 diabetes. In some cases, when diabetes or metabolic syndrome are present for a long time, a reduced incretin effect may be connected to early autonomic neuropathy. Because of this condition, the body may not release enough insulin after meals, causing poor glucose control after eating. Since this relationship is important, it is necessary to assess both the health of nerves and blood glucose levels during clinical assessments. Understanding these interactions can help in developing therapeutic interventions to restore normal pancreatic function and enhance the incretin response, thereby mitigating the risk of glycemic control complications in affected populations, as highlighted in recent studies (Mittal et al., 2016; Meling et al., 2023) (Figure 2.5).

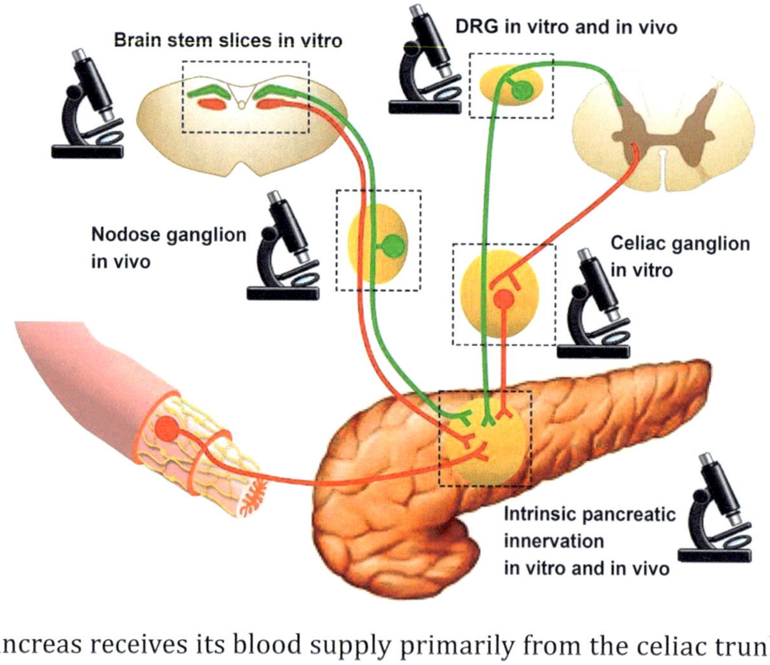

Figure 2.5. The pancreas receives its blood supply primarily from the celiac trunk and the superior mesenteric artery, which facilitate the delivery of essential nutrients and oxygen.

Source: Makhmutova M and Caicedo A (2021) Optical Imaging of Pancreatic Innervation. Front. Endocrinol. 12:663022. doi: 10.3389/fendo.2021.663022

2.2. Mechanism of Insulin Secretion

Insulin secretion is very important for keeping the level of glucose in the body steady. The main part of this process is how pancreatic beta cells react to different glucose levels in the blood. When blood glucose increases, beta cells take it and produce ATP. As ATP rises, the channels that control potassium are closed, which causes the membrane to become less negative. Because of depolarization, calcium channels open and let calcium ions into the cells. The arrival of calcium ions in the cell is a main trigger that leads to the release of insulin into the blood. So, how glucose is processed and how beta cells signal inside the body shows how complex it is to control and secrete insulin for glucose management. Apart from glucose, other things that influence insulin secretion are hormones from the gastrointestinal tract that are released when food is eaten. These hormones, particularly glucagon-like peptide-1 (GLP-1) and glucose-dependent insulinotropic polypeptide (GIP), enhance insulin secretion from beta cells in a glucose-dependent manner. The incretin effect makes insulin release greater than expected from glucose, showing that insulin is regulated in several ways. In obesity and metabolic disorders, the effects of incretins are disrupted, resulting in lower insulin production and thus higher blood glucose. Understanding how incretin hormones amplify the insulin response is crucial for developing interventions aimed at improving glycemic control and counteracting the effects of diabetes and obesity on beta cell function (Lee et al., 2019). Also, the way cells are arranged in the pancreatic islet affects how insulin is secreted. Every islet consists of different endocrine cells that communicate through paracrine and endocrine means, which affects how much insulin is produced. As an illustration, alpha cells make glucagon that can encourage insulin release, while delta cells produce somatostatin that prevents both glucagon and insulin from being released. Because of these many interactions, insulin is secreted only when the body needs it. Insights into the transcriptomes of distinct endocrine cell types have revealed how these cells integrate multiple signals for optimal hormone release (Huising et al., 2019). Studying these interactions between cells gives us useful information for creating better diabetes treatments and for learning more about insulin's functions in different metabolic states and with various diets (Figure 2.6).

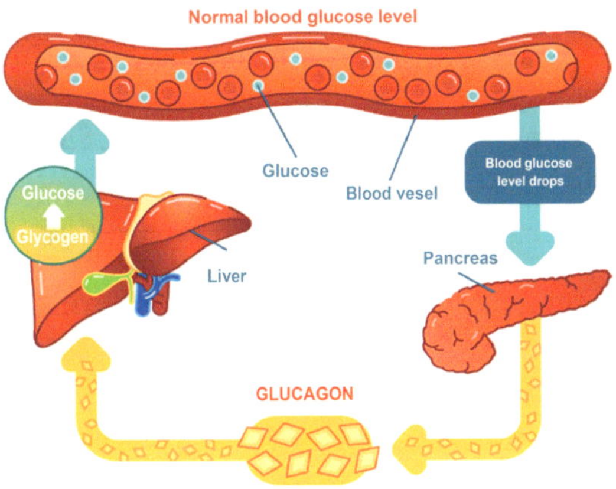

Figure 2.6. The mechanism of insulin secretion is a critical aspect of maintaining glucose homeostasis within the body.

Source: https://www.tandemclinicalresearch.com/wp-content/uploads/2024/04/how-does-glucagon-work.png

2.2.1. Stimuli for Insulin Release

The process of insulin being released from the pancreas is triggered mostly by glucose, amino acids, and fatty acids in the blood. When carbohydrates are consumed, glucose goes up in the blood, which causes the beta cells to start a sequence of metabolic activities. The uptake of glucose via the glucose transporter 2 (GLUT2) leads to an increase in intracellular ATP levels, resulting in the closure of ATP-sensitive potassium channels. As a result of closure, the cell becomes less negative, which opens voltage-gated calcium channels and lets calcium ions enter the cell. Exocytosis of insulin granules relies on an increase in calcium in the cell. Therefore, glucose is the main factor that controls insulin release and underlies insulin's main role in maintaining normal blood sugar levels and metabolism. Apart from glucose, some amino acids and fatty acids are also important for the secretion of insulin. Leucine and arginine help to stimulate insulin release by using different methods. Leucine enables insulin release by boosting the movement of calcium inside cells, and arginine does the same by raising nitric oxide levels. In addition, fatty acids help release insulin by triggering certain metabolic processes. All these stimuli allow the body to respond together, so insulin is released after eating proteins and fats, as well as after eating glucose, to keep the body balanced. The fact that insulin responds to various signals proves how complex the regulations are for insulin secretion during regular nutrient processing. The incretin effect, involving hormones such as glucagon-like peptide-1 (GLP-1) and gastric inhibitory peptide (GIP), amplifies insulin release after meals, demonstrating another layer of regulatory influence. Following the intake of nutrients, these hormones increase the ability of beta cells to respond to glucose and encourage insulin release, which helps to avoid hyperglycemia. This shows how the body responds to food by working together the gastrointestinal system and the pancreas. Studies, for example, those included in the RISE study, explain the role of these hormones in preserving β-cell function and their possible benefits for treating type 2 diabetes. By understanding these stimuli, as indicated in studies assessing β-cell response, such as those cited in Ehrmann et al. (2017) and Gaetano et al. (2019), we can appreciate the multifactorial nature of insulin secretion, especially in the context of metabolic disorders (Figure 2.7).

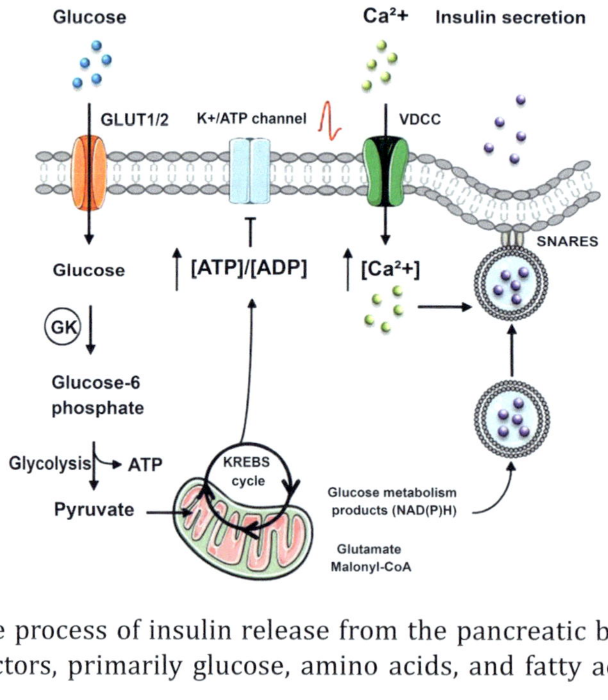

Figure 2.7. The intricate process of insulin release from the pancreatic beta cells is stimulated by various physiological factors, primarily glucose, amino acids, and fatty acids.

Source: Dalle S, Abderrahmani A. Receptors and Signaling Pathways Controlling Beta-Cell Function and Survival as Targets for Anti-Diabetic Therapeutic Strategies. *Cells*. 2024; 13(15):1244. https://doi.org/10.3390/cells13151244

2.2.2. Role of Glucose in Insulin Secretion

Insulin secretion by pancreatic beta cells is closely linked to the role of glucose in keeping the body's metabolism steady. As soon as glucose is absorbed, its levels go up in the blood, making the pancreatic beta cells notice this change through GLUT2 transporters. When glucose is inside beta cells, it increases the amount of ATP and decreases the amount of ADP, which makes the ATP-sensitive potassium channels close. The result of this closure is depolarization of the cell membrane, which makes the voltage-gated calcium channels open. The presence of calcium ions tells the cells to release insulin granules into the bloodstream. Understanding this intricate process is vital, as impaired insulin secretion in response to glucose can lead to metabolic disorders such as type 2 diabetes, highlighting the importance of glucose as a primary stimulus for insulin secretion (Farrugia et al., 2014). It is important to look at the part played by incretin hormones in the relationship between glucose and insulin. These gastrointestinal hormones, chiefly glucagon-like peptide-1 (GLP-1) and glucose-dependent insulinotropic peptide (GIP), significantly enhance insulin secretion in response to oral glucose.

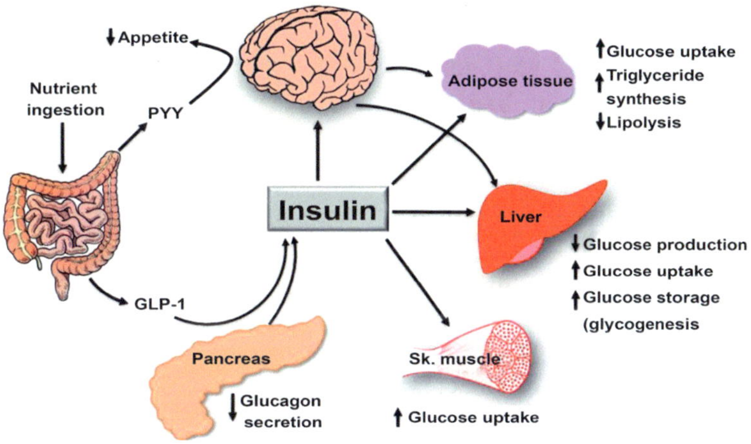

Figure 2.8. The role of glucose in insulin secretion is fundamental to maintaining metabolic homeostasis, primarily executed by the pancreatic beta cells.

Source: https://www.liebertpub.com/cms/10.1089/ars.2017.7046/asset/images/large/figure1.jpeg

They make the beta cells more sensitive to glucose in the body, especially after meals. When a person is obese or insulin resistant, the incretin effect is reduced, and so the body does not secrete enough insulin despite the glucose being high. A reduced response to food is caused by many factors, one of which is that obesity changes the liver's function and reduces the incretin hormones, which can stop GLP-1 from working and lead to higher blood sugar after meals. Thus, a comprehensive understanding of the incretin effect is critical for grasping normal insulin physiology and the pathological alterations seen in type 2 diabetes (Lee et al., 2019). In addition, the fact that pancreatic beta cells sense glucose and respond to neurological and hormonal signals proves that insulin secretion is regulated in many ways. Though glucose is the main signal, other substances called fatty acids, amino acids, and neurotransmitters help control the release of insulin to suit the body's needs. Insulin also acts on lipids and proteins, which helps control the body's overall energy levels. If insulin resistance or an improper incretin response occurs, it highlights how important it is to understand the role of glucose. Therefore, the interplay between glucose levels, beta-cell function, and incretin hormones stands as a cornerstone of both normal physiology and the pathophysiology of metabolic disorders, emphasizing the urgency of research in this critical area (Farrugia et al., 2014) (Figure 2.8).

2.2.3. Influence of Other Hormones on Insulin Release

The way insulin works with other hormones greatly affects the control of glucose metabolism and how much insulin is released. Glucagon is a main regulator that is released by the alpha cells of the pancreas. If blood glucose falls, glucagon causes the liver to release more glucose, which opposes the work of insulin. The relationship is very important because insulin helps cells absorb glucose while glucagon releases glucose when energy is needed. In addition, epinephrine and cortisol hormones raise blood glucose levels when we are stressed by encouraging the breakdown of glycogen stored in the liver into glucose, which in turn stops insulin from being released., further underscore the hormonal intricacies involved in insulin secretion. Gut hormones such as the incretin hormones, primarily glucose-dependent insulinotropic polypeptide (GIP) and glucagon-like peptide 1 (GLP-1), are released when nutrients are eaten and help increase insulin production by the beta cells of the pancreas. These hormones have several roles with insulin: they help release more insulin after meals, but they also play a part in controlling hunger and the production of glucose by the liver. Furthermore, new studies have shown that certain nutritional supplements and what we eat can increase the release of incretins. In fact, studies have shown that taking diabetes-specific oral nutritional supplements may improve post-meal glucose levels by affecting the levels of GIP and GLP-1, which are important for insulin secretion. This research suggests that the type of carbohydrates in a diet can affect both blood glucose and a person's sense of appetite. Some carbohydrates in formulations seem to reduce insulin and GIP and increase GLP-1, suggesting that hormones, hunger, and blood sugar levels are all related. Understanding these interactions further elucidates the multifactorial nature of insulin regulation and the potential for dietary strategies in diabetes management (Dávila et al., 2019; Elamansi et al., 2019) (Figure 2.9).

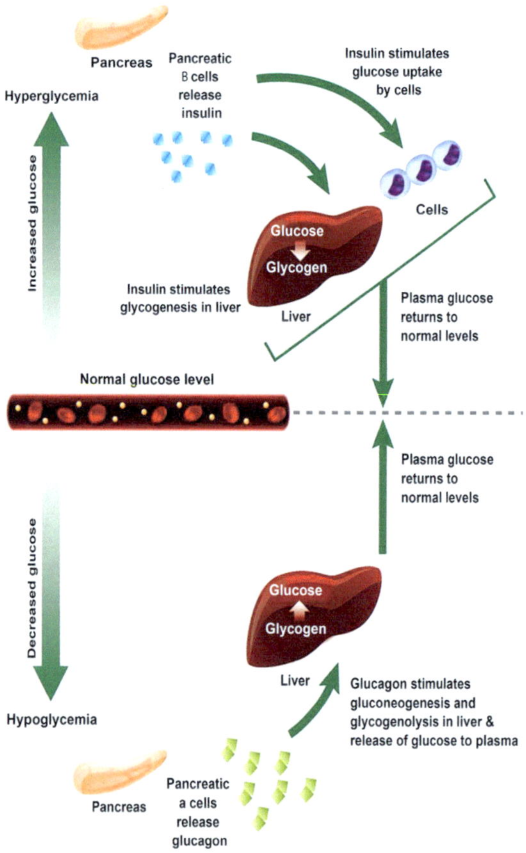

Figure 2.9. When blood glucose levels are low, glucagon stimulates glucose production in the liver, counteracting insulin's effects.

Source: https://www.mayoclinicproceedings.org/cms/10.1016/j.mayocp.2017.12.003/asset/973a4ddf-bb63-4052-b74f-6d50fa979f66/main.assets/gr1_lrg.jpg

2.3. Insulin Action on Target Tissues

Insulin's effect on target tissues is very important for glucose homeostasis and depends on several cellular activities. Following insulin's attachment to its receptor, several internal signaling pathways are set off, which result in major changes in the metabolism of muscle, liver, and adipose tissue. In muscle cells, insulin facilitates the uptake of glucose primarily through the translocation of glucose transporter type 4 (GLUT4) to the cell membrane, which is essential for energy production during physical activity. Likewise, in fat tissue, insulin helps the body build fat by promoting fat storage and stopping the breakdown of stored fat. In the liver, insulin performs several roles, including the regulation of glucose as well as the breakdown of fats. As insulin interacts with hepatic cells, it stops gluconeogenesis, thus lowering the amount of glucose the liver releases after meals. Moreover, insulin helps the liver turn extra glucose into glycogen by increasing the activity of glycogen synthase. Recent studies have highlighted the role of incretin hormones, such as glucagon-like peptide 1 (GLP-1), in enhancing insulin signaling and action in the liver. Understanding how these incretin hormones influence insulin's effects can provide insights into therapeutic strategies for managing conditions such as type 2 diabetes, where insulin action is impaired (Lee et al., 2019). Dipeptidyl peptidase 4 (DPP4) plays a significant role in modulating insulin action and incretin hormone activity, making it a focal point in diabetes research. DPP4 breaks down incretin hormones, which reduces their ability to help insulin be released. It is interesting that DPP4s not only stop these peptides; the peptide fragments left behind can still affect receptors and the body's signaling pathways. For instance, DPP4-cleaved forms of GLP-1 can engage alternative receptors, potentially modifying glucose metabolism in ways previously uncharacterized (Elmansi et al., 2019). For this reason, studying how DPP4 affects insulin signaling helps us understand insulin resistance and points to possible drugs for treating diabetes, making it easier to handle the different aspects of metabolic diseases (Figure 2.10).

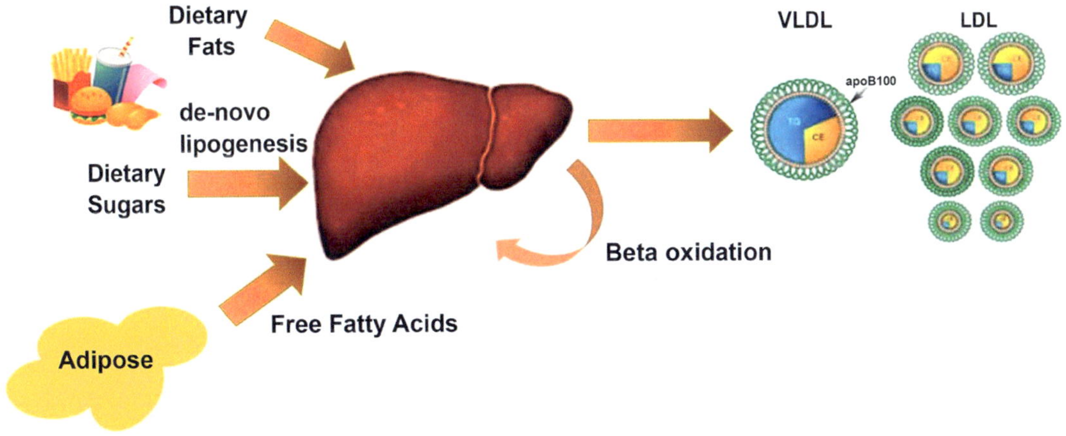

Figure 2.10. In adipose tissue, insulin promotes lipogenesis while inhibiting lipolysis, contributing to fat storage and regulation of energy balance.

Source: Bhat N, Mani A. Dysregulation of Lipid and Glucose Metabolism in Nonalcoholic Fatty Liver Disease. *Nutrients*. 2023; 15(10):2323. https://doi.org/10.3390/nu15102323

2.3.1. Mechanism of Insulin Action on Muscle Cells

Insulin acting on muscle cells is very important for maintaining glucose balance and metabolism. Upon insulin binding to its receptor on the muscle cell membrane, a cascade of intracellular signaling pathways is initiated, predominantly through the insulin receptor substrate (IRS) proteins. This activation leads to the recruitment of phosphoinositide 3-kinase (PI3K) and the subsequent activation of protein kinase B (AKT). The activation of AKT is crucial, as it promotes the translocation of glucose transporter type 4 (GLUT4) to the cell membrane, facilitating glucose uptake from the bloodstream into the muscle cells. This mechanism allows for the storage of glucose in the form of glycogen in muscles, where it can be used as a source of energy for muscle function. Insulin activates pathways that help build protein and stop the breakdown of protein. Notably, the mammalian target of rapamycin (mTOR) pathway is significantly involved in mediating the effects of insulin on protein synthesis.

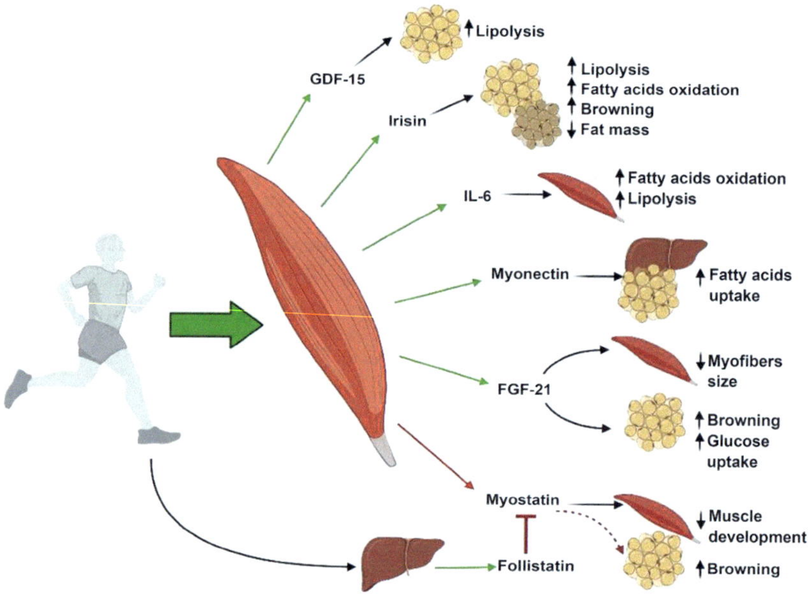

Figure 2.11. Insulin action on muscle cells is a critical component of glucose homeostasis and overall metabolic regulation.

Source: Feraco A, Gorini S, Armani A, Camajani E, Rizzo M, Caprio M. Exploring the Role of Skeletal Muscle in Insulin Resistance: Lessons from Cultured Cells to Animal Models. *International Journal of Molecular Sciences.* 2021; 22(17):9327. https://doi.org/10.3390/ijms22179327

After insulin binds, mTOR is activated, which increases the translation of mRNA to proteins and helps muscles grow and recover from exercise. Moreover, insulins ability to inhibit the breakdown of protein via reduction in the activity of components such as the Forkhead box O (FoxO) transcription factors underscores its essential role in maintaining muscle mass. Such actions are especially important in situations where muscles need to be maintained, such as when you are dieting or getting older, showing the wide effects of insulin signaling on muscles. Interestingly, the interplay between insulin action and incretin hormones, such as glucagon-like peptide-1 (GLP-1), further exemplifies the complexity of metabolic regulation in muscle cells. When we eat, incretins help our bodies secrete more insulin, which improves the body's response to insulin during meals. The positive skeletal effects of GLP-1 receptor agonists (GLP-1RAs) have been recognized, showing potential benefits not only on glucose metabolism but also on bone health, which can indirectly affect muscle function amid metabolic disorders like type 2 diabetes mellitus (Lee et al., 2019) and (Chenu et al., 2017) (Figure 2.11).

2.3.2. Insulin's Effect on Adipose Tissue

Insulin is important for controlling the metabolism of adipose tissue by strongly affecting both lipogenesis and lipolysis. Once insulin is secreted, mainly after eating carbohydrates, it encourages glucose to enter adipocytes and is changed into triglycerides for storage. Insulin does this by activating lipoprotein lipase, which breaks down triglycerides in lipoproteins so that fatty acids are taken up by adipose cells. Insulin's role in adipose tissue is shown by the fact that, when there are extra calories, the surplus glucose is stored as fat instead of being used right away.

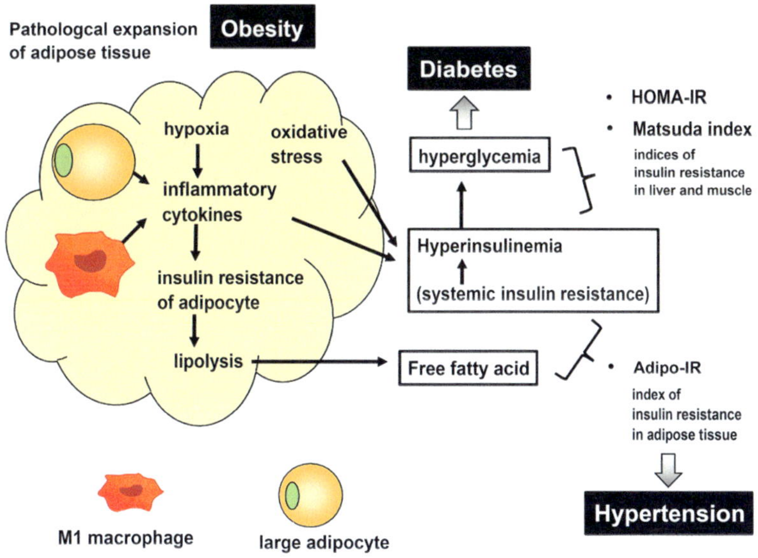

Figure 2.12. Insulin plays a pivotal role in regulating adipose tissue metabolism, exerting significant effects on lipogenesis and lipolysis.

Source: https://media.springernature.com/full/springer-static/image/art%3A10.1038%2Fs41440-023-01263-5/MediaObjects/41440_2023_1263_Figa_HTML.png

Insulin helps create triglycerides from excess glucose, preventing hyperglycemia and storing excess calories in adipose tissues. Besides helping store energy, the relationship between insulin and adipose tissue affects the whole metabolic system. Insulin sensitivity in adipose tissue is very important for keeping blood sugar levels normal and avoiding insulin resistance, which is usually linked to obesity and type 2 diabetes. In healthy people, when insulin increases, it stops fat from being broken down, keeps the amount of free fatty acids low, and supports the uptake of glucose by other tissues. When someone is insulin resistant, the adipose tissue does not react well to insulin, which results in more fat breakdown and an unusual rise in free fatty acids. This dysregulation contributes to elevated plasma glucose levels and may exacerbate systemic insulin resistance, underlining the importance of adipose functional capacity in the broader context of metabolic syndrome and related disorders (Jonathan F Wenk et al., 2013). Insulin's actions on adipose tissue are also influenced by incretin hormones, which shows how different parts of metabolism are linked. Incretins, such as glucagon-like peptide-1 (GLP-1) and glucose-dependent insulinotropic polypeptide (GIP), augment insulin secretion in response to meals while also influencing adipocyte function. In combination with insulin, these hormones help store fats and increase the formation of fat tissue, showing they cooperate in the function of fat cells. Additionally, Dipeptidyl peptidase 4 (DPP4) plays a significant role in modulating the bioactivity of these incretins, with cleaved forms potentially exerting novel, altered effects on adipose tissue function. Understanding these interactions is pivotal for developing therapeutic strategies aimed at improving insulin sensitivity and metabolic health, especially in populations affected by insulin resistance and type 2 diabetes (Figure 2.12).

2.3.3. Role of Insulin in Liver Metabolism

Insulin is essential for the liver's metabolism, as it controls the level of glucose and how energy is stored. When insulin is produced, it enables hepatocytes to take in glucose and convert it to glycogen for storage. The process is necessary to keep blood glucose levels healthy, mainly after meals. To sum up, insulin promotes glycogen formation and also reduces the process of making glucose from non-carbohydrate sources. When there are plenty of nutrients, insulin prevents the liver from releasing glucose, helping energy to be used and stored properly and thus guarding against high blood sugar and its problems.

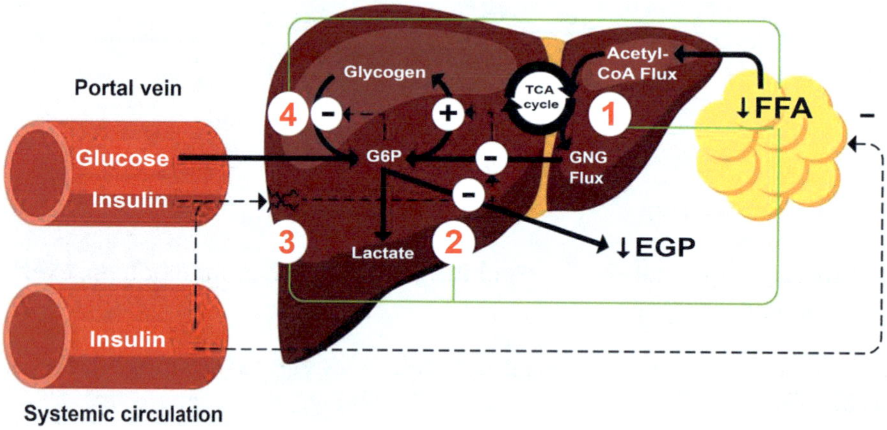

Figure 2.13. Insulin plays a pivotal role in liver metabolism.

Source: https://www.cell.com/cms/10.1016/j.cmet.2021.03.007/asset/6a6e9e93-6a12-45b9-9611-48a3a0a5405e/main.assets/gr2_lrg.jpg

It is important for the liver and metabolism that these processes are well balanced, due to insulin's key role in energy control. The incretin effect also makes insulin's job in liver metabolism more complex, since GLP-1 and GIP hormones increase insulin release after eating. The mechanism increases insulin production and also makes the liver more sensitive to insulin, which helps control its glucose levels. When it comes to obesity and type 2 diabetes, the incretin response usually does not work as well, which results in less insulin sensitivity in the liver and more glucose being produced by the liver. It has been found that obesity can increase DPP4, which breaks down incretin hormones and makes insulin's work in the liver more complicated. As DPP4 activity rises due to obesity-induced changes in liver function, the effectiveness of incretin hormones in augmenting insulin secretion diminishes, leading to a cascade of metabolic disturbances (Lee et al., 2019). It is also important to know the pathways that influence how insulin works in the liver. The release of insulin by the pancreas and the liver's reaction to it are connected, showing that the system needs to work together at different points to keep metabolism balanced. The link is measured with math and advanced measures, such as the Disposition Index, which looks at how insulin is secreted and used, to show β-cell function. However, the pathway of how incretin effects impact β-cell responsiveness remains an area requiring further exploration (Farrugia et al., 2014). Examining these connections between different organs helps us understand the detailed feedback that happens, mainly in cases of insulin resistance and insufficient insulin secretion, which are main features of type 2 diabetes (Figure 2.13).

2.4. Regulation of Insulin Secretion

Maintaining the right level of glucose in the body depends on how insulin is secreted by the body. The main part of this regulation is the pancreatic beta cells, which secrete insulin in a pulsing way depending on glucose levels. This way of secreting insulin is affected by glucose, as well as by various hormones and neurotransmitters. Notably, incretin hormones such as glucagon-like peptide 1 (GLP-1) and glucose-dependent insulinotropic polypeptide (GIP) play a significant role in amplifying insulin release in response to oral glucose intake, a phenomenon known as the incretin effect. GLP-1 and GIP release makes the beta cells more sensitive to glucose, which in turn helps insulin lower blood glucose levels. As a result, knowing how insulin secretion is regulated gives important information about managing diabetes and using incretin-based drugs. The modulation of insulin secretion extends to various substrates that are processed by enzymes that can alter their bioactivity, with dipeptidyl peptidase 4 (DPP4) being a prime example. DPP4 is an enzyme that cuts incretin hormones, making sure they are active and present in the right amounts. New studies are showing that DPP4-cleaved peptides may not be as inactive as we thought, and may have special bioactivities that need further study. By means of DPP4 cleavage, GLP-1 might target different receptors or interact with receptors that were not recognized before, which can influence the outcome of insulin secretion. As the complexity of its role in metabolism is unveiled, it raises critical questions about the conventional understanding of these enzyme functions in metabolic regulation and their implications in the pharmacodynamics of DPP4 inhibitors used in diabetes treatment (Elmansi et al., 2019). In addition, new research shows that obesity can interfere with the incretin effect, resulting in less insulin production and problems with glucose tolerance. The main process involves several organs working together, mainly due to hepatocyte hypoxia and the following expression of HIF-1α. When a person is obese, the liver DPP4 activity goes up, which results in less GLP-1 and less stimulation of insulin release by pancreatic beta cells. Disrupting the normal incretin signaling pathway greatly helps in the development of type 2 diabetes. Investigating these pathways not only enhances our understanding of the multifaceted nature of insulin regulation but also underscores the necessity for targeted interventions that can restore incretin activity and improve metabolic health, therefore paving the way for innovative therapeutic strategies (Lee et al., 2019) (Figure 2.14).

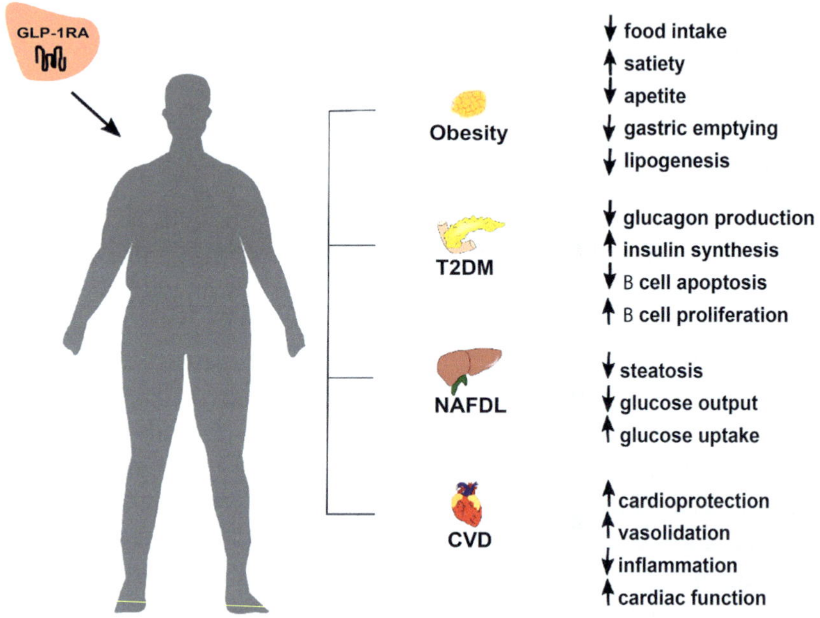

Figure 2.14. Incretin hormones such as glucagon-like peptide 1 (GLP-1) and glucose-dependent insulinotropic polypeptide (GIP) play a significant role in amplifying insulin release in response to oral glucose intake, a phenomenon known as the incretin effect.

Source: Michałowska J, Miller-Kasprzak E, Bogdański P. Incretin Hormones in Obesity and Related Cardiometabolic Disorders: The Clinical Perspective. *Nutrients*. 2021; 13(2):351. https://doi.org/10.3390/nu13020351

2.4.1. Feedback Mechanisms in Insulin Regulation

The way insulin is secreted is closely connected to feedback mechanisms that help maintain balance in the body. The main part of this regulation is the pancreatic beta cells, which react mainly to changes in blood glucose. If the level of glucose increases after we eat, beta cells start to release insulin. It helps to reduce blood glucose by supporting the use of glucose by muscle and adipose tissues. In this case, less insulin is produced when blood sugar goes down, which helps the body balance its use and storage of energy. This process not only prevents hyperglycemia but also ensures that energy reserves are adequately managed, reflecting a finely-tuned system of feedback mechanisms that sustain glucose homeostasis and overall metabolic health (Huising et al., 2019). Apart from glucose, other things also play a role in triggering insulin secretion, which shows how complicated feedback mechanisms can be. Hormonal signals, such as the incretins glucagon-like peptide-1 (GLP-1) and glucose-dependent insulinotropic polypeptide (GIP), play a significant role in facilitating insulin release in response to nutrient absorption. They function by paracrine and endocrine means, which makes beta cells more sensitive to glucose. It is important to note that although incretins raise insulin levels, they also take part in feedback loops that can control insulin action according to the body's condition. For instance, studies indicate that the products generated through the activity of dipeptidyl peptidase 4 (DPP4) can alter the bioactivity of these incretins, suggesting that post-translational modifications further refine feedback mechanisms in insulin regulation, thereby influencing not just insulin secretion but also its effective action (Elmansi et al., 2019). The regulation of glucagon release from alpha cells in the pancreas is also part of the impact of feedback mechanisms. Insulin and glucagon work opposite each other; when insulin goes up, glucagon is suppressed, and this helps maintain the right amount of glucose in the body. On the other hand, when there is not enough glucose in the blood or during fasting, glucagon is released to get glucose from the liver and offset the effects of low insulin. It is very important for blood glucose levels to remain steady, particularly when the body experiences stress due to metabolism. Understanding these interactions, including the influences of incretin peptides and their DPP4-cleaved forms, is essential in grasping how feedback mechanisms not only regulate insulin secretion but also ensure the body's overall metabolic balance and resilience, ultimately affecting long-term health outcomes (Huising et al., 2019) (Figure 2.15).

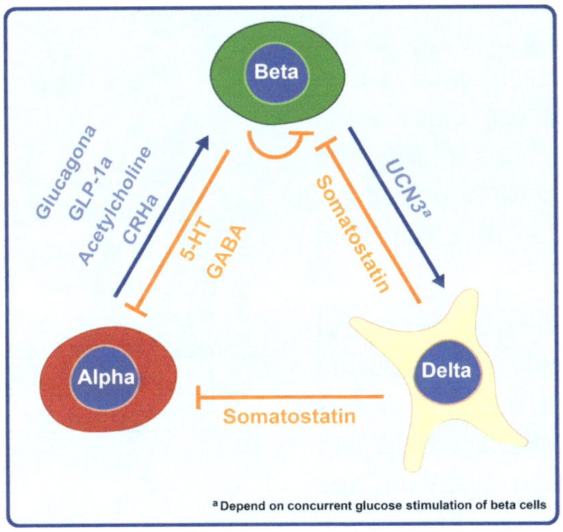

Figure 2.15. The regulation of insulin secretion is intricately tied to feedback mechanisms that ensure homeostasis within the body.

Source: Michałowska J, Miller-Kasprzak E, Bogdański P. Incretin Hormones in Obesity and Related Cardiometabolic Disorders: The Clinical Perspective. *Nutrients*. 2021; 13(2):351. https://doi.org/10.3390/nu13020351

2.4.2. Role of the Autonomic Nervous System

The autonomic nervous system (ANS) plays a crucial role in regulating insulin secretion and action, which are vital components of glucose homeostasis. Both the sympathetic and parasympathetic parts of the ANS have opposite effects on the pancreas. Usually, the sympathetic nervous system blocks insulin secretion by using norepinephrine, but the parasympathetic system, through the vagus nerve, helps insulin release after eating a meal. It allows the body to respond well to different changes in metabolism. Specifically, the incretin effect, which enhances insulin secretion after oral glucose consumption, is significantly influenced by parasympathetic nerve activation and demonstrates the integral connection between the ANS and the pancreatic endocrine response (Meling et al., 2023).

So, studying this relationship helps explain the physical reasons behind metabolic diseases such as type 2 diabetes. Disturbances in the autonomic system may cause serious changes in insulin levels, mainly when someone has diabetes. Autonomic neuropathy, a complication that usually appears late in diabetes, might actually begin earlier and disturb glucose metabolism as well as the actions of incretin hormones. When vagal tone is low, due to problems in the autonomic system, it can lead to poor insulin release and the inability to use glucose, which can make hyperglycemia worse. Moreover, studies highlight the correlation between gastrointestinal glucose handling and autonomic nervous function, with impaired gut sensitivity observed in patients with established diabetes (Meling et al., 2023).

Thus, the ANS does more than control hormones; it plays a key role in regulating metabolism and glucose after meals, which is very important for diabetes management and avoiding its complications. In addition, the fact that both neural and hormonal signals are present in the islets of Langerhans shows that the ANS has many effects on insulin secretion. All the endocrine cells in the pancreatic islet react to signals from neurotransmitters and hormones released by the autonomic system. This way, the body can deal with changes in blood glucose levels in a balanced manner. As an illustration, the alpha and beta cells in the islets use paracrine communication, guided by autonomic signals, so that their actions help maintain healthy glucose levels. Therefore, techniques that boost the autonomic nervous system could help with insulin secretion and control the body's metabolism. To summarize, since the ANS is important for insulin control, diabetes treatment should involve both neural and hormonal approaches (Figure 2.16).

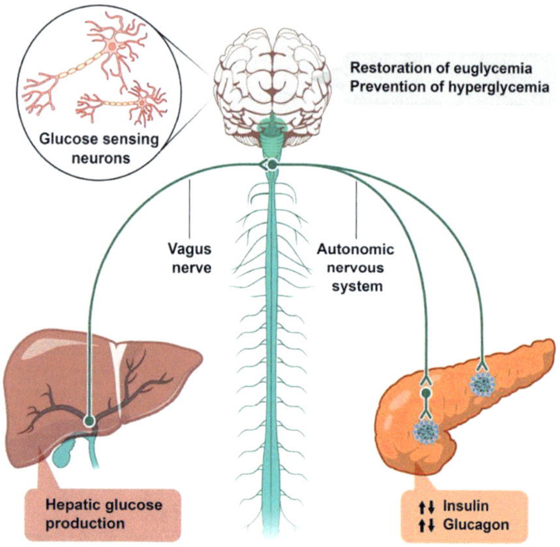

Figure 2.16. Disturbances in autonomic regulation can lead to significant impairments in insulin dynamics, particularly in the context of diabetes.

Source: https://www.cell.com/cms/10.1016/j.cell.2024.06.029/asset/2842281c-1a56-461c-a625-3d122eb5f1ba/main.assets/gr2_lrg.jpg

2.4.3. Impact of Circadian Rhythms on Insulin Secretion

Circadian rhythms, which follow a 24-hour cycle naturally, have a big impact on insulin secretion and other functions in the human body. The release of insulin after eating occurs at the right times to support your body's metabolism all day. It has been found that insulin sensitivity changes more during the day, reaching its highest point in the morning and lowest in the evening. It underlines the fact that the timing of meals and their nutrient balance are important for blood sugar control, mainly in people with diabetes or other glucose problems. The inappropriate timing of carbohydrate-rich meals can lead to destabilized blood glucose levels, exacerbating the risk of metabolic disorders such as type 2 diabetes, thereby illustrating how circadian rhythms shape insulin dynamics and metabolic health overall (Hornemann et al., 2017). Recent research has highlighted the role of incretin hormones, particularly glucagon-like peptide-1 (GLP-1), in the regulation of insulin secretion via circadian mechanisms. When nutrients are eaten, GLP-1 is released from intestinal L-cells and follows a particular daily pattern.

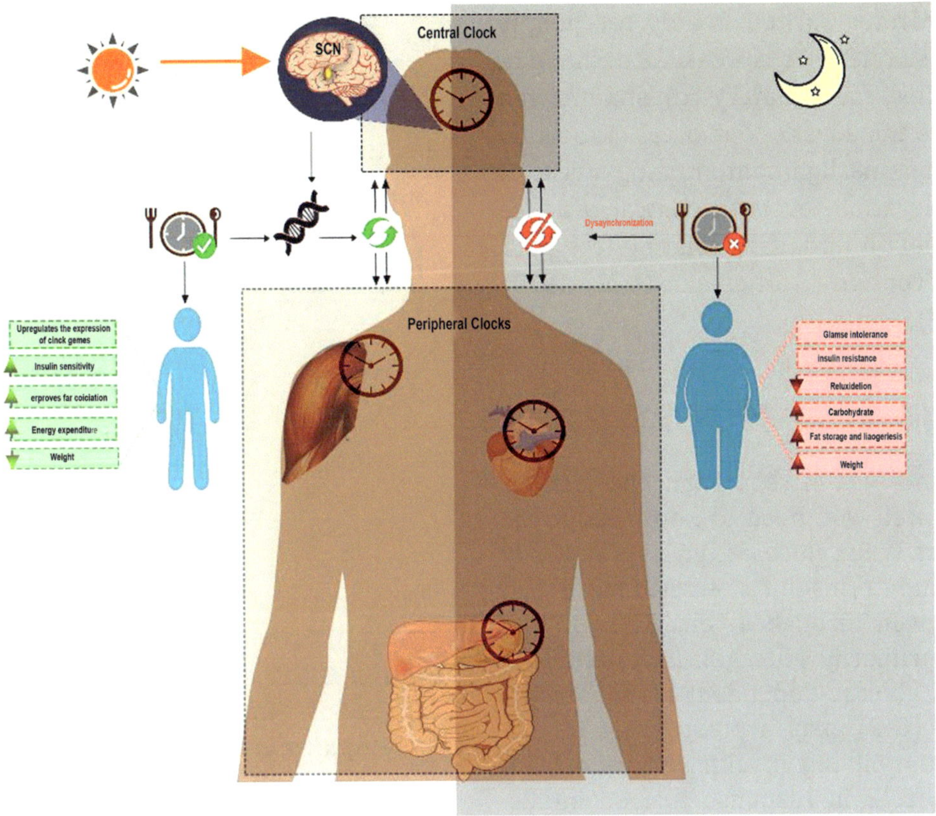

Figure 2.17. Circadian rhythms, the intrinsic biological processes that follow a roughly 24-hour cycle, significantly influence various physiological functions within the human body, including insulin secretion.

Source: BaHammam AS, Pirzada A. Timing Matters: The Interplay between Early Mealtime, Circadian Rhythms, Gene Expression, Circadian Hormones, and Metabolism—A Narrative Review. *Clocks & Sleep*. 2023; 5(3):507-535. https://doi.org/10.3390/clockssleep5030034

The results from mouse studies indicate that GLP-1 is released most at mealtime and this process depends on the core clock gene Bmal1. Mice that do not have Bmal1 have problems with GLP-1 release, suggesting that circadian clocks are linked to incretin hormones. This relationship emphasizes that the timing of food intake can modulate not only insulin secretion but also the actions of incretin hormones, which collectively contribute to glucose homeostasis (Adriaenssens et al., 2020). As a result, studying these rhythms may provide helpful ideas for creating new ways to improve metabolic health. In addition, circadian rhythms strongly affect insulin's ability to help the body take in and store glucose. It is clear from this how and when we eat affects our body's metabolism and increases the risk of metabolic diseases. If meals are timed with an individual's natural body clock, it may help insulin work better and control blood sugar levels. To help with insulin dysregulation, it may be wise to eat carbohydrates earlier, mainly for people whose glucose tolerance is weak. As outlined in various studies, these dietary adjustments can help mitigate the adverse outcomes associated with circadian misalignment, framing a critical area of exploration for both clinical practice and public health initiatives relating to type 2 diabetes prevention (Hornemann et al., 2017) (Figure 2.17).

2.5. The Incretin Effect

To understand insulin regulation and glucose metabolism well, you need to know about the incretin effect. When glucose is given to the body through the mouth, insulin is secreted more than when it is given through a vein. The incretin hormones, primarily glucagon-like peptide-1 (GLP-1) and glucose-dependent insulinotropic polypeptide (GIP), play a pivotal role in this process by amplifying insulin secretion from pancreatic β-cells in response to food intake. It shows that proper β-cell function is vital as it links the process of eating nutrients with the body's metabolic responses. If there is a disturbance in the incretin pathways, it may cause insulin secretion to be impaired, which is a main feature of type 2 diabetes, so it is important to study the molecular aspects of the incretin effect in diabetes. New studies are revealing that the incretin effect is more complicated, especially due to the role obesity plays in metabolic health. Obesity is known to alter the normal physiological responses to incretin hormones, notably by enhancing the degradation of GLP-1 through increased levels of dipeptidyl peptidase-4 (DPP-4) in the liver. As a result of these changes, the levels of GLP-1 in the blood go down, which weakens the incretin effect and the body's insulin response. It can be seen that there are many ways in which liver problems affect β-cells, so this area should be studied further. Critically, understanding these interactions may provide insights into developing therapeutic strategies aimed at reversing the deficits in insulin secretion and action observed in metabolic disorders, particularly for patients struggling with obesity and its related complications (Lee et al., 2019).

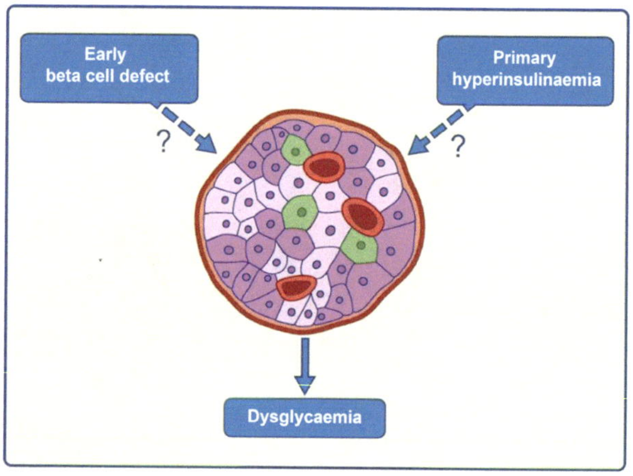

Figure 2.18. Increased hepatocyte HIF-1α expression has been shown to exacerbate the impairments in incretin action, thereby contributing to β-cell dysfunction and glucose intolerance.

Source: https://media.springernature.com/lw1200/springer-static/image/art%3A10.1007%2Fs00125-020-05245-x/MediaObjects/125_2020_5245_Figa_HTML.png

The effects of the incretin system include changes in the whole body's metabolism and liver processes. Recent findings suggest that hypoxia-inducible factors (HIFs) in hepatocytes significantly influence incretin dynamics in states of obesity. For example, when hepatocyte HIF-1α levels increase, it worsens the effects of incretins and leads to problems in the β-cells and glucose intolerance. The way liver oxygen levels affect incretin hormones has been shown to influence insulin control and metabolism of glucose. Future research directed at these mechanisms holds promise for enhancing our understanding of type 2 diabetes and developing interventions that could potentially restore the incretin effect, thereby improving insulin secretion and overall metabolic health (Farrugia et al., 2014) (Figure 2.18).

2.5.1. Definition and Significance of Incretins

Incretins are gastrointestinal hormones that have a key role in controlling insulin release. These hormones, primarily glucagon-like peptide-1 (GLP-1) and gastric inhibitory polypeptide (GIP), are released from the intestinal mucosa in response to food intake. They mainly help by causing the pancreas to release insulin only when blood glucose is high. This process is necessary to maintain normal blood sugar levels and stop post-meal high blood sugar. Knowing what incretins are and what role they play makes it clear how they affect metabolism and why they are important in the management of Type 2 diabetes, where their responses might be reduced. Incretins do more than just help in the secretion of insulin.

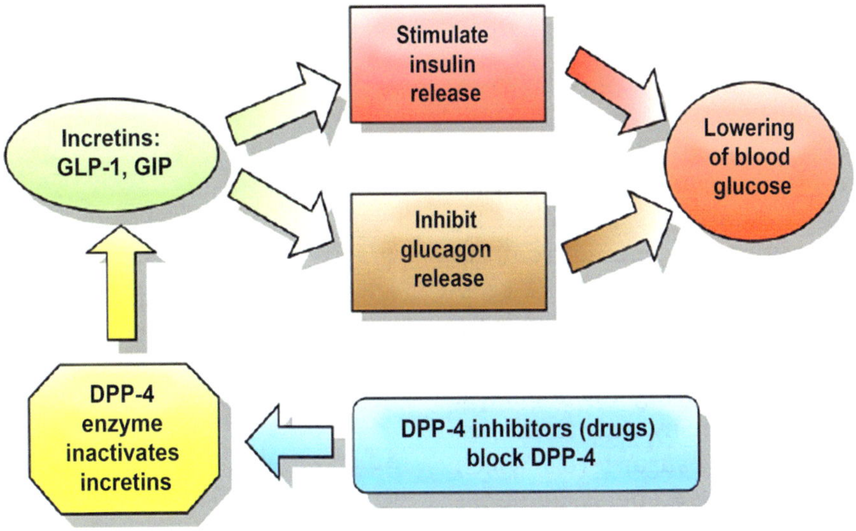

Figure 2.19. Incretins.

Source: https://upload.wikimedia.org/wikipedia/commons/thumb/6/64/Incretins_and_DPP_4_inhibitors.svg/800px-Incretins_and_DPP_4_inhibitors.svg.png

They also take part in slowing down the emptying of the stomach and making people feel full, which helps control blood glucose and appetite. By enhancing the incretin effect, medications such as low-dose gliclazide have shown promise in augmenting beta-cell function and improving glucose sensitivity, thus lowering blood glucose without inducing hypoglycemia, a significant concern in diabetes treatment (Cordiner et al., 2021). Also, the incretin effect is much stronger when nutrients are taken orally, in contrast to when glucose is given intravenously. This quality of incretin hormones proves their importance in handling blood sugar after meals, showing why they are significant for both healthy people and those with diabetes. Recent research keeps pointing out that incretins improve the body's response to insulin and are important for metabolic health during exercise. For instance, post-exercise conditions may lead to a blunted insulin response, implicating a potential involvement of incretin hormones (Glidden et al., 2010). As scientists study further, it is easier to see how incretins are controlled in the body under different conditions. It makes it clear how diet, exercise, and hormones are connected and also points out ways to treat conditions through the incretin pathways. To summarize, knowing how incretins function is important for designing treatments that help insulin work better in cases of Type 2 diabetes (Figure 2.19).

2.5.2. Major Incretin Hormones: GLP-1 and GIP

Incretin hormones, particularly glucagon-like peptide-1 (GLP-1) and glucose-dependent insulinotropic polypeptide (GIP), play a crucial role in enhancing insulin secretion postprandially. When nutrients are taken in, both hormones boost insulin release from the pancreas due to glucose. In the intestine's L-cells, GLP-1 is produced and it not only stimulates insulin but also reduces glucagon and slows down the process of emptying the stomach. Because GLP-1 influences many body functions, it assists in managing blood sugar levels, which is very important for type 2 diabetes. Evidence suggests that the insulinotropic effects of GLP-1 are mediated through its receptor (GLP-1R), which activates intracellular signaling pathways leading to enhanced insulin release, thereby underscoring the importance in the physiology of insulin secretion. Meanwhile, GIP is produced by K-cells in the duodenum and it boosts insulin release, but it is different from GLP-1 in several ways. GIP helps insulin release, but its effect is reduced when blood glucose is high, which shows that the two incretin hormones are complementary. Studies conducted recently show that GIP helps store fat and manage lipid metabolism. Because it acts on the pancreas and beta cells, GIP is an important factor in maintaining balance in metabolic activities. It is important to know that GLP-1 and GIP work with their receptors to explain the incretin effect, which is the stronger insulin response after eating compared to receiving glucose through an IV. GLP-1 and GIP help regulate glucose and also affect the health of beta cells and the body's responses to changes in metabolism.

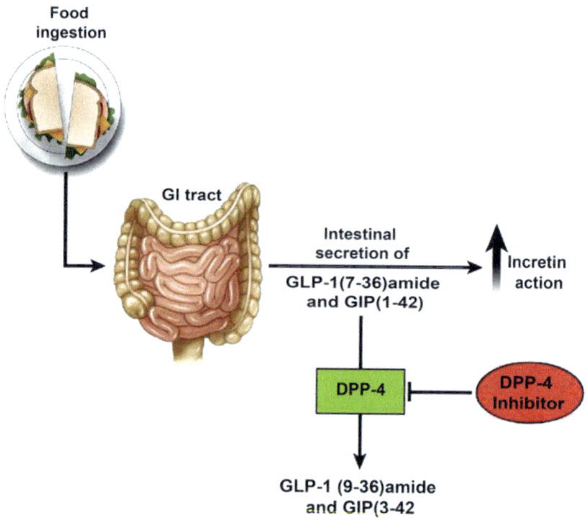

Figure 2.20. Incretin hormones, particularly glucagon-like peptide-1 (GLP-1) and glucose-dependent insulinotropic polypeptide (GIP), play a crucial role in enhancing insulin secretion postprandially.

Source: https://www.gastrojournal.org/cms/10.1053/j.gastro.2007.03.054/asset/42102416-d464-4989-95ca-5da0c03de069/main.assets/gr2_lrg.jpg

Research has shown that the absence of functional GLP-1 and GIP receptors significantly impairs islet adaptations to insulin resistance, as demonstrated by studies on mice lacking these receptors (Flatt et al., 2014). In particular, the mice had less beta cell mass and could not cope well with situations that cause insulin resistance, for example, receiving hydrocortisone. Moreover, these hormones are crucial for maintaining how islets are built and work, which is why they are key in preventing the problems of diabetes.

Therefore, understanding the intricate dynamics of GLP-1 and GIP secretion and action informs therapeutic strategies aimed at enhancing incretin signaling in the management of diabetes and other metabolic disorders while elucidating potential avenues for developing DPP4 inhibitors that address the complexities of incretin biology (Elmansi et al., 2019) (Figure 2.20).

2.5.3. Mechanisms by Which Incretins Enhance Insulin Secretion

When nutrients are eaten, incretins encourage the pancreas to release more insulin. The two primary incretin hormones, glucagon-like peptide-1 (GLP-1) and glucose-dependent insulinotropic polypeptide (GIP), are secreted in response to food intake. As soon as these hormones enter the blood, they attach to certain receptors on pancreatic β-cells, which start a series of internal signals that cause insulin to be released. It makes sure that insulin is released in greater amounts, which helps control blood sugar and avoids high blood sugar episodes. Furthermore, incretins also promote insulin gene expression and β-cell proliferation, suggesting their broader role in preserving pancreatic function over time, particularly in the context of insulin resistance and type 2 diabetes (Lee et al., 2019). Still, the way incretins function is affected by a number of things, like obesity and metabolic conditions.

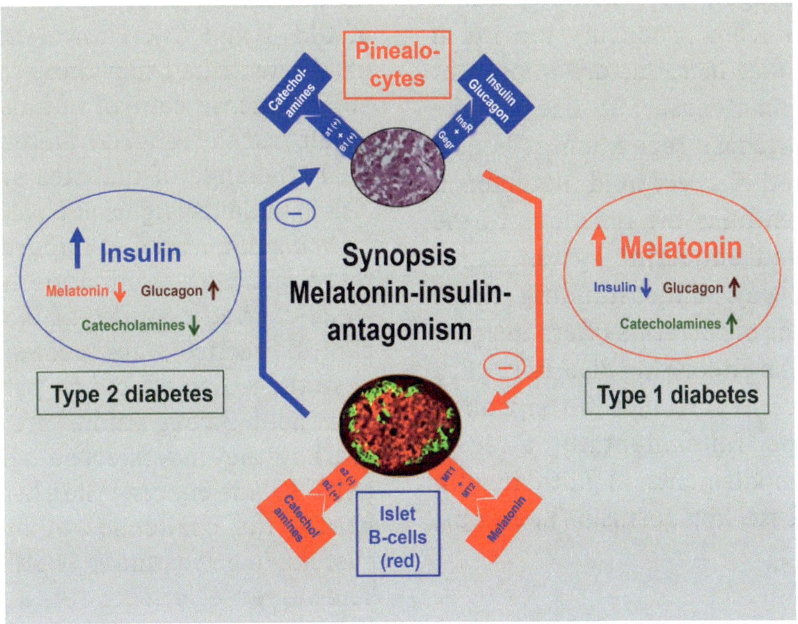

Figure 2.21. Upon entering the bloodstream, these hormones bind to specific receptors on pancreatic β-cells, leading to a cascade of intracellular signaling pathways that ultimately stimulate insulin release.

Source: Peschke E, Bähr I, Mühlbauer E. Melatonin and Pancreatic Islets: Interrelationships between Melatonin, Insulin and Glucagon. *International Journal of Molecular Sciences*. 2013; 14(4):6981-7015. https://doi.org/10.3390/ijms14046981

Research indicates that obesity can disrupt incretin effects due to increased dipeptidyl peptidase 4 (DPP4) activity, which cleaves and inactivates incretin hormones before they can exert their insulinotropic effects. When liver DPP4 rises and sinusoidal blood flow drops due to obesity, the level of GLP-1 in the blood drops too, which makes it less able to stimulate insulin secretion. It proves that there is a strong connection among body weight, hormones, and β-cell function. Studying these connections shows the many layers of glucose metabolism and highlights possible ways to treat it. Targeting DPP4 inhibitors may help restore incretin functionality and reinstate normal insulin secretion patterns, offering a promising approach for metabolic disease management (Elmansi et al., 2019). In addition, incretins influence metabolic pathways that do more than just stimulate insulin, as they also help control the release of glucagon. For example, GLP-1 prevents the liver from producing too much glucose. It shows that incretins are important not only for insulin release but also for the whole process of glucose regulation. It is also believed that incretins affect lipid metabolism and appetite, which links the functions of the gastrointestinal and endocrine systems in a more integrated way. Understanding these multifaceted actions of incretins offers insights into the mechanisms underlying disorders such as type 2 diabetes, where incretin signaling pathways may be fundamentally altered, contributing to impairments in both insulin secretion and glucose homeostasis (Lee et al., 2019) (Figure 2.21).

2.6. Clinical Implications of Insulin Physiology

Insulin physiology affects many metabolic processes and diseases, not just the main one of glucose metabolism. It is very important for medical professionals, mainly diabetes and metabolic disorder specialists, to understand how insulin is secreted and functions. For instance, the incretin effect, which involves hormones such as glucagon-like peptide 1 (GLP-1) and glucose-dependent insulinotropic polypeptide (GIP), enhances insulin secretion in response to oral glucose intake. Because of this, it is important for patients to have a proper incretin response, since its impairment can result in poor blood sugar control. Moreover, the therapeutic targeting of incretin pathways in the development of novel antidiabetic medications highlights the recognition of insulin's complex signaling role, shifting the clinical landscape towards integrated approaches in diabetes management (Elmansi et al., 2019). One of the critical therapeutic advances in diabetes care relates to the understanding of dipeptidyl peptidase 4 (DPP4) inhibitors, which enhance the incretin effect by preventing the degradation of GLP-1 and GIP. Clinical trials and research have established that these inhibitors not only aid in glucose control but also have beneficial cardiovascular effects, thereby addressing the dual challenge of diabetes and cardiovascular risk in patients (Agius et al., 2014). Yet, knowing how insulin works is important to make sure these agents are used properly. The discovery of DPP4-cleaved peptides adds new challenges to clinical practice, since these special ligands may have their own effects on patient responses to treatment. Strong studies are necessary to look into how they may affect both therapy results and possible side effects. When healthcare providers handle the challenges of insulin physiology, customizing treatment is still very important. The diverse effects of antihyperglycemic agents necessitate a personalized approach that considers not only the patient's glycemic control but also their cardiovascular health and overall metabolic profile (Agius et al., 2014). Clinicians should regularly follow new findings about insulin signaling and the incretin effect, as this information will help select and dose medications properly. Besides, learning about the clinical effects of insulin helps doctors use fewer drugs and design better treatment plans for each patient (Figure 2.22).

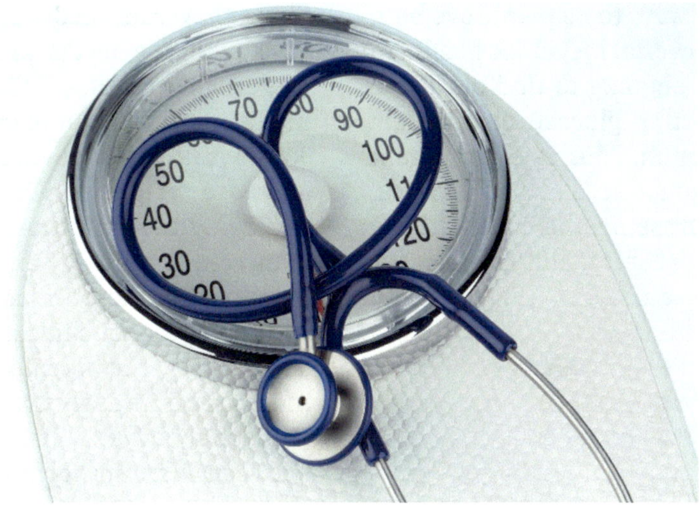

Figure 2.22. The diverse effects of antihyperglycemic agents necessitate a personalized approach that considers not only the patient's glycemic control but also their cardiovascular health and overall metabolic profile

Source: https://www.rgare.com/images/default-source/kc-article-images/cardiorenal-thumb.jpg?sfvrsn=dd56d712_2

2.6.1. Diabetes Mellitus and Insulin Dysregulation

The complexities of diabetes mellitus, particularly type 2 diabetes (T2D), are significantly tied to disruptions in insulin secretion and action. Usually, the pancreatic β-cells secrete insulin when blood glucose levels go up. Still, T2D causes β-cells to gradually lose function, resulting in not enough insulin being made. The main feature of this dysfunction is that insulin is not secreted properly at the beginning and the body is less sensitive to glucose. To evaluate these changes, research such as the Restoring Insulin Secretion (RISE) study has focused on measuring β-cell function through various methodologies, including the assessment of the incretin effect, which tests the body's response to oral glucose compared to intravenous administration. The RISE study underscores the critical importance of understanding these physiological alterations to develop effective interventions aimed at slowing the progression of pancreatic dysfunction in T2D (David A Ehrmann et al., 2017). Further complicating the landscape of T2D is the interplay of incretin hormones, particularly glucagon-like peptide-1 (GLP-1) and glucose-dependent insulinotropic polypeptide (GIP). They help the body release more insulin when glucose levels are high, which improves the way blood glucose is controlled. The lack of the incretin effect in T2D is often linked to problems in managing glucose. For this reason, new antidiabetic drugs called incretin-based therapies have appeared to help address this deficiency. By focusing on augmenting the activity of GLP-1 and GIP, these therapies not only improve insulin secretion but also positively influence insulin sensitivity and may offer neuroprotective benefits, indicating a broader utility of incretin actions beyond glycemic control (Holscher et al., 2016). It is important to consider the relationship between diabetes mellitus and insulin dysregulation in terms of both the body's functions and the types of treatment. The current research points out that making positive changes in β-cell function can help reduce insulin resistance and keep blood sugar levels in control. Medications that work with incretins are among the promising ways to help improve both insulin secretion and overall metabolic health. In addition, studies are ongoing to find out if the same processes affecting glucose metabolism might also affect the brain. Thus, it is paramount to consider both metabolic and neurological outcomes when addressing the multifaceted challenges posed by diabetes mellitus (Holscher et al., 2016; Ehrmann et al., 2017) (Figure 2.23).

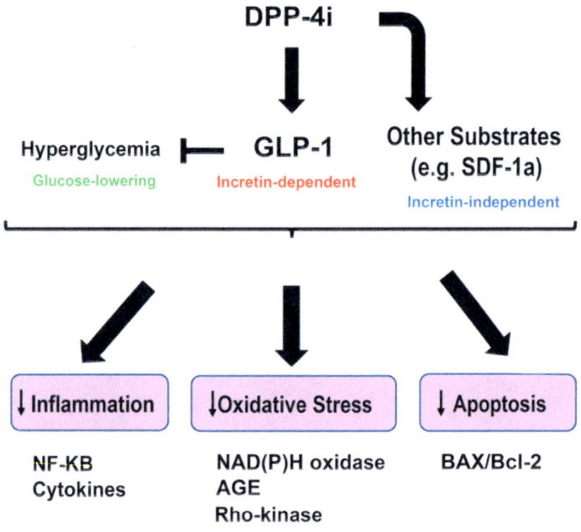

Figure 2.23. Incretin-based medications.

Source: Kawanami D, Matoba K, Sango K, Utsunomiya K. Incretin-Based Therapies for Diabetic Complications: Basic Mechanisms and Clinical Evidence. *International Journal of Molecular Sciences*. 2016; 17(8):1223. https://doi.org/10.3390/ijms17081223

2.6.2. Therapeutic Targets related to Incretin Hormones

In recent years, the therapeutic potential of incretin hormones has garnered significant attention, particularly concerning their role in managing type 2 diabetes mellitus (T2DM). Incretin hormones, including glucagon-like peptide-1 (GLP-1) and glucose-dependent insulinotropic polypeptide (GIP), function to enhance insulin secretion in response to meals, ultimately influencing blood glucose regulation. Since they can encourage insulin release only when glucose levels are high, they are good targets for treating T2DM. For example, when using liraglutide or exenatide, patients with T2DM can improve their blood sugar levels and lose weight, which is very important for managing the condition. As the understanding of incretin physiology expands, the development of innovative incretin-based therapies promises to address unmet clinical needs in diabetes care, showcasing the hormones as pivotal agents in current and future diabetes treatments (Holscher et al., 2016). The detailed link between incretin hormones and insulin shows that more research is needed to explore their uses in treating diseases. It has been found that low GLP-1 secretion is linked to T2DM, so increasing the body's GLP-1 could be a new approach to treating the disease. Some recent studies have looked into encouraging L-cells to release GLP-1, which is a more natural way to treat diabetes compared to the existing drugs. Increasing evidence shows that incretin-based therapies could be useful for neurodegenerative diseases such as Alzheimer's and Parkinson's. These studies suggest that incretin agonists may not only improve metabolic control but also have neuroprotective effects, further emphasizing the need for targeted research into incretin hormones and their multifaceted roles in health (Kappe et al., 2013). Besides, the advancement of incretin-based therapies involves knowing how they function in the body, not only by stimulating insulin release. The combinatorial use of GLP-1 and GIP agonists, alongside newer agents like dipeptidyl peptidase-IV (DPP-IV) inhibitors, has the potential to optimize therapeutic outcomes. They act together to boost the effects of incretin hormones and lower any negative side effects. Because GLP-1 and GIPs are now known to be involved in adipose tissue, gut microbiota, and metabolic balance, using incretin-based therapies could be adapted to each patient's needs, helping personalized medicine. As research continues to uncover the defining characteristics of incretin hormones, they stand poised to revolutionize the therapeutic landscape for diabetes and other related metabolic disorders, highlighting their importance as therapeutic targets in contemporary medicine (Holscher et al., 2016) (Figure 2.24).

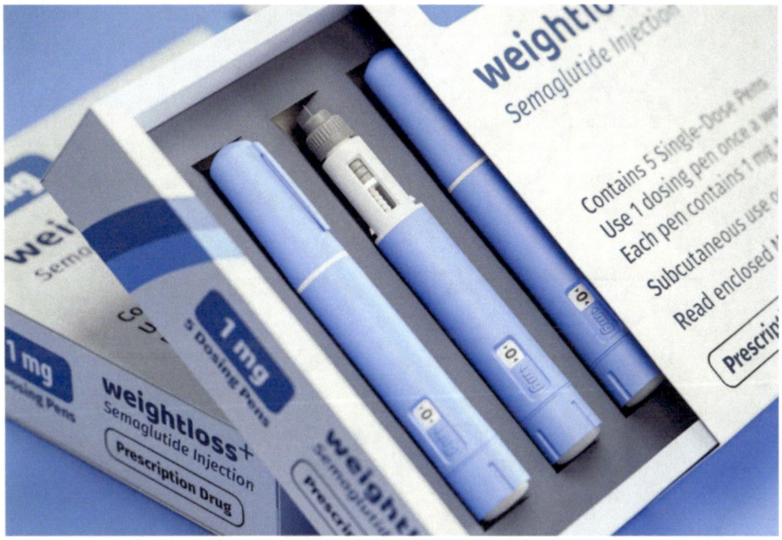

Figure 2.24. Glucagon-like peptide-1 (GLP-1).

Source: https://diatribe.org/sites/default/files/2024-04/semaglutide-istock-2025836701.jpg

2.6.3. Importance of Lifestyle Factors in Insulin Sensitivity

Lifestyle habits are very important for insulin sensitivity, especially since they support the proper functioning of insulin in the body. Frequent exercise makes the body's muscles better at using glucose and increases the body's response to insulin. Doing aerobic and resistance exercises helps increase muscle glucose uptake and also causes the body to lose visceral fat. In addition, research has shown that people who exercise regularly have a lower risk of developing insulin resistance and type 2 diabetes, which proves that prevention is as important as understanding the disease itself. When insulin sensitivity goes up, the body requires less insulin and this helps keep metabolism in good condition. Dietary choices are equally paramount in modulating insulin sensitivity. A diet that contains a lot of whole foods and little refined sugar can help insulin work better by keeping blood glucose under control. There is a link between omega-3 fatty acids, antioxidants, and minerals and better insulin function and less inflammation, which may impact how insulin works. Also, the timing and arrangement of meals can have a major impact on insulin sensitivity, as research demonstrates the benefits of fasting and eating at specific times. They prove that nutrition is vital for metabolic health and question the idea that diet is only used to lose weight, since it mainly helps control insulin and blood glucose levels. There are wider social effects to the relationship between lifestyle and insulin sensitivity, not only personal decisions. The epidemic of type 2 diabetes, characterized by insulin resistance, not only threatens individual health but also poses significant challenges for healthcare systems and economies, as noted in recent studies highlighting the costly complications associated with this condition (Jonathan F Wenk et al., 2013). Seeing how lifestyle factors affect insulin sensitivity is important for both health education and making policies. For obesity and related diseases to be reversed, it is important to introduce effective measures such as community fitness and nutrition programs. Moreover, since certain lifestyle habits can change the risk of insulin resistance, encouraging healthy living could play a key role in diabetes prevention and improving life quality for everyone. When these ideas are applied in healthcare settings, professionals can assist in preventing and controlling metabolic diseases (Figure 2.25).

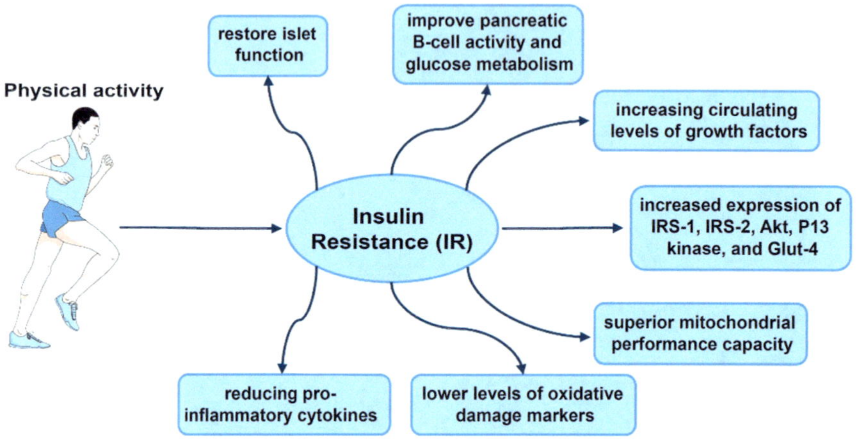

Figure 2.25. Regular physical activity has been shown to enhance the body's muscular ability to utilize glucose and, in turn, improve insulin sensitivity.

Source: Małkowska P. Positive Effects of Physical Activity on Insulin Signaling. *Current Issues in Molecular Biology*. 2024; 46(6):5467-5487. https://doi.org/10.3390/cimb46060327

A CLOSER LOOK

GASTRIC INHIBITORY POLYPEPTIDE (GIP)

Gastric Inhibitory Polypeptide (GIP), also known as glucose-dependent insulinotropic polypeptide, is a hormone produced by the K-cells in the lining of the small intestine, primarily in response to food intake—especially glucose and fat. It mainly helps the pancreas release insulin when blood sugar rises after a meal, helping to control the level of sugar in the blood. GIP does not have a major role in reducing the amount of gastric acid produced by humans. It also supports the process of storing fat by encouraging lipid storage in adipose tissue. GIP, along with GLP-1 (glucagon-like peptide-1), is part of the "incretin" system, which enhances insulin release and is a target in the treatment of type 2 diabetes.

Summary

It is clear from studying how insulin is secreted, works, and interacts with the incretin effect that a detailed knowledge of these processes is needed to progress diabetes care. The role of incretin hormones, particularly glucagon-like peptide 1 (GLP-1) and glucose-dependent insulinotropic polypeptide (GIP), in amplifying insulin release highlights a critical pathway for postprandial glucose regulation. This insight establishes a foundation for therapeutic strategies aimed at enhancing incretin signaling to optimize insulin secretion in patients, particularly those with type 2 diabetes mellitus (T2DM). As research progresses, the challenge remains to fully elucidate the mechanisms through which these hormones exert their effects, including the potential role of DPP4-cleaved peptides in modulating insulin action and overall metabolic health (Elmansi et al., 2019). Insulin signaling and bone health interact, which demonstrates how complicated endocrinology is and how it affects the whole patient. Recent findings indicate that GLP-1 receptor agonists (GLP-1RAs) not only facilitate glycemic control but also demonstrate beneficial effects on bone quality and strength, representing a dual advantage for T2DM management (Chenu et al., 2017). Noticing the risks of diabetes treatments for the skeletal system means doctors should work together, which helps patients live well and reduces their chances of complications. Future studies should aim to clarify the effects of GLP-1RAs on the bones as well as on the body's overall metabolism. To sum up, further research into insulin and the incretin effect creates many chances to improve diabetes treatment. The recognition that DPP4-cleaved peptides may possess distinct bioactive qualities opens the door for innovative treatments that could transcend traditional paradigms of metabolic regulation (Elmansi et al., 2019). Besides, it is clear that GLP-1RAs play a role in controlling blood sugar and bone health, so a variety of treatments should be used in T2DM. Further exploration of these factors can help make diabetes management better and may also change the field of diabetes research and treatment, with better outcomes for those affected.

References

1. Adriaenssens, A. E., Biancolin, A. D., Brubaker, P. L., Chalmers, J., et al. (2020). The core clock gene, Bmal1, and its downstream target, the SNARE regulatory protein secretagogin, are necessary for circadian secretion of glucagon-like peptide-1. https://core.ac.uk/download/288347589.pdf (accessed on 11th June 2025).
2. Agius, R. (2014). An update on pharmacotherapy for type 2 diabetes. https://core.ac.uk/download/46602517.pdf (accessed on 11th June 2025).
3. Elmansi, A. M., Awad, M. E., Eisa, N. H., Kondrikov, D., Hussein, K. A., Aguilar-Pérez, A., Herberg, S., Periyasamy-Thandavan, S., Fulzele, S., Hamrick, M. W., McGee-Lawrence, M. E., Isales, C. M., Volkman, B. F., & Hill, W. D. (2019). What doesn't kill you makes you stranger: Dipeptidyl peptidase-4 (CD26) proteolysis differentially modulates the activity of many peptide hormones and cytokines generating novel cryptic bioactive ligands. *Pharmacology & therapeutics*, *198*, 90–108. https://doi.org/10.1016/j.pharmthera.2019.02.005 (accessed on 11th June 2025).
4. Angarita Dávila, L. C., Aparicio, D., Bermúdez Pirela, V. J., Cisternas, J., et al. (2019). Effect of oral nutritional supplements with sucromalt and isomaltose versus standard formula on glycemic index, entero-insular axis peptides and subjective appetite in patients with type 2 diabetes: A randomized cross-over study. https://core.ac.uk/download/222767716.pdf (accessed on 11th June 2025).
5. Lee, Y. S., Riopel, M., Cabrales, P., & Bandyopadhyay, G. K. (2019). Hepatocyte-specific HIF-1α ablation improves obesity-induced glucose intolerance by reducing first-pass GLP-1 degradation. *Science advances*, *5*(7), eaaw4176. https://doi.org/10.1126/sciadv.aaw4176(accessed on 11th June 2025).
6. Chenu, C., Mabilleau, G., Iepsen, M., & Pereira, M. (2017). Novel skeletal effects of glucagon-like peptide-1 (GLP-1) receptor agonists. https://core.ac.uk/download/132194032.pdf (accessed on 11th June 2025).
7. Cordiner, R. L. M., Mari, A., Pearson, E. R., Tura, A., et al. (2021). The impact of low-dose gliclazide on the incretin effect and indices of beta-cell function. https://core.ac.uk/download/390061164.pdf (accessed on 11th June 2025).
8. De Gaetano, A., Gaz, C., & Panunzi, S. (2019). Consistency of compact and extended models of glucose-insulin homeostasis: The role of variable pancreatic reserve. https://core.ac.uk/download/195776736.pdf (accessed on 11th June 2025).
9. Ehrmann, D. A., Mather, K. J., Nadeau, K. J., Utzschneider, K. M., Savage, P. J., Zeitler, P. S., et al. (2017). Review of methods for measuring β-cell function: Design considerations from the Restoring Insulin Secretion (RISE) Consortium. https://core.ac.uk/download/84832020.pdf (accessed on 11th June 2025).
10. Farrugia, L. P., & Vella, A. (2014). Measuring β-cell function *in vivo* to understand the pathophysiology of type 2 diabetes. https://core.ac.uk/download/46602600.pdf (accessed on 11th June 2025).
11. Flatt, P. R., Moffett, R. C., Thorens, B., Vasu, S., et al. (2014). Role of endogenous GLP-1 and GIP in beta cell compensatory responses to insulin resistance and cellular stress. https://core.ac.uk/download/77179563.pdf (accessed on 11th June 2025).

12. Furman, B., Ong, W. K., & Pyne, N. J. (2010). Cyclic AMP signaling in pancreatic islets. https://core.ac.uk/download/9028568.pdf (accessed on 11th June 2025).

13. Glidden, A. R. (2010). The blunted insulin release after exercise and the relationship with gastric inhibitory polypeptide and glucagon-like peptide-1. https://core.ac.uk/download/38922642.pdf (accessed on 11th June 2025).

14. Gunton, J., & Girgis, C. M. (2012). Pancreatic beta-cell failure in the pathogenesis of type 2 diabetes. In book: A Modern Epidemic: Expert Perspectives on Obesity and Diabetes (pp.87-104)Chapter: Pancreatic beta-cell failure in the pathogenesis of type 2 diabetesPublisher: Sydney University PressEditors: Louise A. Baur, Stephen M. Twigg, Roger S.Magnusson (accessed on 11th June 2025).

15. Holscher, C., Li, L., & Li, Y. (2016). Incretin-based therapy for type 2 diabetes mellitus is promising for treating neurodegenerative diseases. https://core.ac.uk/download/76961787.pdf (accessed on 11th June 2025).

16. Hornemann, S., Kemper, M., Kessler, K., Kramer, M., et al. (2017). A randomized controlled trial. https://core.ac.uk/download/199431430.pdf (accessed on 11th June 2025).

17. Huising, M. O., & Noguchi, G. M. (2019). Integrating the inputs that shape pancreatic islet hormone release. https://core.ac.uk/download/286361735.pdf (accessed on 11th June 2025).

18. Kappe, C. (2013). Molecular regulation of hormone secretion, growth and apoptosis of GLP-1-producing cells. https://core.ac.uk/download/70340438.pdf (accessed on 11th June 2025).

19. Meling, S. V. (2023). *Diabetes Mellitus Type 2; The Incretin Effect and Interaction with The Autonomic Nervous System*. https://core.ac.uk/download/588770247.pdf (accessed on 11th June 2025).

20. Mittal, S. (2016). Pancreas transplantation: Associations with graft failure and measures of function: Pancreas graft failure and function. https://core.ac.uk/download/34074143.pdf (accessed on 11th June 2025).

21. Wenk, J. F., Campbell, K. S., Zhang, X., Liu, Z. Q., et al. (2013). Developing and validating a new comprehensive glucose-insulin pharmacokinetics and pharmacodynamics model. https://core.ac.uk/download/159182601.pdf (accessed on 11th June 2025).

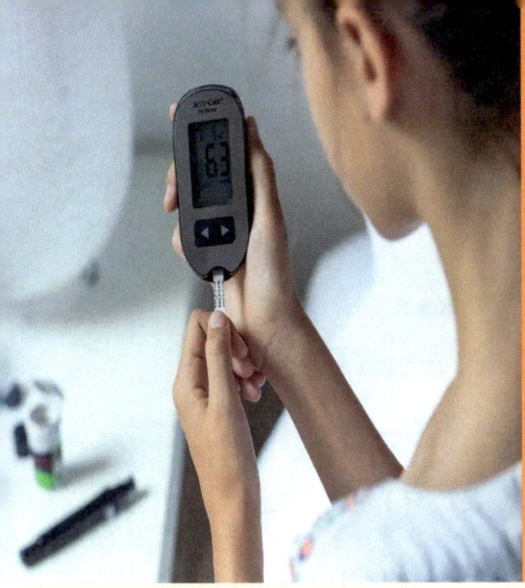

Chapter 3

EPIDEMIOLOGY AND ETIOLOGY OF TYPE 1 DIABETES

Contents

Introduction

The phenomenon of Type 1 Diabetes (T1D) represents one of the most pressing healthcare challenges in the modern world, characterized primarily by autoimmune destruction of insulin-producing beta cells in the pancreas. Although this condition usually appears in children and teens, it can begin at any age. Since the number of cases is rising worldwide, it is clear that cancer is important in public health, so more efforts are needed to study its trends and what causes it. Both social, genetic, and environmental factors are involved in T1D, so it is important to understand the disease by looking at its basic biological processes, not only by analyzing statistics. This type of study explains the people who have T1D and also guides actions to prevent and manage the disease. It is important to study the epidemiology of T1D and how its incidence rate changes in different places and times. It has been found that the number of T1D cases is rising in some populations, which shows that both environment and genetics play a role in these differences. For example, people in northern countries tend to have higher rates, which may suggest that lifestyle, vitamin D, and the immune system are connected. In addition, the number of T1D cases has been increasing lately, so scientists are now looking into possible environmental reasons, such as viruses and what people eat. Since T1D is increasing, studying these patterns is important for developing actions that can lower the number of cases and understand how it affects people and healthcare systems.

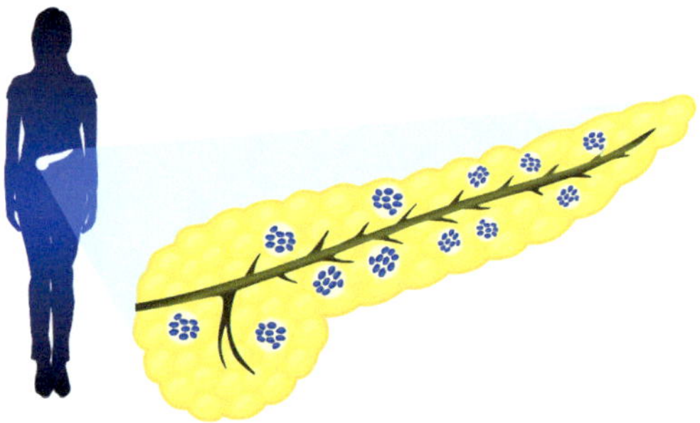

Figure 3.1. Type 1 diabetes (T1D).

Source: https://t1dtoolkit.org/wp-content/uploads/2017/04/Item-2-What-Happens-in-T1D-1-The-Pancreas.png

Along with understanding epidemiology, researchers keep exploring the causes of T1D, showing that it is affected by both genes and the environment. Studies have identified specific susceptibility genes, such as those in the human leukocyte antigen (HLA) region, which interact with environmental triggers to initiate the autoimmune process leading to beta-cell destruction. By looking at genes and environmental factors like viruses or the way people eat, a complete picture of T1D's beginning can be formed. In addition, scientists are focusing on finding out more about these causes and on creating ways to prevent and treat these diseases. Exploring these mechanisms may help improve management and discover new ways for immunotherapy, which would support public health efforts to reduce the effects of Type 1 diabetes on people and communities (Figure 3.1).

3.1. Understanding Type 1 Diabetes

Type 1 diabetes (T1D) represents a complex interplay of genetic susceptibility and environmental triggers, leading to the autoimmune destruction of insulin-producing beta cells in the pancreas. Since there is no insulin in the body, people with this condition must get insulin from outside for the rest of their lives. The epidemiology of T1D requires looking at the number of cases and the population affected by this disease. The rate of multiple sclerosis is higher in Finland and Sweden, which may suggest that both environmental and genetic factors can cause the autoimmune process. Looking into these patterns is very important for public health plans to prevent and detect T1D early, especially in places where it is becoming a major health issue. Moreover, T1D has a multifaceted cause, and researchers have made good progress in finding certain genes related to it. Several genetic areas linked to T1D have been found by genome-wide association studies, meaning that genes play an important role in the disease's development. Still, having these genetic markers does not always mean a person will develop the disease, which points to the importance of viruses or certain foods. As an example, enterovirus has been connected to the development of autoimmune responses that hurt beta cells. With this knowledge, scientists can develop actions that may help people at high risk for T1D avoid the disease, using a wide range of approaches. Apart from genes and the environment, how T1D is handled and its outcomes are influenced by psychological and social elements. Many patients deal with a range of emotions after their diagnosis, such as anxiety, depression, and the constant need to take care of themselves. Since T1D is a long-term condition, people with the disease must monitor their blood sugar closely, which may result in exhaustion and reduced well-being. Family members, friends, and healthcare workers are very important in helping people with diabetes take care of themselves. A better grasp of these psychosocial factors can result in better education and programs, helping to give a more complete approach to diabetes care. Adding psychological support to regular care can help people with T1D stick to their treatment and improve their health, while also giving a better overview of the disease (Figure 3.2).

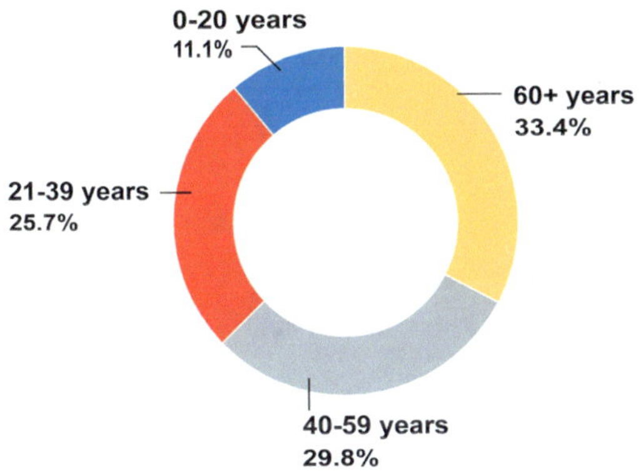

Figure 3.2. Understanding the epidemiology of T1D involves examining the incidence and prevalence of this disease across diverse populations.

Source: https://media.springernature.com/full/springer-static/image/art%3A10.1038%2Fs41574-024-01046-z/MediaObjects/41574_2024_1046_Fig1_HTML.png

3.1.1. Pathophysiology of Type 1 Diabetes

The pathophysiology of Type 1 diabetes is characterized by an autoimmune response that predominantly affects the insulin-producing beta cells of the pancreas. This autoimmune process leads to the selective destruction of these cells, resulting in insufficient insulin production and ultimately, hyperglycemia. Genetic predisposition plays a significant role in the onset of Type 1 diabetes, as individuals with certain human leukocyte antigen (HLA) genotypes are at a greater risk. Environmental factors, such as viral infections and dietary components, may also act as triggers for this autoimmune response. The result of this complex interplay is a profound alteration in glucose metabolism, forcing affected individuals to rely on exogenous insulin for blood glucose regulation, thereby highlighting the critical nature of understanding these underlying mechanisms in the management and prevention of the disease. Once the autoimmune destruction of beta cells begins, various cytokines and autoantibodies are produced, signaling an inflammatory response that further exacerbates the loss of insulin secretion. Specifically, the presence of antibodies to insulin, glutamic acid decarboxylase (GAD), and islet antigen-2 indicates an ongoing immune attack on the pancreatic islets. The progressive loss of beta-cell function leads to a state of absolute insulin deficiency, which manifests clinically as typical symptoms of hyperglycemia, such as polyuria, polydipsia, and weight loss. Furthermore, metabolic derangements induced by insulin deficiency affect the body's ability to utilize glucose and fats properly, resulting in alternative energy pathways, such as ketogenesis. This can lead to the life-threatening condition known as diabetic ketoacidosis (DKA), which necessitates a comprehensive understanding of the metabolic changes accompanying Type 1 diabetes to ensure effective clinical interventions. The long-term consequences of Type 1 diabetes extend beyond the immediate effects of hyperglycemia and insulin deficiency. Chronic exposure to elevated blood glucose levels can lead to microvascular and macrovascular complications, including retinopathy, nephropathy, and cardiovascular diseases. These complications arise not only from poor glycemic control but also from the underlying pathophysiological processes that affect vascular health. For instance, the formation of advanced glycation end products (AGEs) contributes to endothelial dysfunction, thereby enhancing the risk of atherosclerosis and other vascular damages. While advancements in diabetes management have improved outcomes for individuals with Type 1 diabetes, understanding the pathophysiology remains crucial. As ongoing research explores potential immunotherapies and regenerative approaches for beta-cell preservation, it is evident that a multifaceted knowledge base is essential for addressing both the immediate and long-term challenges of this chronic condition (Figure 3.3).

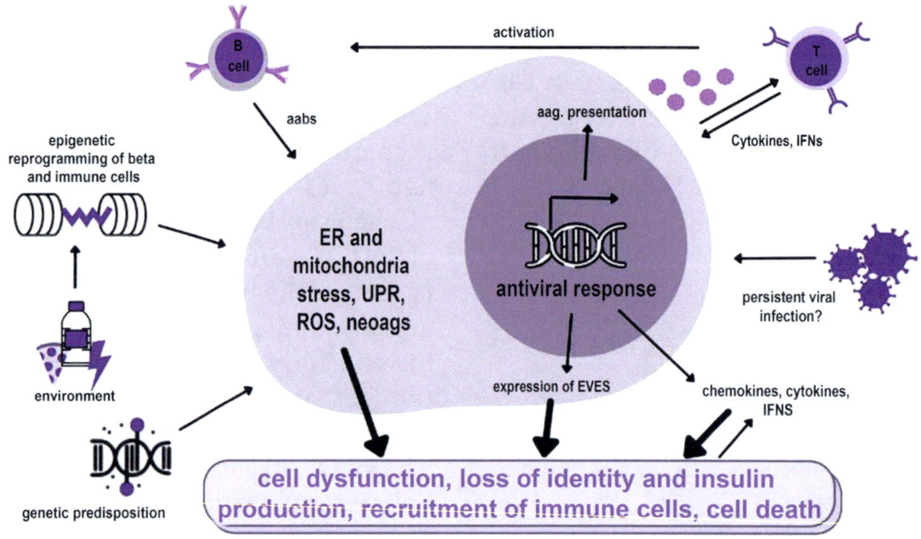

Figure 3.3. The pathophysiology of Type 1 diabetes is characterized by an autoimmune response that predominantly affects the insulin-producing beta cells of the pancreas.

Source: Zajec A, Trebušak Podkrajšek K, Tesovnik T, Šket R, Čugalj Kern B, Jenko Bizjan B, Šmigoc Schweiger D, Battelino T, Kovač J. Pathogenesis of Type 1 Diabetes: Established Facts and New Insights. *Genes*. 2022; 13(4):706. https://doi.org/10.3390/genes13040706

3.1.2. Symptoms and Diagnosis

The symptoms of Type 1 diabetes typically manifest suddenly and can often be severe, distinguishing it from other forms of diabetes. The classic symptoms include polyuria, polydipsia, and polyphagia, indicative of excessive urination, thirst, and hunger, respectively. Patients may also experience rapid weight loss and fatigue owing to the body's inability to utilize glucose effectively due to insufficient insulin production. These clinical signs are usually clear, prompting individuals to seek medical attention. Understanding these symptoms is essential not only for immediate clinical intervention but also for long-term management, as recognizing them can lead to timely diagnosis and treatment, ultimately minimizing complications associated with hyperglycemia and diabetic ketoacidosis, which are particularly dangerous in young, undiagnosed patients. Diagnostic protocols for Type 1 diabetes involve several key laboratory tests to confirm hyperglycemia and evaluate the body's insulin production. The most common initial test is the measurement of fasting plasma glucose levels, where a value of 126 mg/dL or higher indicates diabetes. Additionally, an oral glucose tolerance test and random plasma glucose tests can also support diagnosis. Furthermore, the presence of autoantibodies specific to Type 1 diabetes can be evaluated to distinguish it from Type 2 diabetes. A comprehensive metabolic panel may be employed to assess kidney function, electrolyte balance, and acid-base status, particularly in cases presenting with ketoacidosis. While symptoms guide initial suspicion, precise diagnostic methods are crucial to establishing the etiological framework of Type 1 diabetes and guiding subsequent therapeutic interventions (Kitsiou et al., 2013). Early diagnosis significantly influences the management outcomes of individuals with Type 1 diabetes, as it allows for the prompt initiation of insulin therapy, which is vital for controlling blood glucose levels. Moreover, ongoing monitoring and regular screening for complications such as nephropathy, retinopathy, and cardiovascular issues are crucial components of diabetes care. Effective management requires a multidisciplinary approach, incorporating healthcare professionals such as endocrinologists, diabetes educators, and dietitians. Furthermore, emerging technologies, including continuous glucose monitors and insulin delivery systems, enhance patient autonomy and adherence to treatment regimens. Through a combination of symptomatic awareness and robust diagnostic methodologies, healthcare systems can improve early detection rates and optimize patient outcomes in Type 1 diabetes management, reducing hospitalization rates and enhancing quality of life (Brandt et al., 2008) (Figure 3.4).

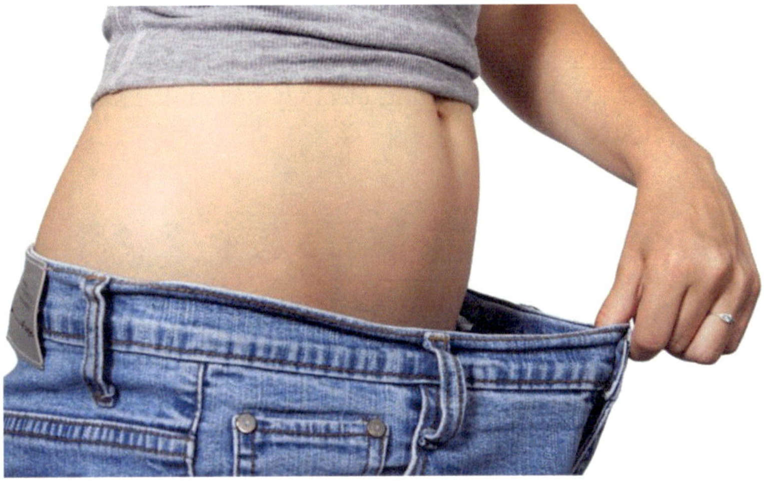

Figure 3.4. Patients may also experience rapid weight loss and fatigue owing to the body's inability to utilize glucose effectively due to insufficient insulin production.

Source: https://www.sugarfit.com/assets/62a75c83a5be9bcdc5bc724c_belly-g1506dba1d_1280_Z2fiE2R.jpg

3.1.3. Differences between Type 1 and Type 2 Diabetes

It is important to know the differences between Type 1 and Type 2 diabetes to understand their effects on public health and the way each condition is distributed. An autoimmune attack on pancreatic beta cells in Type 1 diabetes causes a complete loss of insulin. Most of the time, this condition appears in children or teenagers, but it can also develop in adulthood. On the other hand, Type 2 diabetes is mostly caused by cells in the body not responding well to insulin. Often, this form appears in older people and is linked to being overweight, not exercising, and having certain genes. Since each type of diabetes has its own causes, its distribution among people is not the same. Type 1 is uncommon, making up only 5-10% of all cases, while Type 2 accounts for the majority, or about 90-95%. The reasons behind the development of Type 1 and Type 2 diabetes make their differences easier to understand. The combination of genetic weaknesses, outside triggers, and autoimmune reactions in Type 1 diabetes results in the destruction of cells that make insulin. It has been found that certain HLA genes and other genetic markers linked to Type 1 diabetes make it mostly a condition that runs in families. On the other hand, Type 2 diabetes is caused by both genetic factors and the way someone lives. Many times, it starts with insulin resistance and ends with beta-cell malfunction. It underlines that environmental elements such as diet and exercise are important reasons for the rising number of Type 2 diabetes cases in various populations. Knowing about these differences is necessary to design effective prevention and intervention plans. It is important for public health to consider these factors to handle the diabetes epidemic and adapt its programs accordingly. Since Type 1 diabetes is diagnosed early and must be managed throughout life, more effort should be made to teach young people about autoimmune diabetes. In this case, preventing Type 2 diabetes is mainly about helping people at risk improve their lifestyle. Because of the growing number of Type 2 diabetes cases, it is clear that community health promotion is necessary due to the rise in obesity and inactivity worldwide. Notably, as illustrated in studies examining physical morbidity, emerging patterns suggest a shift in demographic susceptibilities over time, indicating the importance of ongoing research in understanding how these differences evolve across populations (MacLean et al., 2013; Catchpole et al., 2014). These differences in epidemiology and etiology determine the future of research and policies related to diabetes (Figure 3.5).

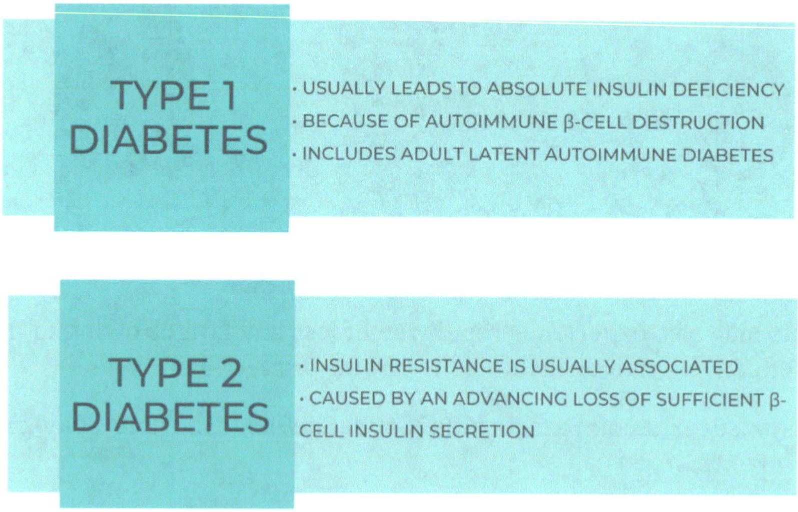

Figure 3.5. Understanding the differences between Type 1 and Type 2 diabetes is vital for grasping the broader implications of these conditions within public health and their respective epidemiological profiles.

Source: Surlari Z, Ciurcanu OE, Budala DG, Butnaru O, Luchian I. An Update on the Interdisciplinary Dental Care Approach for Geriatric Diabetic Patients. *Geriatrics.* 2023; 8(6):114. https://doi.org/10.3390/geriatrics8060114

3.2. Epidemiology of Type 1 Diabetes

The epidemiology of Type 1 diabetes (T1D) presents a complex landscape characterized by variances across geographical regions, age groups, and genetic backgrounds. It has been found that the number of T1D cases is increasing all over the world, with children and young adults in developed countries being most affected. Scandinavian countries have very high numbers of T1D cases, a result of both genetics and exposure to certain environmental elements. On the other hand, African communities have fewer cases of the disease, and its details are not fully understood in many regions. It is very important for public health to understand these patterns so that early diagnosis and treatment can be used to improve patient outcomes. However, the limited data from regions such as Africa necessitate further research to fully comprehend the epidemiological dynamics of T1D across diverse populations (Padoa et al., 2011). Besides location, the age at which Type 1 diabetes starts can be very different for each person. It appears that the age at which African individuals get Alzheimer's is later than the age for Europeans, so researchers are considering what environmental and genetic factors might be involved. According to the trends, the number of cases in Africa is lower, but the later start suggests that the way the disease develops or the genes involved may be different. It is important to understand this, since the age at when T1D is diagnosed can change the way the disease is treated and the patient's long-term results. Clarity on these distinctions can aid healthcare providers in developing more culturally and regionally appropriate prevention and management strategies (Padoa et al., 2011). In addition, Type 1 diabetes is now seen as a chronic autoimmune disease affecting the health of people everywhere. The expenses from this disease are not limited to insulin and monitoring supplies; they also include the costs of long-term problems and lost work productivity. According to research, early detection and treatment of T1D can greatly reduce the complications, which in turn helps reduce the number of deaths and sicknesses. For this reason, knowing the epidemiology of T1D is important for policymakers who need to use resources efficiently and take preventive actions. Enhanced surveillance and data collection efforts across various populations will be integral in addressing the challenges posed by T1D, especially in regions with limited healthcare infrastructure (Padoa et al., 2011) (Figure 3.6).

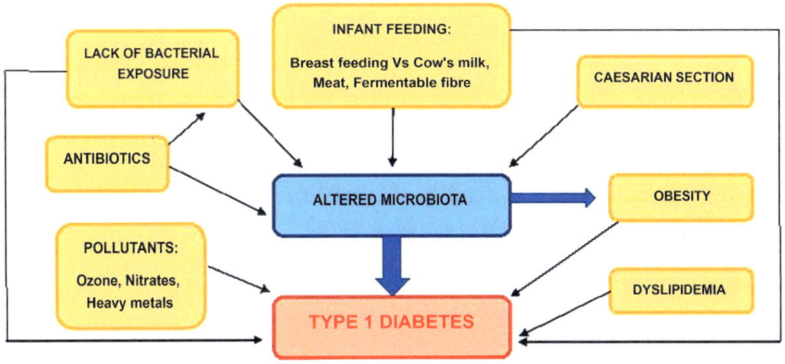

Figure 3.6. The epidemiology of Type 1 diabetes (T1D) presents a complex landscape characterized by variances across geographical regions, age groups, and genetic backgrounds.

Source: Ogrotis I, Koufakis T, Kotsa K. Changes in the Global Epidemiology of Type 1 Diabetes in an Evolving Landscape of Environmental Factors: Causes, Challenges, and Opportunities. *Medicina.* 2023; 59(4):668. https://doi.org/10.3390/medicina59040668

3.2.1. Global Prevalence and Incidence Rates

There are major differences in the number of Type 1 diabetes cases found in different parts of the world. According to data, Type 1 diabetes, which is less frequent than Type 2, can be very serious for those who have it, mainly in places with limited access to healthcare. In different Sub-Saharan African countries, Type 1 diabetes is found in 4 to 12 cases for every 100,000 people. Mozambique had a rate of 4 per 100,000, while Zambia reported 12 per 100,000, which demonstrates that healthcare and testing for these diseases are not the same in both areas. These differences underscore the necessity for extensive epidemiological studies to better understand Type 1 diabetes prevalence and incidence rates, which can significantly influence public health funding and development strategies focused on chronic disease management and prevention (Hall et al., 2011).

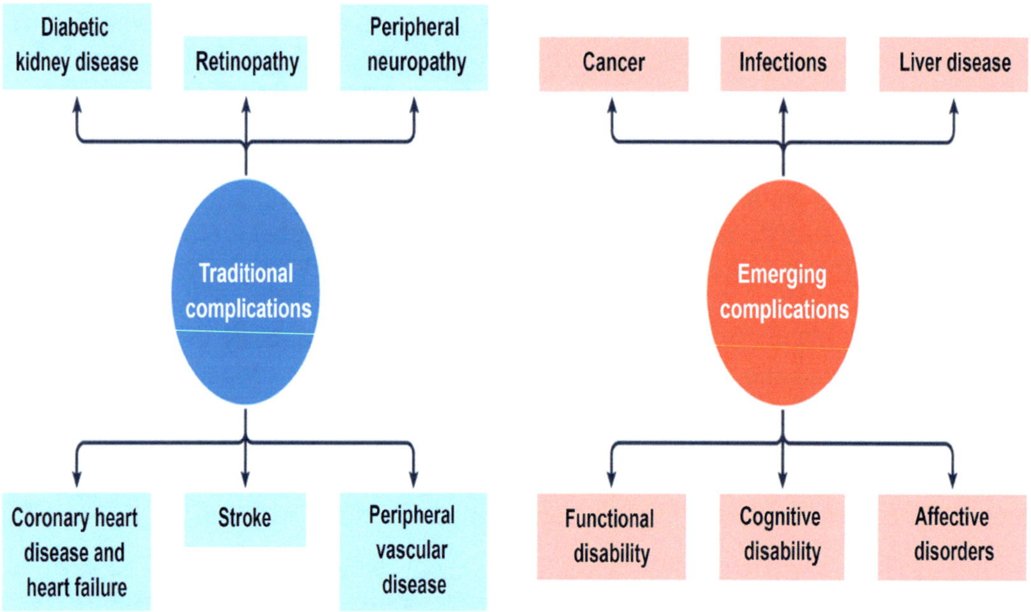

Figure 3.7. Data indicates that Type 1 diabetes, although less common than Type 2, can have severe implications for affected individuals, especially in regions with inadequate healthcare resources.

Source: Surlari Z, Ciurcanu OE, Budala DG, Butnaru O, Luchian I. An Update on the Interdisciplinary Dental Care Approach for Geriatric Diabetic Patients. *Geriatrics.* 2023; 8(6):114. https://doi.org/10.3390/geriatrics8060114

In addition to finding out how common Type 1 diabetes is, it is necessary to study its incidence across the world. Many countries have observed higher numbers of Type 1 diabetes cases, which is worrying both healthcare workers and policymakers. Although the number of cases of Type 1 diabetes is lower than for Type 2, the quick increase in children and teens is a big problem for public health. Therefore, it is necessary to study the factors that may be causing more cases of Type 1 diabetes. The appropriate response to this trend requires concerted efforts to understand these dynamics, particularly in regions where the healthcare infrastructure is insufficient to accommodate the growing number of cases (Kalsi et al., 2013). We should not overlook that Type 1 diabetes adds to the rising number of sick people. As more people are diagnosed with diabetes, they become more likely to experience retinopathy and neuropathy, which may result in major health problems in the future. When there are not enough resources for managing diabetes in some countries, the results are high death rates and poor clinical outcomes. Many people cannot get early treatment for diabetes because of money problems and a shortage of healthcare facilities, which makes the problem worse. As evident from the systematic review, the total annual cost associated with diabetes in regions such as Sub-Saharan Africa reaches an estimated US$67.03 billion, highlighting an urgent need for integrated healthcare strategies that target both communicable and non-communicable diseases, ultimately improving the overall management of Type 1 diabetes (Hall et al., 2011) (Figure 3.7).

3.2.2. Demographic Factors Influencing Prevalence

The number of people with Type 1 diabetes is strongly affected by demographic factors, and there are big differences between different populations. Because Type 1 diabetes usually appears when someone is young, age is a key factor in this disease. It has been found that the number of cases is higher among the younger groups, which means that extra attention and prevention should be given to them. In addition, it has been observed that northern Europe has higher breast cancer rates than southern Europe. Because of these demographic differences, it is important to study the causes of health and how healthcare works in each region, so public health efforts can be directed at Type 1 diabetes.

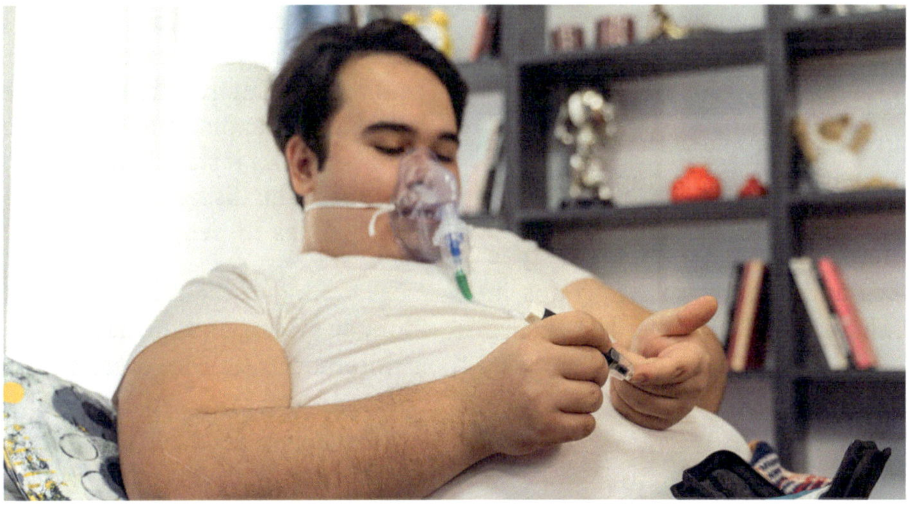

Figure 3.8. Age is one of the most defining demographic elements, as the onset of Type 1 diabetes typically occurs in childhood or early adulthood.

Source: https://diabetesonthenet.com/wp-content/uploads/Young-adult-type-2-diabetes-iStock-1387024489.jpg

The number of people with Type 1 diabetes is affected by gender, which adds an interesting point to its epidemiology. According to research, males are somewhat more likely to develop prostate cancer than females, and this could be due to hormonal and genetic factors in these groups. It makes people wonder about the biological reasons that lead to the difference in risk for men and women. Moreover, some demographic features, for example, family history, social status, and ethnicity, are associated with a person's risk of getting this autoimmune disease. Understanding these factors well is important because it allows healthcare professionals to spot high-risk people and create suitable interventions, which helps patients and the public health in managing Type 1 diabetes. Socioeconomic status (SES) stands out as a significant demographic factor influencing the prevalence of Type 1 diabetes, whereby disparities in health access may exacerbate health outcomes. Those from lower SES groups may not get the right care and management on time, causing their diabetes to become more complicated and affecting their general health. In addition, there are differences in diabetes education and advice for prevention between people of different socioeconomic backgrounds. When SES is combined with ethnicity and place of residence, it becomes easier for risk factors to affect the number of people with diabetes. To sum up, dealing with these demographic factors is essential for creating successful public health policies that help lower the number of Type 1 diabetes cases and make sure all groups in the population have equal access to healthcare (Figure 3.8).

3.2.3. Trends in Type 1 Diabetes Over Time

Over the past few decades, the number of Type 1 diabetes cases has gone up, which has caught the attention of many scientists. It has been observed in epidemiology that the rate of Type 1 diabetes is increasing globally, especially in Scandinavia and North America. Since more cases are being seen, it seems that both genes and the environment are involved, so more research on these factors is required. The fact that incidence rates differ in different areas may mean that people in these areas are exposed differently, have different habits, and experience different early immune events. By knowing these factors, it becomes easier to create public health plans to stop this trend and find those who might develop Type 1 diabetes later on. Also, the age of onset gives important information about the changes happening in Type 1 diabetes. Although it was believed to mostly affect kids and teens, more adults are now being diagnosed with the condition. Adult-onset cases are rising due to a number of reasons, including new ways to diagnose, more awareness, or perhaps an actual rise in these populations. It is now clear that adult-onset Type 1 diabetes can have unique symptoms, which may disrupt the usual ways of managing the disease. As people age, their symptoms or the progression of the disease may change, which makes us question the main causes of the disease. Sorting out these challenges is necessary to create effective management plans for adults with Type 1 diabetes. Environmental elements are very important in explaining the trends seen in Type 1 diabetes. Experts are now looking into what may cause the disease, including diet, infections, and changes in people's daily routines.

Looking at the role of carbohydrates in the immune system and the development of diabetes is interesting because studies have different opinions on this subject. Still, studies have shown that there is little connection between eating different types of macronutrients and the risk of Type 1 diabetes, so more detailed factors should be considered when examining diets. Researchers need to keep including different environmental factors as they study the many aspects of Type 1 diabetes to better understand its patterns and design useful interventions (Figure 3.9).

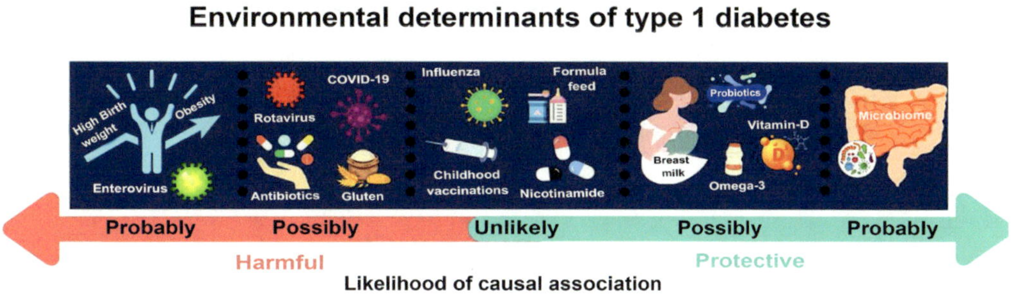

Figure 3.9. Infographic illustrating the key environmental determinants of type 1 diabetes and their likelihood of contributing to causality.

Source: Quinn LM, Wong FS and Narendran P (2021) Environmental Determinants of Type 1 Diabetes: From Association to Proving Causality. Front. Immunol. 12:737964. doi: 10.3389/fimmu.2021.737964

3.3. Genetic Factors in Type 1 Diabetes

The complex interplay of genetic factors significantly contributes to the development of Type 1 Diabetes (T1D), reflecting intricate biological mechanisms that underlie disease susceptibility. Both family and twin studies have found that monozygotic twins are more likely to have T1D together than dizygotic twins, suggesting that genes are very important in causing the disease. It is estimated that 40% of the risk for T1D comes from inherited genes, so only a small number of people with a genetic risk will get the condition. Notably, genetic markers associated with T1D often involve human leukocyte antigen (HLA) genes, which are known to influence immune response and are frequently implicated in autoimmune diseases, including T1D. Identifying these genetic markers is very important, since it helps develop preventative and treatment strategies for at-risk people and increases our knowledge of diabetes epidemiology. In the last few years, new genomic technologies have helped scientists discover the genetic variants linked to T1D, giving us more knowledge about its causes. Comprehensive genome-wide association studies (GWAS) have identified numerous non-HLA genetic loci that contribute to the risk of developing T1D, expanding the genetic landscape of the disease beyond previously established genes. The cystolic fractal gene has been suggested as a possible gene that plays a role in T1D's autoimmune process. Still, these genetic changes do not act by themselves; they are affected by other factors, including viruses and what a person eats, which can be important in causing diabetes. It is important to understand these interactions to see how many different factors are involved in T1D and to follow a comprehensive approach in epidemiology. More analysis of genetics indicates that the family clustering of T1D points to possible environmental factors that work with genetic predispositions. It has been shown through epidemiological studies that having a family history of T1D increases the risk of the disease in offspring, even though the details of the process are not yet clear. It has been found that gestational diabetes and a mother's general metabolic state during pregnancy can change the way diabetes risk genes are expressed in children. Studies point out that changes in the environment inside the womb can alter a person's genetic predisposition, so we should consider both genes and the environment together. They point out that we should pay attention to both genetic and environmental factors when studying Type 1 Diabetes and looking for ways to prevent and treat it (Figure 3.10).

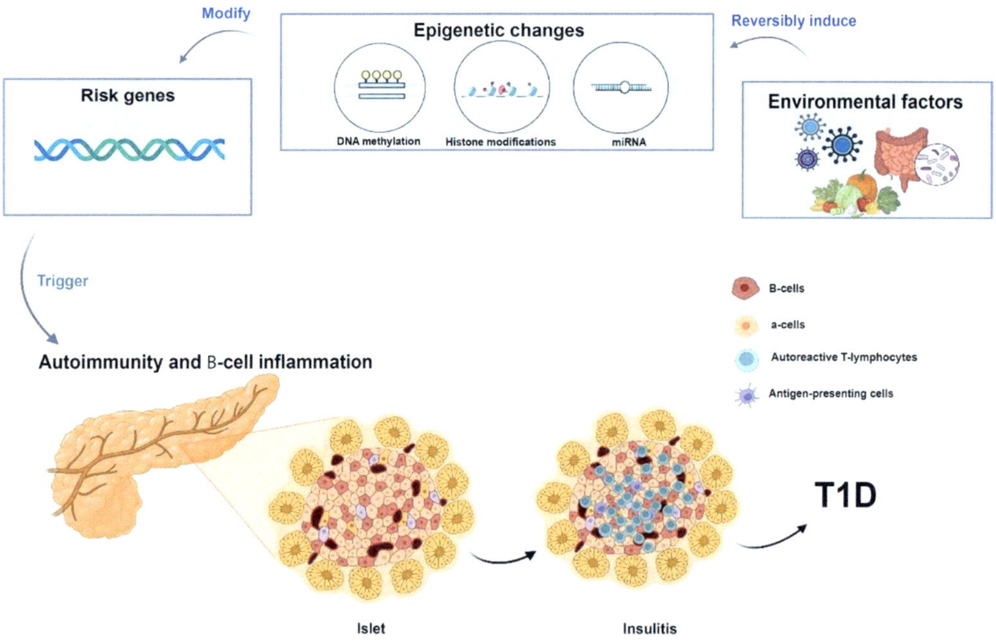

Figure 3.10. The cystolic fractal gene, for instance, has emerged as a candidate gene that may influence autoimmune pathways related to T1D.

Source: Mittal R, Camick N, Lemos JRN and Hirani K (2024) Gene-environment interaction in the pathophysiology of type 1 diabetes. Front. Endocrinol. 15:1335435. doi: 10.3389/fendo.2024.1335435

3.3.1. Role of Family History and Genetics

The intricate relationship between genetics and family history plays a significant role in the epidemiology and etiology of Type 1 Diabetes (T1D). Studies on epidemiology show that individuals with relatives who have T1D, mainly first-degree relatives, are more likely to develop the condition. This familial clustering indicates a genetic predisposition where specific alleles, particularly those related to the human leukocyte antigen (HLA) system, are strongly associated with T1D onset. The more relatives who have the disorder, the higher the risk, which implies that genetics may be the reason for its development. It is also believed that viral infections can interact with genetic factors, which shows that T1D is not only caused by heredity. New findings from genetic research explain that T1D is caused by several different factors. In particular, finding many genetic loci linked to T1D has helped reveal the biological processes involved. As an example, genetic differences in the immune system and pancreas reveal that problems with the immune system are key to the development of these diseases. In addition, research indicates that people with specific risk alleles tend to show different immune activity, which could make them more likely to develop autoimmunity against pancreatic beta cells. It means that knowing the genetic factors of T1D can help find and treat people at risk early, possibly changing the course of the disease for them. A person's family history plays a major role in the development of Type 1 Diabetes. It has been found in several studies that a woman's pregnancy and sibling relationships are important factors in T1D development. The fact that children of mothers with diabetes are more likely to get the condition points to the possible effects of what happened in the womb. Contrarily, research has pointed out that a family history of T1D on the father's or grandparent's side is less related to the disease, which suggests that the mother's genetics and environment are more important. Such findings illuminate the need for comprehensive family history assessments in clinical settings, as they can provide valuable insight into a patient's risk profile and direct proactive monitoring or preventive measures as indicated by familial patterns of diabetes onset (Chircop et al., 2003; Pfister et al., 2011) (Figure 3.11).

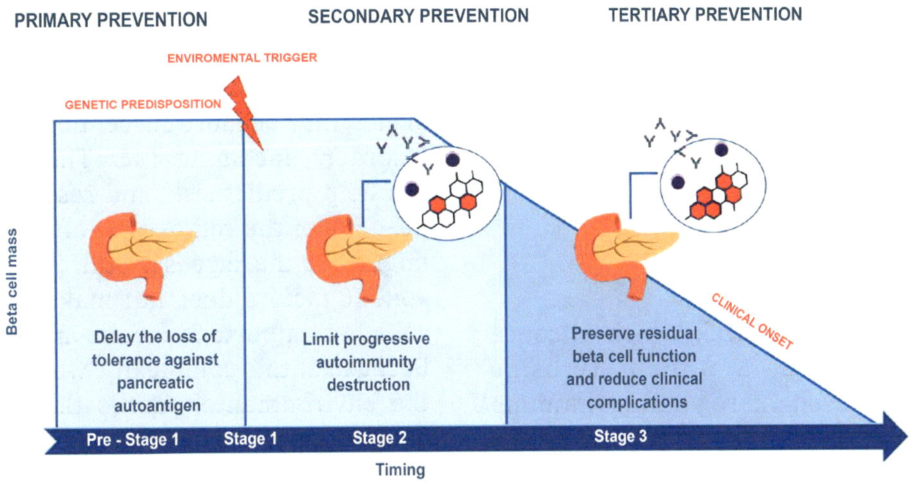

Figure 3.11. Individuals with a family history of T1D, particularly first-degree relatives, exhibit a substantially increased risk of developing the condition.

Source: Ingrosso DMF, Quarta MT, Quarta A, Chiarelli F. Prevention of Type 1 Diabetes in Children: A Worthy Challenge? *International Journal of Environmental Research and Public Health*. 2023; 20(11):5962. https://doi.org/10.3390/ijerph20115962

3.3.2. Specific Genes associated with Type 1 Diabetes

The genetic architecture of Type 1 Diabetes (T1D) is remarkably complex, primarily characterized by the involvement of multiple genes that interact with environmental factors, contributing to disease susceptibility. Among the genes identified, the HLA (human leukocyte antigen) region on chromosome 6 stands out due to its strong association with T1D. For example, having HLA-DR3 or HLA-DR4 alleles seems to raise the risk of diabetes by playing a key part in the autoimmune attack on beta cells in the pancreas. It demonstrates that T1D is influenced by several genes, and the chances of getting it depend on both genetics and the environment. Besides the HLA genes, other genes that are not part of HLA have also been associated with T1D. It is noteworthy that genes such as INS and PTPN22 have been found in several studies to raise a person's risk of developing the disease. When it comes to the INS gene, some specific changes have been linked to differences in insulin production, and these changes may lead to immune-related destruction when certain environmental factors appear. PTPN22 points to the fact that changes in immune regulation can make people more likely to develop autoimmune diseases such as T1D. Since genetics is involved in many ways, it is important to learn about the disease's genetic background and how the immune system works in it. In addition, scientists have started studying common genetic factors that both humans and dogs (for example) have when they develop diabetes.

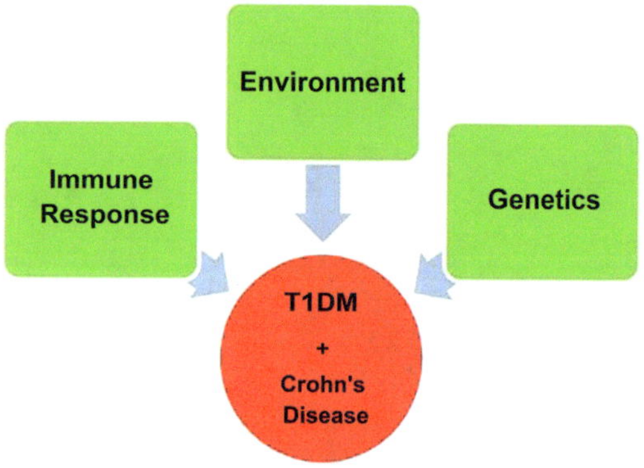

Figure 3.12. Genes like INS, which encodes insulin, and PTPN22, a protein tyrosine phosphatase involved in regulating immune responses, have been identified in various studies as contributing to susceptibility.

Source: Sharp RC, Abdulrahim M, Naser ES and Naser SA (2015) Genetic Variations of PTPN2 and PTPN22: Role in the Pathogenesis of Type 1 Diabetes and Crohn's Disease. Front. Cell. Infect. Microbiol. 5:95. doi: 10.3389/fcimb.2015.00095

A study indicated that certain genes associated with maturity onset diabetes of the adult (MODY) in humans similarly correlate with diabetes in specific dog breeds. It points to the possibility of a similar genetic background and leads us to wonder about the reasons behind diabetes vulnerability in different animals. Also, looking at the common genetic pathways can help explain how diabetes develops in dogs and may lead to special genetic tests for this disease in canines, as well as insights useful for human medicine. The interconnectedness of genetic factors across species enhances our understanding of the complexities underlying Type 1 Diabetes and reinforces the need for multidimensional research strategies to unravel its etiology (Hanley et al., 2009; Catchpole et al., 2014) (Figure 3.12).

3.3.3. Genetic Predisposition Versus Environmental Triggers

Understanding the interplay between genetic predisposition and environmental triggers is crucial in the epidemiology and etiology of Type 1 Diabetes (T1D). Genetic predisposition implies that individuals possessing specific genes, such as certain human leukocyte antigen (HLA) alleles, may be more susceptible to autoimmune disorders, including T1D. These genetic signs can help predict risk, and research shows that 10–15% of the relatives of affected individuals might get the disease. Still, just having these genetic factors does not make T1D inevitable, so other important factors must be involved. Because of this complexity, we should look into the environmental causes that might lead to disease, since they work together with genetics to determine a person's risk. Viral infections are an important environmental factor in the development of T1D, pointing out that this autoimmune disease is caused by several factors. It seems that some viruses, for example, Coxsackie B virus, can act like pancreatic cells, causing the immune system to attack the beta cells that produce insulin. It has been proven by studies that viral infections are linked to T1D, suggesting that environmental factors are important as well as genetics. Besides, the age when someone gets infected with these viruses could be important, since early childhood infections might be more likely to cause the autoimmune process. So, learning about genetic and environmental factors is necessary for creating effective prevention and early detection plans. Although genes are the basis for developing Type 1 Diabetes, it is the combination of these genes and things in the environment that leads to the disease. Investigations done in recent years indicate that what a person eats and the microbes they are exposed to may affect when and if they get T1D. Also, according to studies on autoimmune diseases, the relationship between our genes and the environment is not simple, and several risk factors can increase the likelihood of the disease. As an example, a person who has certain genetic weaknesses can have a much higher risk of getting T1D if they are exposed to certain environmental conditions. Because of this, researchers must take into account that genetic and environmental factors in T1D are related and should not be considered separately (Figure 3.13).

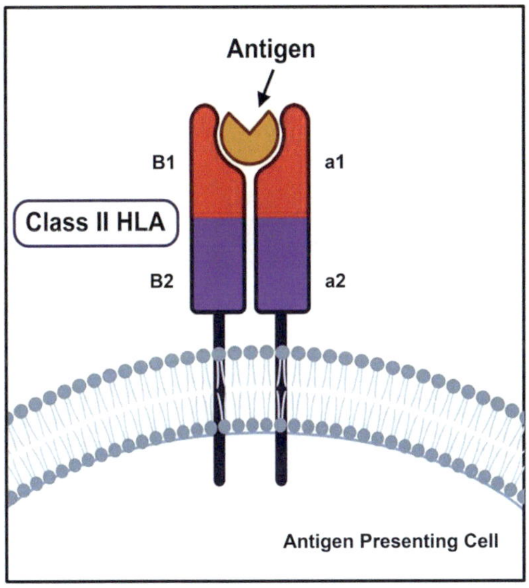

Figure 3.13. Genetic predisposition implies that individuals possessing specific genes, such as certain human leukocyte antigen (HLA) alleles, may be more susceptible to autoimmune disorders, including T1D.

Source: Berryman MA, Ilonen J, Triplett EW and Ludvigsson J (2023) Important denominator between autoimmune comorbidities: a review of class II HLA, autoimmune disease, and the gut. Front. Immunol. 14:1270488. doi: 10.3389/fimmu.2023.1270488

3.4. Environmental Factors in Type 1 Diabetes

The onset of Type 1 Diabetes (T1D) is intricately linked to various environmental factors that interact with genetic predispositions, contributing to the diseases epidemiology. Experts are focusing on how infections caused by viruses such as enteroviruses may lead to autoimmune reactions in the body, resulting in T1D. It has been found through research that infections can start changes in the immune system that destroy the beta cells in the pancreas. The chance of getting T1D is higher if a person is exposed to these viruses during their early years. So, studying these environmental factors can help find ways to prevent the disease, showing the need to look into how viral infections can lead to disease and help identify people at risk and develop treatments for their immune systems. In addition, what a child eats during early life can increase the risk of T1D. A lack of vitamin D in the diet is often considered a possible risk, since new studies suggest that low vitamin D may increase the risk of autoimmune diseases such as T1D. Researchers have also looked at how early gluten is introduced during infancy, as some studies suggest that introducing it early could make people with a genetic risk more likely to develop diabetes. In addition, drinking cow's milk has been connected to this problem, as some researchers think that certain proteins in milk may cause an autoimmune reaction in certain children. Experts are studying what people eat to find times when intervention could decrease the chance of T1D in people who are genetically vulnerable. It is now becoming obvious that environmental pollution plays a significant role in the development of Type 1 Diabetes, showing the link between health and the environment. According to studies, some environmental toxins, like heavy metals and pesticides, could be connected to the development of autoimmune diseases. Such an association is worrying because it could lead to problems with hormones that affect the immune system and insulin production. Moreover, people living in cities are more exposed to pollution, and this has been tied to higher T1D rates, making it necessary to study the connection between health in the environment and disease occurrence. This understanding underscores the importance of environmental policies and proactive measures to reduce harmful exposures, ultimately presenting a broader public health perspective in the fight against Type 1 Diabetes epidemiology and management, as recognized by contemporary research efforts (Brodbelt et al., 2014; Buhagiar et al., 2005) (Figure 3.14).

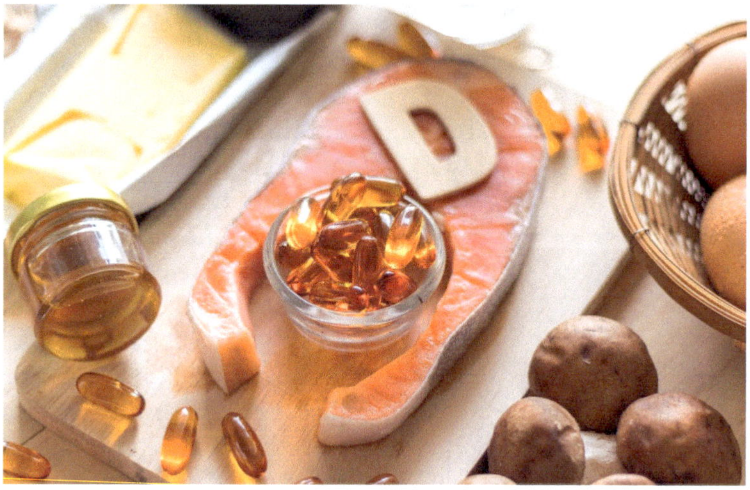

Figure 3.14. A diet deficient in vitamin D is often identified as a potential risk factor, as emerging research suggests a correlation between low vitamin D levels and increased incidence of autoimmune disorders, including T1D.

Source: https://www.news-medical.net/images/news/ImageForNews_777425_17133315331916099.jpg

3.4.1. Role of Viral Infections

Viral infections have garnered significant attention in discussions regarding the etiology of autoimmune diseases, particularly Type 1 Diabetes (T1D). Recent studies show that some viruses might play a role in starting or worsening the autoimmune reactions that lead to T1D. For example, the ways viruses influence the immune system are not well understood. According to studies, viruses may cause the loss of beta cells in the pancreas, which leads to the body attacking itself and causes T1D. As highlighted in previous research, the correlation between viral infections and autoimmune disorders, including T1D, emphasizes the need for further investigation into the exact interplay of genetic predisposition and environmental viral factors as catalysts for disease manifestation). Among the viral infections that may cause T1D, Coxsackie B virus is one that scientists have studied a lot because it is very harmful. Coxsackie B virus can choose and destroy pancreatic beta cells, which then causes the immune system to become active. As a result of this lysis, the immune system may react incorrectly and start attacking the insulin-producing cells in the body. It has been suggested by some studies that enteroviral infections may make people who are genetically susceptible more likely to develop T1D, pointing out how viruses and autoimmune responses are linked. The role of these viral agents in autoimmune diseases necessitates comprehensive epidemiological studies to unravel their impact on T1D incidence rates across different populations and to identify potential preventive strategies (Zanetti et al., 2015). This connection between viral infections and Type 1 Diabetes makes public health officials consider vaccination and early strategies to deal with the disease. Learning about the effects of some viruses on the immune system may help scientists develop vaccines to stop T1D. Studies done recently have pointed out that some viral vaccines can help prevent autoimmune reactions. Paying closer attention to viruses among at-risk people is in line with public health actions to manage viral outbreaks that may relate to the development of T1D. Thus, the intersection of virology and diabetes epidemiology is a burgeoning field, calling for multidisciplinary approaches to ultimately devise preventive measures that could reduce the incidence of Type 1 Diabetes linked to viral infections (Figure 3.15).

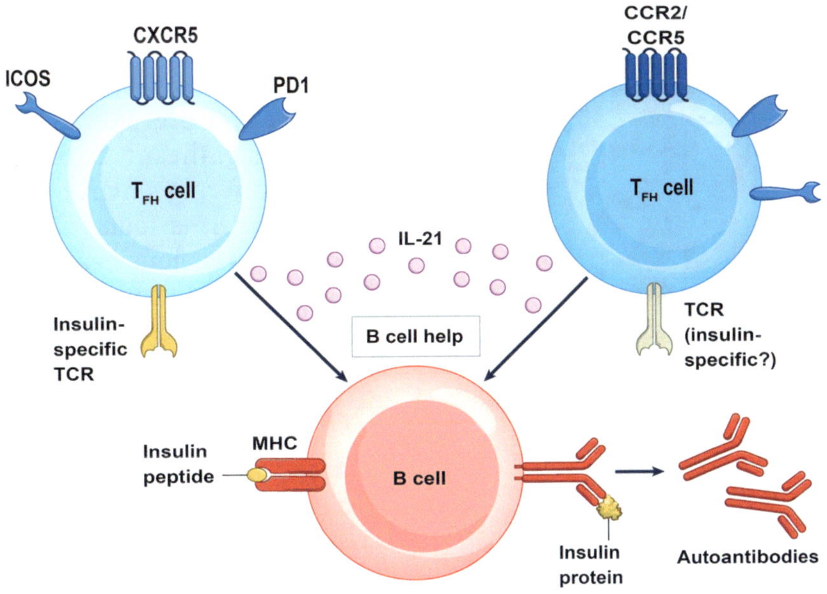

Figure 3.15. Viral infections have garnered significant attention in discussions regarding the etiology of autoimmune diseases, particularly Type 1 Diabetes (T1D).

Source: https://media.springernature.com/lw1200/springer-static/image/art%3A10.1038%2Fs41577-023-00985-4/MediaObjects/41577_2023_985_Fig4_HTML.png

3.4.2. Impact of Diet and Nutrition

The interplay between diet and nutrition is increasingly recognized as a significant factor in the epidemiology and etiology of Type 1 Diabetes (T1D). Current research indicates that what a person eats during early life could play a role in the autoimmune problems that cause T1D. Some people have studied whether eating proteins in cow's milk and gluten can trigger or accelerate T1D in those who are genetically susceptible. Also, when infants are given certain foods may play a role in their chances of getting T1D. New research points out that a careful study of diet and genes can help design preventive strategies for those who are at risk. The changing story highlights why it is important to study epidemiology to find out which dietary elements may lead to T1D. Nutrition plays a big role in managing the metabolic process for people who have T1D. Maintaining a good diet is important for controlling blood glucose and for your general health. Eating a lot of whole grains, fruits, and vegetables improves blood sugar levels and benefits the health of patients. It is also important for caregivers and patients to know how carbohydrates affect insulin levels. Teaching people about healthy eating can make it easier to control diabetes and lower the chances of facing T1D complications.

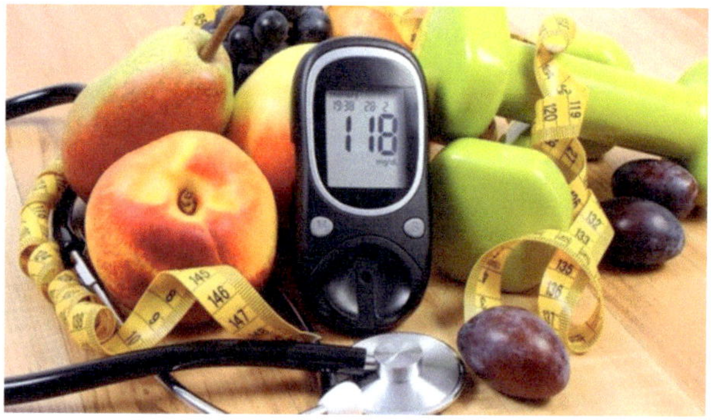

Figure 3.16. A balanced diet is essential for managing blood glucose levels and maintaining overall health.

Source: https://www.hindustantimes.com/ht-img/img/2023/11/15/550x309/_8af76aca-f0e3-11e5-8dad-b4df26f49330_1700058631932.jpg

It is obvious that diet and diabetes are linked, so it is necessary to keep learning and changing habits to maintain good metabolic control and protect health in the long run. How diet affects the bacteria in the gut is also an important topic, especially because it may play a role in immune system control related to T1D. According to recent findings, the gut microbiome is involved in both inflammation and immune response, which are important for the development of T1D. Eating foods that are high in fiber and low in processed sugars may help change the composition of gut microbes and reduce inflammation. In addition, the D-ECCO working group points out that what we eat could be a reason for the rising number of autoimmune disorders. Specifically, conversations surrounding diet not only focus on management but also on its potential role in disease prevention and the maintenance of metabolic health, reinforcing the necessity for future research on nutrition's multifaceted impact in T1D epidemiology (Allan et al., 2017) (Figure 3.16).

3.4.3. Influence of Geographical Location

The influence of geographical location on the incidence and prevalence of Type 1 Diabetes (T1D) is significant, revealing patterns that suggest differing environmental and genetic interactions. It is found that the rates of T1D are higher in regions near the Arctic, especially in Scandinavian countries. This situation is probably caused by several things, such as the amount of sunlight people get, which strongly affects how much vitamin D their bodies produce. It is believed that vitamin D helps control the immune system, so changes in climate and sunlight may play a part in causing T1D. Also, when people move to different areas, their genetic backgrounds and the exposures they had may not work the same way, adding more difficulties to the disease's epidemiology. In some areas, many cases of T1D have been found, which is much higher than what would be expected. Noticing these clusters shows that local environmental aspects, for example, what people eat, city life, and contact with infections, can play a big role in causing T1D. Certain parts of the world may consume more carbohydrates or be exposed to certain pathogens that can disrupt the immune system. Notably, studies have revealed a correlation between increased rates of congenital anomalies and T1D in particular areas, underscoring the complex interplay between genetics, environmental factors, and geographical location (Barbero et al., 2016). Spotting these groups could help public health experts focus on issues in the local diet and lifestyle that might cause T1D. Lastly, the effect of geography is also considered in terms of T1D's social and economic aspects. The way diabetes is managed and the results can change a lot depending on access to healthcare, education, and socio-economic conditions in different regions. In low- and middle-income countries, such as Thailand, the rising prevalence of obesity. a known risk factor for many non-communicable diseases, intersects with geographical influences to exacerbate T1D risks (Luz et al., 2017). It is very important to address these differences to learn more about how geography affects T1Ds. By studying geographical factors completely, more efficient strategies can be created to prevent and treat Type 1 Diabetes, considering the effects of the environment and society (Figure 3.17).

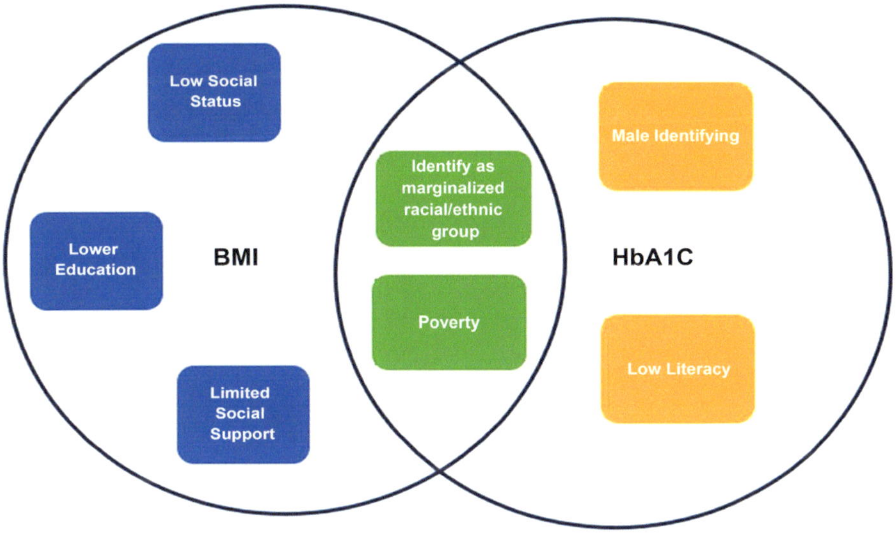

Figure 3.17. Factors such as healthcare access, education, and socio-economic status can vary significantly across regions, affecting the management and outcome of diabetes care.

Source: https://media.springernature.com/lw1200/springer-static/image/art%3A10.1186%2Fs40842-023-00162-5/MediaObjects/40842_2023_162_Fig1_HTML.png

3.5. Immunological Factors in Type 1 Diabetes

The immunological factors contributing to the development of Type 1 Diabetes (T1D) primarily revolve around autoimmune responses that target pancreatic beta cells. Because of a mistake by the immune system, the body treats insulin-producing cells as foreign and sends lymphocytes, mainly T cells, to attack them. Because of the autoimmune response, beta cells are destroyed, which results in an insulin shortage and too much glucose in the blood. Research underscores the role of regulatory T cells (Tregs) in maintaining immune tolerance, suggesting that a deficiency or dysfunction in these cells may foster the conditions conducive to T1D onset. Knowing the immunological factors and pathways related to this disease is important to look for biomarkers that could help detect and stop T1D at an early stage in those who are at risk. Cytokines are important in the immune system of T1D by affecting the balance between inflammation and its control. Elevated levels of pro-inflammatory cytokines, such as interferon-gamma (IFN-γ) and tumor necrosis factor-alpha (TNF-α), have been observed in individuals with T1D, suggesting their contribution to beta cell destruction. At the same time, anti-inflammatory cytokines such as IL-10 are usually not enough to stop the active autoimmune response. If the balance of cytokines is upset, it may lead to an autoimmune attack and continue to cause more inflammation and damage to tissues. As a result, approaches that help restore the balance of cytokines may be useful in regulating the immune system and possibly changing the outcome of T1D in patients. In addition, both genetic factors and environmental exposures play a big role in affecting the immune system related to T1D. Several genetic markers, including certain HLA class II alleles, are associated with a higher chance of developing T1D, proving that these factors greatly affect how the immune system works in each person. Things like viruses or what is eaten can also interact with a person's genes, possibly starting the autoimmune process that attacks beta cells. As an example, viral infections can cause the immune system to attack pancreatic cells, since viral antigens are similar to the pancreas's own antigens. By studying this relationship, we gain more knowledge about T1D and also realize how important it is to research the disease's immunological and epidemiological aspects to develop novel ways to prevent and treat it (Figure 3.18).

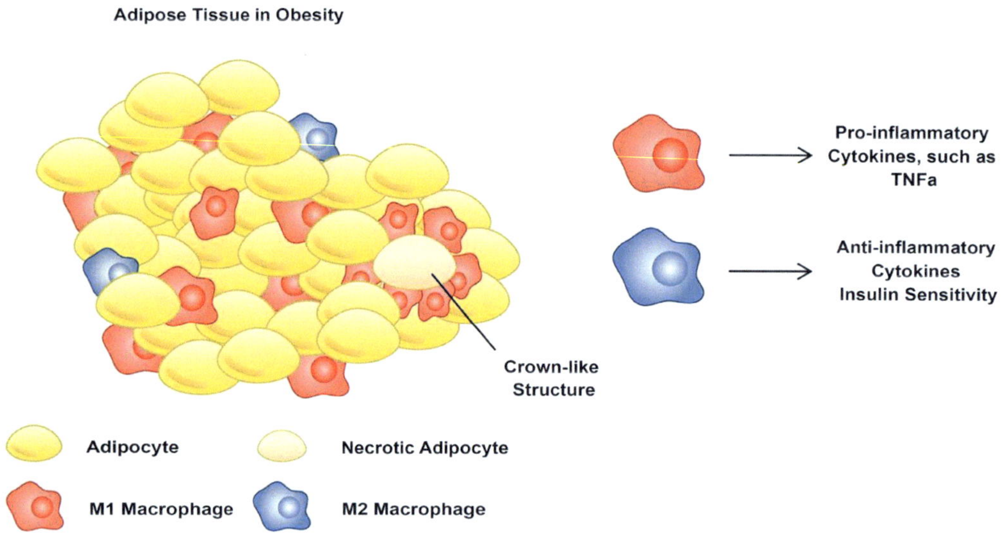

Figure 3.18. Cytokines also play a pivotal role in the immunological landscape of T1D, influencing the balance between pro-inflammatory and anti-inflammatory responses.

Source: Bakinowska E, Krompiewski M, Boboryko D, Kiełbowski K, Pawlik A. The Role of Inflammatory Mediators in the Pathogenesis of Obesity. *Nutrients*. 2024; 16(17):2822. https://doi.org/10.3390/nu16172822

3.5.1. Autoimmune Response and Beta-cell Destruction

The autoimmune response involved in Type 1 Diabetes (T1D) primarily targets the pancreatic beta cells, leading to their destruction. The immune system starts to attack these cells when it thinks they are not part of the body. Genes can make a person more likely to suffer from autoimmune diseases because of the role of certain HLA genotypes. Besides, certain environmental factors, especially viral infections, may worsen this predisposition and lead to autoimmune diseases such as T1D. The exact mechanisms by which viral infections trigger autoimmune responses remain somewhat obscure, as there is a need for more extensive research to elucidate these pathways. It is important to conduct these investigations since learning how environmental factors affect the immune system may help create new ways to prevent and manage T1D. In T1D, beta-cell destruction happens due to the interaction of genes, the environment, and the immune system. When beta cells are lost, insulin production decreases, which leads to too much sugar in the blood and its related problems. Studies have demonstrated that the presence of autoantibodies acts as a biomarker for beta-cell dysfunction and can predict the development of T1D in genetically predisposed individuals (Larsson et al., 2008). The attack on beta cells happens because the immune system does not recognize the body's own cells and starts attacking them. Additionally, research reveals that the period and type of environmental factors, such as infections in the womb, can affect someone's risk of T1D, proving that this disease is influenced by many factors. It is possible to see how the autoimmune response and beta-cell loss happen in T1D by looking at the different stages of immune activity. At first, autoantibodies may be found even though there are no symptoms, which is known as the pre-clinical phase of the disease. This stage can span years, emphasizing the significance of early detection and potential interventions (Larsson et al., 2008). As the disease progresses, the body's immune system becomes stronger, and this causes the blood sugar to rise due to insulin not being produced in sufficient amounts. For this reason, exploring this process helps to identify people who may develop diabetes and supports the development of new treatments that protect beta cells and stop diabetes from occurring. For this reason, it is important to use genetic screening and look at environmental risks when dealing with the epidemiology of T1D (Figure 3.19).

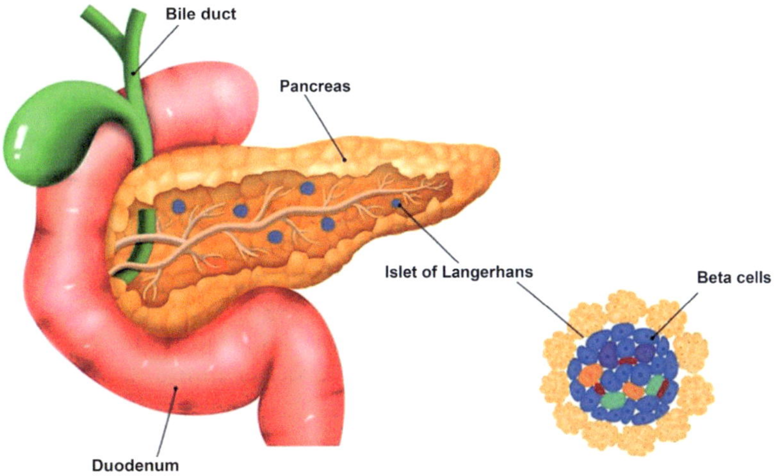

Figure 3.19. The autoimmune response involved in Type 1 Diabetes (T1D) primarily targets the pancreatic beta cells, leading to their destruction.

Source: https://arad.blogs.bristol.ac.uk/files/2024/07/Pancreas-2_high_res-1024x649.png

3.5.2. Role of T-cells and Antibodies

The immune response in the context of Type 1 Diabetes (T1D) is primarily mediated by T-cells and antibodies, which play critical roles in the pathogenesis of the disease. In T1D, a type of T-cell called autoreactive targets beta cells in the pancreas, which results in no insulin being produced. In detail, CD4+ helper T-cells stimulate other immune cells, and CD8+ cytotoxic T-cells are responsible for destroying the pancreatic cells. The intricate balance between regulatory T-cells (Tregs) and effector T-cells is essential, as a dysfunction in this balance can lead to an overt autoimmune attack. Evidence suggests that genetic predispositions often predispose individuals to aberrant T-cell responses, triggering an autoimmune reaction that ultimately results in T1D (Butcher et al., 2019). Antibodies are involved in the autoimmune process of T1D, acting as markers and possibly taking part in the disease development. Many times, GAD65, IA-2, and insulin autoantibodies are found in people before they develop T1D, which suggests the disease is developing due to an autoimmune process. The presence of these antibodies suggests that the immune system is trying to harm the islet cells, showing a major imbalance in both humoral and cellular immunity. Interestingly, some studies have indicated that the levels of certain autoantibodies can correlate with the rate of beta-cell destruction, further illustrating their potential as predictive markers for T1D progression (Czesnikiewicz-Guzik et al., 2017). It proves that antibodies help in both finding out about T1D and understanding the immune system's role in it. The way T-cells and antibodies are involved in T1D reveals how complicated the immune system is and suggests possible treatments. Immunotherapies that aim to restore tolerance, boost the activity of Treg cells, or lower the activity of harmful T-cells are being considered as ways to treat the disease. Also, changing antibody responses using targeted therapies could help control the progression of a disease. Since we now know more about how these immune mechanisms work in T1D, it is clear that more research is necessary to find new treatments for both the symptoms and the causes of the disease. Researchers are exploring the ways T-cells and antibodies work to find new ways to stop or treat T1D (Figure 3.20).

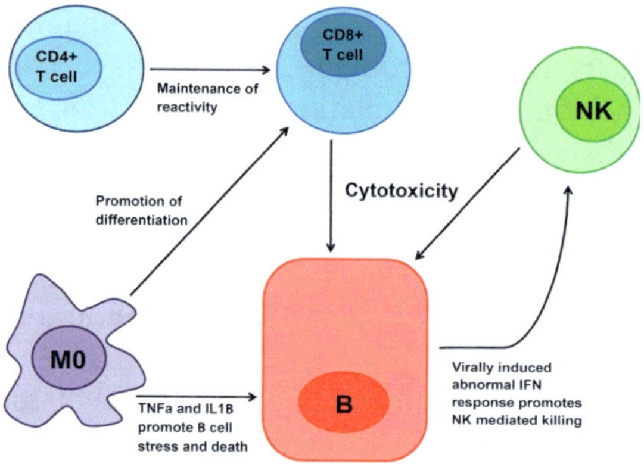

Figure 3.20. The immune response in the context of Type 1 Diabetes (T1D) is primarily mediated by T-cells and antibodies, which play critical roles in the pathogenesis of the disease.

Source: https://www.researchgate.net/publication/259986636/figure/fig1/AS:11431281247415014@1716801459713/Various-immune-cells-are-involved-inT1D-pathogenesis-Cytotoxic-CD8-T-cells-mediate-most.tif

3.5.3. Potential Immunotherapy Approaches

The exploration of potential immunotherapy approaches for Type 1 Diabetes (T1D) is vital due to the disease's autoimmune nature, where the immune system mistakenly targets insulin-producing pancreatic beta cells. One good strategy is to use treatments that alter the immune system to regain tolerance, instead of only suppressing it. New findings show that using antigen-specific treatments can help the immune system identify beta-cell antigens as part of the body, which may lower the attack on these cells. For example, using peptides from insulin or other proteins of beta cells is meant to increase regulatory T cell function, which may result in long-term remission for people recently diagnosed with type 1 diabetes. This approach handles the current treatment issue and also reveals important facts about the immunological processes that cause T1D. Development of immunotherapies is also interesting when it comes to using biological agents like monoclonal antibodies to focus on certain immune processes that lead to T1D. There is growing proof that adjusting the levels of cytokines in the body may help change the disease. For instance, therapies that prevent pro-inflammatory cytokines from working may help control the autoimmune response and make it easier for beta cells to survive. Recently, clinical trials have looked into the effectiveness of anti-CD3 monoclonal antibodies that try to change how T cells function. If these therapies are used right after T1D is diagnosed, they may help delay its progression. For this reason, it is important to understand how these therapies affect inflammation to improve their success and assess the future health of people with T1D. The involvement of the immune system in brain diseases, which includes many connections between the immune system and the brain, could be important for T1D. When researchers explore these relationships more closely, they may find new ways that are helpful in treating diseases. It has been argued that systemic inflammation can affect both metabolism and cognitive function as well as mood in T1D, so it's important to manage the condition in all these areas. Research on anti-inflammatory drugs in neuropsychiatric disorders might help T1D patients by handling autoimmune problems and improving their overall health. Such integrative approaches underscore the evolving understanding of T1D and suggest a future where immunotherapeutic strategies could holistically address both the metabolic and psychological facets of the disease (Zhang, 2011; Cousins et al., 2014) (Figure 3.21).

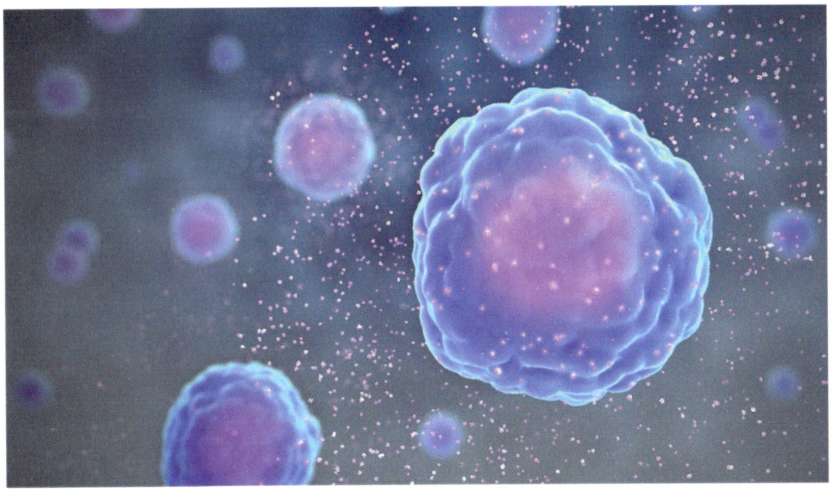

Figure 3.21. Therapies that block pro-inflammatory cytokines may mitigate the autoimmune response and promote an environment conducive to beta-cell survival.

Source: https://upload.wikimedia.org/wikipedia/commons/f/fa/Cytokine_release.jpg

A CLOSER LOOK

HUMAN LEUKOCYTE ANTIGEN (HLA)

Human Leukocyte Antigen (HLA) is a group of proteins found on the surface of most cells in the body, playing a vital role in the immune system. These molecules allow the immune system to tell apart the body's cells from foreign substances by showing protein fragments to immune cells. HLA genes are found on chromosome 6 and they are very variable. Because HLA types play a key role in organ rejection, they are vital in organ transplantation. Certain autoimmune diseases, for example, type 1 diabetes and rheumatoid arthritis, are linked to HLA types.

Summary

It is important to realize that Type 1 diabetes is caused by the interaction of genes, the environment, and the immune system. Studies on the way diseases develop have highlighted that certain genetic changes, such as those in the HLA area, can make some people vulnerable to the disease. In addition, certain viruses and what people eat can trigger the development of these diseases. Since research continues to advance, managing the multiple factors involved in Type 1 diabetes is still necessary for creating prevention strategies. Genetic testing is now used to find people at risk, which reflects how diabetes epidemiology is progressing and helps with targeted actions and prevention for Type 1 diabetes. In addition, considering Type 1 diabetes in relation to glycation processes gives useful information for managing and preventing the disease. Protein glycation linked to oxidative stress could have effects on people with diabetes as well as those who do not have diabetes. Research over time has shown that glycation is linked to a higher risk of chronic diseases in healthy individuals, meaning that changing your lifestyle can help a lot with your metabolic health. What we eat can either make glycation worse or better, which means that managing diet may play a major role in Type 1 diabetes care. Recognizing these relationships can help develop more ways to prevent and manage diabetes by working on people's eating habits and other lifestyle factors. In brief, a good understanding of both the causes and spread of Type 1 diabetes is necessary for making progress in medical research and practice. Using genetic information and lifestyle changes helps in a complete approach to fight the disease. Further studies should aim to explain the role of glycation and oxidative stress in causing Type 1 diabetes. With each new discovery, it may be possible to develop new ways to prevent and treat diseases that mainly affect certain groups. If we join genetics, nutrition, and public health efforts, we can better handle Type 1 diabetes and possibly prevent it, as well as increase the quality of life for those affected by the disease.

References

1. Abraham, A., Hart, A. R., Olsen, A., Tjonneland, A., Racine, A., Trichopoulou, A., et al. (2014). Carbohydrate intake in the etiology of Crohn's disease and ulcerative colitis. https://core.ac.uk/download/29109093.pdf (accessed on 11th June 2025).
2. MacLean, A., Sweeting, H., Egan, M., Der, G., Adamson, J., & Hunt, K. (2013). How robust is the evidence of an emerging or increasing female excess in physical morbidity between childhood and adolescence? Results of a systematic literature review and meta-analyses. *Social science & medicine (1982)*, *78*, 96–112. https://doi.org/10.1016/j.socscimed.2012.11.039(accessed on 11th June 2025).
3. Ahituv, N., Avins, A., Chen, D. C., Eckalbar, T., et al. (2015). A genome-wide association study identifies four novel susceptibility loci underlying inguinal hernia. https://core.ac.uk/download/323078687.pdf (accessed on 11th June 2025).
4. Ala-Korpela, M., Chaturvedi, N., Eastwood, S. V., Forouhi, N. G., et al. (2015). Diabetes risk and amino acid profiles: Cross-sectional and prospective analyses of ethnicity, amino acids and diabetes in a South Asian and European cohort from the SABRE (Southall and Brent REvisited) Study. https://core.ac.uk/download/29411586.pdf (accessed on 11th June 2025).
5. Allan, P., Fiorino, G., Gatti, S., Gerasimidis, K., et al. (2017). Research gaps in diet and nutrition in inflammatory bowel disease. A topical review by D-ECCO Working Group (Dietitians of ECCO). https://core.ac.uk/download/84340703.pdf (accessed on 11th June 2025).
6. Arriola, L., Balkau, B., Barker, A., Barricarte, A., et al. (2014). Common genetic variants highlight the role of insulin resistance and body fat distribution in type 2 diabetes, independent of obesity. https://core.ac.uk/download/77407381.pdf (accessed on 11th June 2025).
7. Atkins, B., Bolivar, S., Buckbinder, L., Collins, J., Corps, J., Crawford, C., et al. (2014). Plantar fasciopathy: Revisiting the risk factors. https://core.ac.uk/download/19936576.pdf (accessed on 11th June 2025).
8. Aulchenko, Y., Baqui, A. H., Bhutta, Z. A., Campbell, O. M., et al. (2011). The case for launch of an international DNA-based birth cohort study. https://core.ac.uk/download/28973486.pdf (accessed on 11th June 2025).
9. Barbero, P., Bidondo, M. P., Gili, J. A., Gimenez, S., et al. (2016). Geographic clusters of congenital anomalies in Argentina. https://core.ac.uk/download/159291453.pdf (accessed on 11th June 2025).
10. Beth, A., Dandouras, I., Garnier, P., Mazelle, C., et al. (2013). "Whose data is it anyway?" The implications of putting small area-level health and social data online. https://core.ac.uk/download/pdf/29026859.pdf (accessed on 11th June 2025).
11. Bharucha, A. E., Bityutskiy, L., Burlen, A., Camilleri, M., Gallagher, J., Hasler, W., Hollowell, M., et al. (2020). Epidemiology and outcomes of gastroparesis, as documented in general practice records, in the United Kingdom. https://core.ac.uk/download/326518073.pdf (accessed on 11th June 2025).
12. Bindman, A. B., Majeed, A., & Weiner, J. P. (2001). Use of risk adjustment in setting budgets and measuring performance in primary care I: How it works. https://core.ac.uk/download/1670616.pdf (accessed on 11th June 2025).

13. Boeschoten, E., Casino, F., Collart, F., Cornet, R., et al. (2012). New primary renal diagnosis codes for the ERA-EDTA. https://core.ac.uk/download/9652512.pdf (accessed on 11th June 2025).

14. Brandt, T., Glaser, M., Strupp, M., Wagner, J., et al. (2008). Downbeat nystagmus: Etiology and comorbidity in 117 patients. https://core.ac.uk/download/12175155.pdf (accessed on 11th June 2025).

15. Brodaty, H., Low, L. F., & Gomes, L. (2025). Australian dementia research: Current status, future directions? https://core.ac.uk/download/pdf/30687280.pdf (accessed on 11th June 2025).

16. Brodbelt, D. C., Church, D. B., Mattin, M. J., McGreevy, P. D., et al. (2014). An epidemiological study of diabetes mellitus in dogs attending first opinion practice in the UK. https://core.ac.uk/download/36777545.pdf (accessed on 11th June 2025).

17. Buhagiar, G. (2005). Rationalisation of the biochemistry laboratory: Which way forwards? https://core.ac.uk/download/46602008.pdf (accessed on 11th June 2025).

18. Butcher, J. P., Henriquez, F. L., Reid, S., Simakou, T., et al. (2019). Alopecia areata: A multifactorial autoimmune condition. https://core.ac.uk/download/293865308.pdf (accessed on 11th June 2025).

19. Catchpole, B., Holder, A. L., Kennedy, L. J., Massey, J., et al. (2014). Searching for "monogenic diabetes" in dogs using a candidate gene approach. https://core.ac.uk/download/157854855.pdf (accessed on 11th June 2025).

20. Chircop, M., Savona-Ventura, C., & Schranz, A. G. (2003). Family history in the etiology of gestational diabetes mellitus and type 2 diabetes. https://core.ac.uk/download/46601850.pdf (accessed on 11th June 2025).

21. Corato, A., Doganci, A., Knueppel, A., Kojima, A., Mqadmi, A., Saxena, A., Zanella, A., et al. (2016). Characterization of the immunophenotype of dogs with primary immune-mediated hemolytic anemia. https://core.ac.uk/download/76980975.pdf (accessed on 11th June 2025).

22. Cousins, L., Deakin, J., Jones, P. B., Khandaker, G. M., et al. (2014). Inflammation and immunity in schizophrenia: Implications for pathophysiology and treatment. https://core.ac.uk/download/42337939.pdf (accessed on 11th June 2025).

23. Czesnikiewicz-Guzik, M., Maciag, A., Maciag, J., Matusik, P., et al. (2017). The effect of the treatment of denture related stomatitis on peripheral T cells and monocytes. https://core.ac.uk/download/74232023.pdf (accessed on 11th June 2025).

24. Czyzyk, A., Sasaki, A., Lowenfels, A. B., Anon, B., Armstrong, B., Balkau, B., et al. (2004). Diabetes status and post-load plasma glucose concentration in relation to site-specific cancer mortality: Findings from the original Whitehall study. https://core.ac.uk/download/1393062.pdf (accessed on 11th June 2025).

25. Hall, V., Henriksen, O., Lohse, N., Thomsen, R. W., et al. (2011). Diabetes in Sub-Saharan Africa 1999–2011: Epidemiology and public health implications. A systematic review. https://core.ac.uk/download/pdf/16666834.pdf (accessed on 11th June 2025).

26. Hanley, A. J., Benyamin, B., Lann, D., Zeggini, E., De Geus, E. J., Mayer, E. J., Liu, G. F., et al. (2009). Bivariate genetic modelling of the response to an oral glucose tolerance challenge: A gene × environment interaction approach. https://core.ac.uk/download/pdf/12937482.pdf (accessed on 11th June 2025).

27. Ho, T. K., Leigh, R. D., & Tsui, J. (2013). Diabetic foot disease and oedema. https://core.ac.uk/download/16219516.pdf (accessed on 11th June 2025).

28. Illanes, E., Mitchell, M. D., & Rice, G. E. (2012). Gestational diabetes mellitus: A positive predictor of type 2 diabetes? https://core.ac.uk/download/pdf/8735629.pdf (accessed on 11th June 2025).

29. Kalsi, J., & Muneer, A. (2013). Erectile dysfunction–An update of current practice and future strategies. https://core.ac.uk/download/29416259.pdf (accessed on 11th June 2025).

30. Kitsiou, A., Caforio, A. L. P., Porta-Sanchez, A., Vahanian, A., Iung, B., Carrera, C., Szymanski, C., et al. (2013). ESC core curriculum for the general cardiologist (2013). https://core.ac.uk/download/55756305.pdf (accessed on 11th June 2025).

31. Larsson, H. (2008). Type 1 diabetes in children–Risk factors and prediction. https://core.ac.uk/download/83739067.pdf (accessed on 11th June 2025).

32. Luz, A., & Teerawattananon, Y. (2017). Obesity in Thailand and its economic cost estimation. https://core.ac.uk/download/93370213.pdf (accessed on 11th June 2025).

33. Pfister, R., Sharp, S., Luben, R., Welsh, P., Barroso, I., Salomaa, V., Meirhaeghe, A., Khaw, K. T., Sattar, N., Langenberg, C., & Wareham, N. J. (2011). Mendelian randomization study of B-type natriuretic peptide and type 2 diabetes: evidence of causal association from population studies. *PLoS medicine*, *8*(10), e1001112. https://doi.org/10.1371/journal.pmed.1001112https://core.ac.uk/download/1437139.pdf (accessed on 11th June 2025).

34. Moore, M. D. (2015). Harnessing the power of difference: Colonialism and British chronic disease research, 1940–1975. https://core.ac.uk/download/43096264.pdf (accessed on 11th June 2025).

35. Padoa, C. J. (2011). The epidemiology and pathogenesis of type 1 diabetes mellitus in Africa. https://core.ac.uk/download/478382958.pdf (accessed on 11th June 2025).

36. Randhawa, G., Sinclair, A. J., Waqar, M., Wilkinson, J., et al. (2016). Meeting the challenge of diabetes in ageing and diverse populations: A review of the literature from the UK. https://core.ac.uk/download/153536478.pdf (accessed on 11th June 2025).

37. Sachdev, P. S. (2025). Is the incidence of dementia declining? https://core.ac.uk/download/pdf/30674873.pdf (accessed on 11th June 2025).

38. Vlassopoulos, A., Bhagwat, S., El-Salem, H., Combet, E., Hao, L., Hodge, A., et al. (2014). Oxidative stress, protein glycation and nutrition–interactions relevant to health and disease throughout the lifecycle. https://core.ac.uk/download/18492207.pdf (accessed on 11th June 2025).

39. Zanetti, A. R., Mele, A., Mariano, A., Galli, C., Spada, E., Taliani, G., Romanò, L., et al. (2015). Clinical, epidemiological and virological features of acute hepatitis B in Italy. https://core.ac.uk/download/153365546.pdf (accessed on 11th June 2025).

40. Zhang, Z. (2011). Neurodegeneration: Potential causes, prevention, and future treatment options. https://core.ac.uk/download/pdf/290265.pdf (accessed on 11th June 2025).

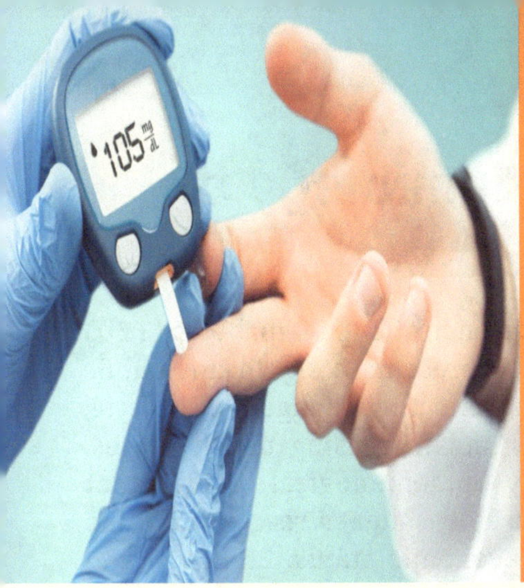

Chapter 4

EPIDEMIOLOGY AND ETIOLOGY OF TYPE 2 DIABETES

Contents

Introduction

The complexity of Type 2 diabetes (T2D) is underscored by its multifactorial nature, which combines genetic predispositions with lifestyle and environmental influences. Around the world, T2D is increasing mostly because of changes in people's eating habits, less exercise, and more obesity. This problem is connected to several issues, for example, insulin resistance and problems with beta cells. It is important to study these factors in the epidemiology of T2D because they are related to its development and spread. Studying family patterns and risk factors for individuals is still helping us understand this disease, which may lead to ways to control and handle it. Many studies have been carried out to examine the factors that lead to Type 2 diabetes, including those from genes and from the environment. It has been found that problems in the womb can increase a person's chances of developing T2D in the future. Notably, recent findings indicate that maternal and sibling family histories of diabetes correlate significantly with both gestational diabetes mellitus (GDM) and subsequent T2D development. Alternatively, the history of a father or grandparent seems to matter less, which suggests a more detailed view of family risks. These insights emphasize the importance of considering both genetic heritability and environmental exposures, particularly during critical developmental windows, in the investigation of T2D etiology (Chircop et al., 2003). Recent evidence also highlights the potential role of biological factors, such as B-type natriuretic peptide (BNP) levels, in the onset of T2D. It appears from studies that having higher BNP levels is linked to a lower chance of diabetes, suggesting that the BNP system could play a role in regulating glucose and insulin. Since NT-pro-BNP is linked to T2D, it is important to study these markers because they can teach us about the disease and its risks. It is also necessary to keep learning about this relationship to discover its causes and look for new cures. Ultimately, understanding both the epidemiology and etiology of Type 2 diabetes will enhance strategies for prevention and management, paving the way for improved health outcomes (Pfister et al., 2011) (Figure 4.1).

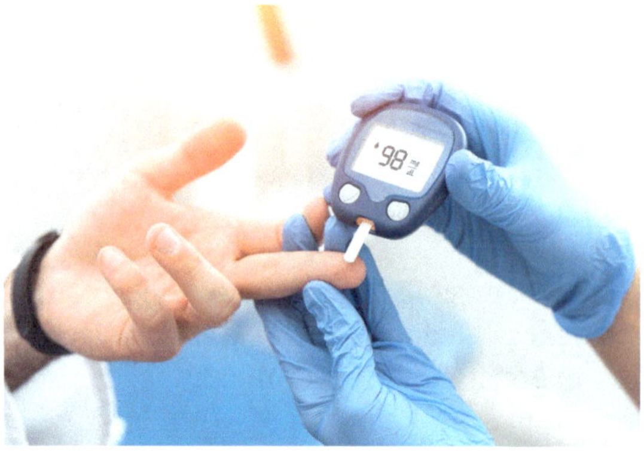

Figure 4.1. Type 2 diabetes (T2D).

Source: https://www.ox.ac.uk/sites/files/oxford/field/field_image_main/shutterstock_1439349791.jpg

4.1. Epidemiology of Type 2 Diabetes

The rising prevalence of Type 2 diabetes (T2D) across the globe presents a significant public health concern, reflecting changes in lifestyle, dietary habits, and increasing obesity rates. It is shown by epidemiological studies that some groups are at a higher risk of T2D due to their socio-economic status, ethnicity, and their environment. Asian and Hispanic people are affected more than Caucasians, which may mean that genes and lifestyle are connected in some way. This shows that it is important to use public health measures that meet the needs of different population groups. Moreover, the problem of T2D is made worse by its connection to several other illnesses, such as heart diseases and metabolic disorders, so it is important to use an integrated method in research and healthcare to decrease the number of cases and improve patients. The link between NT-pro-BNP and T2D points out the need to recognize and study such biological markers, as they can give us useful knowledge about the disease and its risk. In addition, it is important to keep studying this relationship to understand its causes and find new treatments. Ultimately, understanding both the epidemiology and etiology of Type 2 diabetes will enhance strategies for prevention and management, paving the way for improved health outcomes (Pfister et al., 2011). According to these findings, using genetics can improve how people are grouped for risk assessment and the development of unique public health strategies. In addition to genetics, things that happen in the womb can have a major effect on the epidemiology of T2D as seen in different groups of people. Research indicates that a maternal history of diabetes correlates strongly with the development of gestational diabetes mellitus (GDM) and later T2D in offspring, emphasizing the importance of the prenatal environment in shaping long-term metabolic health (Chircop et al., 2003). Since family plays a role, early actions should consider both genetic and environmental factors in a person's upbringing. Therefore, understanding the way T2D spreads requires looking at genetic, environmental, and social factors, which allows for a better response to the diabetes epidemic (Figure 4.2).

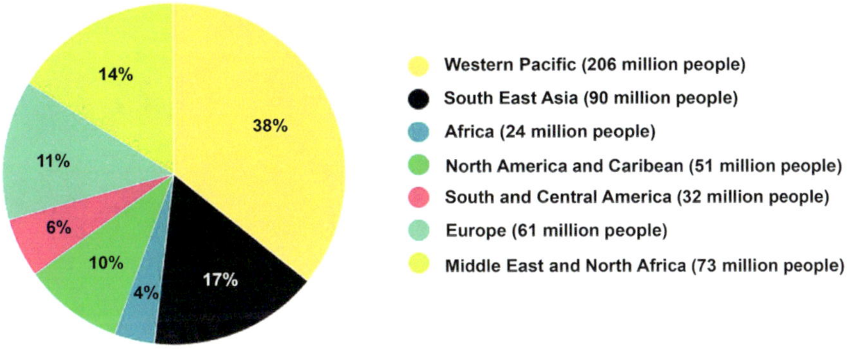

Figure 4.2. The rising prevalence of Type 2 diabetes (T2D) across the globe presents a significant public health concern, reflecting changes in lifestyle, dietary habits, and increasing obesity rates.

Source: Chandrasekaran P, Weiskirchen R. The Role of Obesity in Type 2 Diabetes Mellitus—An Overview. *International Journal of Molecular Sciences*. 2024; 25(3):1882. https://doi.org/10.3390/ijms25031882

4.1.1. Global Prevalence and Incidence Rates

The global prevalence of type 2 diabetes (T2D) has surged dramatically over the past few decades, positioning it as a major public health concern worldwide. It has been found that the number of adults with diabetes increased from 108 million in 1980 to 422 million in 2014. In countries where income is low or moderate, this pattern is more obvious because changes in lifestyle and city life are leading to obesity, which is a main risk for T2D. Nearly all the diabetes cases in Sub-Saharan Africa are now type 2 diabetes. Estimates indicate that population prevalence rates range from 1% in rural Uganda to as high as 12% in urban Kenya, highlighting the considerable disparities in diabetes prevalence influenced by geographical and socioeconomic factors (Hall et al., 2011). The reason for more T2D cases is that genes, the environment, and people's lifestyles are affecting each other. Urban growth leads more people to live a sedentary lifestyle and eat more calories, which increases the number of obese people. It is being reported that diabetes is now appearing in people in their 30s and 40s, rather than in their older years. As a result of this trend, healthcare systems encounter numerous difficulties and people often deal with the long-term effects of cardiovascular disease and other conditions. Furthermore, the interaction of diabetes with infectious diseases, particularly in regions like Sub-Saharan Africa, complicates management strategies and escalates healthcare costs, necessitating a robust response from public health authorities (Hall et al., 2011). It is even more difficult to handle the global T2D problem because many cases go undetected and treatment is not always available. Many people with diabetes have not been diagnosed, which leads to poor health and a lower quality of life. Among certain populations, it was found that more than 40% of people with diabetes had not realized they had the disease, showing that there is a big problem with screening and education. Also, when people are unable to get tests, affordable care, or regular check-ups, it results in bigger health differences and more possible complications. As observed in Sub-Saharan Africa, where treatment costs can be prohibitively high, the total annual cost of diabetes is estimated at US$67.03 billion, emphasizing the urgent need for comprehensive healthcare strategies that address both communicable and non-communicable diseases in a coordinated manner (Hall et al., 2011) (Figure 4.3).

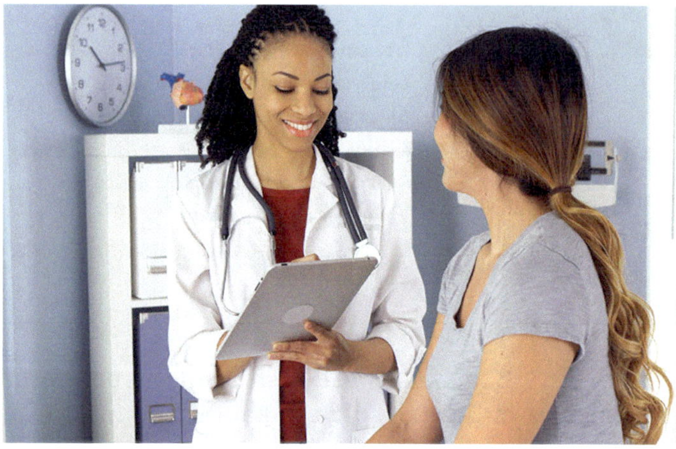

Figure 4.3. Barriers to accessing diagnostic tools, affordable treatment, and continuous monitoring exacerbate health disparities and increase the risk of complications.

Source: https://www.ruralhealthinfo.org/assets/2632-9902/healthcare-access-tw.jpg

4.1.2. Demographic Factors Influencing Prevalence

Factors such as age, gender, ethnicity, and socioeconomic status have a big impact on the number of cases of type 2 diabetes. Age stands out, since the chance of getting type 2 diabetes goes up as you get older, usually due to changes in metabolism and lifestyle that come with aging. For example, people over the age of 45 are much more likely to develop this condition, which means public health should focus on older people. It is also noticed that men may be more likely to have diabetes than women, which might be related to how their bodies carry fat. It is very important to understand these age and gender factors when making health policies for people at risk of type 2 diabetes. Type 2 diabetes is also strongly affected by a person's ethnicity. African Americans, Hispanics, and Native Americans are more likely to have diabetes than Caucasian people. It is often connected to both a person's genes and the obstacles they face because of their social and economic status, such as not having enough healthcare or education. For instance, people from these risky ethnic groups might struggle to get medical advice or healthy foods on time, which can increase their chances of getting diabetes. In addition, the way people eat and live has a major impact on why diabetes is more common among some racial and ethnic groups than others. It is very important to understand these factors well if we want to create effective strategies for different groups. People's economic and social backgrounds are important in determining the frequency of type 2 diabetes. Those who come from low-income families usually have a greater chance of getting the disease because they face difficulties in getting healthcare, healthy food, and chances to exercise. It is found that individuals with less income and education tend to be more obese, which greatly increases their chances of getting type 2 diabetes. When people are stressed financially, it can cause mental health issues, which may encourage them to make unhealthy choices, leading to more diseases. This information shows that tackling socioeconomic problems is important for cutting down on type 2 diabetes. Providing equal access to health resources and teaching people about diabetes risk factors may help reduce the effects of social and economic differences on the number of diabetes cases (Figure 4.4).

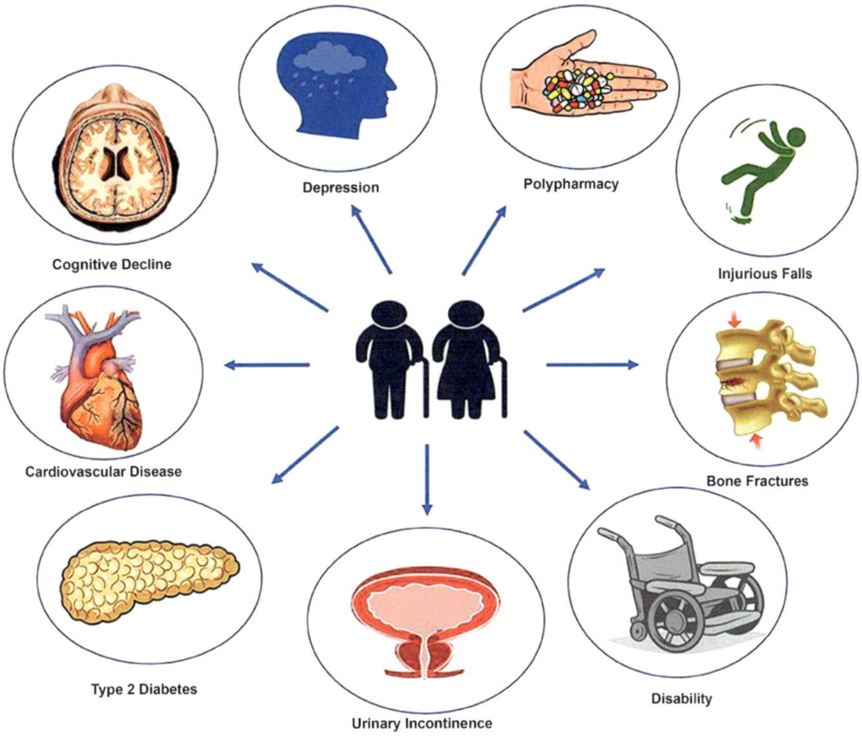

Figure 4.4. Age is particularly notable, as the risk of developing type 2 diabetes increases with advancing years, often attributed to metabolic changes and lifestyle factors associated with aging.

Source: Longo M, Bellastella G, Maiorino MI, Meier JJ, Esposito K and Giugliano D (2019) Diabetes and Aging: From Treatment Goals to Pharmacologic Therapy. Front. Endocrinol. 10:45. doi: 10.3389/fendo.2019.00045

4.1.3. Trends in Type 2 Diabetes over the Past Decades

The rate of Type 2 diabetes has changed a lot in the last several decades, along with changes in lifestyle, food choices, and socioeconomic conditions. The number of people who are obese, which is often a precursor to Type 2 diabetes, has increased significantly because of the rise in processed foods containing a lot of sugar and fat. In particular, studies have found that obesity rates around the world have almost tripled since 1975 and this has led to a rise in diabetes cases in developed countries. More children and adolescents are being diagnosed with Type 2 diabetes, which was not common in the past because it usually affected older people. The population changes lead to challenges for healthcare systems everywhere, so there is a need for special public health efforts to prevent and manage this chronic condition. In addition, the number of Type 2 diabetes cases is strongly affected by both social and environmental changes. Since urbanization causes people to be less active, it adds to the health issues linked to Type 2 diabetes. In several low- and middle-income countries, the fast development of industries and cities has encouraged environmental changes that make people eat unhealthy foods and exercise less. Because of these determinants, there are not enough healthcare resources for those who are most at risk of diabetes. The fact that diabetes is more common among people with low income proves that we must focus on the medical and social aspects of health. If these gaps are not closed, the number of Type 2 diabetes cases will probably keep increasing. Also, better knowledge of the causes of Type 2 diabetes has led to new ways of diagnosing and treating it. Since it is now clear that many factors contribute to diseases, healthcare professionals are taking a more detailed approach to their work. With the progress of endocrinology, scientists are now looking into what causes people to be more likely to develop Type 2 diabetes. New studies have established that insulin resistance is strongly tied to the rise in the disease, so it is important to address the problem early and make healthy lifestyle changes. Still, pharmaceutical progress keeps being made to help control blood sugar, but it is not enough unless people also focus on preventing health problems. Using this approach is a major trend in diabetes care, pointing to a move toward caring for patients more fully and preventing this health issue worldwide (Figure 4.5).

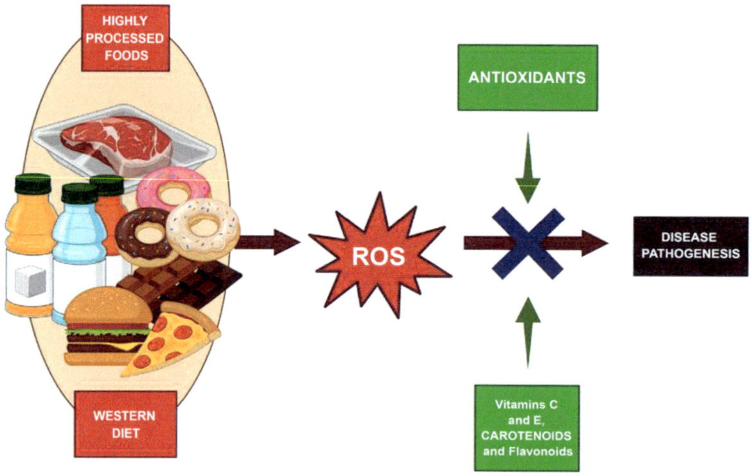

Figure 4.5. In many low- and middle-income countries, rapid industrialization and urban sprawl have facilitated environmental changes that promote unhealthy eating habits and reduced physical activity levels.

Source: Clemente-Suárez VJ, Beltrán-Velasco AI, Redondo-Flórez L, Martín-Rodríguez A, Tornero-Aguilera JF. Global Impacts of Western Diet and Its Effects on Metabolism and Health: A Narrative Review. *Nutrients*. 2023; 15(12):2749. https://doi.org/10.3390/nu15122749

4.2. Risk Factors for Type 2 Diabetes

Understanding the risk factors for Type 2 Diabetes (T2D) is crucial for both prevention and management strategies. Lifestyle factors such as not being active enough, being overweight, and eating unhealthy are some of the most important ones. Eating many refined carbs and sugars is linked to weight gain, and this is a major risk for the disease. Besides, staying inactive for long periods increases the chances of insulin resistance, which can lead to T2D. It has been found that cutting down on calories and exercising more can greatly reduce the number of T2D cases in people at high risk. This points out that changing people's behavior is a key strategy for reducing the number of T2D cases in the public health sector. A person's genes can also greatly increase the risk of developing T2D. Changes in genes that control lipid metabolism and insulin sensitivity may make a person more vulnerable. According to research, there is a link between the BNP system and T2D, which means that some genes may affect a person's risk of developing the disease. Notably, elevated levels of N-terminal pro-B-type natriuretic peptide (NT-pro-BNP) have been shown to correlate with a decreased risk of T2D, indicating a complex interaction between genetic factors and metabolic processes (Pfister et al., 2011). Therefore, considering genetic differences as well as lifestyle plays a key role in designing effective risk assessments and treatment plans for each person. Factors such as people's economic situation and the level of urbanization can also raise the risk of T2D. In many low- and middle-income countries, fast urbanization causes people to eat less healthy foods and become less physically active as they depend more on machines for transportation. Highlighting this issue, research in sub-Saharan Africa emphasizes the need for context-specific epidemiological studies to better understand the unique challenges faced by these populations (Adebamowo et al., 2016). By integrating genomic data with lifestyle and environmental assessments, initiatives like the Human Heredity and Health in Africa (H3Africa) project aim to shed light on the multifaceted epidemiology of T2D. By studying this topic so thoroughly, we can develop better public health plans and improve the impact of actions taken to fight the disease (Figure 4.6).

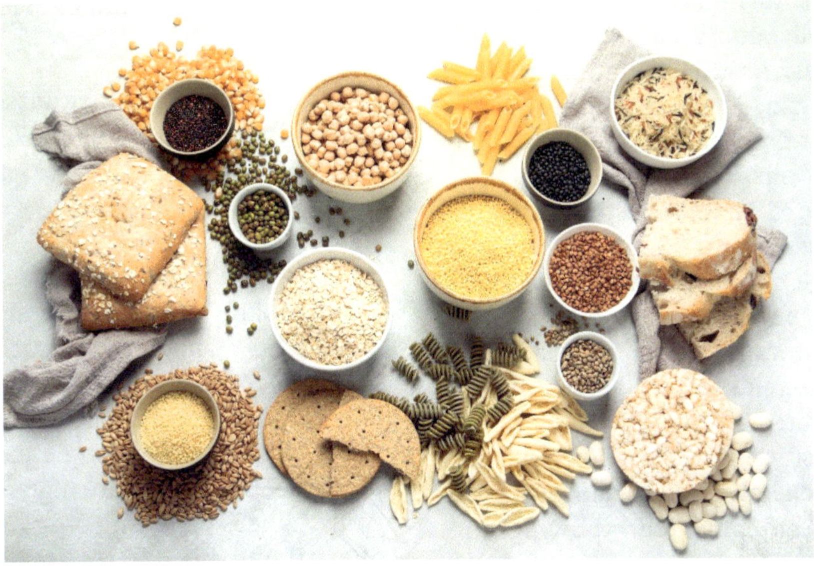

Figure 4.6. Diets high in refined carbohydrates and sugars contribute to weight gain, which is a primary risk factor for the disease.

Source: https://www.news-medical.net/images/news/ImageForNews_784373_17199653671039100.jpg

4.2.1. Genetic Predisposition

Genetic predisposition is very important in explaining the causes and spread of Type 2 diabetes. Although it is accepted that diet and exercise play a role, studies have found that particular genes can also affect a person's chances of getting the disease. It has been found that a person's risk of autism is often linked to their family history, especially with their mother and siblings. It is clear from research that having a mother or siblings with diabetes raises the chances of a person getting gestational diabetes and later developing Type 2 diabetes. This finding underscores the complex interaction between genetic factors and environmental influences, suggesting that genetic predisposition may act as a foundation upon which lifestyle factors exert further impact on disease development (Chircop et al., 2003). In addition, looking into how genes and macronutrients interact has revealed new insights into the causes of Type 2 diabetes. The EPIC-InterAct study and similar studies have tried to find out how genes and the types of food people eat work together to cause diabetes. At the beginning, people thought that certain genes might change the link between diet and diabetes, but the study found no proof of this. Therefore, it seems that genes do not have a major effect on how diet affects the development of diabetes. These findings challenge simple deterministic views of genetics in Type 2 diabetes, emphasizing the necessity of a multifaceted approach that incorporates both genetic and lifestyle factors in preventive strategies (Agudo et al., 2018). Genetic predisposition for Type 2 diabetes has important effects on how public health strategies are planned and implemented. Knowing how genetics and behavior are linked can guide the development of special programs for people who are more at risk. As an example, those with a family background of diabetes could be advised to pay more attention to their health and make changes in their lifestyle and eating habits. It is possible to create health education programs that help people understand their family's risks and learn how to prevent them. Noticing genetic predisposition does not take away from personal choice in health matters, but helps in finding more personal solutions to the growing number of Type 2 diabetes cases in many populations (Figure 4.7).

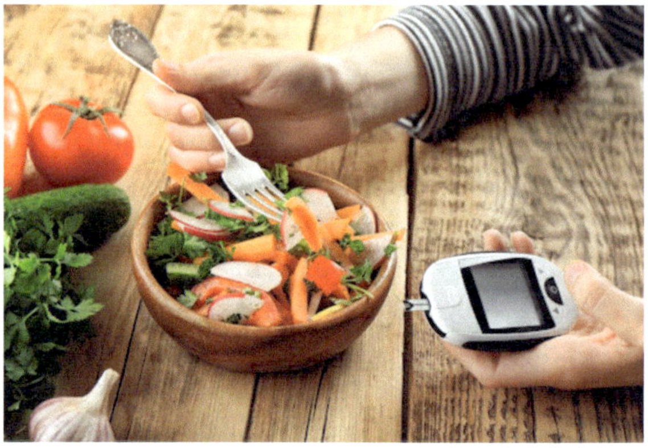

Figure 4.7. Individuals with a strong family history of diabetes might benefit from increased monitoring and proactive lifestyle modifications aimed at weight management and dietary improvements.

Source: https://cdn.squats.in/kc_articles/e70fb0dbfb4f85f37460045d72ef7438.jpeg

4.2.2. Lifestyle Factors (Diet, Physical Activity)

When looking at the causes and spread of type 2 diabetes, what people eat and how active they are is very important. Insulin sensitivity and how glucose is metabolized are greatly affected by the way people eat. Eating a lot of processed foods that are high in carbs increases your chances of getting type 2 diabetes through obesity and insulin resistance. Eating a diet rich in whole foods, low glycemic index carbs, and healthy fats has been found to lower these risks. Besides affecting metabolism, the diet also interacts with genes, which makes it harder to understand how lifestyle affects the onset of diabetes. For this reason, it is very important to understand the role of diet in preventing type 2 diabetes. How active you are plays a major role in reducing your chances of getting type 2 diabetes. Being physically active regularly helps your body use insulin well and manage your weight, which decreases the chances of metabolic issues. Researchers routinely find that not being physically active increases the chances of getting type 2 diabetes. In fact, doing just a little more physical activity each day can greatly improve your health. Moderate activities such as walking and cycling can help maintain blood sugar and reduce the risk of diabetes. The benefits of exercise and diet working together are very important, since they both play a role in shaping a person's metabolic health. For this reason, public health strategies should focus on helping people exercise more and choose a healthier diet to prevent diabetes. In addition, new studies indicate that our lifestyle may affect our dietary needs at the genetic level, mainly in terms of vitamin D levels and the amount of carbohydrates we consume. A study focused on Asian Indians demonstrated that metabolic genetic risk scores (GRS) interact with dietary habits, particularly carbohydrate consumption, to influence vitamin D levels, which are crucial for metabolic regulation. People who follow a low-carbohydrate diet and have fewer metabolic risk alleles had significant increases in their 25-hydroxyvitamin D levels. Therefore, personalized nutrition for diabetes may be useful, since people with different genes could require different diet plans. As such, integrating genetic insights into public health dietary recommendations could enhance the effectiveness of lifestyle interventions aimed at reducing the prevalence of type 2 diabetes and promoting overall health (Kitsiou et al., 2013; Alathari et al., 2020) (Figure 4.8).

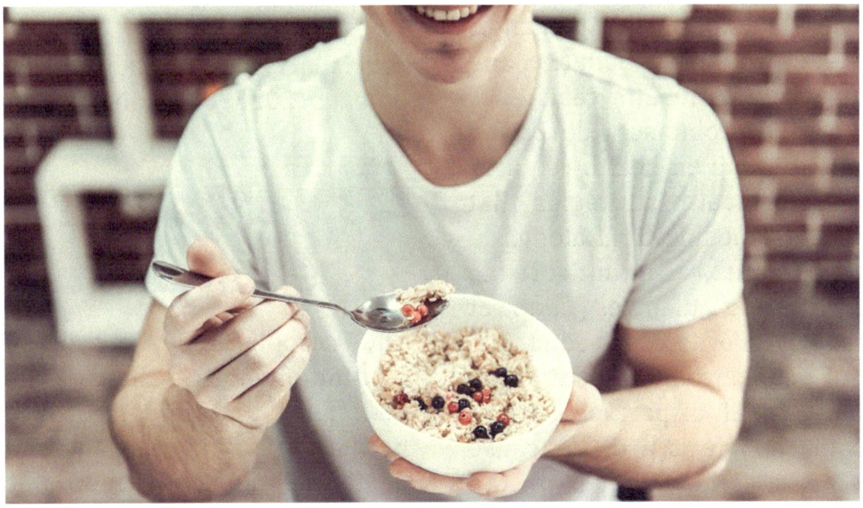

Figure 4.8. High-carbohydrate diets, often rich in processed foods, are linked to increased risk factors for type 2 diabetes, including obesity and insulin resistance.

Source: https://integrishealth.org/-/media/blog/2023/oyh_food-and-diabetes.ashx?revision=b81b42ba-537a-49d9-99f4-69118f3c9af4

4.2.3. Environmental Influences (Socioeconomic Status, Urbanization)

To understand how the environment affects Type 2 diabetes, it is necessary to look into socioeconomic status, which is closely connected to health outcomes. People from lower socioeconomic backgrounds usually deal with more stress, not enough food, and fewer healthcare options. Because of such hardships, people tend to eat unhealthy foods and exercise less, which are major causes of

Type 2 diabetes. Also, people in economically disadvantaged situations often deal with more health issues, and the lack of community organization can prevent them from using health-promoting resources. Notably, recent research emphasizes that economic inequities directly correlate with increased incidences of chronic diseases, including Type 2 diabetes, thereby underscoring the critical relationship between economic status and metabolic health outcomes within various populations (Badpa et al., 2024). An increase in urbanization is another important factor that affects the rate of Type 2 diabetes. When people move from rural to urban areas, their way of living can become unhealthy. While cities provide easy access to supermarkets, they are usually full of fast-food places and have less space for recreation. The existence of "food deserts" in cities makes it harder for low-income people to get nutritious foods. In addition, living in cities usually means dealing with more pollution and stress, which may lead to insulin resistance and various metabolic problems. Addressing urbanization's implications on health requires comprehensive public health strategies that consider environmental modifications alongside community wellness initiatives to mitigate the risks associated with Type 2 diabetes (Badpa et al., 2024). Different levels of access to education and healthcare for people from different social classes can increase health disparities. Lack of resources for some people is a major cause of preventable health issues, shown by the rise in serious health events when healthcare is not easily available. Several studies using Structural Equation Modeling have shown that socioeconomically disadvantaged people often cannot manage their diabetes well because they are less able to take part in healthy habits. Because of these barriers, individuals from low socioeconomic groups are more likely to develop diabetes and other long-term diseases. By addressing these inequitable structures and investing in healthier urban environments, community resilience can be enhanced, ultimately aiming to reduce the prevalence of Type 2 diabetes in vulnerable populations across diverse geographic regions, reinforcing the need for inclusive health policies (Smith et al., 2007) (Figure 4.9).

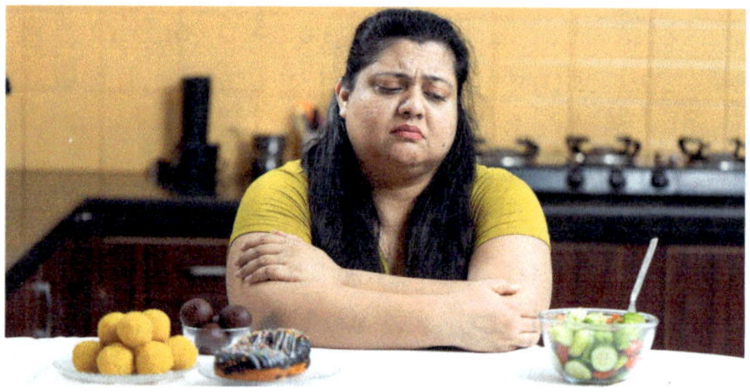

Figure 4.9. The phenomenon of "food deserts" in urban environments further complicates dietary options, particularly for economically disadvantaged populations who may lack access to nutritious foods.

Source: https://geimshospital.com/wp-content/uploads/2025/04/Diabetes-Causes.jpg

4.3. Pathophysiology of Type 2 Diabetes

The pathophysiology of Type 2 Diabetes (T2D) is fundamentally characterized by insulin resistance and impaired insulin secretion. Because of insulin resistance, muscle, liver, and fat tissues do not take up glucose effectively and produces more glucose in the liver. As a result of this resistance, there is more glucose in the blood, which makes the pancreas secrete more insulin. Still, with time, the beta cells get tired and no longer work properly, resulting in not enough insulin being produced. It is believed that genetic reasons, obesity, and a lack of physical activity are important factors in causing insulin resistance, which proves that T2D is a disease with many causes. Since metabolic and endocrine problems are linked in diabetes, this makes the disease more complex and important to study in diabetes epidemiology. Also, inflammation plays a major role in T2D because constant low-level inflammation is known to cause insulin resistance and problems with beta cells. Adipose tissue, particularly in the presence of obesity, releases pro-inflammatory cytokines such as tumor necrosis factor-alpha (TNF-α) and interleukin-6 (IL-6), which interfere with insulin signaling pathways. This situation worsens the metabolic problems in T2D, which results in more insulin resistance and poorer blood sugar control. The relationship between inflammation and insulin resistance links to findings on B-type natriuretic peptide (BNP), which suggest an inverse association between BNP levels and the risk of developing T2D. Understanding these mechanisms provides critical insights into potential therapeutic targets for managing and preventing T2D, as indicated in various studies (Pfister et al., 2011). Besides insulin resistance and inflammation, T2D is greatly affected by genetics. Changes in certain genes responsible for glucose and insulin functions have been linked to the disease. Remarkably, the variant rs198389 in the BNP locus is related to a lower chance of T2D, probably by changing BNP levels and the processes linked to them. The more research is done, the more likely it is that genetics and epidemiology will lead to personalized medicine for T2D. The role of genetic, environmental, and lifestyle factors in T2D shows how important it is to study the condition as a whole. By addressing these elements, public health strategies can be better tailored to mitigate the impact of this pervasive metabolic disorder (Kitsiou et al., 2013) (Figure 4.10).

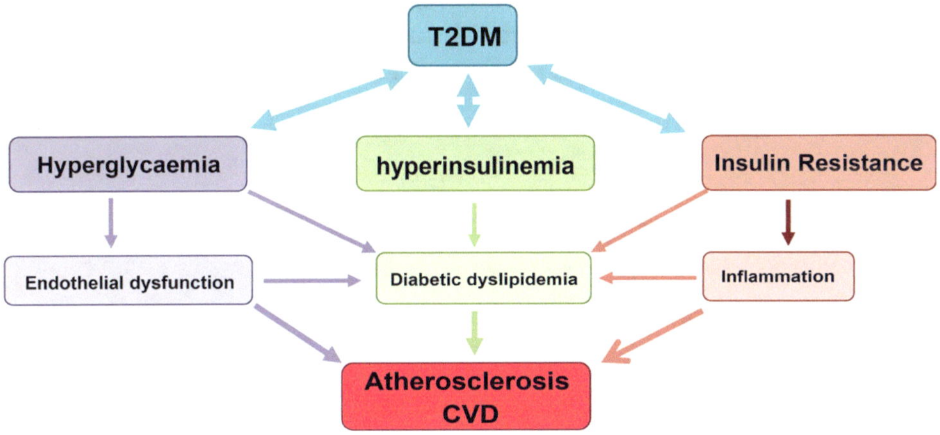

Figure 4.10. The pathophysiology of Type 2 Diabetes (T2D) is fundamentally characterized by insulin resistance and impaired insulin secretion.

Source: https://pub.mdpi-res.com/ijms/ijms-21-06275/article_deploy/html/images/ijms-21-06275-g006.png?1598767316

4.3.1. Insulin Resistance Mechanisms

The mechanisms of insulin resistance play a pivotal role in the epidemiology and etiology of Type 2 Diabetes (T2D), influencing the diseases onset and progression. When the liver, muscle, and adipose tissue do not respond well to insulin, insulin resistance happens. Because of this impairment, blood glucose rises, which causes hyperglycemia. In particular, the rise of insulin resistance is related to obesity, not being active, and certain genes. It has been found that cytokines and adipokines produced by adipose tissue can disrupt the way insulin works. As a result, the interplay between these biological mechanisms manifests as decreased metabolic efficiency, thereby significantly increasing the risk of T2D in affected populations (Pfister et al., 2011). Changes in genes have been linked to the process of insulin resistance, pointing to the role of many factors in the risk of T2D. New studies have found certain genetic changes that are linked to insulin resistance and secretion, giving us more knowledge about the condition's causes. It was found that a genetic score linked to insulin resistance was also linked to lower insulin sensitivity, which suggests that genes can impact metabolism on their own, apart from body weight. Even in those who are not obese, insulin resistance can happen because of excess fat in the wrong places and its negative impact on metabolism, showing that T2D is caused by several factors. As demonstrated in various studies, understanding these genetic components helps elucidate how insulin resistance operates at a cellular level and informs targeted prevention strategies (Arriola et al., 2014). In addition, insulin resistance in T2D affects more than just genetics and lifestyle choices and impacts the health of the population. Insulin resistance among people with metabolic syndrome is linked to other heart disease risks, which makes the health problems more serious for the population. Since insulin resistance is linked to hypertension, dyslipidemia, and obesity, it is very important to focus on preventing and treating T2D. Strategies that work on improving insulin sensitivity by changing lifestyle habits or using drugs could help lower the number of T2D cases. If insulin resistance is tackled, healthcare systems can reduce the risk of other health problems and help the population live healthier lives. The need for continued research on the underlying mechanisms of insulin resistance remains essential for devising effective public health strategies aimed at curbing the growing T2D epidemic (Pfister et al., 2011) (Figure 4.11).

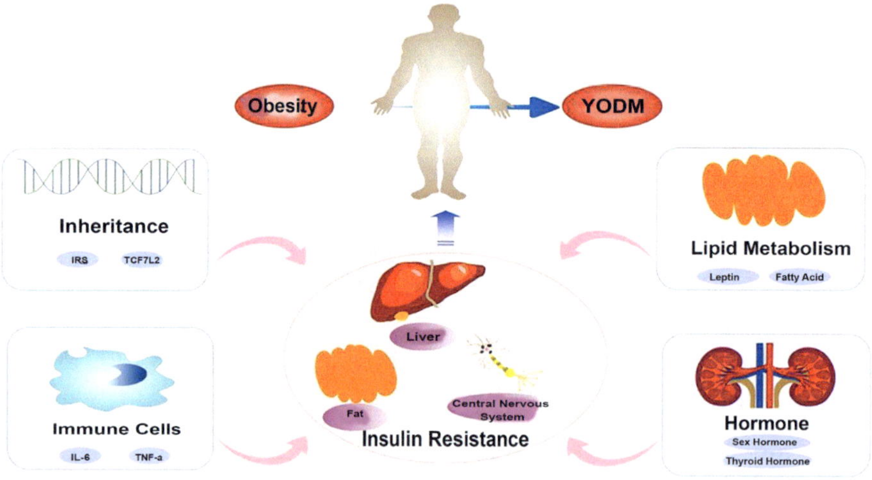

Figure 4.11. The mechanisms of insulin resistance play a pivotal role in the epidemiology and etiology of Type 2 Diabetes (T2D), influencing the disease's onset and progression.

Source: Jia Q, Zhang Y, Zhang B and An X (2024) Reassessing type 2 diabetes in adolescents and its management strategies based on insulin resistance. Front. Endocrinol. 15:1377918. doi: 10.3389/fendo.2024.1377918

4.3.2. Role of Pancreatic Beta Cells

Pancreatic beta cells play a crucial role in regulating blood glucose levels and maintaining metabolic homeostasis, which are fundamental in the context of type 2 diabetes (T2D). The main task of these cells found in the islets of Langerhans is to produce and release insulin when blood glucose levels go up. Insulin helps the body's muscles and fat cells absorb glucose, which lowers the blood sugar level after eating. If there are not enough beta cells or if they do not produce enough insulin, it causes glucose metabolism to become disordered, which is a main feature of T2D. Therefore, the disease's pathophysiology depends on beta cells, so they are important in both explaining the epidemiology and the causes of T2D. Genetic and environmental factors together contribute to the decrease in beta cell function in people who may develop T2D. According to research, some genetic factors may change how insulin signaling happens and how well beta cells adapt. It has been found that some genetic variants are related to a higher risk of T2D, proving that genetics can greatly affect the function of beta cells. In addition, issues such as being overweight and not exercising enough make beta cells work less effectively by causing insulin resistance. The fact that genetics and environmental factors affect T2D in different ways proves that the disease is complex and requires attention to beta cell changes in its management and prevention. Taking care of beta cells could be a useful approach for treating diabetes. New studies are pointing out that the mechanisms that control beta cells are essential for understanding the development of T2Ds. According to research, inflammation, oxidative stress, and lipotoxicity can both reduce the function and survival of beta cells. It has been shown that chronic low-grade inflammation, caused by pro-inflammatory cytokines, is related to less beta cell mass and insulin secretion problems. Besides, when there are more free fatty acids, it adds to the stress on beta cells and leads to their decline. Knowing these mechanisms helps us better understand T2D and shows ways to protect the function of beta cells. When we understand what leads to beta cell failure, we can find new ways to prevent and treat T2D, which in turn helps patients deal with this common disease (Figure 4.12).

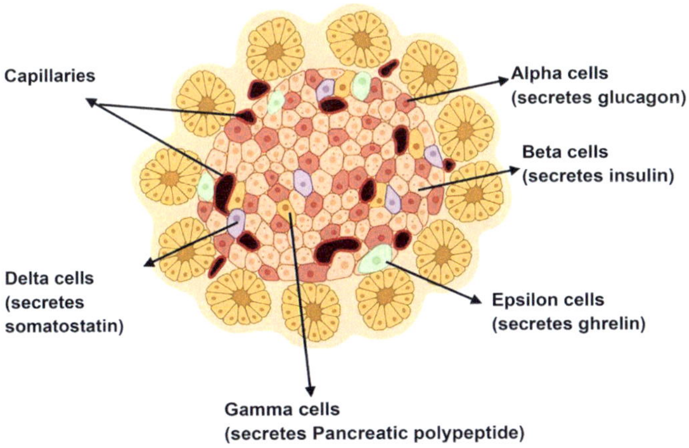

Figure 4.12. Pancreatic beta cells play a crucial role in regulating blood glucose levels and maintaining metabolic homeostasis, which are fundamental in the context of type 2 diabetes (T2D).

Source: Carroll J, Chen J, Mittal R, Lemos JRN, Mittal M, Juneja S, Assayed A, Hirani K. Decoding the Significance of Alpha Cell Function in the Pathophysiology of Type 1 Diabetes. *Cells*. 2024; 13(22):1914. https://doi.org/10.3390/cells13221914

4.3.3. Impact of Obesity on Glucose Metabolism

Obesity is fundamentally linked to the dysregulation of glucose metabolism, serving as a significant risk factor for the development of type 2 diabetes mellitus (T2D). Too much fat in the body, mainly visceral fat, causes chronic inflammation and makes the body resistant to insulin. Pro-inflammatory cytokines and free fatty acids build up, which interfere with the usual functions of insulin. If insulin resistance occurs, the pancreas tries to make up for it by secreting more insulin. In the end, this way of handling blood sugar does not work, leading to higher blood glucose and the development of T2D. Furthermore, the interplay between genetic predispositions and environmental factors, such as sedentary lifestyles and dietary habits, exacerbates this relationship, highlighting the need for comprehensive strategies targeting obesity to mitigate T2D risk (Pfister et al., 2011).

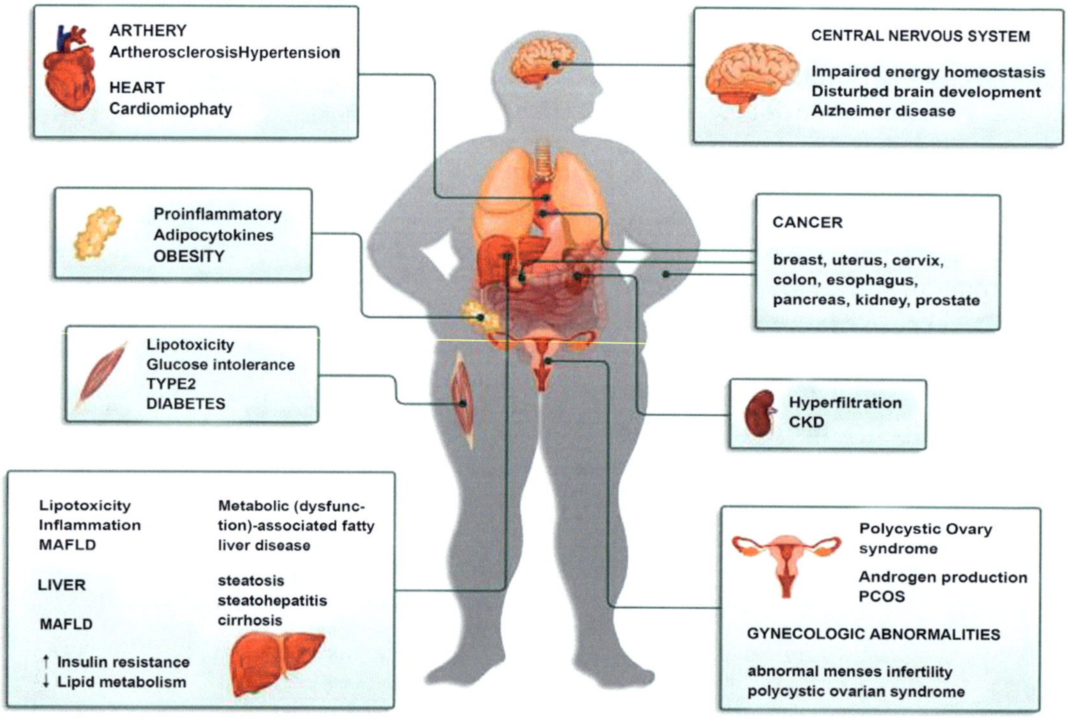

Figure 4.13. The metabolic disturbances associated with obesity extend beyond insulin resistance, impacting further mechanisms involved in glucose homeostasis.

Source: https://media.springernature.com/lw685/springer-static/image/art%3A10.1038%2Fs41392-022-01073-0/MediaObjects/41392_2022_1073_Fig4_HTML.png

The problems in metabolism caused by obesity affect more than insulin resistance and impact additional parts of glucose regulation. It has been found that adipose tissue stores extra energy and also contributes to metabolic regulation by releasing hormones such as leptin and adiponectin. Leptin is mainly made by adipocytes and helps control hunger and the use of energy. Alternatively, low amounts of adiponectin in obese people lead to problems with glucose metabolism since it has anti-inflammatory and insulin-sensitizing effects. These hormonal problems can make it easier for obese people to develop T2D. Moreover, the relationship between obesity and abnormal glucose metabolism is often compounded by factors such as genetic variations affecting insulin action and secretion, reinforcing the importance of individualized approaches to prevention and treatment (Arriola et al., 2014). Due to the obvious link between obesity and glucose problems, programs that help with weight loss should be considered to prevent T2D. Eating a healthy diet and exercising more can greatly improve how insulin works and control blood sugar levels. In addition, using medications for weight loss and behavioral therapy has been found to help people with high risk for T2D by both improving their metabolic health and lowering the rate of T2D. Telling the public about the risks of obesity is important for early actions that can change the course of certain diseases. As research continues to uncover the mechanistic pathways linking obesity and glucose metabolism, an integrative understanding can facilitate the development of targeted strategies aimed at curtailing the T2D epidemic (Pfister et al., 2011) (Figure 4.13).

4.4. Etiological Theories of Type 2 Diabetes

The phenomenon of Type 2 Diabetes (T2D) emerges from a complex interplay of genetic, environmental, and lifestyle factors, encapsulated within several etiological theories. Genetic predisposition is important because some alleles and polymorphisms may increase a person's risk of getting T2D. As more studies are done, it appears that having variations in the FTO gene is linked to obesity, a main risk factor for T2D. It provides an understanding of how some populations are more likely to be affected by certain environmental factors because of their genes. Gaining knowledge about these genetic factors is necessary because it helps create special ways to prevent T2D by using both lifestyle changes and new drugs. The role of the environment is very important in the development of Type 2 Diabetes, especially since it is tied to both society and personal habits. T2D is becoming more common because of urbanization and changes in people's diets. As people eat more processed foods with lots of sugars and fats and move less, the rate of obesity has gone up. Therefore, studying both local and worldwide economic situations, as suggested by many studies, may help reveal ways to better understand T2D epidemiology. Moreover, the role of socio-economic status as a determinant of health cannot be overstated; disparities in access to health education and nutritious food are tightly woven into the fabric of T2D risk, further emphasizing the need to analyze socio-economic factors within a broader epidemiological framework (Leung et al., 2010). Moreover, the impact of social factors and their ties to biological systems have become a well-known aspect of what leads to Type 2 Diabetes. According to epigenetic research, long-term effects on health and wealth from the past may result in people developing T2D.

In other words, the belief that better living conditions over the years can affect our biological makeup underlines why we should consider the long-term effects of socio-economic factors on health. Since T2D is more common among some groups, it is necessary to pay attention to those who suffer from the disease due to social and economic inequalities. Consequently, effective prevention strategies should not only target lifestyle changes but also advocate for policies aimed at addressing systemic health inequities, thereby fostering a comprehensive approach to T2D management and prevention (Balasubramanyam et al., 2007) (Figure 4.14).

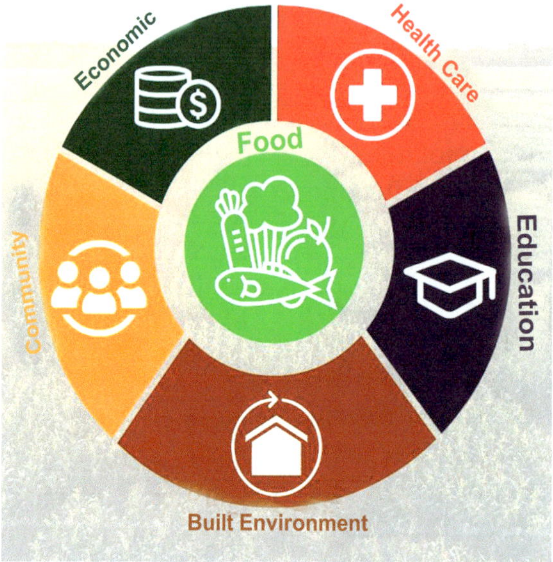

Figure 4.14. The role of socio-economic status as a determinant of health cannot be overstated; disparities in access to health education and nutritious food are tightly woven into the fabric of T2D risk

Source: https://www.aboundfoodcare.org/wp-content/uploads/2022/06/HubSpoke-Post.png

4.4.1. The Role of Inflammation

Chronic inflammation plays a pivotal role in the development and progression of Type 2 Diabetes (T2D). It is now acknowledged that an improper activation of the immune system may cause metabolic problems in addition to protecting from pathogens. Adipose tissue is especially affected by this, as too much fat in the tissue causes inflammation. The presence of TNF-alpha and interleukin-6 sends pro-inflammatory messages, which make the body resistant to insulin. As a result, this connection between inflammation and metabolism proves that systemic inflammation worsens and reflects the environment that increases the risk of T2D. Learning how inflammation and glycation are connected gives us a better idea of the causes of T2D. When there is inflammation, the process called glycation increases and worsens metabolic problems. Elevated levels of glycated hemoglobin (HbA1c) are often observed in T2D patients, marking the importance of glycation in disease diagnosis and management. New studies on epidemiology indicate that having high blood sugar levels is not the only thing that increases the risk of chronic diseases in inflammatory situations. The link between metabolic health and chronic inflammation is shown by the important role of inflammation and oxidative stress. Therefore, it is important to conduct more research to explain these pathways and how they affect T2D treatments. The way diet, inflammation, and T2D are related should be carefully studied. Eating lots of antioxidant-rich foods, fruits, and vegetables can help reduce chronic inflammation. Eating a lot of processed foods and sugar may lead to faster development of T2D by triggering inflammation in the body. This way of thinking about food points out the link between nutrition and inflammation and also fits into the overall picture of disease prevention. With more research, it is obvious that inflammation plays a key role in lifestyle interventions. Future research should focus on clarifying these interactions, contributing to comprehensive dietary guidelines aimed at reducing T2D risk and enhancing overall metabolic health (Kitsiou et al., 2013) (Figure 4.15).

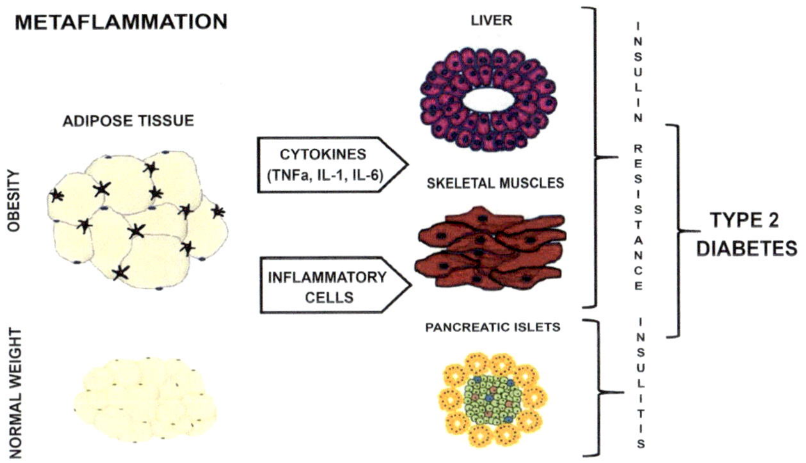

Figure 4.15. Chronic inflammation plays a pivotal role in the development and progression of Type 2 Diabetes (T2D).

Source: Kuryłowicz A, Koźniewski K. Anti-Inflammatory Strategies Targeting Metaflammation in Type 2 Diabetes. *Molecules*. 2020; 25(9):2224. https://doi.org/10.3390/molecules25092224

4.4.2. The Gut Microbiome and Its Influence

The gut microbiome plays a pivotal role in human health, influencing various physiological processes that are linked to the pathogenesis of type 2 diabetes (T2D). Because it consists of many microorganisms, the gut microbiome is important for digestion, absorbing nutrients, and protecting the immune system. Any changes in the balance of microbes have been linked to conditions like obesity and insulin resistance, which increase the risk of T2D. It is now being studied more often how changes in gut microbiota may influence the development of T2D by affecting fat storage and blood sugar control. When we know how these interactions work, we can find ways to prevent or treat T2D by changing the gut microbiota. For this reason, understanding the relationship between the gut, the brain, and the microbiome is still a main focus in diabetes research. Many ideas have been suggested to show how the gut microbiome might lead to insulin resistance, which is a main symptom of type 2 diabetes. The composition of gut microbiota can affect the production of short-chain fatty acids (SCFAs) through the fermentation of dietary fibers, which are known to enhance insulin sensitivity and reduce inflammation. In addition, if gut bacteria are not balanced, it can increase the permeability of the intestines, letting lipopolysaccharides and other inflammatory substances into the blood, which raises inflammation throughout the body and affects metabolism. It is important to realize that adding prebiotics and probiotics to your diet may help change the mix of bacteria in your gut and improve its health. As a result of these changes, individuals may become stronger against T2D, stressing the significance of treating health holistically by paying attention to diet and gut health. In addition, research is showing that the gut microbiome could be a useful target for preventing and managing T2D. It has been found recently that some types of diets can change the balance of gut bacteria, which improves the way our bodies use energy. The D-ECCO working group delves into the intricate relationship between diet and microbiome, suggesting structured nutritional therapy may play a role in not only the management of inflammatory bowel disease but also in mitigating the risk of T2D (Allan et al., 2017). Additionally, the application of fecal microbiota transplantation (FMT) and the administration of specific probiotics are being investigated as novel strategies for attenuating insulin resistance and promoting metabolic health (Cotter et al., 2014). The results highlight the importance of more research on using the gut microbiome to support the current efforts to treat type 2 diabetes (Figure 4.16).

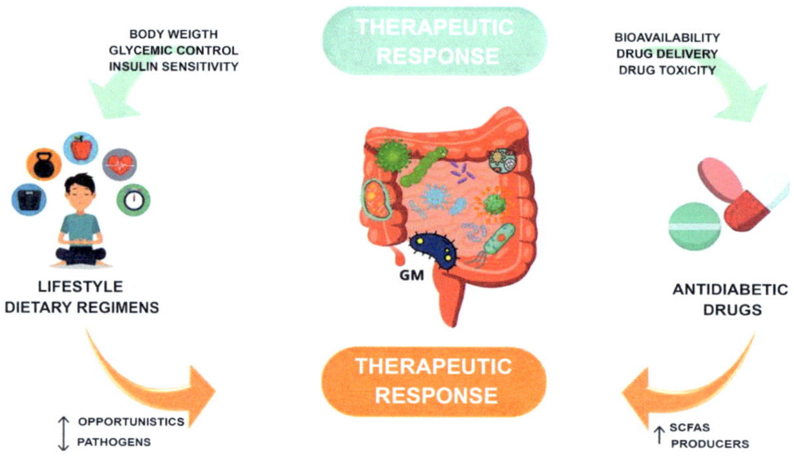

Figure 4.16. The gut microbiome plays a pivotal role in human health, influencing various physiological processes that are linked to the pathogenesis of type 2 diabetes (T2D).

Source: https://www.thelancet.com/cms/10.1016/j.ebiom.2023.104821/asset/af3ed81e-661d-48d3-914b-98d6ab9859c4/main.assets/gr2_lrg.jpg

4.4.3. The Impact of Endocrine Disruptors

The significance of endocrine disruptors in the context of type 2 diabetes is an area of increasing concern among researchers and public health officials. These chemical substances interfere with hormone systems, which can lead to various adverse health outcomes, including metabolic disorders. The workshop held in Parma, Italy, focused on understanding environmental metabolic disrupting chemicals and their relationship with obesity and metabolic syndrome. One of the workshop's primary objectives was to review the existing data, primarily from animal models and epidemiological studies, to ascertain how these disruptors contribute to obesity and, subsequently, to the rising prevalence of type 2 diabetes. By broadening the definition of obesogens to include metabolic disruptors, it becomes crucial to explore the implications of these chemicals in altering the body's metabolic responses, thus shedding light on their potential role in the diabetes epidemic (Janesick et al., 2015). In addition to their impact on obesity, endocrine disruptors are also implicated in the more nuanced interactions between hormonal systems and diabetes development. Evidence suggests that synthetic chemicals that mimic estrogen can lead not only to increased fat accumulation but also to insulin resistance, a core characteristic of type 2 diabetes. These environmental exposures often occur during critical developmental windows, which could amplify their long-term effects on metabolic health. The relationship between hormone-sensitive conditions, such as type 2 diabetes, and various endocrine disruptors warrants further exploration. By examining these interactions through an integrated and systems thinking approach, researchers can identify potential preventive strategies that address both environmental and lifestyle factors contributing to the disease (Plant et al., 2016). Understanding how endocrine disruptors affect insulin sensitivity and glucose metabolism is vital for developing comprehensive prevention and intervention strategies. The use of a multidisciplinary approach, as highlighted in recent research, facilitates a better grasp of these complex interactions between environmental chemicals and metabolic disease processes. Identifying knowledge gaps concerning the effects of endocrine disruptors could lead to more focused research efforts, informing public health recommendations and regulatory policies. Moreover, as the prevalence of type 2 diabetes continues to rise globally, assessing the impact of these metabolic disruptors becomes an imperative task. Through ongoing research, it is possible to establish a new framework for understanding the multifaceted influences of endocrine disruptors, advancing our knowledge and potentially mitigating the increasing burden of type 2 diabetes (Janesick et al., 2015) (Figure 4.17).

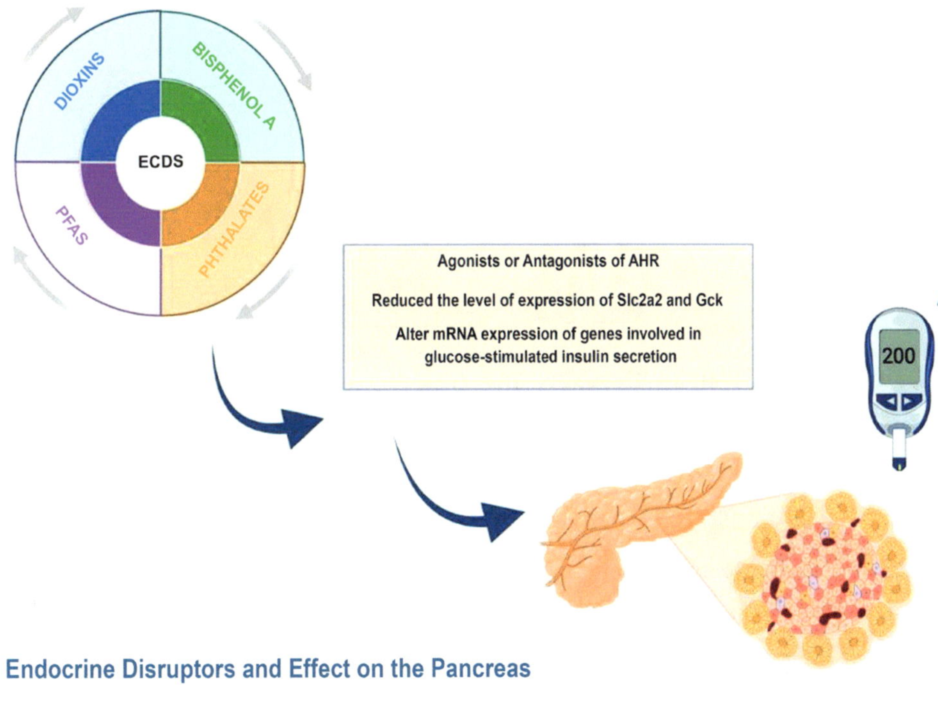

Figure 4.17. The significance of endocrine disruptors in the context of type 2 diabetes is an area of increasing concern among researchers and public health officials.

Source: Keskesiadou G-N, Tsokkou S, Konstantinidis I, Georgaki M-N, Sioga A, Papamitsou T, Karachrysafi S. Endocrine-Disrupting Chemicals and the Development of Diabetes Mellitus Type 1: A 5-Year Systematic Review. *International Journal of Molecular Sciences*. 2024; 25(18):10111. https://doi.org/10.3390/ijms251810111

4.5. Complications Associated with Type 2 Diabetes

The challenges caused by Type 2 diabetes are of great concern because they seriously affect both people's lives and the healthcare system. Among these complications, cardiovascular disease (CVD) emerges as one of the most critical. Those with Type 2 diabetes are twice to four times more likely to get heart disease than people who do not have diabetes. The reason for this increased risk is mainly related to insulin resistance, obesity, and dyslipidemia, all of which make atherosclerosis worse. Managing cardiovascular risk factors as soon as possible helps patients with Type 2 diabetes avoid deaths from CVD.

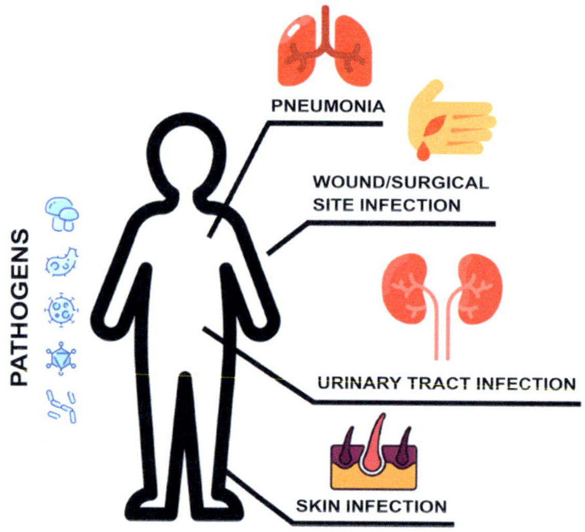

Figure 4.18. Diabetes significantly increases the risk of various infections, including pneumonia and tuberculosis, particularly in regions with limited healthcare resources.

Source: Pari B, Gallucci M, Ghigo A, Brizzi MF. Insight on Infections in Diabetic Setting. *Biomedicines*. 2023; 11(3):971. https://doi.org/10.3390/biomedicines11030971

For this reason, healthcare services should focus on screening for heart problems and educating patients to reduce the risks, which helps improve patient outcomes in diabetes management. Retinopathy, nephropathy, and neuropathy are major complications that Type 2 diabetes patients must deal with. Among working-age adults, diabetic retinopathy is the main reason for preventable blindness due to damage to the retinal blood vessels. Reports indicate that patients with diabetes can experience rates of retinopathy complications ranging from 7% to 63%, depending on the population studied (Hall et al., 2011). In the same way, diabetic nephropathy can result in end-stage renal disease and may require either dialysis or a kidney transplant. Neuropathy in the peripheral nerves can bring about pain, leave people disabled, and increase the chance of foot ulcers and amputations. Since these microvascular complications are so common, it is necessary to regularly check patients and use management strategies that involve strict blood sugar control and teaching them about preventive care. Besides problems in blood vessels, the way Type 2 diabetes and infectious diseases interact should be considered in public health. In places where healthcare is not widely available, diabetes raises the likelihood of getting infections such as pneumonia and tuberculosis. It is a matter of concern, and it becomes more challenging in Sub-Saharan Africa, as both diabetes and infectious diseases are hard to manage together. The economic burden of diabetes, estimated at $67.03 billion annually in the region, can hinder access to necessary diagnostic and treatment tools, thereby exacerbating complications (Hall et al., 2011). In addition, the high price of diabetes care and the shortage of required medical tools lead to poor results. It is important to deal with these challenges together to reduce the number of complications linked to Type 2 diabetes, showing the need for health interventions that last (Figure 4.18).

4.5.1. Cardiovascular Diseases

Cardiovascular diseases (CVD) and type 2 diabetes (T2D) are intricately interconnected, often sharing common risk factors that amplify the likelihood of developing both conditions. It is clear how this relationship works through insulin resistance, inflammation, and dyslipidemia, which are important in developing T2D and also lead to heart problems. Various studies have proven that people with T2D are more likely to suffer from heart problems due to metabolic changes. Moreover, since the relationship works both ways, taking care of one condition may lead to better results in the other. For this reason, it is important to understand the effects of CVD and T2D when making strategies to prevent and treat these conditions. Studying the biochemical links between CVD and T2D gives us important knowledge about their relationship.

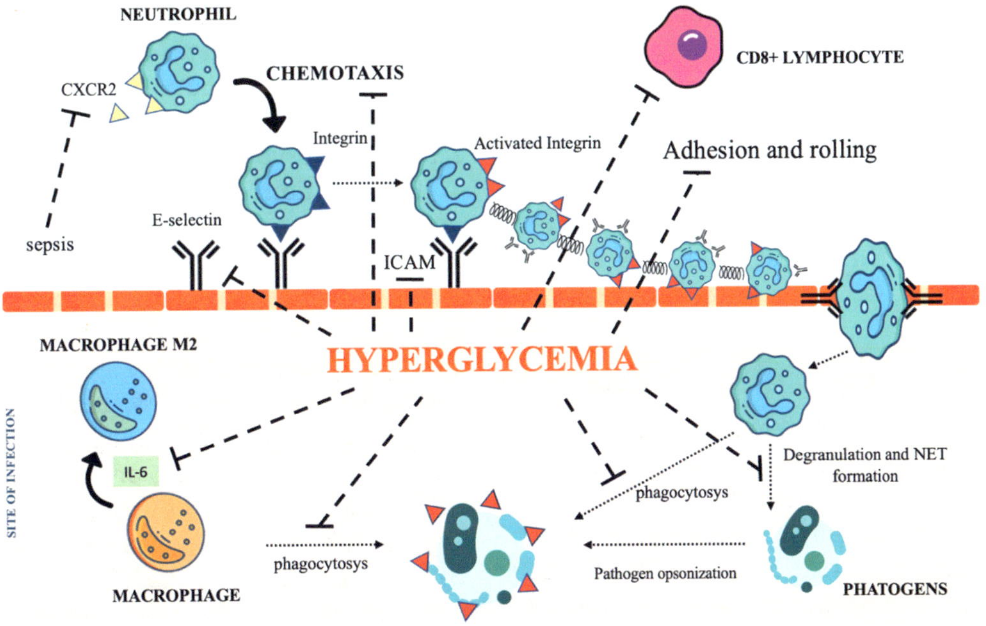

Figure 4.19. Cardiovascular diseases (CVD) and type 2 diabetes (T2D) are intricately interconnected, often sharing common risk factors that amplify the likelihood of developing both conditions.

Source: Pari B, Gallucci M, Ghigo A, Brizzi MF. Insight on Infections in Diabetic Setting. *Biomedicines*. 2023; 11(3):971. https://doi.org/10.3390/biomedicines11030971

For instance, the role of B-type natriuretic peptide (BNP) has emerged as a significant area of research, as lower levels of BNP have been correlated with an increased risk of T2D. One particularly relevant study highlighted a 21% decreased risk of incident T2D per standard deviation increase in NT-pro-BNP levels, after adjusting for various confounding factors such as age, sex, and body mass index (Pfister et al., 2011). This means that the BNP system may play a role in causing T2D. In addition, researchers understand that more studies are needed to learn how BNP affects both T2D and heart health, which could lead to better treatments. The results prove that treating both cardiovascular and metabolic diseases at the same time is highly necessary. Doctors and other health workers should focus on early detection and assessment of risks for people with T2D and heart problems. Also, making changes to your diet, exercising more, and managing your weight can be very important for lowering the risks of CVD and T2D. The relationship between these diseases points out opportunities to improve both cardiovascular health and diabetes outcomes at the same time. Ultimately, a holistic understanding of cardiovascular diseases within the context of T2D is essential for enhancing patient care and developing effective public health initiatives (Kitsiou et al., 2013) (Figure 4.19).

4.5.2. Neuropathy and Its Effects

Neuropathy is a major problem that happens in Type 2 diabetes and has a big effect on the lives of people everywhere. The main reason for this disease is prolonged high blood sugar, which leads to problems with the nerves as the disease develops. The most common way this condition appears is peripheral neuropathy, and people with this usually feel numbness, tingling, and pain in their arms and legs. Loss of sensation can lead to more injuries and infections, since the neuropathic condition makes them worse. Because people with diabetes are at risk for foot ulcers, it is important to know how neuropathy is connected to them and to manage the situation with regular foot checks and patient information on self-care. Besides the physical symptoms, neuropathy also leads to mental and social difficulties for people with Type 2 diabetes. Many people with chronic pain or neuropathy often go through emotional distress, anxiety, and depression. When people can't do their daily routines and fear losing a limb to diabetes, they may choose to isolate themselves and live with less happiness. In managing diabetes, a strong focus is placed on approaches that help with both body and mind. Being aware that better pain management, healthy lifestyle changes, and mental health support can enhance the outcomes of diabetic patients with neuropathy and its results. In addition, neuropathy plays a major part in the development of diabetes-related complications. The process of diabetic neuropathy involves many factors, including decreased blood flow, changes in nerve tissues, and the lasting results of inflammation. New studies suggest that the relationship between these factors may result in serious conditions like diabetic foot ulcers, which can be very dangerous and may need amputation. We should look for ways to manage neuropathy that control the symptoms and also handle infections and slow healing. Overall, a comprehensive understanding of neuropathy is pivotal for implementing preventive measures and enhancing quality of life for individuals with Type 2 diabetes, given its intricate relationship with myriad diabetic manifestations, such as those presented in Ho et al. (2013) and Brandt et al. (2008) (Figure 4.2).

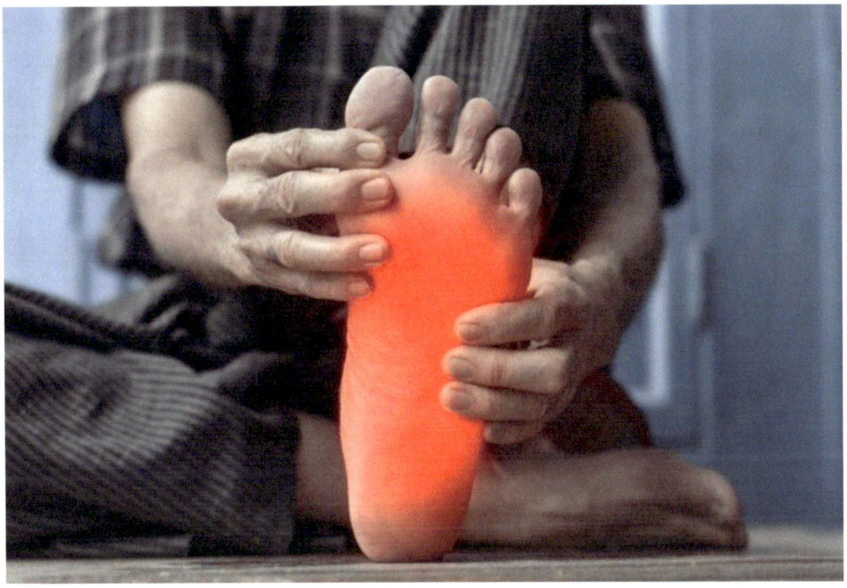

Figure 4.20. Neuropathy is a significant complication associated with Type 2 diabetes, impacting the quality of life for millions of individuals worldwide.

Source: https://premierneurologycenter.com/wp-content/uploads/sites/436/2024/07/shutterstock_2175261423-768x512.jpg.optimal.jpg

4.5.3. Kidney Disease and Diabetic Nephropathy

Diabetic nephropathy is a common problem for people with type 2 diabetes, since it affects the kidneys and causes more illness and death in those who have it. Usually, the disease causes the kidneys to work less and less, often resulting in end-stage renal disease, which requires dialysis or a kidney transplant. It has been found through epidemiology that between 20% and 40% of people with diabetes will get diabetic nephropathy, and the risk increases with the length of diabetes and poor glycemic control. Besides, what leads to this disease are hyperglycemia-related oxidative stress, inflammation, and changes in blood flow to the kidneys, which end in glomerulosclerosis. Spotting and managing hypertension and dyslipidemia at an early stage is important for keeping diabetic nephropathy at bay in patients with type 2 diabetes. It is important to use advanced tools and biomarkers to help find and manage diabetic nephropathy early on. Current studies have found proteomic biomarkers that not only describe the disease's development but can also be used to predict its future development. They may be used to spot people at risk for serious kidney disease and plan their treatment accordingly. Still, these proteomic markers are not widely used in clinical practice because many studies do not have enough validated data and enough participants. For these biomarkers to be used properly in medicine, both academic and business sectors should cooperate, and there should be stronger regulations to ensure the studies are powerful enough. This progress could change how kidney disease in diabetic patients is managed, making the outcomes better. Because diabetic nephropathy is a major form of kidney disease, it greatly affects healthcare systems everywhere, especially since type 2 diabetes is becoming more common. It is important to pay close attention to kidney function and changes in the disease when caring for people with diabetes. The development of standardized primary renal diagnosis (PRD) codes, in alignment with international guidelines, could facilitate better tracking and management of diabetic nephropathy within clinical settings, as suggested by the ERA-EDTA Registry. They would not only help patients receive better care but also assist in research that looks into the causes and spread of kidney disease in diabetic people. In the end, a better understanding of the link between type 2 diabetes and kidney problems will help design special preventive and treatment plans for this increasing health issue (Figure 4.21).

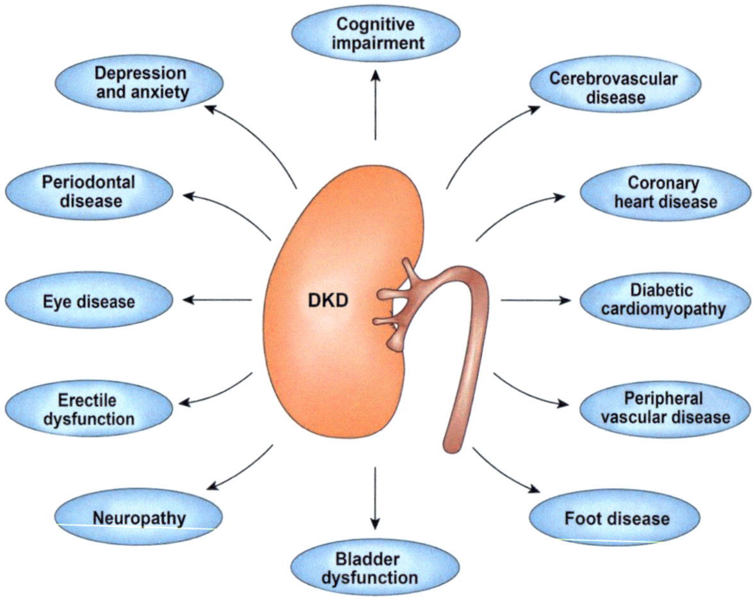

Figure 4.21. Diabetic nephropathy, a common complication of type 2 diabetes, significantly impacts the kidneys and contributes to increased morbidity and mortality among affected individuals.

Source: https://media.springernature.com/lw1200/springer-static/image/art%3A10.1038%2Fnrdp.2015.18/MediaObjects/41572_2015_Article_BFnrdp201518_Fig7_HTML.jpg

A CLOSER LOOK

GESTATIONAL DIABETES MELLITUS (GDM)

Gestational Diabetes Mellitus (GDM) is a type of diabetes that develops during pregnancy, usually in the second or third trimester. It happens when the body does not make enough insulin for pregnancy, which causes the blood sugar to rise. The condition usually ends after childbirth, but it raises the chances of high birth weight, preterm birth, and developing type 2 diabetes in the future for both mother and child. A person with diabetes is advised to check their blood sugar, follow a healthy diet, exercise regularly, and sometimes use insulin therapy. It is very important to diagnose problems early and look after them properly for a healthy pregnancy.

Summary

In synthesizing the epidemiological and etiological understanding of Type 2 Diabetes (T2D), it becomes evident that this multifaceted disease presents significant public health challenges, particularly in diverse demographic contexts. Because T2D is becoming more common globally, it is clear that public health strategies should be in place. As mentioned in several studies, both genes and lifestyle play a role in increasing the chances of T2D. Furthermore, emerging research, including findings on B-type natriuretic peptide (BNP) levels, suggests potential pathways through which biological markers may influence the risk of developing T2D, highlighting the complexity of its etiology (Pfister et al., 2011). So, knowing these different factors helps create effective strategies to control the increasing number of cases of this metabolic disorder. Socio-economic problems and weak health systems make the T2D epidemic worse in Sub-Saharan Africa. The systemic literature review reveals alarming statistics; T2D prevalence ranges from 1% to 12% in varying populations, indicating not only a significant public health crisis but also a pressing need for robust data to inform health policy (Hall et al., 2011). Since both diabetes and infections are common, healthcare should focus on treating both types of diseases at the same time. Besides, it is difficult for many people to get the help they need because of limited resources and high prices, which results in more deaths among those affected. It is important to deal with these barriers to reduce the effects of T2D in these areas. To summarize, the reasons behind T2D are related to genes, the environment, and socio-economic factors, so public health should address the issue from several angles. Further research is essential to elucidate the mechanisms underlying T2D, as recent studies suggest potential causal roles of biological markers like BNP in disease pathogenesis (Pfister et al., 2011). It is important for policymakers to include diabetes management in overall healthcare plans, most especially in places dealing with both diabetes and infectious diseases. The high economic costs associated with uncontrolled diabetes further advocate for preventive measures that could alleviate future healthcare expenditures while improving population health outcomes (Hall et al., 2011). It will be very important to use comprehensive methods to address T2D and support healthier communities.

References

1. MacLean, A., Sweeting, H., Egan, M., Der, G., Adamson, J., & Hunt, K. (2013). How robust is the evidence of an emerging or increasing female excess in physical morbidity between childhood and adolescence? Results of a systematic literature review and meta-analyses. *Social science & medicine (1982)*, *78*, 96–112. https://doi.org/10.1016/j.socscimed.2012.11.039(accessed on 11th June 2025).
2. Adebamowo, C., Balde, N., Ekoru, K., Hennig, B. J., et al. (2016). H3Africa multi-center study of the prevalence and environmental and genetic determinants of type 2 diabetes in sub-Saharan Africa: Study protocol. https://core.ac.uk/download/145317836.pdf (accessed on 11th June 2025).
3. Afshar, M., Farhud, D., & Golalipour, M. J. (2006). Epidemiologic aspects of neural tube defects in South East Iran. https://core.ac.uk/download/52205121.pdf (accessed on 11th June 2025).
4. Agudo, A., Ardanaz, E., Aune, D., Boeing, H., et al. (2018). Interplay between genetic predisposition, macronutrient intake and type 2 diabetes incidence: Analysis within EPIC-InterAct across eight European countries. https://core.ac.uk/download/84340703.pdf (accessed on 11th June 2025).
5. Alathari, B. E., Anjana, R. M., Bodhini, D., Jayashri, R., et al. (2020). A nutrigenetic approach to investigate the relationship between metabolic traits and vitamin D status in an Asian Indian population. https://core.ac.uk/download/323052747.pdf (accessed on 11th June 2025).
6. Allan, P., Fiorino, G., Gatti, S., Gerasimidis, K., et al. (2017). Research gaps in diet and nutrition in inflammatory bowel disease. A topical review by D-ECCO Working Group (Dietitians of ECCO). https://core.ac.uk/download/84340703.pdf (accessed on 11th June 2025).
7. Amendola, G., Bicocchi, R., Borgia, G., Brambilla, L., et al. (2018). Epidemiology and microbiology of skin and soft tissue infections: Preliminary results of a national registry. https://core.ac.uk/download/196288595.pdf (accessed on 11th June 2025).
8. Arriola, L., Balkau, B., Barker, A., Barricarte, A., et al. (2014). Common genetic variants highlight the role of insulin resistance and body fat distribution in type 2 diabetes, independent of obesity. https://core.ac.uk/download/77407381.pdf (accessed on 11th June 2025).
9. Aulchenko, Y., Baqui, A. H., Bhutta, Z. A., Campbell, O. M., et al. (2011). The case for launch of an international DNA-based birth cohort study. https://core.ac.uk/download/28973486.pdf (accessed on 11th June 2025).
10. Badpa, M. (2024). Long-term exposure to environmental factors and risk of metabolic disorders in children. https://core.ac.uk/download/613738917.pdf (accessed on 11th June 2025).
11. Balasubramanyam, M., & Mohan, V. (2007). Diabetes in 2007 – What are the promises & challenges? https://core.ac.uk/download/33800035.pdf (accessed on 11th June 2025).
12. Boeschoten, E., Casino, F., Collart, F., Cornet, R., et al. (2012). New primary renal diagnosis codes for the ERA-EDTA. https://core.ac.uk/download/9652512.pdf (accessed on 11th June 2025).
13. Brandt, T., Glaser, M., Strupp, M., Wagner, J., et al. (2008). Downbeat nystagmus: Etiology and comorbidity in 117 patients. https://core.ac.uk/download/12175155.pdf (accessed on 11th June 2025).

14. Brodbelt, D. C., Church, D. B., Mattin, M. J., McGreevy, P. D., et al. (2014). An epidemiological study of diabetes mellitus in dogs attending first opinion practice in the UK. https://core.ac.uk/download/36777545.pdf (accessed on 11th June 2025).

15. Brooks, B. (2013). Obesity and diabetes: The enemies within. https://core.ac.uk/download/41237912.pdf (accessed on 11th June 2025).

16. Catchpole, B., Holder, A. L., Kennedy, L. J., Massey, J., et al. (2014). Searching for "monogenic diabetes" in dogs using a candidate gene approach. https://core.ac.uk/download/157854855.pdf (accessed on 11th June 2025).

17. Chircop, M., Savona-Ventura, C., & Schranz, A. G. (2003). Family history in the etiology of gestational diabetes mellitus and type 2 diabetes. https://core.ac.uk/download/46601850.pdf (accessed on 11th June 2025).

18. Cotter, P. D., Guinane, C. M., O'Toole, P. W., Walsh, C. J., et al. (2014). Beneficial modulation of the gut microbiota. https://core.ac.uk/download/45656343.pdf (accessed on 11th June 2025).

19. Hall, V., Henriksen, O., Lohse, N., Thomsen, R. W., et al. (2011). Diabetes in Sub-Saharan Africa 1999–2011: Epidemiology and public health implications. A systematic review. https://core.ac.uk/download/pdf/16666834.pdf (accessed on 11th June 2025).

20. Heerspink, H. J. L., Mischak, H., & Pena, M. J. (2016). Proteomics for prediction of disease progression and response to therapy in diabetic kidney disease. https://core.ac.uk/download/84148392.pdf (accessed on 11th June 2025).

21. Ho, T. K., Leigh, R. D., & Tsui, J. (2013). Diabetic foot disease and oedema. https://core.ac.uk/download/16219516.pdf (accessed on 11th June 2025).

22. Janesick, A., Mantovani, A., Suvorov, A., Cohn, B. A., Angle, B. M., et al. (2015). Parma consensus statement on metabolic disruptors. https://core.ac.uk/download/42131375.pdf (accessed on 11th June 2025).

23. Kalsi, J., & Muneer, A. (2013). Erectile dysfunction–An update of current practice and future strategies. https://core.ac.uk/download/29416259.pdf (accessed on 11th June 2025).

24. Kitsiou, A., Caforio, A. L. P., Porta-Sanchez, A., Vahanian, A., Iung, B., Carrera, C., Szymanski, C., et al. (2013). ESC core curriculum for the general cardiologist (2013). https://core.ac.uk/download/55756305.pdf (accessed on 11th June 2025).

25. Leung, G. M., & Schooling, C. M. (2010). A socio-biological explanation for social disparities in non-communicable chronic diseases: The product of history? https://core.ac.uk/download/37953763.pdf (accessed on 11th June 2025).

26. Pfister, R., Sharp, S., Luben, R., Welsh, P., Barroso, I., Salomaa, V., Meirhaeghe, A., Khaw, K. T., Sattar, N., Langenberg, C., & Wareham, N. J. (2011). Mendelian randomization study of B-type natriuretic peptide and type 2 diabetes: evidence of causal association from population studies. *PLoS medicine*, *8*(10), e1001112. https://doi.org/10.1371/journal.pmed.1001112(accessed on 11th June 2025).

27. Phillips, L. (2023). Lifelong health and well-being in men born with hypospadias. https://core.ac.uk/download/570950836.pdf (accessed on 11th June 2025).

28. Plant, J., Stanley, E., & Voulvoulis, N. (2016). Environmental chemical exposures and breast cancer. https://core.ac.uk/download/77011572.pdf (accessed on 11th June 2025).

29. Smith, H. (2007). Social pathogenic sources of poor community health. https://core.ac.uk/download/236295739.pdf (accessed on 11th June 2025).

30. Vlassopoulos, A., Bhagwat, S., El-Salem, H., Combet, E., Hao, L., Hodge, A., et al. (2014). Oxidative stress, protein glycation and nutrition–interactions relevant to health and disease throughout the lifecycle. https://core.ac.uk/download/18492207.pdf (accessed on 11th June 2025).

31. Weis, N. (2020). Low carbohydrate ketogenic diet versus aerobic physical activity in the management and treatment of type 2 diabetes: A review paper. https://core.ac.uk/download/304683154.pdf (accessed on 11th June 2025).

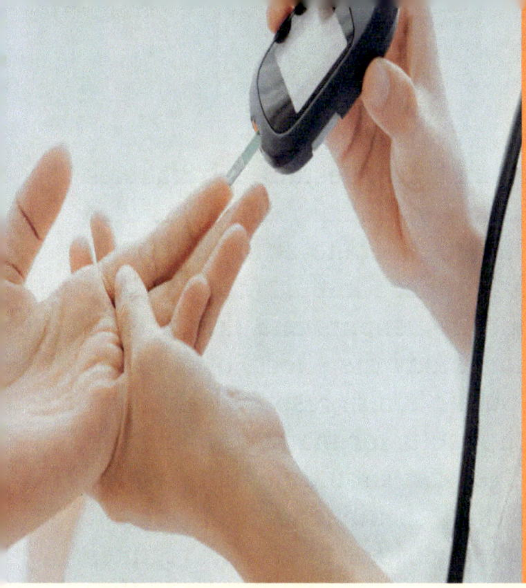

Chapter 5

OTHER TYPES OF DIABETES

Contents

Introduction

To understand diabetes, one must first learn about its different forms, since they are very different in how they develop and how they are treated. While Type 1 and Type 2 diabetes are the most widely known types, several other forms, such as gestational diabetes and latent autoimmune diabetes in adults (LADA), also warrant attention. Every type of cancer brings its own problems for those who have it and for healthcare systems that treat them. Since about 100 million people around the world have diabetes, it is clear that different types of the disease must be addressed quickly. Treatment approaches often revolve around optimal glycemic control to prevent or delay complications, necessitating a multifaceted understanding of these diabetes types (Ambrosiadou et al., 2000). When we pay attention to various forms of diabetes, we can provide better care for patients and develop effective public health plans. Since diabetes has many aspects, it is clear that both inherited, environmental, and lifestyle elements can increase a person's risk of the disease. For instance, gestational diabetes presents unique health risks during pregnancy, not only influencing maternal health but also increasing the likelihood of developing Type 2 diabetes later in life (DeGaetano et al., 2019). In the Australian Capital Territory, public health efforts are now putting more importance on early detection and treatment of diabetes in pregnancy, considering both the benefits and the costs to healthcare services. Using sophisticated models, researchers can now study the effects of diabetes on the body and how this affects both medical care and the use of public health resources. It helps us understand better how to improve the quality of care and health results for many people. With ongoing research, it is becoming more obvious that diabetes management should be adjusted for each type of the disease. The use of decision tree learning algorithms in diabetes management shows how technology is being used more in healthcare. By analyzing various treatment regimes through these algorithms, healthcare providers can support personalized treatment plans that cater to individual patients' needs and circumstances (Ambrosiadou et al., 2000). Also, research on diabetes in pregnancy continues to encourage interventions that put more focus on positive outcomes for patients. Being aware of the various forms of diabetes, health professionals can come up with better strategies to treat affected individuals (Figure 5.1).

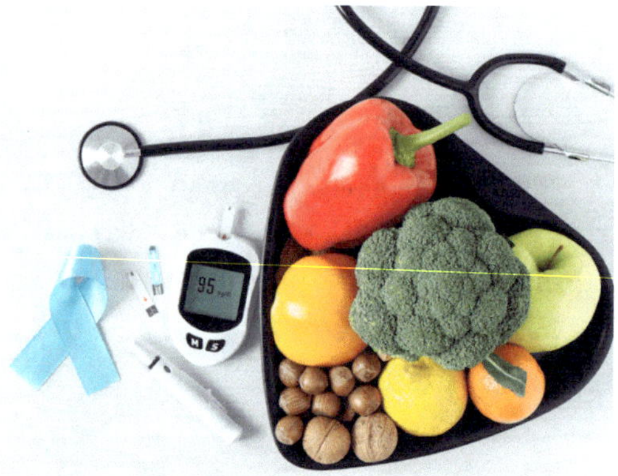

Figure 5.1. Treatment approaches often revolve around optimal glycemic control to prevent or delay complications, necessitating a multifaceted understanding of these diabetes types

Source: https://www.circufiber.com/cdn/shop/articles/Circufiber_Ultimate_Guide_to_Diabetes_Prevention_Strategies_and_Benefits_1_1600x.png?v=1708714212

5.1. Gestational Diabetes

Gestational diabetes mellitus (GDM) represents a unique form of diabetes that occurs during pregnancy, characterized by glucose intolerance that develops or is first recognized during this period. The situation can harm the mother's health and also endanger the baby while it is growing. Women with GDM usually face problems such as heavier babies and a greater chance of a cesarean delivery. It is important to note that GDM may cause lasting health problems; women who have GDM are more likely to get type 2 diabetes later in life. This chronic risk highlights the importance of proper screening and management strategies during and after pregnancy, particularly among populations that may be more susceptible, such as Latina women, as evidenced by current research (Althavale et al., 2015). Because GDM requires effective solutions, researchers have studied different ways to change lifestyles and use medicines. It appears that making changes to diet, increasing exercise, and checking blood sugar help both mothers and their babies achieve better results. Specifically, studies indicate that lifestyle modifications can reduce the prevalence of large-for-gestational-age infants, a common complication associated with GDM (Alsweiler et al., 2018). Still, these procedures must be carefully considered because some evidence shows they may carry risks. As an example, efforts to change lifestyle habits could result in more cases of labor induction, showing how complicated it is to treat GDM. New methods, including specially designed health communication programs, are being used to assist women with GDM, mainly among those from diverse cultures. These interventions aim to promote adherence to the Diabetes Prevention Program (DPP) and incorporate culturally relevant strategies that resonate with the experiences of postpartum women. For instance, the STAR MAMA initiative focuses on using health coaching and support networks to foster behavior change among postpartum Latina mothers, addressing both emotional and practical aspects of managing diabetes (Althavale et al., 2015). Taking culture into account is necessary since the usual management methods may not help people from different backgrounds who have GDM. With more research, it may be possible to find better ways to help women and their children enjoy better health (Figure 5.2).

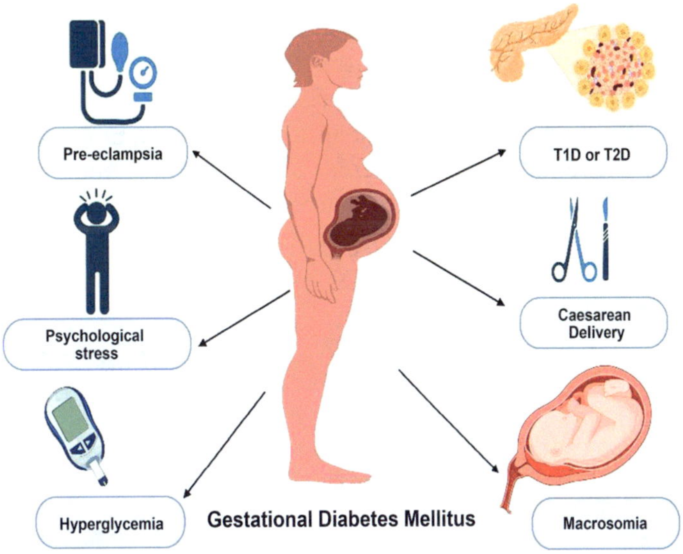

Figure 5.2. Gestational diabetes mellitus (GDM) represents a unique form of diabetes that occurs during pregnancy, characterized by glucose intolerance that develops or is first recognized during this period.

Source: Mittal R, Prasad K, Lemos JRN, Arevalo G, Hirani K. Unveiling Gestational Diabetes: An Overview of Pathophysiology and Management. *International Journal of Molecular Sciences.* 2025; 26(5):2320. https://doi.org/10.3390/ijms26052320

5.1.1. Definition and Risk Factors

It is necessary to clearly define and organize diabetes types, especially the ones that are not as widely known as Type 1 and Type 2. Diabetes Mellitus (DM) is defined as a syndrome characterized by chronic hyperglycemia resulting from defects in insulin secretion, insulin action, or both. According to recent discussions, correctly identifying and classifying diabetes is very important for learning about the reasons behind it and choosing the best treatments. It is notable that different causes can result in diabetes, which affects the way diabetes is managed and the outcomes for patients. Consequently, looking at the symptoms of DM as well as the factors that cause it to develop and worsen helps create a clear picture of the disease. The causes of diabetes are also many and difficult to understand. Although obesity, lack of exercise, and irregular eating habits are tied to Type 2 diabetes, other forms, such as diabetes caused by pancreatic disease, need a careful review of risk factors. As an example, when dogs get exocrine pancreatic disease, it can lead to diabetes, making one wonder if similar situations occur in humans. A person's chances of getting diabetes are higher if they have a family history of the disease. These risk factors collectively underscore the need for comprehensive screening and early interventions, particularly for populations most at risk, as early diagnosis can dramatically alter prognosis and management of the disease (Wu et al., 2016). Along with other traditional risk factors, a person's economic status and ability to get healthcare play a major role in diabetes. Because they may not have enough money, people from lower socio-economic groups can find it challenging to get healthy food, preventive medical care, and diabetes education, which puts them at greater risk of diabetes. In addition, living in cities and being exposed to some pollutants can make these risks more serious. Studies that were supported by funding mechanisms point out that using several disciplines is important for understanding the relationship between these factors in diabetes. By integrating knowledge about these diverse influences, the healthcare community can better direct efforts toward prevention, early detection, and effective management strategies across all types of diabetes, thereby improving health outcomes for affected populations (Wu et al., 2016) (Figure 5.3).

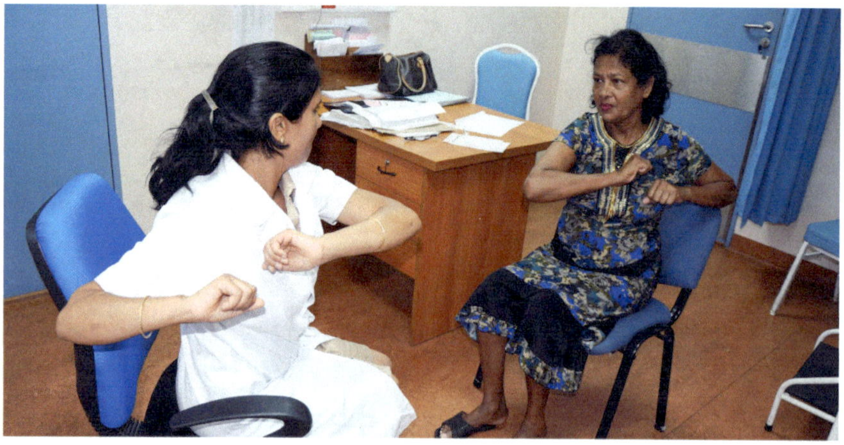

Figure 5.3. Individuals from lower socio-economic backgrounds may encounter barriers such as limited access to nutritious food, preventative healthcare services, and diabetes education programs, thereby increasing their vulnerability to developing diabetes.

Source: https://ncdalliance.org/sites/default/files/news/diabetes-masthead.jpg

5.1.2. Impact on Pregnancy and Fetal Health

It is necessary to manage diabetes properly in pregnancy because it may impact the baby's health and the mother's wellbeing. Specifically, conditions such as gestational diabetes mellitus (GDM) have been shown to elevate the risk of both maternal and neonatal complications, including preeclampsia and preterm birth. New studies show that focusing on the maternal microbiome could help reduce these dangers. Probiotic treatments have shown that they might reduce the chance of preeclampsia and GDM by changing the balance of bacteria in the body. While findings in this area have not yet provided conclusive results, the exploration of microbial factors represents a promising avenue for potentially mitigating adverse effects on pregnancy and fetal health, indicating the need for further investigation into the connections between the microbiome and gestational complications (Dunn et al., 2019). If a mother has high blood sugar, it can be very harmful to the fetus by affecting its growth through DNA methylation. It appears that modifications in fetal DNA methylation, especially in leptin genes, are related to how much glucose is in a mother's blood during pregnancy. Such changes can impact neonatal leptin levels as well as affect a child's risk of being overweight. Scientists have found that the levels of sugar in the mother's blood affect certain parts of the baby's DNA, which may lead to increased fat storage. It is therefore very important to control blood sugar levels during pregnancy to avoid problems for the mother and child. Consequently, understanding the epigenetic mechanisms at play offers a new perspective on how maternal health directly affects fetal development and may dictate obesity risk later in life (Bouchard et al., 2020). Effects of diabetes during pregnancy can be seen in the baby's health now and in the future. If a mother's blood sugar is not well controlled, her baby may face issues such as premature birth, having a low birth weight, and an increased risk of metabolic disorders. If a child is exposed to a mother's high blood sugar, they are more likely to develop obesity and type 2 diabetes. This shows that it is important to handle diabetes well and early on during pregnancy. Improving the rules for healthcare and spreading knowledge about diabetes in pregnant women could be important for the health of both the mother and the baby. Ensuring that diabetic women receive proper care during their pregnancy can thus mitigate risks and promote healthier futures for their children, making diabetes management an essential pillar of maternal care strategies (Dunn et al., 2019; Bouchard et al., 2020) (Figure 5.4).

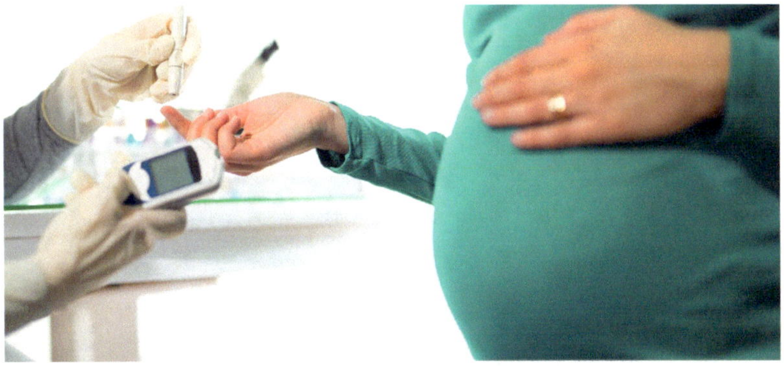

Figure 5.4. The management of diabetes during pregnancy is critical due to its potential effects on fetal development and maternal health.

Source: https://www.sitarambhartia.org/wp-content/uploads/2017/10/GDM-1170x520@2x.jpg

5.1.3. Management and Long-Term Implications

Proper management of diabetes, mainly type 2 diabetes, is necessary since it can affect health in the long run. It is important to use several approaches, including sticking to medicine, making healthy lifestyle changes, and interacting with the doctor. Setting goals is an important method in diabetes care, as it encourages patients and doctors to work together. As mentioned in recent studies, this process enables patients to share their main concerns and what they want to achieve, which helps set their treatment goals. It is very important to understand how these interactions, which depend on patient and doctor roles, expectations, and ways of communicating, work. A well-structured consultation that focuses on these considerations may significantly enhance the effectiveness of goal-setting, paving the way for improved health outcomes and long-term adherence to management plans (Ford et al., 2020). The effects of diabetes management go further than just health, since many people still fail to take their medication as directed. People with type 2 diabetes usually take several medications, including antidiabetic drugs, blood pressure medications, and statins, which can make their care more difficult. It is found that patients may not follow treatment plans for many reasons, both on purpose and by accident. For instance, as the number of medications prescribed increases, so does the likelihood of intentional nonadherence, particularly regarding statin use (Bundy et al., 2010). It is important to understand these behaviors, as it helps create interventions that support patients in sticking to their treatment plan for a long time and enjoy better health. Also, management approaches for diabetes should consider the mental and social aspects of the disease. Teaching patients, supporting their feelings, and clear communication can greatly affect how they deal with their treatment plans. When healthcare providers involve patients in setting goals, it helps reduce the stress of taking many medications. Adding behavioral techniques to regular medical care helps patients follow their treatment and also better explains what it is like for them to live with diabetes. This holistically oriented approach acknowledges that long-term health outcomes are shaped not only by physiological factors but also by emotional and psychological well-being, emphasizing the importance of comprehensive management in the treatment of other types of diabetes (Ford et al., 2020) (Figure 5.5).

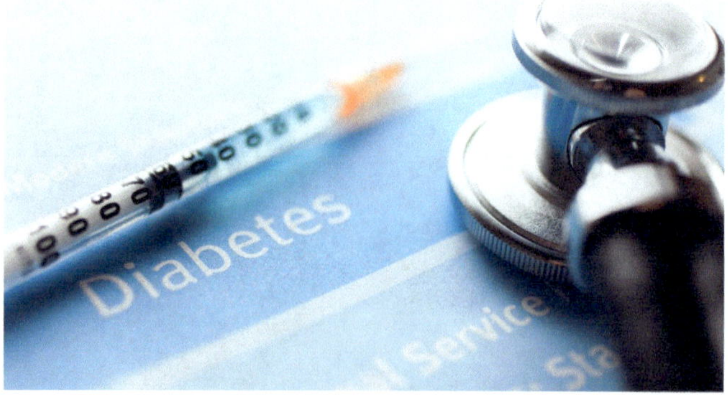

Figure 5.5. Effective management of diabetes, particularly other types such as type 2 diabetes, is crucial due to its long-term health implications.

Source: https://nutritionsource.hsph.harvard.edu/wp-content/uploads/2024/11/AdobeStock_62404725.jpeg.

5.2. LADA (Latent Autoimmune Diabetes in Adults)

LADA, which is short for Latent Autoimmune Diabetes in Adults, is a kind of diabetes that is different from Type 1 and Type 2 because it brings unique challenges. Most cases of this condition appear in adults who are over 30 and at first display resistance to insulin, much like Type 2 diabetes. Still, the disease develops slowly by damaging the insulin-producing beta cells in the pancreas with the body's own immune system. Therefore, many individuals might be given the wrong diagnosis of Type 2 diabetes since their symptoms and early treatment reactions are alike, resulting in ineffective care. It is important for healthcare providers to become aware of the features and testing methods of LADA so that they can identify and treat the condition accurately and on time.

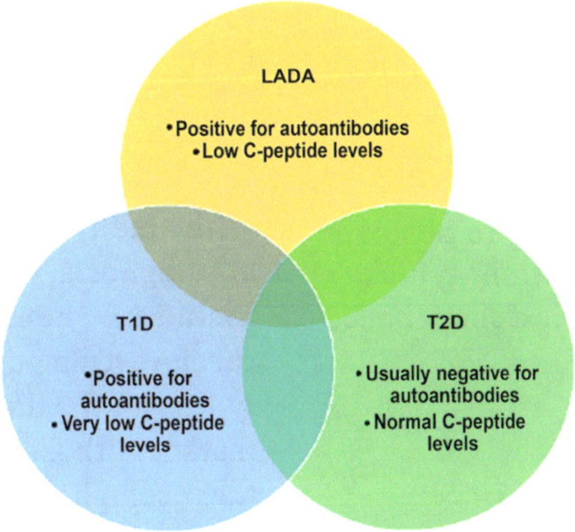

Figure 5.6. Latent autoimmune diabetes in adults.

Source: https://higherlogicdownload.s3.amazonaws.com/AADE/UploadedImages/jTfx2VRESk2hViPEDWQJ_Picture1.png

The way LADA affects the body helps explain why it is called a hybrid form of diabetes, as it shows signs of both Type 1 and Type 2 diabetes. Unlike typical Type 2 diabetes, where beta-cell function is primarily impaired due to insulin resistance, LADA patients face autoimmune beta-cell destruction, often indicated by the presence of specific islet autoantibodies such as GAD (glutamic acid decarboxylase) antibodies. These autoantibodies play an important role in clinical practice since their presence can help diagnose LADA in people who have unusual symptoms or do not respond to oral drugs. Consequently, understanding these underlying mechanisms aids in distinguishing LADA from other types of diabetes, thereby refining treatment protocols that align with the true nature of the disease (Shankarappa et al., 2024). Managing LADA is still a main concern in the wider field of diabetes care. At first, the condition was mistaken for Type 2 diabetes, and patients continued to have increasing blood sugar despite treatment with oral medicines, so insulin was needed. There are also notable risk factors associated with LADA, such as low body mass index (BMI) and a family history of autoimmune diseases, which further underline the need for personalized treatment approaches. So, it is important for doctors to use lifestyle changes and drugs that are suitable for people diagnosed with LADA. Holistic management not only addresses immediate glycemic control but also mitigates the long-term complications associated with inadequate diabetes management, thus enhancing overall patient quality of life (Shrivastav et al., 2024) (Figure 5.6).

5.2.1. Characteristics and Differences from Type 1 and Type 2

The distinction between Type 1 and Type 2 diabetes lies fundamentally in the etiology and pathophysiology of each condition. Type 1 diabetes is primarily characterized by autoimmune destruction of insulin-producing beta cells in the pancreas, leading to absolute insulin deficiency. This condition typically manifests in childhood or adolescence, hence the term juvenile diabetes.

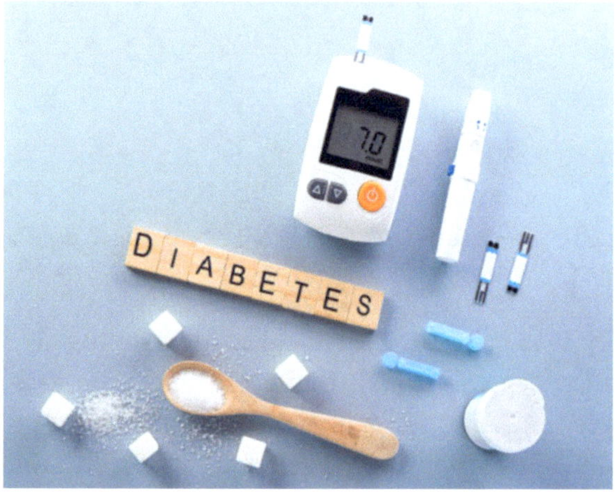

Figure 5.7. The distinction between Type 1 and Type 2 diabetes lies fundamentally in the etiology and pathophysiology of each condition.

Source: https://mandayahospitalgroup.com/wp-content/uploads/2024/05/diabetes.jpg

On the contrary, Type 2 diabetes arises from insulin resistance, where the body's cells fail to respond effectively to insulin, coupled with a relative insulin deficiency over time. Age, obesity, and sedentary lifestyle significantly influence the development of Type 2 diabetes, making it more commonly diagnosed in adults. Understanding these physiological differences is crucial for proper diagnosis, treatment, and management of diabetes, as misclassification can lead to inappropriate therapeutic strategies that may compromise patient health outcomes. The clinical manifestations and long-term complications of Type 1 and Type 2 diabetes also diverge significantly. Individuals with Type 1 diabetes often present with acute symptoms such as unexplained weight loss, polyuria, and polyphagia, requiring immediate insulin therapy to prevent life-threatening ketoacidosis. Conversely, Type 2 diabetes develops insidiously, with many patients being asymptomatic at diagnosis. The long-term complications, including neuropathy, nephropathy, and cardiovascular diseases, are prevalent in both types, yet the onset and severity can differ. For instance, those with Type 2 may experience these complications earlier due to the protracted period of undiagnosed hyperglycemia. These differences underscore the importance of tailored management approaches, considering the distinctive challenges and characteristics inherent to each type, ultimately guiding healthcare providers toward improved patient care. Furthermore, the demographic and socio-economic factors surrounding the prevalence of Type 1 and Type 2 diabetes highlight noteworthy disparities. Research indicates a significant rise in Type 2 diabetes prevalence among various ethnic groups, particularly in locations such as New Zealand, where barriers to achieving good glycemic control are compounded by socio-cultural and psychological issues affecting lifestyle and diet (Sanderson et al., 2005). In California, data illustrating disparities in diabetes prevalence among different population groups reveal that access to comprehensive medical care plays a pivotal role in management outcomes (Diamant et al., 2003). Therefore, it is critical for healthcare systems to address these inequities through targeted educational programs and culturally sensitive interventions, ensuring that all individuals, regardless of background, receive optimal support in managing their diabetes. This holistic approach will not only enhance clinical outcomes but also contribute to reducing the overall burden of diabetes within diverse communities (Figure 5.7).

5.2.2. Diagnosis Challenges

The complexities surrounding the diagnosis of diabetes, particularly non-traditional types such as LADA (Latent Autoimmune Diabetes in Adults) and MODY (Maturity-Onset Diabetes of the Young), present significant challenges for healthcare providers. Because the symptoms of these forms of diabetes are like those of type 2 diabetes, it is often very hard to tell them apart. If a diagnosis is wrong or delayed, the treatment given may make the patient's condition worse. In addition, the fact that symptoms vary from person to person makes it difficult to diagnose them. It is very important for healthcare practitioners to notice these small details to provide timely and correct care to patients. Addressing these challenges necessitates an approach grounded in continuous education and enhanced awareness of the diverse manifestations of diabetes among medical professionals, thereby improving diagnostic accuracy and outcomes for patients with atypical forms of the disease (Pope et al., 2008).

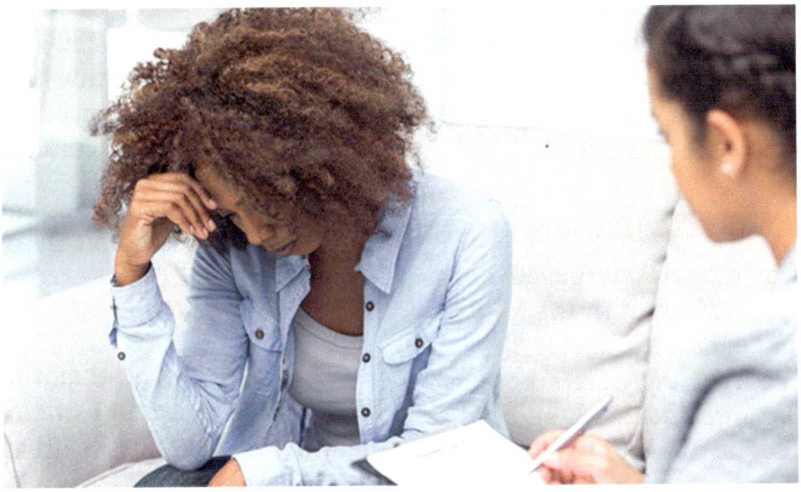

Figure 5.8. Patients facing challenges in the diagnosis of their diabetes often report a variety of coping difficulties in the aftermath of their medical encounters.

Source: https://www.niddk.nih.gov/-/media/Images/Blog/Stress_Article_2_600x350.jpg

It is also difficult to identify some types of diabetes because there are no standard guidelines for diagnosis. While type 1 and type 2 diabetes are well-known and have standard ways to diagnose them, LADA and MODY are usually not diagnosed as carefully. Since the goals are not clear, both patients and healthcare providers may not know what to do, resulting in incomplete treatment. Moreover, practices that focus on performance payments for improving healthcare quality, such as those described in recent studies, may inadvertently prioritize immediate outcomes over nuanced understanding of less common diabetes types (Pope et al., 2008). As a result, medical experts should support and design new ways to diagnose these conditions so that every patient gets the right care for their situation. Patients who have trouble getting a diagnosis for their diabetes say they have several difficulties coping after their medical appointments. Researchers found that many adults, after leaving the hospital, had difficulties understanding their condition and managing it. Having diabetes misunderstood or misdiagnosed often leads to more stress and doubt in a person's life. Many patients mention that they want to talk more with healthcare providers and learn more about their type of diabetes, which could help them overcome these difficulties. Improving how diagnoses are made helps healthcare systems give patients a better experience and better results, encouraging them to take care of their health ahead of problems. Better communication between patients and providers encourages people with non-traditional diabetes to better manage their condition (Figure 5.8).

5.2.3. Treatment Strategies

The management of diabetes is based on a combination of approaches that fit the kind of diabetes and the patient's own needs. Type 1 diabetes is different from the others because it needs regular insulin injections since the body cannot produce it. It may be necessary to have daily injections or use an insulin pump to control blood sugar levels. In most cases, type 2 diabetes is handled by changing your diet and exercising more. At times, oral drugs are used to boost the body's response to insulin or to increase the amount of insulin produced. In the end, a treatment plan created by healthcare professionals helps control blood sugar and prevents many diabetes complications. When a woman has gestational diabetes, a more complicated approach to treatment is needed because the condition usually improves after giving birth. Usually, the management of this condition requires checking blood sugar levels regularly and modifying the diet to keep glucose levels down while ensuring the baby's health. If changes in lifestyle do not help enough, insulin therapy is often given to secure the health of the mother and the fetus.

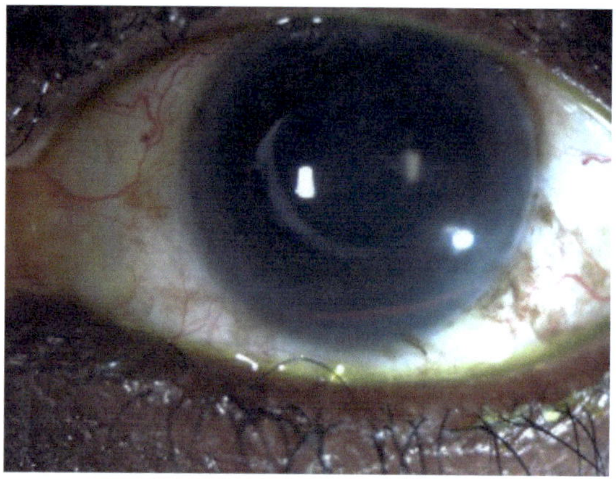

Figure 5.9. Neovascular glaucoma (NVG), resulting from proliferative diabetic retinopathy, requires a combination of therapeutic options due to its challenging nature.

Source: https://eyewiki.org/w/images/thumb/b/be/Ectropion_Uveae_and_Hyphema_in_NVG.jpg/320px-Ectropion_Uveae_and_Hyphema_in_NVG.jpg

Automated information systems are now being used more often, which may help healthcare providers identify and handle gestational diabetes. They help doctors manage patients better and educate them so they can follow the recommended treatment plans for safer pregnancies and after. Besides, diabetes-related issues may call for new approaches to treatment. For instance, neovascular glaucoma (NVG), resulting from proliferative diabetic retinopathy, requires a combination of therapeutic options due to its challenging nature. The usual treatment approach for NVG is panretinal photocoagulation, anti-VEGF injections, anti-glaucoma eye drops, and surgery when it is required. It is very important to catch and treat the disease early to save vision and stop the neovascularization process that is a part of the condition. These nuanced treatment strategies highlight the importance of comprehensive management protocols tailored to the varying presentations of diabetes and its related complications, ensuring that patients receive optimal care throughout the course of their illness (Tang et al., 2023; Sonia et al., 2023) (Figure 5.9).

5.3. MODY (Maturity Onset Diabetes of the Young)

Maturity Onset Diabetes of the Young (MODY) represents a distinct category of diabetes that typically manifests during adolescence or early adulthood, distinguishing it from the more prevalent types such as Type 1 and Type 2 diabetes. This condition is mainly defined by the fact that it is caused by changes in one gene, which results in the malfunction of pancreatic β-cells. MODY covers several types, and some of them, such as HNF1A and HNF4A, are linked to mutations that can have a big effect on insulin production. Unlike Type 1 diabetes, where insulin therapy is often required from diagnosis, many individuals with MODY may have sufficient endogenous insulin production and can be effectively managed without insulin treatment, highlighting the importance of genetic diagnosis for appropriate therapeutic strategies (Kavvoura et al., 2018).

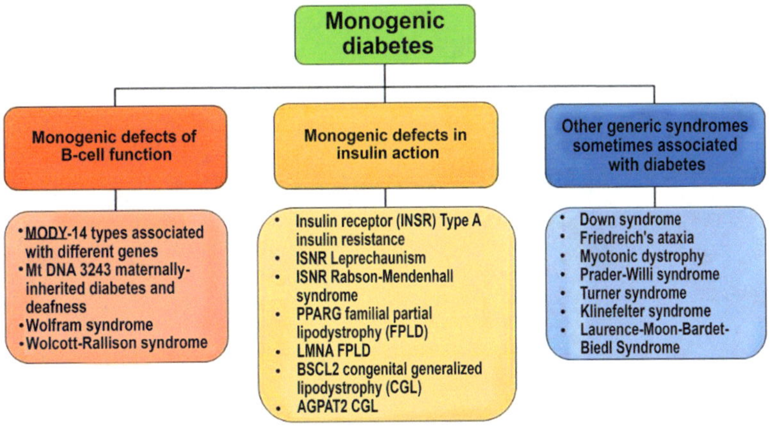

Figure 5.10. Maturity Onset Diabetes of the Young (MODY) represents a distinct category of diabetes that typically manifests during adolescence or early adulthood, distinguishing it from the more prevalent types such as Type 1 and Type 2 diabetes.

Source: Skoczek D, Dulak J, Kachamakova-Trojanowska N. Maturity Onset Diabetes of the Young—New Approaches for Disease Modelling. *International Journal of Molecular Sciences.* 2021; 22(14):7553. https://doi.org/10.3390/ijms22147553

Because many people do not know about MODY, they might be wrongly diagnosed with Type 1 or Type 2 diabetes. As a result, managing and treating MODY is made more difficult because the condition requires special care. It seems that monogenic diabetes, including MODY, is more common than previously thought, especially in children. For instance, a systematic study in the U.K. revealed that approximately 2.5% of patients under the age of 20 had monogenic diabetes, with a significant portion remaining undiagnosed (Colclough et al., 2016). This proves that healthcare professionals should recognize MODY more often, as quick genetic testing can help people with this condition live better and longer. MODY points out that diabetes is caused by genes and stresses the role of personalized medicine in treating it. Pharmacogenetics is very important for this condition; for example, certain subtypes, such as those caused by HNF1A and HNF4A mutations, react well to sulfonylurea drugs. Type 1 diabetes is different because patients with this type need insulin to survive. Besides, because MODY is genetic, screening family members can help identify similar risks and allow everyone to be monitored for their health. The integration of genetic understanding into clinical practice emphasizes the evolution of diabetes treatment paradigms and the necessity of a nuanced approach to diabetes management in light of various types, including MODY (Kavvoura et al., 2018) (Figure 5.10).

5.3.1. Genetic Basis and Inheritance Patterns

More and more, it is understood that genetics plays a key role in explaining the different types of diabetes. Lately, scientists have found that several genes are involved in the development of type 1 and type 2 diabetes. For instance, type 1 diabetes is primarily linked to autoimmune processes influenced by genetic predispositions, particularly involving the human leukocyte antigen (HLA) genes.

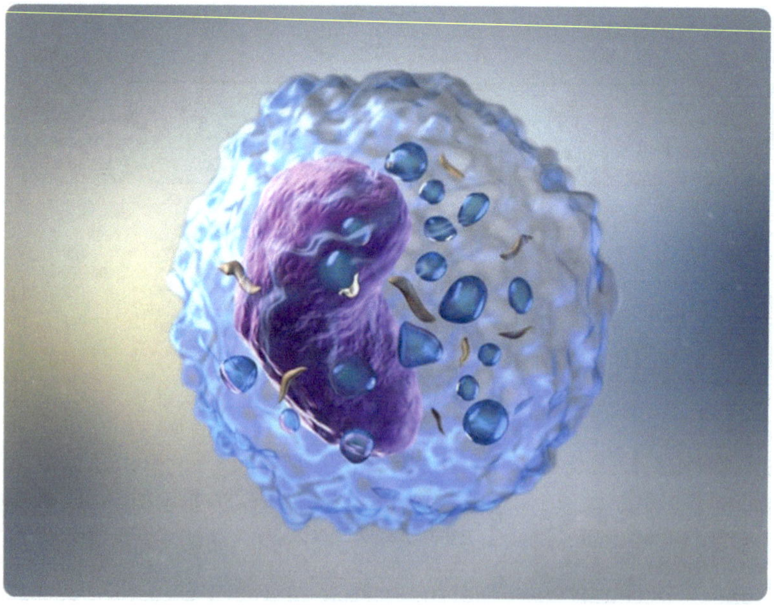

Figure 5.11. Human leukocyte antigen (HLA) genes.

Source: https://www.news-medical.net/image-handler/picture/2018/5/shutterstock_395448409.jpg

They are important for the immune system's actions and their effect on insulin-producing pancreatic beta cells. In contrast, the genetic causes of type 2 diabetes are more complicated and are usually affected by several risk alleles that change insulin sensitivity and the function of beta cells. The interplay of these genetic components underscores the necessity of recognizing genetic variability when diagnosing and treating different forms of diabetes, which remains a prominent focus in ongoing research initiatives (Clifford R Jack et al., 2018). There is complexity in how diabetes is inherited, as it can happen through Mendelian or polygenic routes. Monogenic forms of diabetes, such as maturity-onset diabetes of the young (MODY), arise from single-gene mutations, while polygenic forms result from the cumulative effects of numerous genetic variants, each contributing small effects. To illustrate, research on MODY found that a person's family background is very important, since these inherited features can cause the disease to appear in later generations. Type 2 diabetes is usually passed down in a way that depends on many factors, including the way someone lives and eats. Because of its many hereditary aspects, it becomes necessary for clinicians to assess a patient's family history in detail. As studies go on, it becomes clear that precision medicine based on a person's genes is necessary for diabetes. This idea is in line with new diabetes management strategies that consider a patient's genetic background when choosing treatment and care. For instance, the American Diabetes Association suggests using genetic testing in clinical settings to help design treatments that focus on a person's genetic risks. These progresses suggest that genetic findings can help us understand diabetes better and improve the outcomes for patients. As investigations into the genetic factors influencing diabetes continue to advance, they remain pivotal in unraveling the complexities associated with this diverse group of metabolic disorders (Clifford R Jack et al., 2018) (Figure 5.11).

5.3.2. Symptoms and Age of Onset

The way the symptoms of diabetes appear and the age at which they begin are important for learning about the disease and how to treat it. Usually, type 1 diabetes is found in children or teenagers and appears all of a sudden with symptoms such as increased thirst, more frequent urination, and weight loss without explanation. These acute symptoms can progress rapidly, necessitating immediate medical intervention to prevent severe complications, including diabetic ketoacidosis (DKA). On the other hand, Type 2 diabetes usually affects people as they get older and brings about symptoms such as tiredness, blurry vision, and slow healing of wounds. The gradual start of these conditions can cause them to be diagnosed late, which may lead to major health problems such as heart disease and nerve damage, so it is important to detect and manage them early in groups of people with specific ages and symptoms. It is also clear from research that metabolic factors may change when diabetes begins and the symptoms it causes. People who have metabolic syndrome and show signs of obesity and hypertension may develop Type 2 diabetes earlier. It is notable that research reveals that people with abnormal triglyceride levels often have increased depressive symptoms after the age of 12, possibly showing a link between unhealthy metabolism and diabetes. This association underlines the critical need to monitor not only glucose levels but also the broader metabolic landscape, particularly in at-risk populations where mental health may compound the risks related to diabetes progression (Michael et al., 2017). In addition, knowing about these connections can guide efforts to treat both metabolic and psychological health problems. Besides biological reasons, the time when diabetes develops is largely affected by the environment and social conditions. Being diagnosed with Type 1 diabetes often leads to special psychosocial issues for children and adolescents. Prompt diagnosis is necessary since it affects how they live and how they deal with others who are not affected by the disease. Because there are many health issues common in older people, the early signs of Type 2 diabetes can be easily missed. Furthermore, individuals with lower socioeconomic status may have limited access to preventive healthcare and education about the disease, further exacerbating the onset and management challenges encountered by diverse populations (Marchetti, 2019). Thus, dealing with these social and environmental issues can help public health manage diabetes and apply early interventions for people of all ages (Figure 5.12).

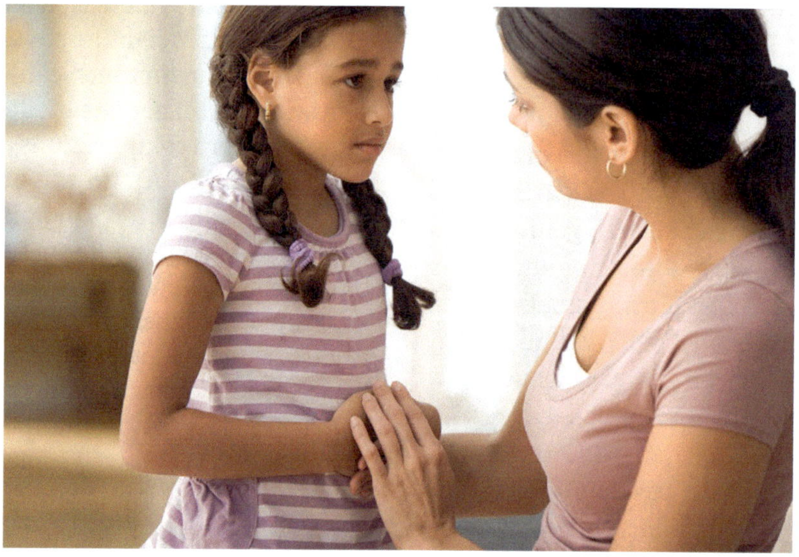

Figure 5.12. Type 1 diabetes, typically diagnosed in childhood or adolescence, often manifests suddenly with symptoms such as excessive thirst, frequent urination, and unexplained weight loss.

Source: https://www.breakthrought1d.org/wp-content/uploads/2023/05/type-1-diabetes-symptoms.jpg

5.3.3. Management and Treatment Options

Managing and treating different forms of diabetes calls for an approach that takes into account each patient's needs, the reasons behind the disease, and any other health conditions. If diabetes is a factor in sudden hearing loss, the treatment must be adjusted to deal with these extra issues. For instance, when a diabetic patient suddenly loses hearing, it is necessary to choose medications that do not worsen their condition. Selecting the wrong treatments could make a person's health worse, so it is important to use treatments that fit each person's needs. Effective glycemic control not only aids in diabetes management but also plays a crucial role in preventing or mitigating associated complications, which highlights the interconnectedness of diabetes management and overall health outcomes (Badiu et al., 2019). Managing diabetes is greatly affected by cultural factors, mainly in populations with many cultures. People of Indian origin often let their social and cultural background impact the way they understand diabetes and follow their treatment plans. Studies point out that cultural backgrounds can affect the way people choose their foods, work out, and feel about taking medicine. For this reason, healthcare providers should use culturally sensitive methods when talking about treatment options with patients to make sure the plans are in line with their beliefs. By doing so, healthcare professionals can empower patients to take an active role in their healthcare decisions, reducing resistance to lifestyle changes and improving adherence to treatment protocols (Tresslor, 2008). Also, using technology to handle diabetes has brought about new ways to monitor and treat the disease. Continuous glucose monitoring (CGM) systems and insulin pumps provide patients with real-time data, empowering them to make informed decisions about their health. Thanks to these new tools, it is now easier to manage blood sugar and respond quickly to any changes in a patient's needs. Since diabetes can be very different for each person and responds differently to treatment, such tools can help doctors provide better care and help patients keep their blood sugar under control. Along with other approaches, technology helps complete the best strategies for managing diabetes (Figure 5.13).

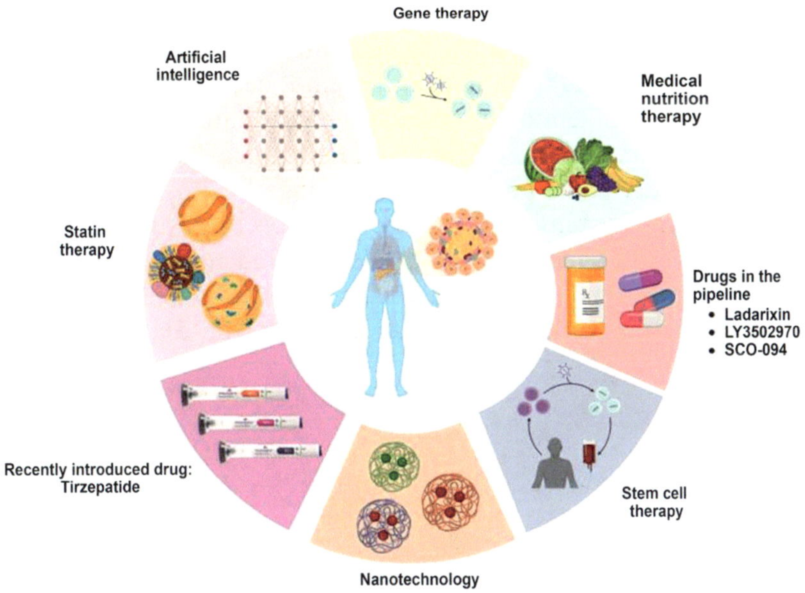

Figure 5.13. Management and treatment options for various types of diabetes require a nuanced approach that considers individual patient needs, underlying causes, and comorbidities.

Source: https://media.springernature.com/m685/springer-static/image/art%3A10.1038%2Fs41366-023-01369-3/MediaObjects/41366_2023_1369_Fig1_HTML.png

5.4. Other Rare Forms of Diabetes

Researchers and doctors find it difficult to diagnose and treat rare types of diabetes. Conditions such as Maturity Onset Diabetes of the Young (MODY) and Wolfram syndrome are among those classified as atypical types of diabetes. Many times, MODY is mistaken for either Type 1 or Type 2 diabetes because of how much it looks like them. Most of the time, this genetic disorder is noticed during adolescence or early adulthood because it is caused by changes in genes responsible for insulin production. Unlike the other two types of diabetes, MODY calls for a special way of managing it by doing genetic tests and giving personalized care. Such differentiation is vital in improving patient outcomes and understanding the broader implications of diabetes pathology as highlighted in recent studies, including those examining autoimmune DM types and pancreatic disease associations (Gilor et al., 2016). Another notable rare form of diabetes is associated with genetic syndromes such as Williams-Beuren syndrome (WS). People with this condition experience developmental delays, heart defects, and problems with glucose metabolism. According to recent studies, people with WS are likely to have insulin resistance and problems with their beta cells, which is similar to what happens in type 2 diabetes. Since many people in this group have impaired glucose metabolism, it is necessary to screen them often and act early to stop complications. This research points out that diabetes is more complicated than previously thought and calls for individualized ways of managing it. By acknowledging the intricate relationship between genetic factors and metabolic dysfunction, researchers are better equipped to address the multifaceted nature of diabetes, emphasizing early diagnosis and targeted therapies (Bedeschi et al., 2017). There is also a growing recognition of diabetes that occurs due to other endocrinopathies or conditions such as Cystic Fibrosis (CF) and its related diabetes, often referred to as Cystic Fibrosis-related diabetes (CFRD). When the pancreas is damaged, it cannot secrete enough insulin and this is the cause of this type of diabetes. Unlike most forms of diabetes, CFRD is found mainly in people with CF who are teenagers or adults, making their treatment much more difficult. Since the disease is different, the treatment must focus on keeping the lungs healthy and controlling blood sugar. In addition, learning about the systemic effects of cystic fibrosis on glucose metabolism can help in creating new treatments that handle the main disease and its metabolic problems. Increased awareness and research on these rare forms of diabetes can improve detection and health outcomes for affected individuals, thus enhancing the overall discourse on diabetes management (Gilor et al., 2016) (Figure 5.14).

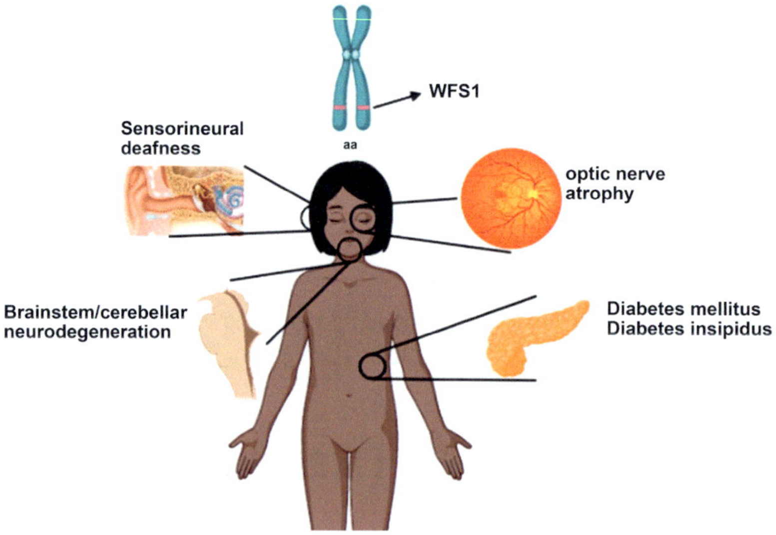

Figure 5.14. Wolfram syndrome.

Source: https://endocrinology.wustl.edu/files/2023/03/Untitled-design-13.png

5.4.1. Description of Conditions like Wolfram Syndrome

Wolfram Syndrome, which is also called DIDMOAD syndrome, is a rare disease that links diabetes and problems with the nervous system. The main feature of this condition is diabetes mellitus that often appears in childhood, together with other problems like vision loss and hearing impairment. The disease happens because of changes in the WFS1 gene, which makes the protein wolframin needed for the endoplasmic reticulum. At the onset, Wolfram Syndrome reveals issues in many systems, including metabolic and neurological systems, which show how diabetes management is related to the worsening of neurological symptoms. In particular, patients find it hard to keep their blood sugar levels under control, which makes it important to discuss this syndrome when talking about different types of diabetes. The causes of Wolfram Syndrome give us important knowledge about diabetes-related conditions. Research suggests that the pathology of Wolfram Syndrome includes disturbances in the endoplasmic reticulum (ER) and mitochondrial dysfunction, which contribute to neuronal degeneration and systemic symptoms. These disturbances trigger the unfolded protein response (UPR), leading to increased stress and neuronal loss, implications that resonate with other diabetes-related conditions as well, particularly those with a neurodegenerative component. Also, neuroimaging research shows that brain changes happen early on, which may connect changes in myelination to the clinical symptoms of the disease. Knowing about these mechanisms is important for diabetes management in many hereditary and degenerative conditions, because it points out the relationship between metabolic and neurological health. Besides, Wolfram Syndrome demonstrates the way genetics can contribute to diabetes and neurological problems. The syndrome proves that diabetes is connected to other health complications and may be a sign of more serious underlying problems. The discovery that the WFS1 gene plays a major role in the disease means that looking at genetic factors is very important for finding treatments. The latest research on WFS1 in oligodendrocytes during brain development points to possible ways to treat myelination problems found in other similar conditions. As researchers continue to investigate the intricacies of Wolfram Syndrome, they may uncover novel insights applicable not only to this specific case but also to other types of diabetes, as both scientific and clinical communities strive to delineate the multifactorial nature of these diseases (Dougherty et al., 2019) (Figure 5.15).

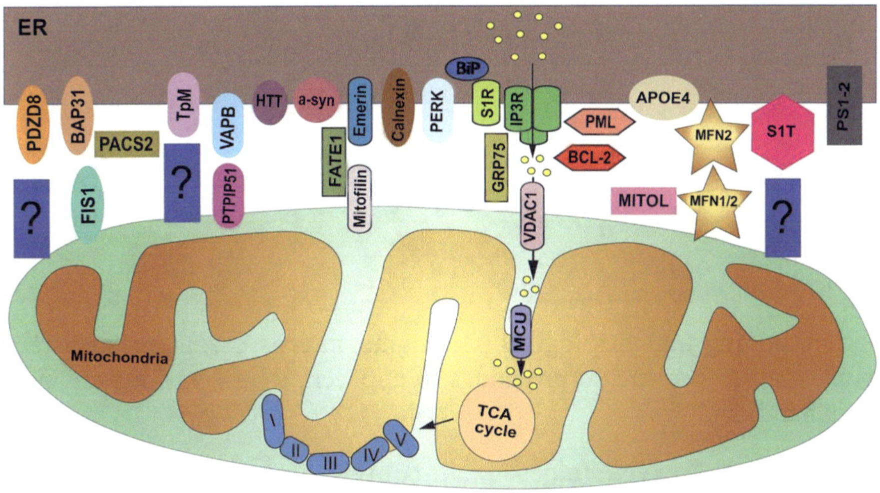

Figure 5.15. The pathology of Wolfram Syndrome includes disturbances in the endoplasmic reticulum (ER) and mitochondrial dysfunction, which contribute to neuronal degeneration and systemic symptoms.

Source: https://media.springernature.com/full/springer-static/image/art%3A10.1038%2Fs41419-018-0406-3/MediaObjects/41419_2018_406_Fig1_HTML.jpg

5.4.2. Impact on Patients and Families

Diabetes has many aspects that go beyond the body and greatly influence both the patients and their families. In the case of Latent Autoimmune Diabetes in the Young (LADA), the discovery of such a complex form of the disease can be particularly overwhelming for families. A child's development can be impacted greatly by the diagnosis, so both the affected child and their caregivers need to adapt quickly. Families have to deal with the emotions of living with diabetes, worrying about the future and getting used to managing the condition every day. The case report on a 10-year-old girl with LADA illustrates this struggle, elucidating how diabetes impacts family dynamics and highlighting the necessity for comprehensive support structures to mitigate emotional distress and strengthen familial resilience (Galea et al., 2015). It is very important for families to put effective support systems in place while managing diabetes. Organizations like the International Diabetes Federation (IDF) provide essential resources aimed at enhancing patient care and supporting families. The framework they offer includes insulin, equipment for blood glucose monitoring, and helpful educational services for families dealing with diabetes. They help people with diabetes get immediate medical care and also ensure that diabetes care lasts over time, which benefits the entire family. When families have access to appropriate resources, they are better positioned to navigate the complexities of the condition, leading to improved health outcomes for the patient and decreased emotional burden for caregivers (Sigfrid et al., 2015).

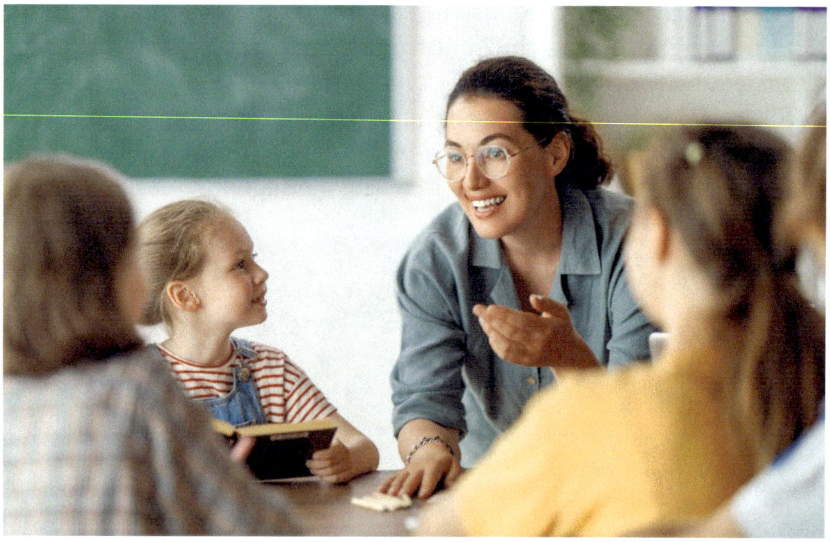

Figure 5.16. Understanding the sociological paradigms, microsystems, mesosystems, exosystems, and macrosystems, enables healthcare providers to appreciate how various environmental factors influence family dynamics.

Source: https://www.simplypsychology.org/wp-content/uploads/bronfenbrenner-classroom-applications.jpeg

The effects of diabetes on families' mental and emotional well-being are very significant. Looking after chronic illnesses, such as diabetes, is a constant task and this can cause stress, anxiety, and make people feel isolated, affecting both patients and their families. Often, caregivers have to take on new duties in healthcare, leading to more stress and possible exhaustion. Healthcare providers can understand how environmental factors play a role in family life by knowing about microsystems, mesosystems, exosystems, and macrosystems. By adopting a holistic approach that considers these systems, healthcare professionals can better support both patients and families, leading to more effective management of diabetes and improved overall well-being for those affected (Galea et al., 2015) (Figure 5.16).

5.4.3. Research and Future Directions

The landscape of diabetes research is rapidly evolving, particularly in the context of various nontraditional diabetes forms, such as maturity-onset diabetes of the young (MODY) and latent autoimmune diabetes in adults (LADA). With more evidence backing up these subtypes, researchers are now paying more attention to what makes them work. Genomic and proteomic studies have become very important for both identifying diabetes types and predicting the course and response to treatment.

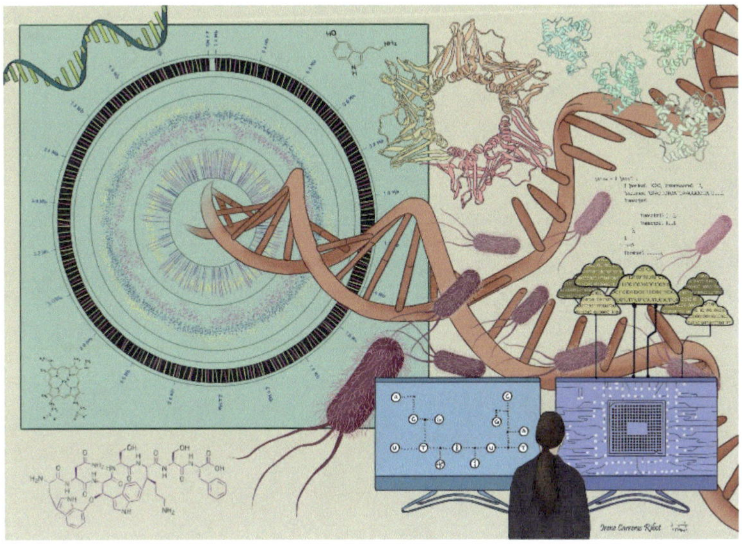

Figure 5.17. Numerous biomarkers have been identified, yet the complexity of CMD mechanisms calls for comprehensive strategies that go beyond traditional approaches.

Source: Krassowski M, Das V, Sahu SK and Misra BB (2020) State of the Field in Multi-Omics Research: From Computational Needs to Data Mining and Sharing. Front. Genet. 11:610798. doi: 10.3389/fgene.2020.610798

The emergence of exploratory-descriptive designs in transition research, such as those documented in recent literature, highlights a critical need for continuous inquiry into the nuances of diabetes management across diverse populations (Arksey et al., 2018). In the future, researchers should use different theories to better explain the factors that affect diabetes, which will help improve understanding and lead to better treatments. As research progresses, the intersection of diabetes and cardiometabolic diseases (CMD) emerges as a crucial area for exploration. Although many biomarkers have been found, the complexity of CMD means that a complete strategy is needed that goes beyond what is usually done. Reports indicate that integrating multi-omics data, comprising genomics, metabolomics, and other domains, has immense potential to yield insights into disease pathways and identify robust biomarkers (Argano et al., 2019). In the future, scientists should study these biomarkers to determine how they can be used in personalized treatment plans for diabetes patients. Using this approach could lead to improved treatment results and fewer cases of diabetes for people from different groups. Gender is also beginning to play a noticeable role in how diabetes develops, and this area needs more research. Learning how gender differences influence diabetes can improve the way doctors treat the disease. Recent calls for the integration of gender medicine into diabetes research highlight the need for a more nuanced approach that considers both biological and cultural factors (Argano et al., 2019). Further studies ought to examine how gender differences in diabetes can affect both the types of diabetes and the success of various treatment methods. Adding a gender perspective to diabetes research helps design strategies that are more understanding of each person's health needs, which may improve health and well-being for all patients (Figure 5.17).

A CLOSER LOOK

CHRONIC HYPERGLYCEMIA

Chronic hyperglycemia means that someone's blood glucose levels stay high for a long time, which is common in people with uncontrolled diabetes. Long-term effects of this condition may harm the eyes, kidneys, nerves, and blood vessels. Some of the symptoms are thirst, more frequent urination, tiredness, and blurred vision. If not treated, high blood sugar over a long period can cause diabetic retinopathy, nephropathy, neuropathy, and cardiovascular disease. Taking care of your health by changing your lifestyle, using the right medicine, and getting checked regularly is necessary to prevent these problems.

Summary

It is important to realize that the other types of diabetes show a lot of variety and complexity. Although most people focus on Type 1 and Type 2 diabetes, gestational diabetes and other uncommon forms should not be overlooked because of their major health effects. Because diabetes is affected by many factors, it is important to understand every type of diabetes in detail. Specifically, lifestyle modifications such as diet and exercise have been shown to mitigate the risk of developing Type 2 diabetes, suggesting that preventive measures can be vital in targeting at-risk populations and ultimately improving public health outcomes (Asadi et al., 2016). As a result, it is necessary to concentrate on education and awareness to deal with and control different types of diabetes. Besides those who have diabetes, families, healthcare systems, and the entire community can be affected by this disease. For instance, neonates born to mothers with pregestational diabetes face a heightened risk of severe birth injuries, an outcome that not only affects individual families but also adds strain to healthcare resources (Gissler et al., 2021). This approach points out that early care and management are important in maternal health, showing why specific healthcare policies are needed. Better care during pregnancy for women with diabetes can greatly reduce the risk for their babies and help improve the health of people over the years. Because of this, it is still very important to solve the educational and healthcare issues related to diabetes. To summarize, considering other types of diabetes makes it obvious that different approaches are needed for different groups. With better knowledge of diabetes, healthcare providers will be able to give interventions that meet the specific challenges of each type of diabetes. More research is being done to understand what affects diabetes, stressing the need for personalized care in both preventing and handling the disease. If researchers, healthcare practitioners, and patients join forces, we can design strategies that deal with the many issues of diabetes and enhance the lives of those who have it.

References

1. Gilor, C., Niessen, S. J., Furrow, E., & DiBartola, S. P. (2016). What's in a Name? Classification of Diabetes Mellitus in Veterinary Medicine and Why It Matters. *Journal of veterinary internal medicine, 30*(4), 927–940. https://doi.org/10.1111/jvim.14357 (accessed on 11th June 2025).
2. Akbarnia, B., Ames, C., Bess, S., Burton, D., et al. (2016). The health impact of symptomatic adult spinal deformity: Comparison of deformity types to United States population norms and chronic diseases. https://core.ac.uk/download/323069856.pdf (accessed on 11th June 2025).
3. Alsweiler, J., Brown, J., Crowther, C. A., Downie, M., et al. (2018). Treatments for women with gestational diabetes mellitus: An overview of Cochrane systematic reviews. https://core.ac.uk/download/187724799.pdf (accessed on 11th June 2025).
4. Althavale, P., Fisher, L., Gonzalez-Mendez, E., Handley, M., et al. (2015). Applying the COM-B model to creation of an IT-enabled health coaching and resource linkage program for low-income Latina moms with recent gestational diabetes: The STAR MAMA program. https://core.ac.uk/download/323074056.pdf (accessed on 11th June 2025).
5. AMBROSIADOU, B. V.; Vadera, S.; SHANKARAMAN, Venky; Goulis, D.; and Gogou, G.. Decision Support Methods in Diabetic Patient Management by Insulin Administration Neural Network vs. Induction Methods for Knowledge Classification. (2000). *Proceedings of the ICSC Symposium on Neural Computation 2000: May 23-26, Berlin*. 852-858. **Available at:** https://ink.library.smu.edu.sg/sis_research/1147 (accessed on 11th June 2025).
6. Anto, N., Bastiaens, H., Chow, E., Griffiths, F., et al. (2007). Understanding the diversity and dynamics of living with diabetes: A feasibility study focusing on the case. https://core.ac.uk/download/1387204.pdf (accessed on 11th June 2025).
7. Argano, V., Balistreri, C. R., Giarratana, R. M., Lio, D., et al. (2019). On the road to accurate biomarkers for cardiometabolic diseases by integrating precision and gender medicine approaches. https://core.ac.uk/download/268910274.pdf (accessed on 11th June 2025).
8. Arksey, H., Arnett, J., Aseltine, R., Bozick, R., Côté, J., et al. (2018). A scoping review of transitions, stress, and adaptation among emerging adults. https://core.ac.uk/download/228028474.pdf (accessed on 11th June 2025).
9. Asadi, F., Fallahzadeh, H., & Rahmanian, M. (2016). Determining the factors related to diabetes type II with mixed logistic regression. https://core.ac.uk/download/143844355.pdf (accessed on 11th June 2025).
10. Aslam, F., & Kulasena, H. (2017). To identify and examine the different causes of liver disease in Sri Lanka. https://core.ac.uk/download/293755106.pdf (accessed on 11th June 2025).
11. Wu, P., Kwok, C. S., Haththotuwa, R., Kotronias, R. A., Babu, A., Fryer, A. A., Myint, P. K., Chew-Graham, C. A., & Mamas, M. A. (2016). Pre-eclampsia is associated with a twofold increase in diabetes: a systematic review and meta-analysis. *Diabetologia, 59*(12), 2518–2526. https://doi.org/10.1007/s00125-016-4098-x(accessed on 11th June 2025).
12. Badiu, D. C., Burcea-Dragomiroiu, G. T. A., Gherghiceanu, F., Hainarosie, R., et al. (2019). Management options in the sudden hearing loss of a diabetic patient. https://core.ac.uk/download/216811037.pdf (accessed on 11th June 2025).
13. Bedeschi, M. F., Grancini, V., Lalatta, F., Lunati, M., et al. (2017). Impaired glucose metabolism

in subjects with the Williams-Beuren syndrome: A five-year follow-up cohort study. https://core.ac.uk/download/141696869.pdf (accessed on 11th June 2025).

14. Bouchard, L., Breton, E., Cardenas, A., Fortin, M., et al. (2020). Mediation analysis supports a causal relationship between maternal hyperglycemia and placental DNA methylation variations at the leptin gene locus and cord blood leptin levels. https://core.ac.uk/download/323081505.pdf (accessed on 11th June 2025).
15. Bundy, C. E., Elliott, R. A., Gibson, M., New, J. P., et al. (2010). Intentional and unintentional non-adherence in community dwelling people with type 2 diabetes: The effect of varying numbers of medicines. https://core.ac.uk/download/30639328.pdf (accessed on 11th June 2025).
16. Colclough, K., Cox, J., Ellard, S., Fraser, F. C., et al. (2016). Systematic population screening, using biomarkers and genetic testing, identifies 2.5% of the U.K. pediatric diabetes population with monogenic diabetes. https://core.ac.uk/download/42553606.pdf (accessed on 11th June 2025).
17. DeGaetano, A., Ferrara, A., Gaetano De, A., Hayes, A., Topp, B., Athukorala, C., Knight-Agarwal, C. R., et al. (2019). Multi-scale simulation modeling for prevention and public health management of diabetes in pregnancy and sequelae. http://arxiv.org/abs/1905.02552 (accessed on 11th June 2025).
18. Denaxas, S., Hemingway, H., & Papez, V. (2017). Evaluating openEHR for storing computable representations of electronic health record phenotyping algorithms. https://core.ac.uk/download/111007267.pdf (accessed on 11th June 2025).
19. Diamant, Allison & Babey, Susan & Brown, E & Chawla, Neetu. (2003). Diabetes in California: Nearly 1.5 million diagnosed and 2 million more at risk. Policy brief (UCLA Center for Health Policy Research). 1-8. (accessed on 11th June 2025).
20. Dougherty, J., Hershey, T., Marshall, B., Neyman, C., et al. (2019). Developmental hypomyelination in Wolfram syndrome: New insights from neuroimaging and gene expression analyses. https://core.ac.uk/download/322802313.pdf (accessed on 11th June 2025).
21. Dunn, A. B., Hanson, L., Leslie, S., Vandevelde, A., et al. (2019). Through the microbial looking glass: Premature labor, preeclampsia, and gestational diabetes: A scoping review. https://core.ac.uk/download/228028393.pdf (accessed on 11th June 2025).
22. Ford, J., Lenaghan, E., Murdoch, J., Salter, C., et al. (2020). The "unknown territory" of goal-setting: Negotiating a novel interactional activity within primary care doctor-patient consultations for patients with multiple chronic conditions. https://core.ac.uk/download/323057198.pdf (accessed on 11th June 2025).
23. Galea, M. (2015). Sociological framework applied to a case report of diabetes in adolescence. https://core.ac.uk/download/46603524.pdf (accessed on 11th June 2025).
24. Gissler, M., Huttunen, T. T., Kekki, M., Koukkula, O., et al. (2021). Severe birth injuries in neonates and associated risk factors for injury in mothers with different types of diabetes in Finland. https://core.ac.uk/download/534019709.pdf (accessed on 11th June 2025).
25. Jack, C. R., Bennett, D. A., Blennow, K., Carrillo, M. C., Dunn, B., Budd Haeberlein, S., Holtzman, D. M., et al. (2018). NIA-AA research framework: Toward a biological definition of Alzheimer's disease. *Alzheimer's & Dementia, 14*, 535–562. https://doi.org/10.1016/j.jalz.2018.02.018 (accessed on 11th June 2025).

26. Kavvoura, F. K., & Owen, K. (2018). Monogenic diabetes. https://core.ac.uk/download/346568875.pdf (accessed on 11th June 2025).
27. Kealey, S. (2011). Continual evolution: The experience over three semesters of a librarian embedded in an online evidence-based medicine course for physician assistant students. https://core.ac.uk/download/84118460.pdf (accessed on 11th June 2025).
28. Marchetti, A. L. (2019). Building prediction models for dementia: The need to account for interval censoring and the competing risk of death. https://scholarworks.indianapolis.iu.edu/items/9ce8f985-808b-48ac-9307-15f0392a90a4(accessed on 11th June 2025).
29. Michael, J. R. (2017). The relations of metabolic syndrome to anxiety and depression symptoms in children and adults. https://core.ac.uk/download/84397711.pdf (accessed on 11th June 2025).
30. Miller, J. F., Piacentine, L., & Weiss, M. (2008). Coping difficulties after hospitalization. https://core.ac.uk/download/213057283.pdf (accessed on 11th June 2025).
31. Pope, G., Kautter, J., Aggarwal, J., Trisolini, M., & Leung, M. (2008). The Medicare Physician Group Practice Demonstration: Lessons learned on improving quality and efficiency in health care. https://core.ac.uk/download/71353237.pdf (accessed on 11th June 2025).
32. Sanderson, L. (2005). Attitudes to food and lifestyle choices in women with well-controlled and poorly-controlled type 2 diabetes mellitus from different ethnic groups: A pilot study. https://core.ac.uk/download/148643450.pdf (accessed on 11th June 2025).
33. Shankarappa, R. S., & Kumar, N. M. (2024). Latent autoimmune diabetes of adults presenting as recurrent diabetic ketoacidosis. *International Journal of Medical Science and Clinical Research Studies.* https://www.semanticscholar.org/paper/887bc6a604566c876b5d1e7f816d17146c02a7ad (accessed on 11th June 2025).
34. Shrivastav, R., Koshti, S. V., Singh, A., & Tasgaonkar, R. (2024). Current treatment options for diabetes: A review. *International Journal of Innovative Science and Research Technology (IJISRT).* https://www.semanticscholar.org/paper/0e86c1737e621094e19fc01ce7e69b8c8e84233c (accessed on 11th June 2025).
35. Sigfrid, L., McKee, M., Eeles, M., Atkinson, S., & Atkinson, Z. (2015). From surviving to thriving: Evaluation of the International Diabetes Federation Life for a Child Program. https://core.ac.uk/download/80510988.pdf (accessed on 11th June 2025).
36. Sonia, J., Jayachandran, P., Md, A. Q., Mohan, S., Sivaraman, A. K., & Tee, K. (2023). Machine-learning-based diabetes mellitus risk prediction using multi-layer neural network no-prop algorithm. *Diagnostics, 13.* https://www.semanticscholar.org/paper/11ed0eabcff0d521ce43bfde1548f8526e3badbe (accessed on 11th June 2025).
37. Tang, Y., Shi, Y., & Fan, Z. (2023). The mechanism and therapeutic strategies for neovascular glaucoma secondary to diabetic retinopathy. *Frontiers in Endocrinology, 14.* https://www.semanticscholar.org/paper/a5df124d538cc74ed0b8a5dc29ae5845d7ecbf40 (accessed on 11th June 2025).
38. Tollen, L. (2008). Physician organization in relation to quality and efficiency of care: A synthesis of recent literature. https://core.ac.uk/download/71353828.pdf (accessed on 11th June 2025).
39. Tresslor, S. K. (2008). "It's a whole package": Type 2 diabetes and what it means for the body, life and self of people of Indian origin in New Zealand. https://core.ac.uk/download/157568844.pdf (accessed on 11th June 2025).

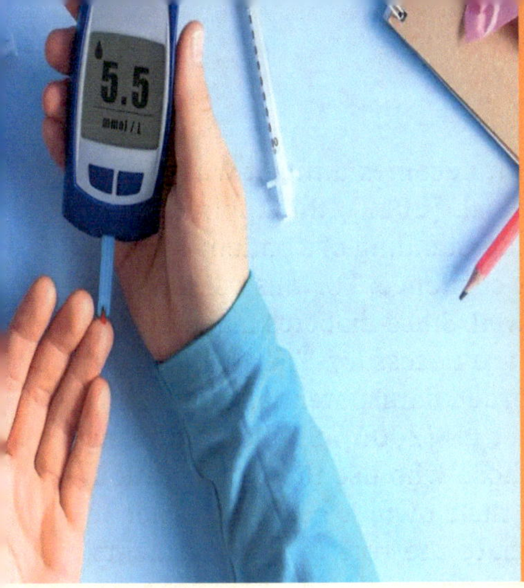

Chapter 6

DIABETES CONTROL AND ITS MEASUREMENT

Contents

Introduction

It is important to discuss diabetes control and its measurement to understand how common and complicated this chronic condition is. All over the world, diabetes mellitus impacts many people and results in various health issues that need strict control. To look after patients properly, doctors rely on different assessment methods to choose the best treatment and modify their approach for each patient. Along with altering the patient's lifestyle and giving medications, it is very important to monitor their condition closely. Various methods of checking blood sugar enable doctors to pay close attention to diabetics and protect them from the problems that can arise from poor diabetes management. Managing diabetes calls for an approach that includes medical examinations and what patients say about their health. A number of monitoring tools have been suggested, and each one is different in its strengths and weaknesses. Using both basic and advanced glucose-monitoring tools, doctors can see how a patient's blood sugar is changing with time. It becomes difficult when these techniques are not integrated properly. As outlined in Willems et al. (2012), the application of complementary monitoring procedures can significantly enhance understanding of a patient's health, although balancing accuracy and practicality remains a persistent challenge. For this reason, it is important to choose the best mix of tools to help manage diabetes well. Since diabetes management keeps evolving, it is clearer than ever that regular measurements are necessary. The variations in measurement protocols can lead to significant discrepancies in recorded data, potentially impacting treatment decisions and health outcomes, as highlighted in Bilo et al. (2006). Studies are being carried out to make these methods more reliable and helpful for those who use them. In addition, when patients understand their condition and keep track of it on their own, it becomes easier to control diabetes. If patients learn about their disease and appreciate the role of measurements, they can work together with their healthcare providers. The information in this chapter prepares readers to explore the various ways diabetes is controlled and how it is measured (Figure 6.1).

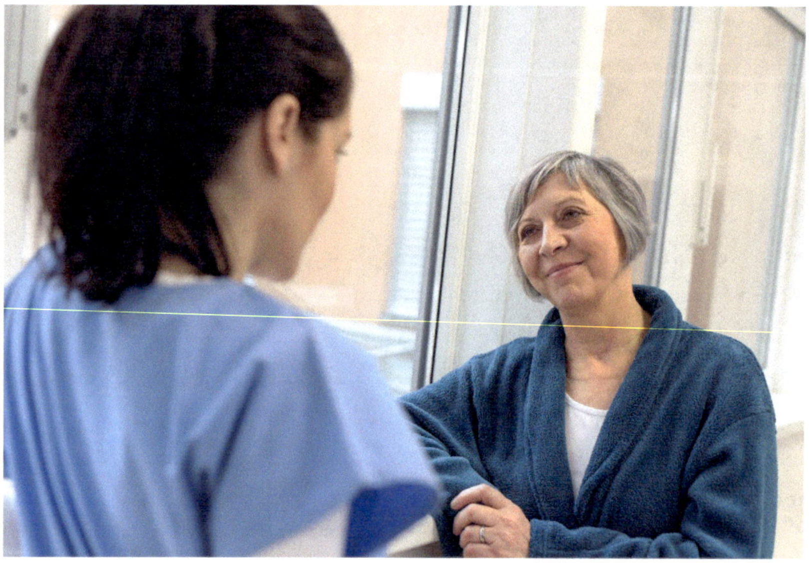

Figure 6.1. Understanding diabetes management involves a multifaceted approach that incorporates both clinical assessments and patient-reported outcomes.

Source: https://aihcp.net/main/wp-content/uploads/2024/04/cbi-0216-022_001_100115-scaled.jpg

6.1. Importance of Blood Glucose Monitoring

Managing diabetes well requires checking blood glucose levels often, as it shows how well the blood sugar is being controlled. The main goal of blood glucose monitoring is to help people keep track of their glucose levels and make prompt changes to their diet, drugs, and exercise. Quick feedback from the loop helps to stop acute complications such as low or high blood sugar, as these issues can seriously harm a person if they are not treated fast. In addition, knowing about one's glucose levels encourages patients to care for themselves and stick to their treatment plans. As noted, adequate monitoring is indispensable in mitigating the risks of long-term complications associated with diabetes, such as kidney failure and cardiovascular disease, highlighting the integral role monitoring plays in overall health maintenance (Willems et al., 2012). Besides supporting immediate health, monitoring blood glucose is now a major part of managing diabetes in the future. Fasting glucose tests are an old method to diagnose diabetes, but they only show a single picture of blood sugar and not any changes over time. Therefore, the transition towards utilizing glycated proteins, such as Hemoglobin A1c (HbA1c) and glycated albumin (GA), has become increasingly prevalent. They show the typical blood glucose level for a long period, making it easier to assess how well diabetes is being managed. Research has shown that the adoption of such indicators offers numerous advantages, including high accuracy and the ability to account for variability in measurements, reinforcing their importance in comprehensive diabetes management (Abdolrahim et al., 2017). Thus, it is important to use these methods regularly for patients who want to manage their condition well. In addition, checking blood glucose is helpful for patients to learn more and take better care of themselves. When individuals know what their blood glucose readings mean, they can take action and spot anything that might affect their health. Because of this, patients are better able to decide on healthy habits such as eating well and exercising, which may help control their blood sugar levels. For instance, continuous glucose monitoring systems give a lot of information that helps doctors make specific plans for each patient's glucose levels. Using technology to monitor patients has made it easier and more suitable for each person to manage diabetes. In short, blood glucose monitoring helps people with diabetes in many ways, making their lives better than before (Figure 6.2).

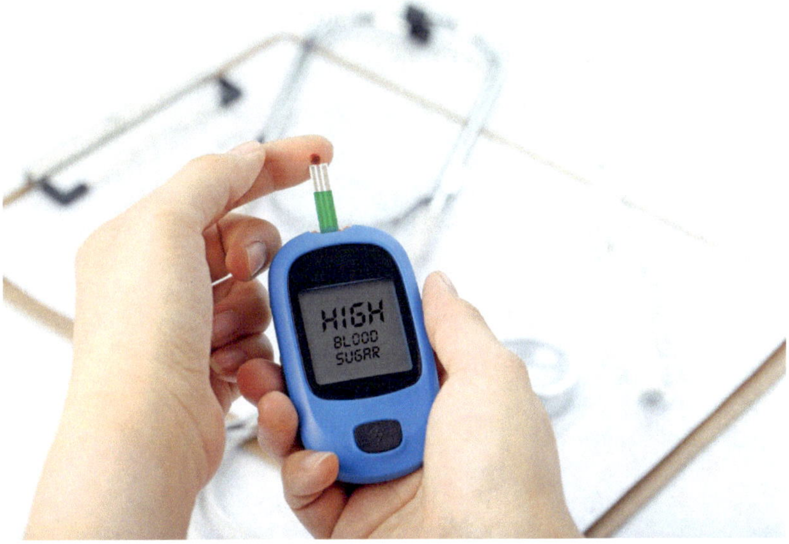

Figure 6.2. The primary purpose of blood glucose monitoring is to provide individuals with real-time data about their glucose levels, thereby facilitating timely adjustments in diet, medication, and physical activity.

Source: https://www.hiranandanihospital.org/public/uploads/blogs/1745312473.jpg

6.1.1. Daily Management of Diabetes

To manage diabetes well each day, one should follow a healthy diet, exercise regularly, and keep track of blood sugar levels. Those with diabetes must pay attention to how many carbohydrates they eat, since this affects their blood sugar levels. Following dietary recommendations, having meals that contain whole grains, fruits, and vegetables can improve glycemic control. In addition, doing physical activity that matches your skills is necessary for improving insulin sensitivity and avoiding diabetes-related issues. A combination of healthy eating and regular exercise makes it easier to handle diabetes each day and supports good health in the long run. One of the main difficulties people with diabetes encounter daily is called therapeutic inertia, which hinders them from reaching their best blood sugar levels. When doctors do not alter treatment even though glycemic targets are not met, this is known as therapeutic inertia and can lead to treatment that is not effective for a long time. It is especially worrying for type 2 diabetes patients, as studies reveal that just half of them manage to control their blood sugar levels, despite the availability of newer drugs. Therapeutic inertia can be tackled by teaching patients consistently and taking action when needed by healthcare providers. By recognizing and overcoming the factors contributing to this inertia, healthcare teams can significantly improve diabetes management in their patients, enhancing both immediate and long-term health outcomes (Rodriguez et al., 2024). Taking care of diabetes every day is not only up to the patient; it also requires the help of several healthcare professionals. Taking care of diabetes requires the efforts of doctors, nurses, pharmacists, and diabetes educators. It is important for teams to cooperate so they can create and carry out personalized management plans that consider what each patient is going through. The complexity of managing diabetes, particularly in older adults with multimorbidity, underscores the importance of tailored approaches that prioritize quality of life and functional ability (Umegaki, 2024). When doctors and nurses communicate, patients tend to follow their treatment plans, which helps control blood sugar and achieve better health (Figure 6.3).

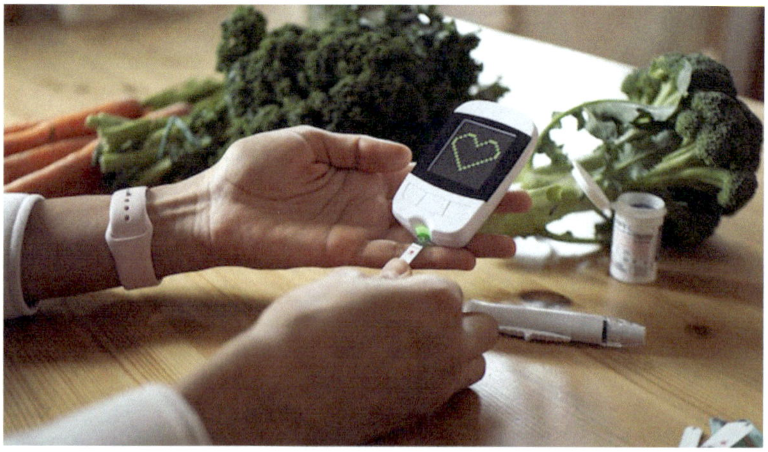

Figure 6.3. Individuals with diabetes must be vigilant about their carbohydrate intake, as this directly influences their blood sugar control.

Source: https://akm-img-a-in.tosshub.com/indiatoday/images/story/202209/Health-Diabetes.jpg?VersionId=5pCH1d6xxcGcemHsHp0q0s1U70SMp0ar&size=690:388

6.1.2. Prevention of Complications

Problems in diabetes management can be avoided mostly by controlling blood sugar well. Chronic hyperglycemia is a primary contributing factor to the development of systemic vascular complications associated with diabetes mellitus (DM), underlining the necessity for individuals to sustain their blood glucose levels within target ranges. Adhering to current guidelines that recommend personalized treatment goals based on glycated hemoglobin (HbA1c) levels can significantly mitigate the risks of complications. To manage their diabetes well, patients should gain new knowledge and check their blood sugar levels regularly with a meter. The regular evaluation of metabolic parameters is essential, as it not only aids in adjusting therapeutic strategies but also empowers patients to take an active role in their health management, ultimately paving the way for improved long-term outcomes and reduced complication rates (Biryukova, 2024). Self-monitoring of blood glucose (SMBG) is a critical component of diabetes prevention strategies, facilitating proactive management of blood sugar levels. Often, checking blood sugar levels makes it easier to manage diabetes and reduces the risk of problems caused by hypoglycemia. Mobile apps that work with glucose meters make it easier for people to monitor their blood sugar since they can get quick feedback and look at their past results. In addition, if patients are aware of their glucose levels, they can decide on the best way to eat and live. As evidenced by ongoing research, patients who engage consistently in SMBG display an overall reduction in the prevalence of long-term complications related to diabetes, underscoring the pivotal role of education in diabetes self-management (Sindi et al., 2023).

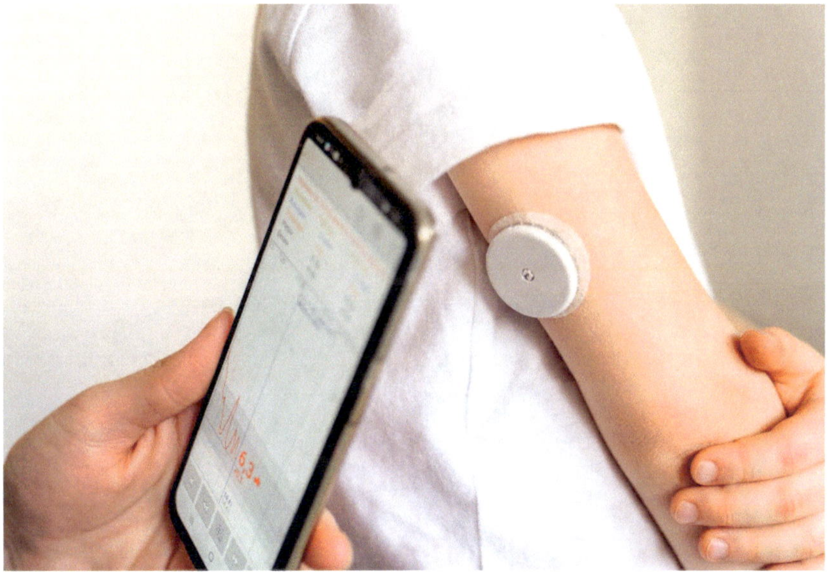

Figure 6.4. Self-monitoring of blood glucose (SMBG) is a critical component of diabetes prevention strategies, facilitating proactive management of blood sugar levels.

Source: https://aptivamedical.com/wp-content/uploads/2021/12/system-of-continuous-monitoring-of-glucose-on-childs-arm-picture-id1367251295.jpg

Apart from managing blood sugar and doing SMBG, it is important to focus on other possible complications, including microalbuminuria, in diabetes care. Microalbuminuria is an early sign that kidney problems might develop because of repeated hyperglycemia. Studies done recently have shown that children with high HbA1c levels are more likely to develop microalbuminuria, showing the link between blood sugar and kidney health. This means that doctors should check for microalbuminuria regularly and keep working to control blood sugar levels. Educating patients about the importance of maintaining metabolic targets will not only reduce the incidence of microalbuminuria but will also contribute to lower rates of long-term complications associated with diabetes, reinforcing the need for a holistic approach to diabetes care (Sindi et al., 2023) (Figure 6.4).

6.1.3. Role in Treatment Adjustments

Managing diabetes well requires frequent changes in treatment plans, considering glycemic control, any other health problems, and the patient's reaction to treatment. To check how well diabetes is controlled, doctors mainly use hemoglobin A1c levels, which reflect blood glucose over a longer period. Yet, using real-time blood glucose monitoring can give useful information about daily changes, which helps doctors make more accurate treatment decisions. In such a case, patients with high blood sugar after meals might need to change their insulin doses or choose healthier foods. As a result, it is important for doctors to monitor patients well, since this helps them create the right treatment plans and manage diabetes more effectively. In addition, when hypertension and insulin resistance are also present, diabetes treatment needs to be changed so that the glycemic control drugs function properly.

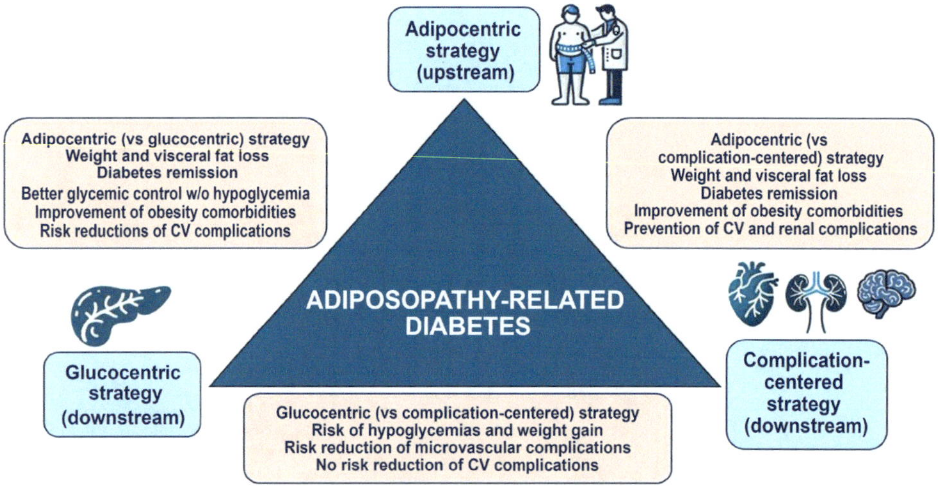

Figure 6.5. Adjustments in diabetes treatment must consider the presence of comorbid conditions such as hypertension and insulin resistance, which can impact the efficacy of glycemic control medications.

Source: Gorgojo-Martínez JJ. Adipocentric Strategy for the Treatment of Type 2 Diabetes Mellitus. *Journal of Clinical Medicine.* 2025; 14(3):678. https://doi.org/10.3390/jcm14030678

It has been found that people with type 2 diabetes often develop hypertension and issues in their blood vessels. Therefore, since hypertension and diabetes are linked, a team of healthcare professionals should check both blood sugar and blood pressure levels at the same time. With better knowledge of these conditions, doctors can prescribe antihypertensive drugs that will not affect how diabetes is managed. For example, information sourced from studies indicates that certain antihypertensive strategies may be influenced by the presence of diabetes (Hughes et al., 2022). For this reason, it is very important to address these related health problems to help patients get better treatment and results. In addition, teaching patients how to manage their condition plays a key role in making changes to treatment. Providing patients with the ability to monitor their health can encourage them to take their treatment and improve their blood sugar levels. Teaching patients about carbohydrate counting, insulin, and the importance of checking blood sugar can greatly help them adjust their treatment plans. Technology-based strategies, for example, mobile apps and continuous glucose monitoring, have shown they can help people make prompt changes to their treatment plans. Furthermore, understanding the psychosocial factors that motivate or hinder self-management can enhance patient engagement in their treatment (D'Elia et al., 2022). To summarize, creating a positive environment for patient education plays a key role in making it possible to review and adjust treatments regularly, which helps control diabetes (Figure 6.5).

6.2. Common Measurement Techniques

The way diabetes is measured has improved a lot as experts learn more about the disease and its importance to monitor closely. In the past, fasting plasma glucose and random plasma glucose were the main ways to diagnose diabetes. Still, these methods mainly show a single picture of blood sugar and don't share details about long-term glucose control. Recognizing this limitation, healthcare professionals have shifted toward measuring glycated proteins, particularly hemoglobin A1c (HbA1c), which captures the average blood glucose levels over a prolonged period. The transition to HbA1c not only enables better prognostic insights but also aligns with a broader array of diabetic management strategies aimed at minimizing complications associated with erratic glycemic control, such as cardiovascular disease and chronic kidney failure (Abdolrahim et al., 2017). In addition to HbA1c, glycated albumin (GA) has emerged as an important marker for monitoring diabetes, particularly for certain patient populations. GA is less affected by things that shorten red blood cell life, so it may give more reliable results than HbA1c when hemoglobin variants or erythropoietic factors are present. Common laboratory methods to measure these glycated proteins include high-performance liquid chromatography (HPLC) and immunoassay techniques, which offer substantial accuracy and reproducibility. Moreover, recent studies emphasize innovative approaches like the use of dried blood spots for HbA1c testing, which presents practical advantages in terms of cost and accessibility (Delavari et al., 2011). Different ways of measuring heart function prove that it is important to use the best techniques for each patient and their needs. The strength of assessing glycemic control relies on regular improvements in the methods used for measurements. Tests done on dried blood spots have shown good results, meaning they could be a good alternative to standard methods. According to studies, the results from dried blood samples are very similar to those from conventional blood tests, proving that they can be trusted in outpatient care. Since setting up labs is not always necessary, having different ways to measure could motivate more patients to follow their diabetes plans. Overall, employing a tailored approach to diabetes measurement techniques not only improves individual patient outcomes but also enhances public health strategies aimed at controlling this prevalent chronic condition effectively (Delavari et al., 2011) (Figure 6.6).

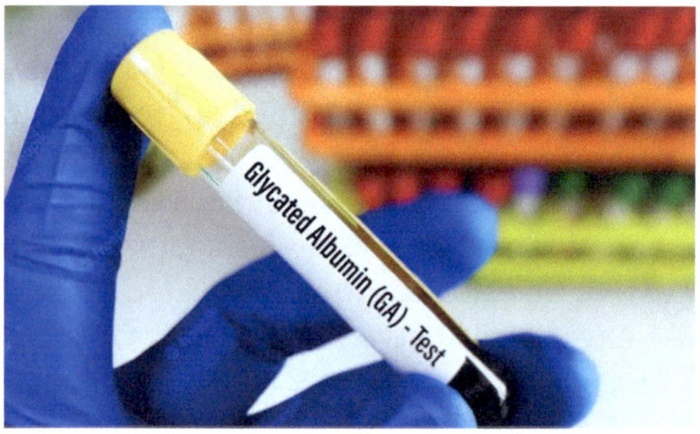

Figure 6.6. Glycated albumin (GA) tests.

Source: https://medicaldialogues.in/h-upload/2023/05/05/208867-glycated-albumin.webp

6.2.1. Self-monitoring of Blood Glucose (SMBG)

The role of self-monitoring of blood glucose (SMBG) in diabetes management is critical for achieving optimal glycemic control. Checking their health frequently helps people with diabetes decide on their diet, activity, and any needed changes to their medicines. It is very important to keep metabolic targets under control, because high blood sugar for a long time can lead to complications such as heart disease and nerve damage. According to the current guidelines, SMBG should be used based on a patient's treatment and personal requirements. This necessity underscores the importance of therapeutic training, enabling patients to correctly interpret their glucose readings and implement necessary lifestyle changes that reinforce their health outcomes (Biryukova, 2024). New devices for checking glucose levels have made it easier to control diabetes lately. Today, people living with diabetes can use glucose meters at home since there are many choices available. Accuracy and simplicity are the key factors when selecting a glucose meter, so that everyone can use it without much difficulty. Patients can also use mobile apps on these devices to manage their diabetes and play a bigger role in looking after it. These technological advancements serve not only to streamline the process of SMBG but also to facilitate a proactive approach to maintaining desired glycemic levels (Biryukova, 2024). Furthermore, the evolving landscape of diabetes care now includes comparisons of SMBG with continuous glucose monitoring (CGM) systems, which have been shown to offer significant advantages in certain populations. Studies show that CGM is linked to a lasting decrease in HbA1c compared to SMBG, and this is associated with fewer chances of having acute diabetic events and long-term complications. Using a microsimulation model, CGM was found to be more cost-effective than SMBG for people with type 2 diabetes on basal insulin, since it led to fewer hospitalizations from severe hypoglycemia and diabetic ketoacidosis. It appears that SMBG is still a main part of diabetes control, but CGM may help patients achieve better results and lower costs (Figure 6.7).

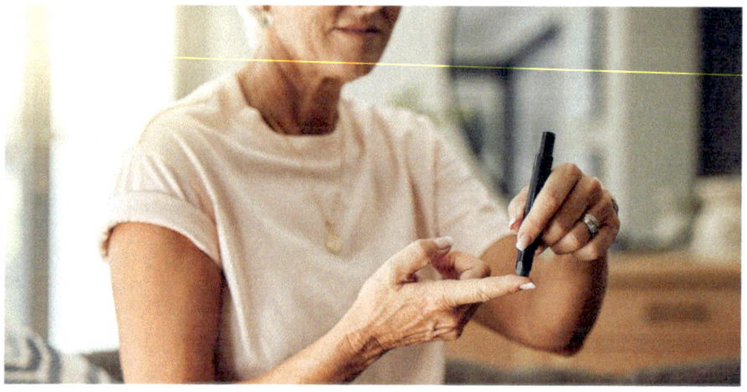

Figure 6.7. Regular monitoring allows individuals with diabetes to make informed decisions regarding their dietary intake, physical activity, and medication adjustments.

Source: https://diabetes-m.com/wp-content/uploads/2023/05/self-management-1200x600.jpg

6.2.2. Continuous Glucose Monitoring (CGM)

The advent of Continuous Glucose Monitoring (CGM) represents a significant advancement in diabetes management, particularly for individuals with Type 1 Diabetes Mellitus (T1DM). Traditional blood glucose monitoring methods, primarily self-monitoring of blood glucose (SMBG), have long been used to track glucose levels. Even so, they do not provide a lot of details since they only check glucose levels at certain times. CGM systems check the glucose level in the fluid outside cells, so users can notice any irregularities in their blood sugar. Being able to check blood sugar in real time helps people choose the right insulin and food for managing their blood sugar. Evidence suggests that CGM can effectively reduce HbA1c levels and improve overall diabetes management, underscoring its potential as an essential tool in the arsenal against diabetes (Thalia, 2025). Apart from helping people track their glucose levels, CGM systems make life better for adolescents and children with T1DM. Since diabetes care is stressful, continuously monitoring blood sugar reduces some of the anxiety that comes with its changes. CGM makes it easier to avoid low blood sugar, since the systems usually alert users when glucose levels are decreasing.

Sharing CGM data on different devices makes it easier for families and caregivers to cooperate in managing diabetes. Furthermore, CGM data allows healthcare providers to make more personalized adjustments to treatment plans, fostering a more supportive management environment for patients (Emmanuel, 2025). Although CGM technology is helpful, getting it used by many is still difficult due to issues with cost and access. Many people find it hard to pay for CGM systems and their supplies since this can be very expensive, especially in areas where healthcare is not well developed. Besides, the complicated nature of using CGM can discourage some patients from using it. Healthcare providers and patients have to figure out how to use CGM in their usual routines. Besides, users are concerned about the inaccuracy of some sensors and the need to calibrate them often. To achieve the best results from CGM in diabetes management, these challenges must be dealt with. Innovations in affordability, education, and technology may pave the way for broader acceptance and enhanced diabetes control in the long term (Thalia, 2025) (Figure 6.8).

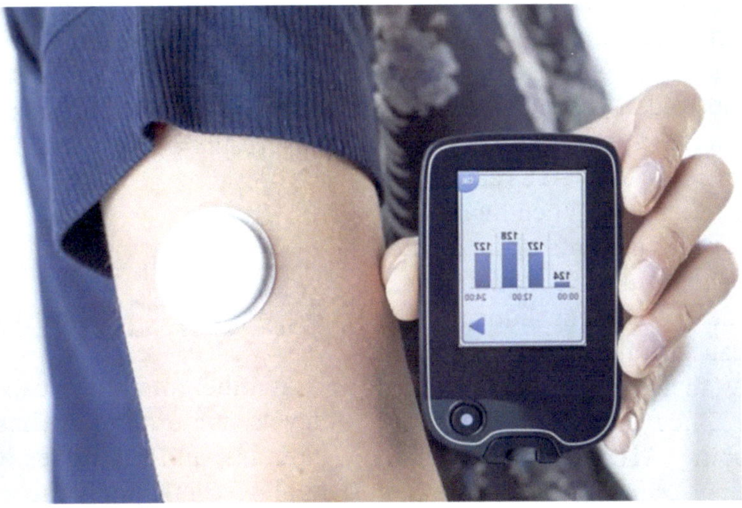

Figure 6.8. The advent of Continuous Glucose Monitoring (CGM) represents a significant advancement in diabetes management, particularly for individuals with Type 1 Diabetes Mellitus (T1DM).

Source: https://medicaldialogues.in/h-upload/2022/10/11/187560-flash-glucose-monitoring.webp

6.2.3. A1C Testing

Managing diabetes well depends on measuring glycemic control, and A1C testing is very important in this process. The A1C test shows the average blood glucose levels from the past two to three months by checking the amount of glycated hemoglobin. Having a long-term outlook is important since it helps healthcare providers see if treatment plans are working and make the needed changes. A higher A1C level increases the chance of getting diabetes-related issues such as cardiovascular disease and neuropathy. As a result, the A1C test helps find diabetes and also guides the care team in managing the disease for the patient's benefit. The relevance of A1C testing expands beyond conventional diabetes as it is being explored in conditions like gestational diabetes mellitus (GDM), where its diagnostic accuracy remains under scrutiny (Kahraman et al., 2025). Studies have proven that A1C levels play a key role in assessing treatment success in different groups of people. In a study involving pregnant women, A1C values were compared with traditional glucose tolerance tests to assess gestational diabetes, revealing potential limitations of A1C in certain subgroups (Kahraman et al., 2025). This shows that A1C testing is useful, but its results need to be looked at closely since every person's case is different. It is also necessary for patients to learn about their A1C results and how to handle their diabetes. When healthcare professionals aim to help patients manage their blood sugar, they should always explain what their A1C levels mean for them. Education is very important because it often helps patients be satisfied and follow the recommended changes in their lifestyle. Since diabetes treatments are always developing, A1C testing should be included with other approaches to manage the condition. The combination of A1C testing with technologies such as continuous glucose monitoring (CGM) offers a more rounded view of glucose variability and overall control. New educational programs highlight that counting carbs is an effective approach for managing blood sugar in people with Type 1 diabetes, and A1C is an important indicator to watch in dietary situations. Knowing what A1C testing can and cannot do, healthcare providers can provide interventions that best fit each patient's needs. Overall, A1C testing is important in diabetes care, as it helps doctors decide on treatment and supports better health results (Figure 6.9).

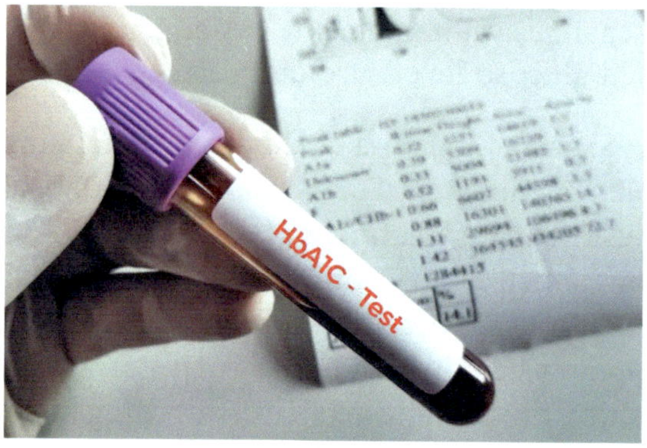

Figure 6.9. The A1C test, which measures the percentage of glycated hemoglobin in the blood, provides insights into average blood glucose levels over the preceding two to three months.

Source: https://img.lb.wbmdstatic.com/vim/live/webmd/consumer_assets/site_images/article_thumbnails/BigBead/hba1c_blood_test_bigbead/1800x1200_hba1c_blood_test_bigbead.jpg?resize=750px:*&output-quality=75.

6.3. Factors Affecting Blood Glucose Levels

A number of things can affect blood glucose levels, for example, what you eat, how active you are, and hormones. Carbohydrates with a high glycemic index cause blood glucose to rise very quickly. When blood sugar spikes, it can be very harmful for people with diabetes since it can upset their metabolic balance. On the other hand, a diet that includes a lot of fiber and not much processed sugar helps maintain steady blood sugar levels by making digestion and absorption slower. In addition, being physically active on a regular basis improves the body's ability to use glucose. The way diet and exercise affect blood glucose levels shows that lifestyle is very important for managing diabetes, so it is necessary to teach patients about their diet and encourage them to exercise regularly. Managing blood glucose depends a lot on emotional and psychological health. High levels of stress for a long time can make the body release hormones that increase blood glucose by promoting the creation of glucose in the liver. Besides, when people are anxious or depressed, they tend to eat less healthily and exercise less, which makes it even more difficult for them to handle diabetes. If these psychological factors are understood, it becomes easier to manage diabetes since addressing mental health can improve following treatment plans and making healthy lifestyle changes. As a result, healthcare providers should manage diabetes by looking after the patient's blood sugar as well as their mental health to ensure the best possible results. Besides, age and genetics play a major role in how individuals handle blood glucose, since they affect glucose processing in the body. When people grow older, their metabolism can slow down and their bodies become less sensitive to insulin, which may result in higher blood glucose levels and an increased chance of getting diabetes. Therefore, regular check-ups and preventive actions should be given special attention to middle-aged people with a family background of diabetes. It seems that older people may have difficulties managing diabetes because of reduced mobility or mental issues that make it hard to maintain a steady blood sugar level. By recognizing the multifaceted nature of these influencing factors, healthcare systems can better tailor educational programs and interventions aimed at distinct age groups, thereby improving the overall management and control of diabetes within the population (Pasupathi et al., 2011; Cachia et al., 2016) (Figure 6.10).

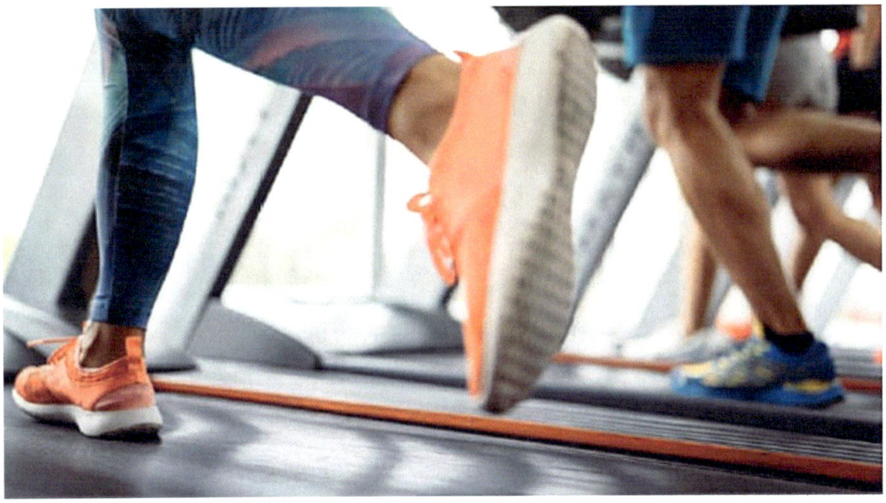

Figure 6.10. Blood glucose levels are significantly influenced by a variety of factors, including dietary habits, physical activity, and hormonal regulation.

Source: https://img.lb.wbmdstatic.com/vim/live/webmd/consumer_assets/site_images/article_thumbnails/reference_guide/controlling_spikes_through_diet_and_exercise_ref_guide/650x350_controlling_spikes_through_diet_and_exercise_ref_guide.jpg

6.3.1. Diet and Nutrition

Taking care of diet and nutrition is very important for diabetes as it greatly affects blood sugar control and health. Both patients and healthcare providers need to know how certain diets can influence blood glucose levels. For individuals with diabetes, tailored nutritional approaches, such as the Mediterranean diet, have demonstrated particular efficacy in preserving kidney function, a crucial concern considering the heightened risk of chronic kidney disease (CKD) in diabetic patients. The Mediterranean diet is characterized by its balance of healthy fats, moderate carbohydrates, and rich sources of fiber, which have been linked to improved glucose regulation and a lower decline in kidney function in those with concomitant obesity and type 2 diabetes mellitus (T2DM; Podadera-Herreros et al., 2024). So, it is important to have diet plans that control blood sugar and address other issues such as obesity. On top of this, it's important to realize that using medications for diabetes is not enough; dietary changes are equally necessary for reaching glycemic targets. Research indicates that appropriate medical nutrition therapy can lead to significant reductions in glycated hemoglobin (HbA1c) levels, thereby lessening the risk of long-term complications associated with diabetes. Evidence suggests that regular dietary intervention can beneficially influence weight management and improve metabolic health (Yeh et al., 2023).

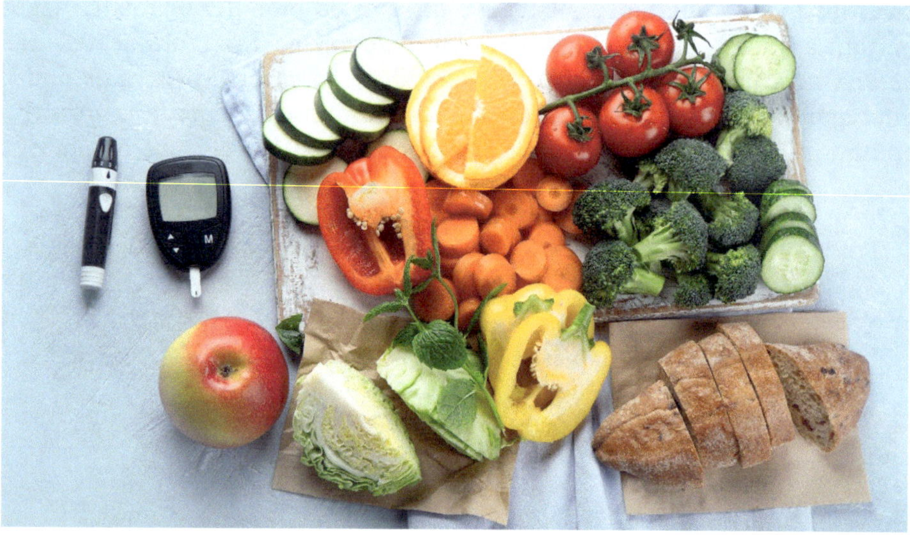

Figure 6.11. Diet and nutrition are pivotal components in the management of diabetes, significantly influencing glycemic control and overall health outcomes.

Source: https://www.news-medical.net/images/news/ImageForNews_757635_16933948141623635.jpg

Individuals with T2DM usually have to pay attention to their carbohydrate intake and insulin doses, so it is important to teach them about nutrition. Involving dietitians in a patient's care can lead to improved eating habits and lasting lifestyle changes that fit the person's needs. It is important to note that diet in diabetes management means eating healthy and paying attention to what foods are chosen. To manage diabetes well, it is recommended to eat more non-starchy vegetables, cut down on sugars, and pick whole foods instead of processed ones. Additionally, it is crucial to assess individual dietary needs, taking into account factors such as age, body weight, and cultural preferences while also recognizing barriers to dietary changes (Yeh et al., 2023). Such nutrition plans allow patients to control their diabetes and reduce the chances of developing diabetic kidney disease. For this reason, teaching patients about healthy diets and giving them meal plans is vital for controlling diabetes and achieving better results (Figure 6.11).

6.3.2. Physical Activity

Being physically active is very important for controlling and preventing Type II diabetes. Taking part in regular exercise helps control weight and also makes the body more sensitive to insulin, which improves how glucose is handled. This way of controlling diabetes highlights the need to do both aerobic and resistance exercises. These activities may result in a significant decrease in hemoglobin A1c levels, which are important for checking how well glucose is controlled over time. From what is known in the literature, people who exercise regularly have fewer diabetes-related complications, which shows that physical activity is important for diabetes management. Using various exercise types shows a complete approach, since every type brings its own benefits that suit each person's health, helping manage diabetes. Although it is clear how physical activity helps manage diabetes, obesity and not being active enough make diabetes care more difficult. The high level of obesity in some jobs greatly increases the chances of developing Type II diabetes. As an illustration, those who are employed in the road and rail industries, which require a lot of sitting, are more likely to be obese. It is important to encourage physical activity in these particular groups. Organizing activities such as fitness programs and giving information on healthy living can bring about important changes. As highlighted in studies, effective health promotion initiatives that incentivize active living have shown measurable successes, ultimately enhancing the well-being of workers while addressing the mounting societal burden of chronic diseases like diabetes (Naweed et al., 2015). In addition, making physical activity part of your daily life is necessary to maintain your health, mainly for those who may develop diabetes. Opting for walking or cycling over driving can greatly help you become more physically active. Besides, starting community programs for group exercise can help people find support, making staying fit more pleasant and lasting. Since diabetes is influenced by many factors, controlling it calls for an approach that supports people and also creates an environment that promotes physical activity. As emerging research points to the broader implications of habitual physical activity on metabolic health, including its association with lower prevalence rates of prediabetes and diabetes, it is imperative to prioritize physical activity as a fundamental component in public health strategies aimed at diabetes prevention and management (Africano et al., 2018) (Figure 6.12).

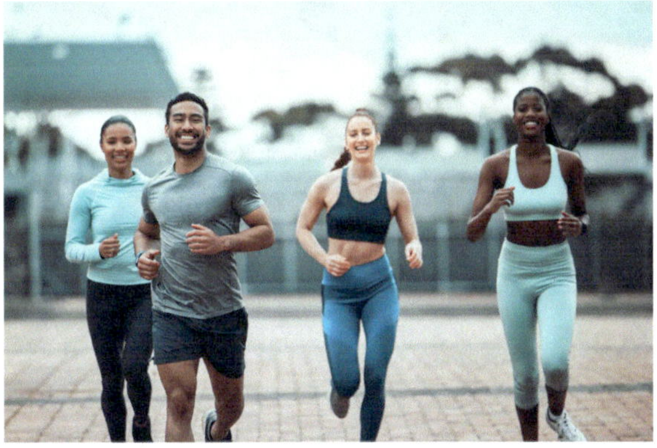

Figure 6.12. Regular engagement in physical activity not only aids in weight management but also enhances insulin sensitivity, allowing for improved glucose metabolism.

Source: https://forumhealth.com/wp-content/uploads/2022/11/iStock-1366052585.webp

6.3.3. Stress and Illness

Diabetes management is greatly affected by the strong relationship between stress and illness.

Stress is a reaction to tough situations that can greatly influence a person's health. It has been noticed that increased stress in people with diabetes often leads to poor blood sugar control, mainly due to hormonal changes that lower insulin sensitivity. It is very important to know how stress plays a role in diabetes management when planning care strategies. It has been found that ongoing stress can cause changes in metabolic processes, which may affect blood glucose levels and make it harder to manage diabetes. So, realizing how stress affects diabetes helps doctors understand patients' results and underlines the importance of stress-reduction strategies in diabetic care. Moreover, the study of postprandial glucose (PPG) levels provides valuable insights into the role of stress in diabetes management. PPG helps show how well the body handles glucose after meals and gives a wider view of insulin and macronutrient metabolism. In older people, how much they can do, how they take care of themselves, their sleep, and their stress can all have a major impact on PPG. Yet, studies reveal that these factors might not be directly linked to PPG in elderly diabetics, suggesting that other things are also involved.

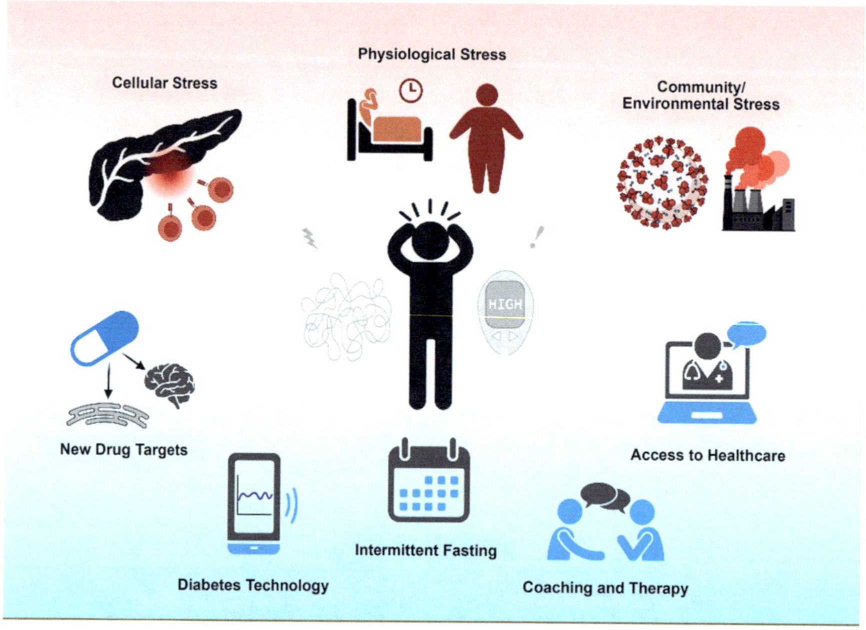

Figure 6.13. Understanding how stress contributes to the management of diabetes is critical for developing comprehensive care strategies.

Source: https://static.cambridge.org/binary/version/id/urn:cambridge.org:id:binary:20231213100637195-0135:S2059866123006465:S2059866123006465_fig1.png?pub-status=live

The identification of additional predictive factors in determining PPG levels underscores the necessity of a holistic approach to diabetes care that considers not only physiological but also psychosocial elements impacting health outcomes, thereby bridging the gap between stress and glycemic control in diabetes management (Manungkalit et al., 2019). The implications of stress on diabetes management are further underscored by studies linking stress to elevated hemoglobin A1c (HbA1c) levels, particularly among specific demographics such as women. It was found that many stressed women had unusual blood sugar levels, which might make them more likely to get diabetes. Because of this relationship, it is important to handle stress when caring for people with diabetes. When healthcare providers add stress management to treatment, it may help patients better control their blood sugar and enjoy better health. Also, the connection between stress and blood glucose levels has important effects on programs that try to prevent and control diabetes. A more profound understanding of this relationship can inform the design of targeted programs that empower individuals to cope with stress more effectively, thereby enhancing their capacity to manage diabetes successfully (Figure 6.13).

6.4. Challenges in Diabetes Control

The main difficulty in controlling diabetes is that the disease has many different aspects. Diabetes is best managed by taking medicine, eating healthy foods, being physically active, and checking blood sugar levels regularly. Many patients struggle to keep up with these changes, which results in unstable blood sugar and possible health problems. Besides, dealing with a chronic disease is very difficult for patients emotionally. Many patients mention having anxiety and depression, and these feelings may lead to more health problems and prevent them from taking their medicine as directed. Therefore, to manage diabetes well, we must consider mental and emotional health as well as physical health, since this aspect is usually not addressed in clinical settings. Having access to healthcare resources is a major problem in controlling diabetes.

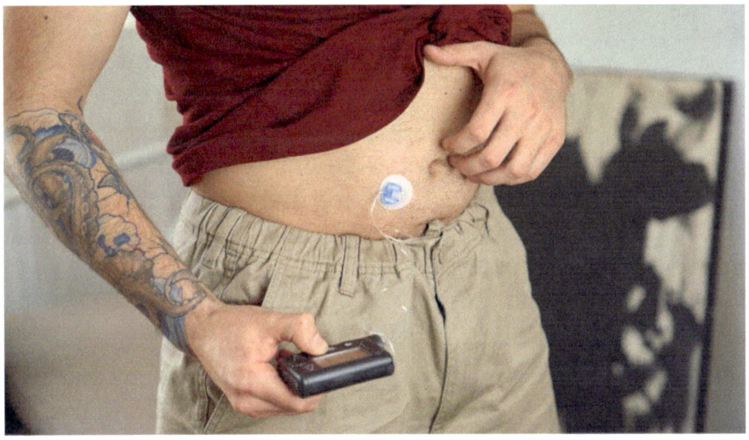

Figure 6.14. Patients often face difficulties in maintaining these lifestyle changes, leading to erratic glucose levels and potential complications.

Source: https://post.medicalnewstoday.com/wp-content/uploads/sites/3/2022/06/diabetes-monitor-1296x728-header-1024x576.jpg

In several low-income regions, patients have to deal with a shortage of healthcare professionals, expensive diabetes medicine, and not enough information on how to manage their diabetes. Besides, people with low health literacy find it more difficult to understand their condition, which adds to the difficulties of managing it themselves. Since support is not tailored to different groups, many people with diabetes are not given the care and knowledge they require. Therefore, these factors in the system are connected to worse health and higher long-term expenses for healthcare. To solve these problems, healthcare systems should introduce plans that make care more accessible and help people learn how to handle their diabetes better. It is very important to detect chronic diseases early and keep monitoring them regularly. According to studies, it is important to know about hypertension and increased blood glucose levels to control diabetes effectively. Yet, studies have revealed that awareness about diabetes has gone down among some groups of middle-aged people over the years. Even with better ways to control blood pressure, the decline in diabetes management shows that there is a big need for more diabetes education. With no proactive steps, including thorough screening, some people may not know their risk, which makes it harder to stop the disease. Addressing this issue involves not only reinforcing education about diabetes but also integrating awareness initiatives in communities to ensure that preventive strategies are targeting those most at risk (Cachia et al., 2016) (Figure 6.14).

6.4.1. Adherence to Treatment Plans

Following the treatment plan is very important for managing diabetes well. Many patients find it challenging to follow the complicated diabetes treatment that requires them to check their blood sugar, change their diet, and take their medicines regularly. Therefore, when people don't follow their treatment plan, their blood glucose levels may become uncontrolled and put them at greater risk of major health issues. Studies indicate that for medication management to succeed, healthcare providers and patients should work together, mainly when they are trying to follow a treatment plan. When clinical pharmacists use motivational interviewing to help patients, it has shown positive results in improving how well patients follow their treatment plans. (Bosworth et al., 2010) This proactive approach integrates patient education, monitoring, and tailored interventions, which collectively enhance the likelihood that patients will follow their treatment plans consistently. Support systems and educational programs for patients are also very important when it comes to adherence. Since many people with diabetes do not know how to manage their condition well, education forms an important part of their treatment. It is important for patients to realize why they should follow their medication, diet, and exercise plans. Programs in the community that give access to coaching and peer guidance can encourage people to follow their treatment plans. Also, when care plans are created with patients, they are more likely to take part in managing their health. It makes people more likely to obey and also encourages them. Targeted help that matches patients' needs and situations can greatly boost their involvement in treatment, resulting in better clinical results. (McCarthy et al., 2009) Moreover, technology has emerged as a powerful tool in promoting adherence to treatment plans for diabetes management. Mobile applications, glucose monitoring devices, and telehealth have made a big difference in how patients deal with their health plans. They remind patients, allow them to track their progress, and make it possible to communicate with doctors in real time. Experts say that these technologies help patients stick to their treatment plans by letting them view their health information and respond quickly. Using technology with traditional methods helps overcome the problems related to sticking to treatment. When patients can get help and information quickly, healthcare providers can help them become more involved in their diabetes care and lower the risk of complications (Figure 6.15).

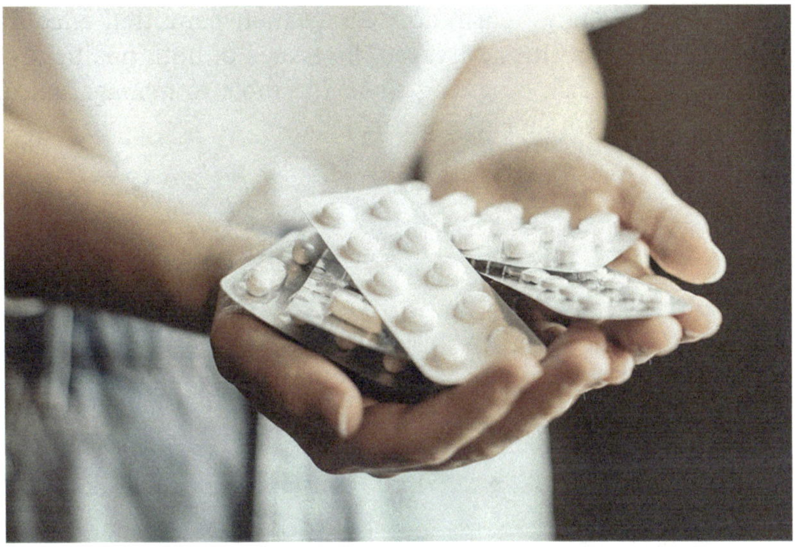

Figure 6.15. Patients must understand the importance of adhering to medication regimens, dietary recommendations, and exercise routines.

Source: https://cdn.careindeed.com/medication%20management.png

6.4.2. Access to Healthcare Resources

Taking care of diabetes is much easier when healthcare resources are available. If there is not enough access to healthcare, people with diabetes encounter many obstacles to controlling their blood sugar levels and getting the necessary preventive care. The level of a person's income often affects their ability to visit medical centers, buy medications, and get information about managing diabetes. Researchers have found that people from lower socioeconomic groups usually encounter more obstacles that make it harder for them to manage their disease. The fact that some people do not have equal access to healthcare points to the need for major changes in the system. Improving infrastructure and resources in underprivileged communities allows healthcare systems to help patients recover better from diabetes and lowers the rate of diabetes complications among them, which supports public health efforts to reduce the disease's impact. In addition, differences in geography make it harder for some people to manage their diabetes. Healthcare services in rural regions of Pakistan and similar countries may not be adequate, so people do not receive timely help when they need it. It is found that diabetes is more common in these underserved areas because people there deal with extra obstacles, such as not having enough transportation and few healthcare workers. It becomes much easier for lifestyle factors, such as not being active and eating badly, to increase the risk of diabetes when healthcare resources are not available. Therefore, it is necessary to use specialized programs, update policies, and reach out to communities to help more people with diabetes get the healthcare they require. Health education and the ease of getting healthcare resources are also very important for controlling diabetes. Those who do not know much about their disease or who do not see the importance of regular check-ups and treatment are more prone to have negative health consequences. Good educational programs can help patients choose healthy lifestyles and follow the treatment plan. In fact, knowing how diet and exercise affect blood sugar can help a lot in controlling it. According to recent studies, helping people who are more likely to suffer from diabetes learn more about their condition encourages them to take care of their health. When public health addresses the issues of both healthcare and education, it can more easily support those at risk by giving them the tools to manage and measure diabetes, which helps the community as a whole (Figure 6.16).

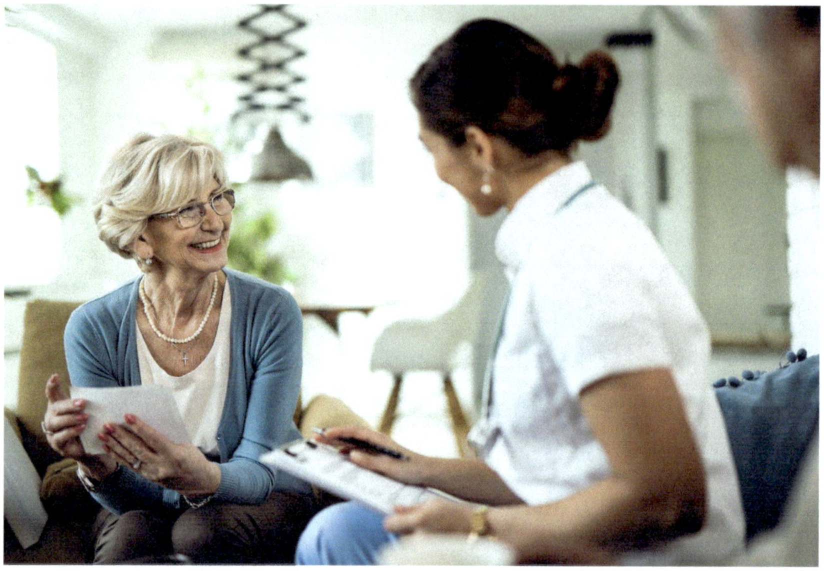

Figure 6.16. Effective educational programs can empower patients to make informed lifestyle choices and adhere to treatment regimens.

Source: https://miro.medium.com/v2/resize:fit:1400/1*pSz81D-lwLgMSdrI1hzFjA.jpeg

6.4.3. Psychological Factors

Although medications and changes in diet are important, psychological aspects are also very important in managing diabetes. Being emotionally well helps patients stick to their diabetes plan; however, stress and anxiety may prevent them from taking care of themselves regularly. As an illustration, people under a lot of stress could skip healthy eating, which can cause their blood glucose to fluctuate. It has also been found that stress can lead to higher HbA1c levels for female patients, which means that diabetes care should consider mental health as well. Addressing the psychological dimensions of diabetes management is essential for effective treatment outcomes, as unmanaged emotional stress can exacerbate the challenges of living with diabetes and hinder overall health and well-being (Thielman et al., 2019). Another factor that affects managing diabetes is how people see their weight and body image, which is most common among children and adolescents. Among younger people, dealing with diabetes can be made more difficult by the influence of society and self-esteem issues. When psychological factors are not considered, interventions to promote healthy habits usually fail. A school-based program designed to combat obesity, for example, demonstrated a surprising increase in participants' body mass index (BMI) instead of the expected decrease. This outcome underlines the considerable influence of psychological factors on health behavior change; if students do not perceive themselves positively or are not motivated, even well-structured education can fail to effect meaningful change in obesity-related risk factors, including those for diabetes (Thielman et al., 2019). In addition, the relationship between psychology and diabetes is also seen in patients' social and environmental settings. When people in a community have economic problems or lack healthy food, they may feel more stressed and this can lead to difficulties managing diabetes. Among women in a particular community, 58.3% of those with stress also had abnormal blood glucose, which clearly showed a link between stress and physical health. This research points out that intervention strategies should help people with diabetes as well as consider the social and environmental influences on their condition. Such an integrated approach can facilitate better health outcomes by fostering resilience and coping mechanisms among diabetes patients (Figure 6.17).

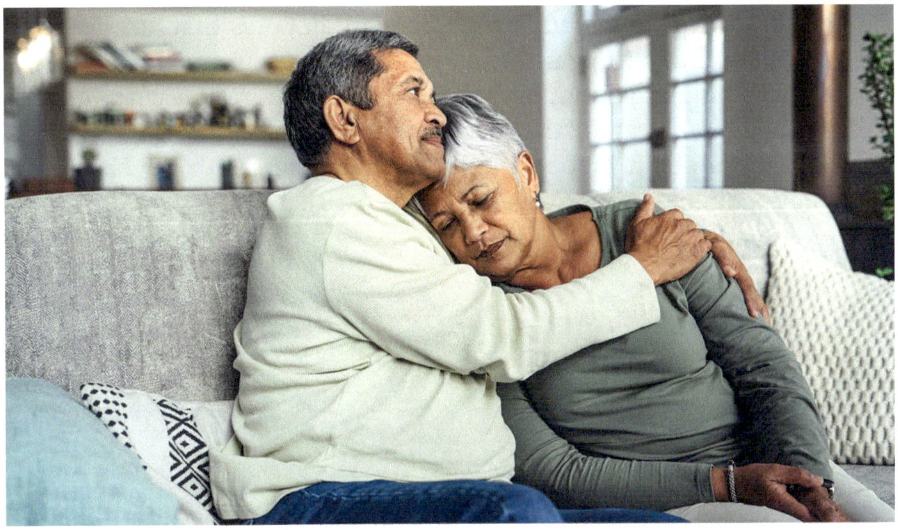

Figure 6.17. Addressing the psychological dimensions of diabetes management is essential for effective treatment outcomes, as unmanaged emotional stress can exacerbate the challenges of living with diabetes and hinder overall health and well-being

Source: https://www.cdc.gov/diabetes/images/library/features/GettyImages-1357522267.jpg

6.5. Advances in Diabetes Management

Lately, new developments in managing diabetes have allowed people to control their blood glucose levels much better. Continuous glucose monitoring (CGM) systems, for instance, offer real-time data that allows patients and healthcare providers to make timely decisions regarding insulin administration and dietary choices. Instead of the old fingerstick method, these devices now use advanced sensors to help create a record of blood sugar levels and make it easier to predict and prevent hypo- or hyperglycemic events. With these innovations, people with diabetes can be more proactive and take part in their own care. In addition, the combination of mobile health applications and CGM technology gives people the chance to use data to improve their routines. They indicate a major change towards diabetes care that puts the patient's comfort and freedom first. At the same time, new technology has appeared, the pharmaceutical sector has helped improve diabetes management with new drugs. Recent research has expanded the repertoire of diabetes medications beyond traditional insulin therapies to include glucagon-like peptide-1 (GLP-1) receptor agonists and sodium-glucose cotransporter-2 (SGLT-2) inhibitors. Using these drugs improves blood sugar levels and helps protect the heart and kidneys, which greatly improves the health of diabetic patients. Research that stresses the use of combination therapies has proven helpful in treating complex cases that call for several types of treatment. As seen in the studies funded by various pharmaceutical companies, including those supported by de Bruin et al. (2015), there is a significant emphasis on adherence to treatment protocols, which is understood to be crucial for transforming diabetes management paradigms. Besides new drugs and technology, animal models are now more important in diabetes research. In the past, using dogs helped create many diabetes treatments, including pancreatic islet transplantation and immunosuppressive methods needed for their effectiveness. Lately, researchers have started using monoclonal antibody therapies in people and have expanded their studies to include primates with diabetes that has been induced. Moving on, diabetes that occurs naturally in pets owned by clients can give valuable insights, leading to innovations that resemble human patient responses. The collaboration with industry partners, as highlighted by Adin et al. (2017), can further accelerate these research efforts. The use of different models helps us learn more about diabetes and gives us chances to develop useful treatments, which can improve how patients are managed (Figure 6.18).

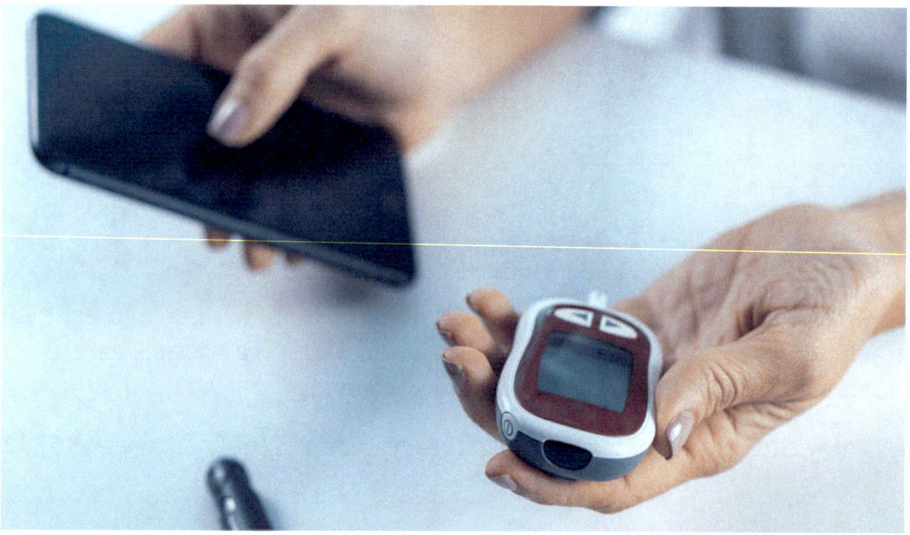

Figure 6.18. The integration of mobile health applications with CGM technology has created avenues for personalized insights, allowing individuals to adjust their routines based on data analytics.

Source: https://cdn.sigma.software/wp-content/uploads/2024/08/blog-integrated-diabetes-management-app.png

6.5.1. Technological Innovations

Diabetes management has advanced a lot because of new technologies that make it easier for people to care for themselves. One important progress is that mobile apps give users instant updates and personalized advice about their health. For young adults with type 1 diabetes, the integration of such technology has proven critical in supporting better health-related quality of life (HRQOL). It has been found that using mobile devices for diabetes management helps young patients understand their treatment better, encouraging them to follow the treatment plan. The best applications are not limited to tracking; they adjust to a person's way of life and habits, providing a personalized method of managing diabetes. Therefore, fostering the involvement of young patients in the design and implementation of these technologies is essential, as their feedback can lead to enhancements that resonate with their specific needs and challenges (Adaji et al., 2013). In addition to mobile applications, continuous glucose monitoring (CGM) systems represent a significant technological leap in diabetes management. Such devices make it possible for people to check their glucose levels without pricking their fingers, which lowers their need for traditional tests. CGMs supply real-time data, which helps patients decide on insulin and what to eat at any given time. Getting feedback quickly can help patients handle their condition better and, as a result, reduce the chances of complications in the future. As healthcare systems keep changing, including CGMs in diabetes care plans has proven to be effective. The ProvenCare model showcases how physician-led groups can enhance clinical outcomes while streamlining resource use, illustrating the potential benefits of adopting innovative monitoring technologies in treatment protocols (McCarthy et al., 2009). Besides, telehealth has become more important in diabetes care due to the COVID-19 pandemic and the rise of technology. With telehealth platforms, patients are able to keep in touch with their caregivers, even if they cannot go to the doctor in person. This way of managing diabetes is helpful for people who do not have many specialized diabetes services nearby. Taking part in virtual consultations and getting personal advice on diabetes, medicines, and lifestyle changes encourages people to be more involved in their health. Through telehealth and similar technologies, patients can manage their diabetes plans and enjoy a helpful relationship with their medical team (Figure 6.19).

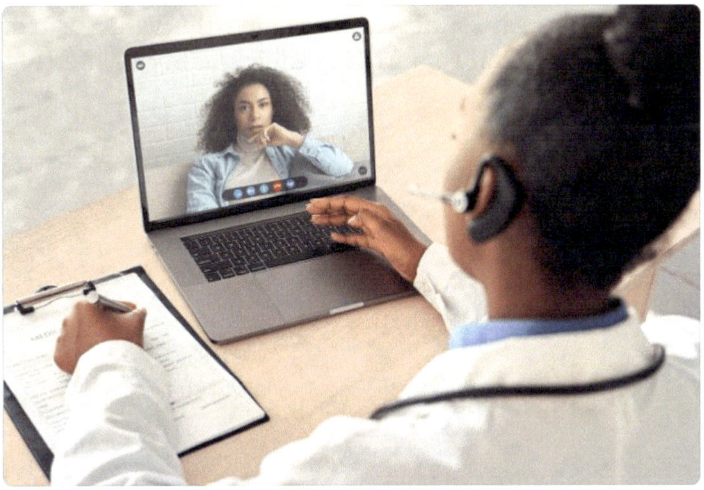

Figure 6.19. Telehealth platforms allow patients to maintain regular contact with healthcare providers, ensuring continued support and guidance regardless of physical distance.

Source: https://i0.wp.com/www.geneca.com/wp-content/uploads/2023/08/0ffba2ac-68be-4d2d-8191-d4e7e4004dbf.png?fit=710%2C476&ssl=1

6.5.2. New Medications and Therapies

The introduction of new drugs and treatments is very important for the better management of diabetes. Among the most notable advancements are the novel classes of antidiabetic agents, such as sodium-glucose cotransporter-2 inhibitors (SGLT2 inhibitors) and glucagon-like peptide-1 receptor agonists (GLP-1 RAs). These drugs lower blood glucose and also help protect the heart and kidneys, dealing with the various problems linked to diabetes. Their special ways of working help people lose weight and play a big role in managing diabetes. Since new research reveals the long-term effects and safety of these drugs, healthcare providers can develop treatment plans that suit each patient, leading to better results and better compliance. Besides, using personalized medicine in diabetes care is changing the way patients are treated. Considering genetics, the patient's way of life, and other current conditions, healthcare professionals can ensure the best use of drugs for each patient. For example, choosing drugs that fit an individual's genetic profile can help them work better and have fewer side effects, which is very important for elderly people with several health problems. Personalized treatment approaches are necessary to help patients get the most suitable therapies for their health. Concerning anticoagulation therapy in other contexts, as outlined in Capi et al. (2018), similar personalized approaches could enhance diabetes management by identifying the best medication and dosage for every individual based on their unique characteristics. Pharmacists working together with other healthcare professionals is a major new approach to diabetes management. Having pharmacists in healthcare teams has been found to help patients get the best results from their medicines. Collaborative models, such as those described in Awdishu et al. (2019), emphasize the importance of interprofessional cooperation in managing chronic conditions like diabetes. When pharmacists, physicians, and other healthcare providers work closely together, these models make it easier to review and adjust medications, which improves following the prescribed treatment. In daily work, pharmacists inform patients about recent treatments, watch their results, and look after possible side effects, helping to manage diabetes in the long run. The continuous progress of such strategies highlights the value of teamwork in supporting people with diabetes for a long time and improving their quality of life (Figure 6.20).

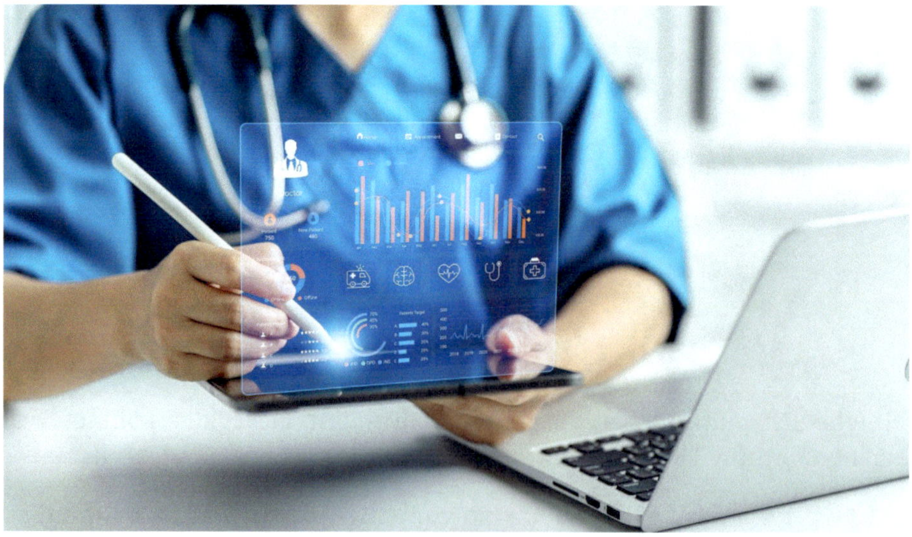

Figure 6.20. Pharmacist-led collaborative care models also represent a significant innovation in diabetes management.

Source: https://media.licdn.com/dms/image/v2/D4D12AQEsNiJDroIcaw/article-cover_image-shrink_720_1280/B4DZbnuttbG8AM-/0/1747644509692?e=2147483647&v=beta&t=FW8plnB01HA7RMnSclaEWt2iLg8rEmPptLMVHx-dvp0

6.5.3. Education and Support Programs

Support and education are very important for managing diabetes and improving patient outcomes. They are made to provide people with the skills and understanding needed to use self-management methods. When diet, exercise, taking medications, and checking blood sugar levels are included, education can greatly help control diabetes. It appears that structured education for patients can help control blood sugar levels and lower the chances of diabetes complications. Moreover, they allow patients to talk about what they go through, which encourages them to be responsible and stay motivated. Yet, although these programs may greatly benefit diabetes management, some people are not able to use them because of issues such as access and differences in quality. The use of innovative approaches, for example, nurse-led tele-coaching, proves that modern methods can make diabetes management programs more effective. Studies show that tele-coaching is an affordable way to improve health results, mainly for people with uncontrolled blood sugar. In one study examining a nurse-led tele-coaching program, participants experienced notable gains in Quality Adjusted Life Years (QALYs), illustrating the program's effectiveness in promoting better health. Furthermore, the cost-effectiveness study showed that extra support could lead to major long-term improvements, proving that these programs are important for healthcare. By facilitating ongoing communication and support, tele-coaching empowers patients to actively engage in their diabetes management, leading to improved self-efficacy and health outcomes over time (Aertgeerts et al., 2016). Another important part of education and support programs is the way pharmacists take part in collaborative care. Improving the use of medicines and helping patients learn more about them are now important parts of pharmacy practice. Pharmacists can help more than usual by joining teams that focus on diabetes care from all angles. With their knowledge in managing drugs, they can help patients follow their treatment plan and feel better about it. It has been found that involving pharmacists in diabetes care helps patients get better care and access to specialized information. When pharmacists collaborate with healthcare professionals, they contribute to a holistic approach to diabetes management that emphasizes education, resource utilization, and support for lifestyle changes, ultimately leading to better health outcomes for patients (Awdishu et al., 2019) (Figure 6.21).

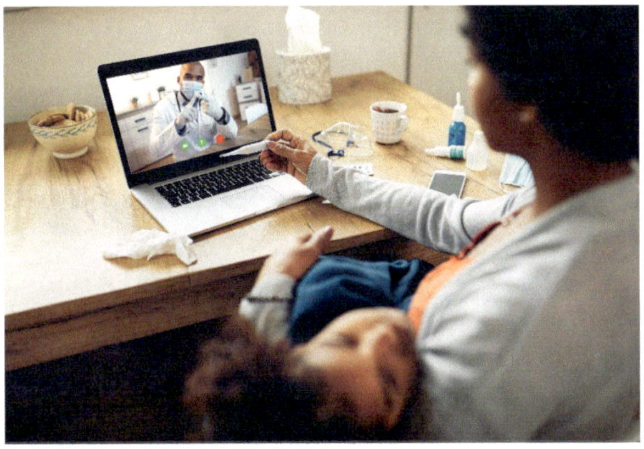

Figure 6.21. The integration of innovative models, such as nurse-led tele-coaching, demonstrates how modern approaches can enhance education and support programs for diabetes management.

Source: https://publichealth.jhu.edu/sites/default/files/2024-07/closeup-mother-having-video-call-with-pediatrician-while-measuring-daughter-s-temperature-home.jpg

A CLOSER LOOK

HEMOGLOBIN A1C

Hemoglobin A1c (HbA1c) is a blood test that measures the average blood glucose levels over the past two to three months. It reflects the percentage of hemoglobin (a protein in red blood cells) that is coated with glucose. Having an HbA1c below 5.7% is normal, between 5.7% and 6.4% means prediabetes, and 6.5% or more points to diabetes. It is usually used to detect diabetes and to check how diabetes is being managed in people who have it. Blood sugar tests are done daily, but HbA1c gives a longer overview of glucose levels to help decide on treatment.

Summary

The management of diabetes, particularly type 2 diabetes mellitus (T2DM), necessitates a comprehensive understanding of various strategies aimed at improving patient outcomes. A key focus in recent research has been the effectiveness of dietary interventions, notably very low-calorie diets (VLCDs) and low-energy liquid-formula diets (LELDs). There is no major difference in weight loss between people with and without T2DM when using these diets. It was found that the average weight loss was only -1.2 kg, and both groups showed similar rates of weight loss, meaning that these diets can be helpful for obesity management in people with or without diabetes. The potential to achieve substantial weight loss targets of over 15-20% captivates interest in clinical practice and offers pathways for further research into personalized dietary solutions for diabetes control (Harris et al., 2017). Besides focusing on what people eat, diabetes management also includes making lifestyle changes and upgrading healthcare services. Businesses are now more important than ever in finding solutions for sustainable health, mainly in regions where diabetes management is greatly needed. Techniques used by companies in many industries show that it is possible to improve the lifestyle and health of people with diabetes. Organizations that develop and evaluate business strategies for these communities can improve their competitiveness and help public health at the same time. This synergy between economic gain and health initiatives highlights the multifaceted dimensions of diabetes control, creating a platform for holistic development and empowerment within vulnerable populations (Wendel et al., 2012). In the end, checking diabetes control includes various measures that help determine if patients follow their treatment plans and if the management approach is effective. Hemoglobin A1c levels, checking blood glucose often, and changes in weight are important for both patients and their doctors to follow progress. The use of technology like continuous glucose monitors and mobile health apps makes the measurements more accurate and motivates people to take part in their health. Since diabetes is becoming more common around the world, it is very important to have effective ways to measure the disease, as they help both doctors and patients address the problem promptly and prevent further complications.

References

1. Abdolrahim, M., Jazayeri, H. E., Rabiee, M., Rajab, A., et al. (2017). Evaluation of glycated albumin (GA) and GA/Hba1c ratio for diagnosis of diabetes and glycemic control: A comprehensive review. https://core.ac.uk/download/213086982.pdf (accessed on 11th June 2025).
2. Adaji, A., Berg, M., Hennink, M., Holloway, K., et al. (2013). Ideas and enhancements related to mobile applications to support type 1 diabetes. https://core.ac.uk/download/12681435.pdf (accessed on 11th June 2025).
3. Adin, C. A., & Gilor, C. (2017). The diabetic dog as a translational model for human islet transplantation. https://core.ac.uk/download/323071786.pdf (accessed on 11th June 2025).
4. Aertgeerts, B., Annemans, L., Goderis, G., Nobels, F., et al. (2016). Delivering diabetes education through nurse-led tele coaching: Cost-effectiveness analysis. https://core.ac.uk/download/84044503.pdf (accessed on 11th June 2025).
5. Africano, S., Bachand, A. M., Benka-Coker, M. L., Brook, R. D., et al. (2018). Exposure to household air pollution from biomass-burning cookstoves and HbA1c and diabetic status among Honduran women. https://cupola.gettysburg.edu/cgi/viewcontent.cgi?article=1079&context=healthfac (accessed on 11th June 2025).
6. Awdishu, L., Singh, R. F., Saunders, I., Yam, F. K., Hirsch, J. D., Lorentz, S., Atayee, R. S., Ma, J. D., Tsunoda, S. M., Namba, J., Mnatzaganian, C. L., Painter, N. A., Watanabe, J. H., Lee, K. C., Daniels, C. D., & Morello, C. M. (2019). Advancing Pharmacist Collaborative Care within Academic Health Systems. *Pharmacy (Basel, Switzerland)*, *7*(4), 142. https://doi.org/10.3390/pharmacy7040142(accessed on 11th June 2025).
7. Baker, G., Burton, N. W., Estabrooks, P., Foster, C., et al. (2010). Recruiting hard-to-reach populations to physical activity studies: Evidence and experiences. https://core.ac.uk/download/9032156.pdf (accessed on 11th June 2025).
8. Bilo, H. J. G., Groenier, K. H., Houweling, S. T., Kleefstra, N., et al. (2006). Pitfalls in blood pressure measurement in daily practice. https://core.ac.uk/download/pdf/12919819.pdf (accessed on 11th June 2025).
9. Biryukova, E. V. (2024). Therapeutic avenues and prospects of blood glucose self-monitoring, the essential component of diabetes mellitus management. *Clinical Review for General Practice*. https://www.semanticscholar.org/paper/ffcae33c440c662c0f14138e89ce36948aebb884 (accessed on 11th June 2025).
10. Bosworth, H. B., Heisler, M. M., Hofer, T. P., Hogan, M. M., et al. (2010). Study protocol: The Adherence and Intensification of Medications (AIM) study–a cluster randomized controlled effectiveness study. https://core.ac.uk/download/pdf/8472048.pdf (accessed on 11th June 2025).
11. C. K. (Chut), B., S. A. (Sabariah), H., L. A. (Lily), J., et al. (2017). Do stressed women have abnormal glucose level? https://core.ac.uk/download/480549937.pdf (accessed on 11th June 2025).
12. Cachia, J., Calleja, N., & Sammut, A. (2016). Investing in the health of the 41–60-year-old: Reaping the return in the 60+ population? https://core.ac.uk/download/46603884.pdf (accessed on 11th June 2025).

13. Capi, M., Koverech, A., Lionetto, L., Martelletti, P., et al. (2018). Changing the approach to anticoagulant therapy in older patients with multimorbidity using a precision medicine approach. https://core.ac.uk/download/188826888.pdf (accessed on 11th June 2025).

14. Willems, Annelies, Pascale Smets, Isabel Van de Maele, Sophie Vandenabeele, and Sylvie Daminet. 2012. "Monitoring of Diabetic Dogs." *VLAAMS DIERGENEESKUNDIG TIJDSCHRIFT* 81 (4): 195–204.(accessed on 11th June 2025).

15. de Bruin, M., Grégoire, J. P., Guillaumie, L., Guénette, L., et al. (2015). Effectiveness and content analysis of interventions to enhance oral antidiabetic drug adherence in adults with type 2 diabetes: Systematic review and meta-analysis. https://core.ac.uk/download/42130668.pdf (accessed on 11th June 2025).

16. Delavari, A., Heshmat, R., Keshtkar, A., Larijani, B., et al. (2011). Glycated hemoglobin measurements from dried blood spots: Reliability and relation to results obtained from whole blood samples. https://core.ac.uk/download/52204830.pdf (accessed on 11th June 2025).

17. D'Elia, M. P. B., Cassiano, D., Espósito, A., & Miot, H. (2022). Concerning the characterization of metabolic syndrome in epidemiologic studies. Comments on "metabolic syndrome in melasma: A case–control study." *Journal of Cosmetic Dermatology, 21.* https://www.semanticscholar.org/paper/7ce4fbe1d6bfc50be2480e224e71f4e2de92e646 (accessed on 11th June 2025).

18. Emmanuel, M. K. (2025). Exploring the effectiveness of continuous glucose monitoring in improving quality of life and reducing hypoglycemic episodes in children with type 1 diabetes: A narrative review. *IDOSR Journal of Applied Sciences.* https://www.semanticscholar.org/paper/c437aeadd2062d09ba0c94758ba4b4ae4a923a5e (accessed on 11th June 2025).

19. Ewers, B., Blond, M. B., Bruun, J. M., & Vilsbøll, T. (2024). Comparing the effectiveness of different dietary educational approaches for carbohydrate counting on glycemic control in adults with type 1 diabetes: Findings from the DIET-CARB Study, a randomized controlled trial. *Nutrients, 16.* https://www.semanticscholar.org/paper/b4360b6904000b7abadd2341b322e3fb010be8bf (accessed on 11th June 2025).

20. Frank, J. R., Son, D., Szafranski, K., & Poon, Y. (2024). Continuous glucose monitoring for self-management of diabetes in people living with type 2 diabetes mellitus on basal insulin therapy: A microsimulation model and cost-effectiveness analysis from a US perspective with relevance to Medicaid. *Journal of Managed Care & Specialty Pharmacy.* https://www.semanticscholar.org/paper/4cd2ac2da15f4d09377f2694fe534e806180597d (accessed on 11th June 2025).

21. Gauthier, A. K., Sims-Kastelein, K., Takach, M., & Kaye, N. (2010). Strengthening primary and chronic care: State innovations to transform and link small practices. https://core.ac.uk/download/71355266.pdf (accessed on 11th June 2025).

22. Gkrinia, E. M. M., & Belančić, A. (2025). A narrative review on the risk factors and healthcare disparities of type 2 diabetes. *Diabetology.* https://www.semanticscholar.org/paper/dbdf8289a9268b0b26711222311d46e8a2984746 (accessed on 11th June 2025).

23. Harris, L., Lean, M. E. J., Leslie, W. S., Taylor, R., et al. (2017). Weight losses with low energy formula diets in obese patients with and without type 2 diabetes: Systematic review and meta-analysis. https://core.ac.uk/download/77600838.pdf (accessed on 11th June 2025).

24. Hughes, A., Eastwood, S. V., Tillin, T., & Chaturvedi, N. (2022). Antihypertensive medication use and its effects on blood pressure and hemodynamics in a tri-ethnic population cohort:

Southall and Brent Revisited (SABRE). *Frontiers in Cardiovascular Medicine, 8.* https://www.semanticscholar.org/paper/a58105d285ea43ac5a784e5bec5673d1d3ada36a (accessed on 11th June 2025).

25. Jamali, Y. A., Pechuho, T., Ali, M., & Mughal, A. A. (2025). Association of risk factors with diabetes mellitus in rural areas of Nawabshah City: A case-control study. *Journal of Health, Wellness and Community Research.* https://www.semanticscholar.org/paper/dc0b4b6fe6ea26514d562432ea24aaef0f17c75a (accessed on 11th June 2025).

26. Kahraman, N. C., Baran, G. K., Celik, O. Y., Aslanova, S., Mehrasa, I. O. U., Gurer, D. M., Çağlar, A., et al. (2025). Utility of maternal A1c measurement in the second trimester for the diagnosis of gestational diabetes mellitus. *BMC Pregnancy and Childbirth, 25.* https://www.semanticscholar.org/paper/276e8f867a924a14c0f482360a7150a14694c030 (accessed on 11th June 2025).

27. Kasture, S., Mondkar, S. A., Khadilkar, A., Gondhalekar, K., Sethi, A., & Khadilkar, V. (2024). Dynamic muscle function parameters in Indian children and adolescents with type 1 diabetes mellitus: A case-control study. *Indian Journal of Endocrinology and Metabolism, 28*, 201–207. https://www.semanticscholar.org/paper/64ae5c83cc0a5a23734fff6d924ef82d146e8112 (accessed on 11th June 2025).

28. Manungkalit, M., & Sari, N. P. (2019). Predictors of post prandial glucose level in diabetic elderly. https://media.neliti.com/media/publications/300706-predictors-of-post-prandial-glucose-leve-3dbe36d0.pdf (accessed on 11th June 2025).

29. McCarthy, D., & Mueller, K. (2009). Organizing for higher performance: Case studies of organized delivery systems. https://core.ac.uk/download/71353606.pdf (accessed on 11th June 2025).

30. McCarthy, D., Wrenn, J., & Mueller, K. (2009). Geisinger Health System: Achieving the potential of system integration through innovation, leadership, measurement, and incentives. https://core.ac.uk/download/71351432.pdf (accessed on 11th June 2025).

31. Mitchell, S. E., Kallen, M. A., Troost, J. P., De La Cruz, B. A., Bragg, A., Martin-Howard, J., Moldovan, I. A., et al. (2024). Four new patient-reported outcome measures examining health-seeking behavior in persons with type 2 diabetes mellitus (REDD-CAT): Instrument development study. *JMIR Diabetes, 9.* https://www.semanticscholar.org/paper/b140631db4d717e0f115bf1c959fbc845c2c1bf8 (accessed on 11th June 2025).

32. Naweed, A., & Chapman, J. (2015). Health initiatives to target obesity in surface transport industries: Review and implications for action. https://core.ac.uk/download/pdf/30671333.pdf (accessed on 11th June 2025).

33. Pasupathi, P., Rao, Y. Y., Farook, J., Subramaniyam, S., Ponnusha, B. S., & Ambika, A. (2011). The combinational effect of cardiac and biochemical markers in diabetic patients with cardiovascular disease. *International Journal of Current Biomedical and Medical Sciences.* https://core.ac.uk/download/pdf/14681.pdf (accessed on 11th June 2025).

34. Podadera-Herreros, A., Arenas-de Larriva, A. P., Gutierrez-Mariscal, F., Alcalá-Díaz, J., Ojeda-Rodríguez, A., Rodríguez-Cantalejo, F., Cardelo, M., et al. (2024). Mediterranean diet as a strategy for preserving kidney function in patients with coronary heart disease with type 2 diabetes and obesity: A secondary analysis of CORDIOPREV randomized controlled trial. *Nutrition & Diabetes, 14.* https://www.semanticscholar.org/paper/676284cbcdf6daeebfb40fbc8be1e8a301093565 (accessed on 11th June 2025).

35. Rein, A., DeCoudres, B., Fairbrother, G., Kennedy, H., Sabharwal, R., & Singer Cohen, R. (2012). Evaluation design and technical assistance opportunities: Early findings from the Beacon Community Program evaluation teams. https://core.ac.uk/download/71358114.pdf (accessed on 11th June 2025).

36. Rodriguez, P., San Martin, V. T., & Pantalone, K. (2024). Therapeutic inertia in the management of type 2 diabetes: A narrative review. *Diabetes Therapy, 15*, 567–583. https://www.semanticscholar.org/paper/0459f1784e58febe67a9d6509cbb8c803407e893 (accessed on 11th June 2025).

37. Sindi, F., Pabuti, A., & Rini, E. A. (2023). The relationship between metabolic control status and microalbuminuria in pediatric diabetes mellitus patients at Dr. M. Djamil General Hospital, Padang, Indonesia. *Bio Scientia Medicina: Journal of Biomedicine and Translational Research.* https://www.semanticscholar.org/paper/4b0e1cff3ba8768fe7cd40b492cefdbce4812cff (accessed on 11th June 2025).

38. Thalia, O. P. (2025). Impact of continuous glucose monitoring (CGM) vs self-monitoring of blood glucose (SMBG) on glycemic control in adolescents with type 1 diabetes. *IDOSR Journal of Scientific Research.* https://www.semanticscholar.org/paper/ed8589c1db72cde75fcf8713dfceb0e495d94c22 (accessed on 11th June 2025).

39. Thielman, L. (2019). The impact of a school-based program on diabetes and cardiovascular risk factors. https://core.ac.uk/download/215463837.pdf (accessed on 11th June 2025).

40. Umegaki, H. (2024). Management of older adults with diabetes mellitus: Perspective from geriatric medicine. *Journal of Diabetes Investigation, 15*, 1347–1354. https://www.semanticscholar.org/paper/8cede7a7293660b6034a0c3a1c3782c77c729372 (accessed on 11th June 2025).

41. Wendel, C., Hills, G., & Borgonovi, V. (2012). Shared value in emerging markets: How multinational corporations are redefining business strategies to reach poor or vulnerable populations. https://core.ac.uk/download/71360050.pdf (accessed on 11th June 2025).

42. Yeh, Y., Yen, F., & Hwu, C. (2023). Diet and exercise are a fundamental part of comprehensive care for type 2 diabetes. *Journal of Diabetes Investigation, 14*, 936–939. https://www.semanticscholar.org/paper/653167f8b211bf19df461600dbbb84eb420c8044 (accessed on 11th June 2025).

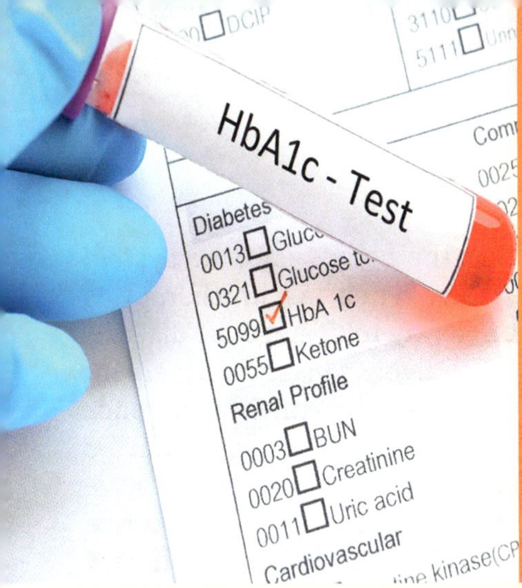

Chapter 7

MANAGEMENT OF TYPE 1 DIABETES

Contents

Introduction

The management of Type 1 Diabetes (T1D) represents a multifaceted challenge that impacts not only physiological health but also psychological well-being. Since there are many adolescents with T1D, we should be aware of the unique ways to manage their condition. A good way to manage diabetes is to regulate blood sugar, choose a proper diet, use insulin, and seek support from others. Significantly, studies show that adolescents with T1D tend to face heightened psychosocial stressors, for instance, parent-child conflict and the need for increased independence, that make disease care challenging (Ellis et al., 2016). Moreover, current research highlights gender disparities in the management of cardiovascular risk factors, emphasizing an urgent need for gendered strategies that consider sex differences (Aguayo et al., 2024). Overall, these facts indicate that a comprehensive strategy is needed to manage T1D throughout the years.

7.1. Insulin Therapy

The main reason for using insulin therapy in Type 1 diabetes is that the body's immune system attacks and destroys pancreatic beta cells, leaving no insulin available. When insulin therapy is combined with strong diabetes education, patients often improve their ability to manage the disease. For instance, a study indicated that diabetes education contributes positively to self-management and insulin-making skills, underscoring its essential role in enhancing patient treatment adherence and clinical outcomes (Elif Ünsal Avdal et al., 2024). In addition, insulin in the treatment helps maintain blood sugar levels and prevents major problems caused by diabetes. Notably, comprehensive management protocols, such as self-monitoring of blood glucose, have been found to be effective in both elderly and non-elderly patients, highlighting the therapy's broad applicability and efficacy in various demographic groups (Sugihara et al., 2013) (Figure 7.1).

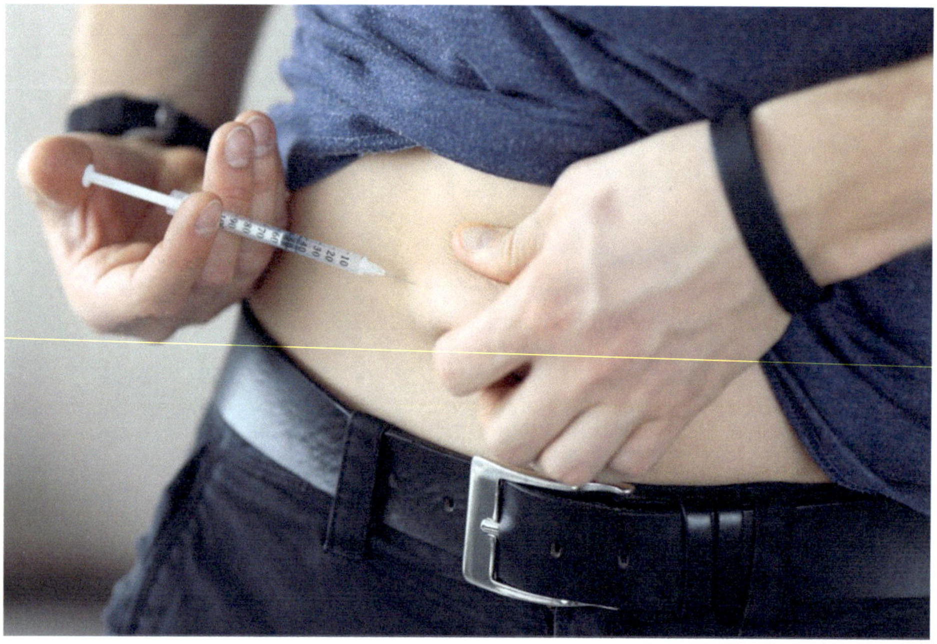

Figure 7.1. Insulin therapy serves as a cornerstone in the management of Type 1 diabetes, primarily due to the autoimmune destruction of pancreatic beta cells that leads to absolute insulin deficiency.

Source: https://www.pharmacyplanet.com/media/wysiwyg/type-1-diabetes.jpeg

7.1.1. Types of Insulin Available

To manage Type 1 diabetes well, it is important to know all the different types of insulin available. Insulin is sorted into four groups depending on how quickly it works: rapid-acting, short-acting, intermediate-acting, and long-acting. When a rapid-acting insulin such as insulin aspart is used, it works fast and is usually given before meals to control high blood sugar after meals. Long-acting insulins, like insulin detemir and insulin glargine, provide a steady basal insulin level and are administered once daily or twice daily, thus facilitating better overall metabolic control (Amiel et al., 2017). Additionally, the choice of insulin regimen may impact patient outcomes; for example, insulin detemir administered twice daily has shown the highest cost-effectiveness in long-term studies (Amiel et al., 2017). In addition, poor blood sugar control before surgery can cause blood sugar problems during the procedure, which is why it is important to give insulin based on the patient's needs (Figure 7.2).

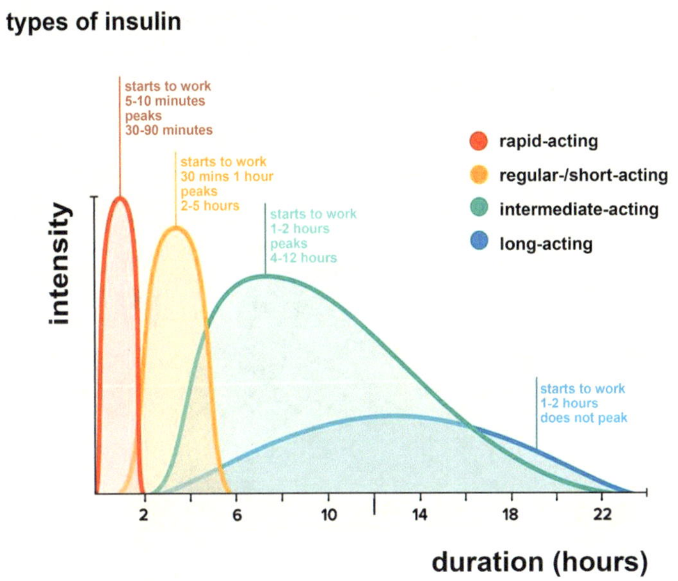

Figure 7.2. Insulin can be categorized into various types based on their duration of action: rapid-acting, short-acting, intermediate-acting, and long-acting.

Source: https://i0.wp.com/images-prod.healthline.com/hlcmsresource/images/topic_centers/2019-3/11371-types-of-insulin-1296x960-body.jpg?w=1155&h=2016

7.1.2. Insulin Delivery Methods (Injections, Pumps)

Effective management of Type 1 diabetes (T1DM) often hinges on the choice of insulin delivery method, with multiple daily injections (MDIs) and insulin pumps being the predominant options. Many people use MDIs because they are flexible, but studies have shown that insulin pumps might offer better control of blood sugar. For instance, one trial demonstrated that those using pumps experienced a significant reduction in glycated hemoglobin (HbA1c) levels compared to MDI users, although the overall cost-effectiveness of pumps remains contentious (Amiel et al., 2017). Additionally, insulin delivery systems are advancing, with continuous glucose monitoring (CGM) technologies helping to improve the accuracy in dosing insulin and patient outcomes. The potential advantages of CGMs are promising, but limitations such as cost and ease of use limit their adoption (Bergenstal et al., 2017). Patients have to decide between injections and pumps by considering their needs, daily habits, and how they would like to control their diabetes.

7.1.3. Importance of Insulin Dosing

Taking the right amount of insulin is very important for Type 1 Diabetes, since it affects blood sugar levels and the chances of complications. To give the right dose, you should look at blood sugar, the amount of carbohydrates eaten, and how much exercise is done. Continuous glucose monitoring

(CGM) systems have enhanced the management of Type 1 Diabetes by providing real-time data, which aids in determining appropriate insulin dosages to prevent hypo- or hyperglycemic episodes (Facchinetti, 2016). Moreover, studies have demonstrated that specific insulin regimens, such as insulin detemir, can optimize outcomes, offering significant improvements in quality-adjusted life years (QALYs) and overall cost-effectiveness compared to other insulin therapies (Amiel et al., 2017). So, using the right insulin for each patient is good for their health and demonstrates why different treatments are needed for diabetes (Figure 7.3).

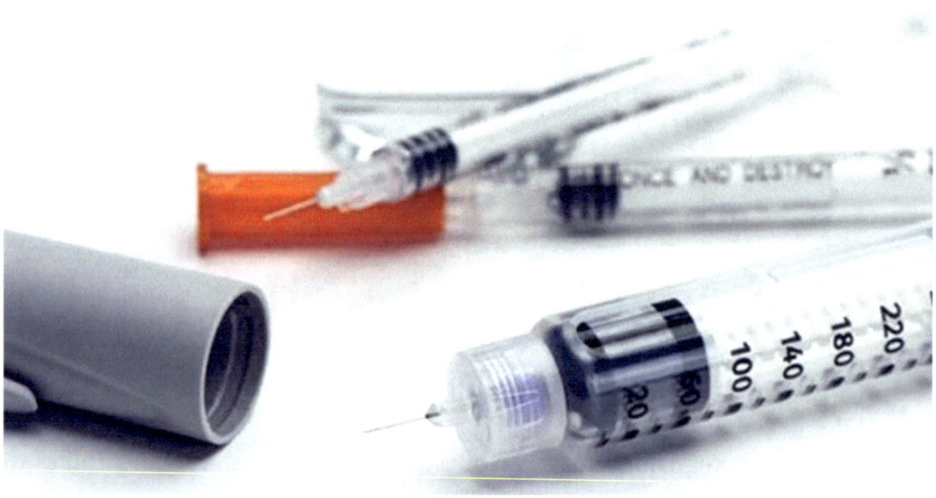

Figure 7.3. Accurate dosing requires careful consideration of various factors, including blood glucose levels, carbohydrate intake, and physical activity.

Source: https://glucare.health/wp-content/uploads/2024/07/Blog-banner.jpg

7.1.4. Monitoring Blood Glucose Levels

Blood glucose monitoring is very important for people with Type 1 diabetes, especially when they are physically active. Regularly assessing blood glucose helps in identifying patterns that may emerge due to varying exercise intensities, as research indicates that different exercises affect glucose levels distinctly; for instance, moderate-intensity aerobic exercise typically reduces blood glucose, while vigorous exercise may induce a spike (Zaharieva et al., 2019). In addition, the incorporation of continuous glucose monitoring (CGM) technology enables real-time recording of interstitial glucose levels, offering vital information to be utilized for the modification of insulin regimens before and after physical activity in order to avoid the risk of hypoglycemia (Zaharieva et al., 2019). Overall, employing an individualized method of managing blood sugar and being attentive to it enables individuals with diabetes to exercise safely and enhances their sports life and performance.

7.1.5. Adjusting Insulin Based on Food Intake

For type 1 diabetes to be managed well, insulin dosages should be adjusted according to the amount of carbohydrates eaten and how they affect blood sugar. The amount of insulin needed by a person changes because foods and their timing can be different, and everyone's metabolism is different. As an example, a meal with lots of complex carbohydrates may call for a different insulin dose than one with lots of simple sugars, which is why recent studies stress the importance of adjusting insulin based on the type of carbs. Also, controlling both what is eaten and insulin doses is important for avoiding complications, since well-managed blood sugar can help stop or delay diabetic nephropathy. As diabetes management continues to intersect with dietary innovation, implementing effective behavioral and nutritional strategies will remain instrumental in enhancing patient outcomes and promoting sustained metabolic health (Ambrosiadou et al., 2000; Iacobini et al., 2017) (Figure 7.4).

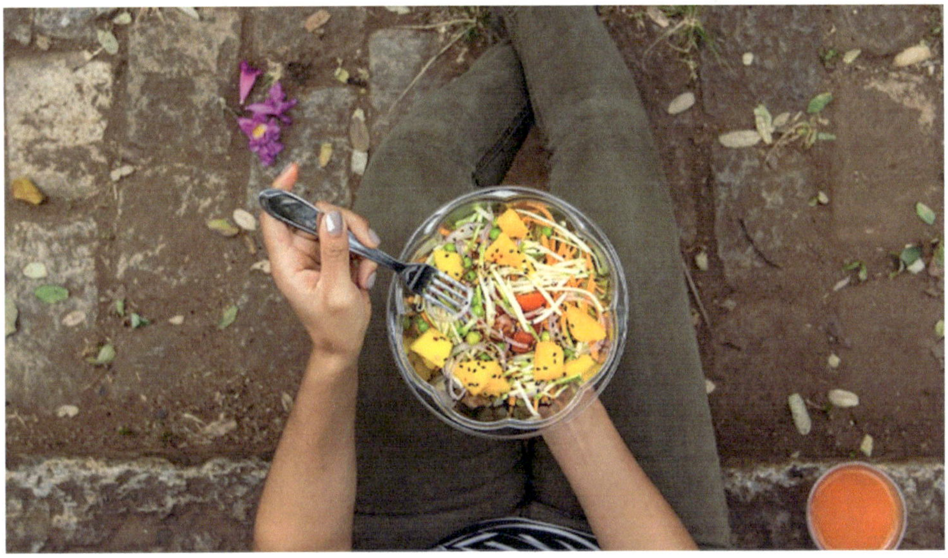

Figure 7.4. Effective management of type 1 diabetes necessitates precise adjustments in insulin dosages based on food intake, underscoring the importance of understanding carbohydrate ratios and glycemic responses.

Source: https://i0.wp.com/post.healthline.com/wp-content/uploads/2020/12/Walmart_Type-1-Diabetes-Diet.jpg?w=1155&h=1528

7.1.6. Managing Insulin During Exercise

For those with type 1 diabetes, exercise brings both benefits and difficulties, mainly when it comes to insulin management. Doing physical activity can change how insulin works in the body and may cause blood glucose levels to change, so people with diabetes should adjust their insulin doses to avoid hypoglycemia. Strategies, for example, reducing basal insulin delivery before, during, and after exercise, as reported by McAuley and colleagues, could optimize glucose control and reduce the risk of hypoglycemic events (Thabit et al., 2016). It is also suggested to include supplementary intake of carbohydrates before the exercise to normalize blood glucose levels during the performance of the activity (Błaszczak et al., 2024). Because athletes can monitor their glucose levels all the time, they can choose the right insulin dose while they are exercising. For this reason, adjusting insulin based on a person's needs and knowing how exercise affects the body are important for managing diabetes.

7.1.7. Risks of Insulin Therapy (Hypoglycemia, etc.)

Managing Type 1 Diabetes by using insulin can be dangerous, mainly because hypoglycemia is a serious risk for patients. Hypoglycemia is commonly mentioned as a reason why patients find it hard to control their blood sugar, and severe episodes can increase the risk of major heart problems, eye diseases, and death. In fact, insulin treatment is a notable predictor of hypoglycemia, leading to symptomatic episodes that can occur as frequently as twice a week in the context of Type 1 diabetes (Castaneda et al., 2016). Moreover, patients who experience recurrent hypoglycemic events may develop defective counter-regulation, diminishing their ability to recognize such episodes, which can be life-threatening (Castaneda et al., 2016). As the intensity of insulin dosage increases to achieve glycemic targets, the risks for adverse events such as weight gain and hypoglycemia heighten, calling for careful monitoring and patient education in the implementation of insulin therapy (Castaneda et al., 2016) (Figure 7.5).

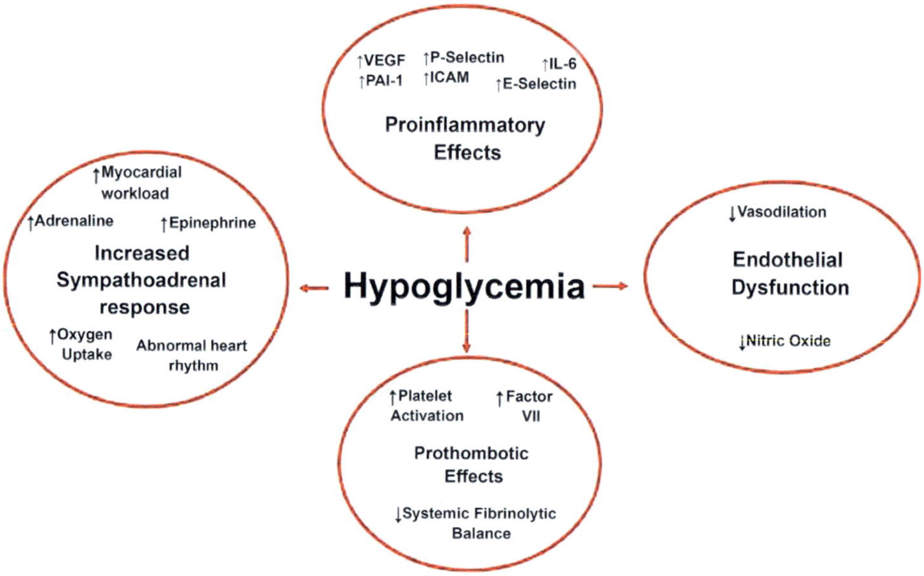

Figure 7.5. Hypoglycemia is often cited as a rate-limiting factor that hinders patients from achieving optimal glycemic control, with severe episodes linked to an increased risk of major macrovascular events, microvascular complications, and mortality rates.

Source: Ali AAG, Niinuma SA, Moin ASM, Atkin SL, Butler AE. The Role of Platelets in Hypoglycemia-Induced Cardiovascular Disease: A Review of the Literature. *Biomolecules.* 2023; 13(2):241. https://doi.org/10.3390/biom13020241

7.1.8. Innovations in Insulin Therapy

Thanks to new insulin treatments, people with Type 1 Diabetes find it much simpler to manage their condition. New fast-acting insulin and continuous insulin delivery systems have helped control blood sugar levels much better. For this reason, patients receive the correct amount of medicine that suits them. In addition, insulin delivery devices, including pens and smart pumps, utilize technology that allows for point-of-care glucose monitoring and computerized insulin dosing adjustments that allow for enhanced patient self-management (Curtis et al., 2006). A recent innovation in the field is the advancement of inpatient-patient-managed OPAT or S-OPAT, which has proven to be effective in improving self-management and lowering HbA1c levels in diabetic patients (Ganguly, 2018). All these developments help Type 1 Diabetes patients manage their health better and achieve better health results.

7.1.9. Patient Education on Insulin Management

Efficient patient education on the use of insulin is important for T1DM patients in managing their daily health care and avoiding complications. Those who are well-educated about insulin therapy, how much to administer, when to take it, and what types are available can choose what is best for them. Recent technological progress, including continuous glucose monitoring and new forms of insulin preparations, reinforces the value of incorporating technology into educational programs to enable more effective self-management behavior and increased metabolic control (Association et al., 2018). In addition, organized education programs may help to confront obstacles confronted by patients, including the fear of taking insulin and dealing with rapidly changing glucose levels, consequently improving the quality of life (Aleppo et al., 2019). Education of patients by physicians regarding diabetic control prevents both low and high blood sugar (Figure 7.6).

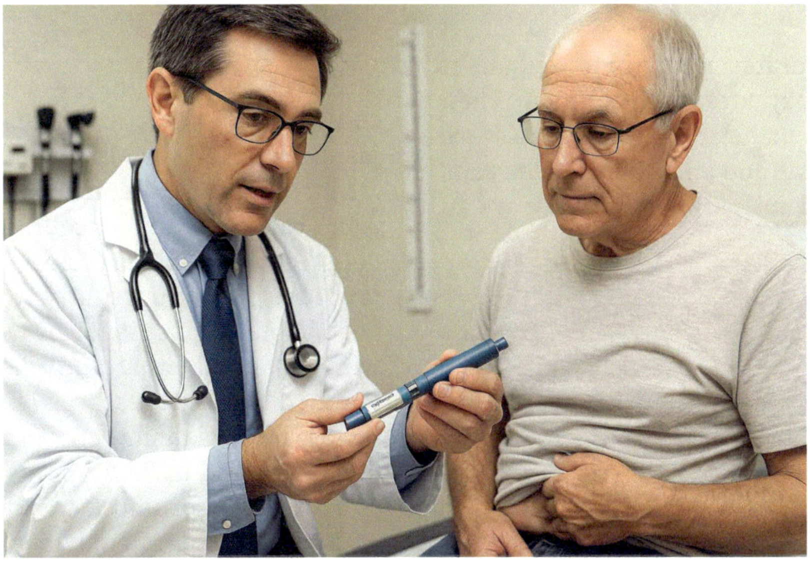

Figure 7.6. Understanding insulin therapy, including dosages, timing, and types of insulin, empowers patients to make informed decisions about their care.

Source: https://www.diabetesincontrol.com/wp-content/uploads/2025/05/compressed_insulin_glargine_image.jpg.

7.2. Nutrition and Lifestyle Management

Type 1 diabetes is best managed when nutrition and lifestyle are carefully managed, as they play a major role in blood sugar control and general health. Following a diet high in nutritious foods may help individuals control their blood glucose and avoid diabetes-related complications. It is shown by studies that regular exercise helps with weight control and makes insulin work better. In addition, the success of the process is influenced by networks and healthcare professionals. For example, research indicates that nurse support is key to the success of obese and overweight patients in maintaining weight loss, says Nicky Kim (Kime et al., 2013). Interventions also show that culturally specific interventions, especially among high-risk populations like postpartum Latina women, can be effective in inducing dietary and lifestyle modifications consistent with diabetes prevention strategies (Althavale et al., 2015). These broad strategies are essential for the effective management of diabetes.

7.2.1. Role of Carbohydrates in Diabetes Management

Because carbohydrates affect blood sugar, it is important to pay attention to them when managing type 1 diabetes. Carbohydrates are changed into glucose and enter the bloodstream, so it is important to know how they work to control diabetes.

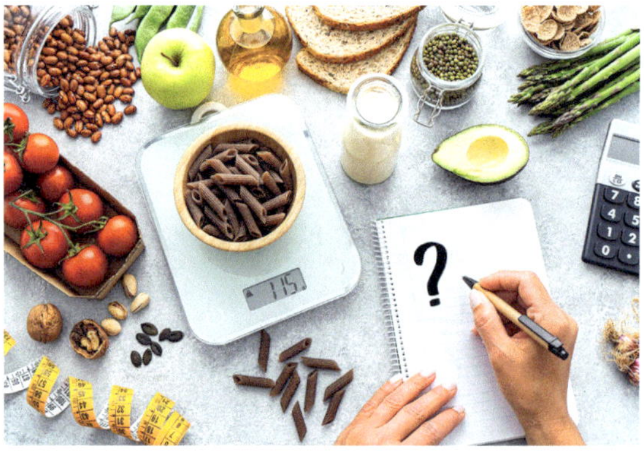

Figure 7.7. The management of type 1 diabetes necessitates a careful consideration of carbohydrate intake, as carbohydrates directly influence blood glucose levels.

Source: https://tcoyd.org/wp-content/uploads/2024/03/how-many-carbs_1100x733-1.jpg

Research indicates that consistent carbohydrate counting can aid individuals in predicting insulin needs and maintaining stable blood glucose levels, reducing the risk of complications associated with uncontrolled hyperglycemia (Rajagopal et al., 2023). Additionally, dietary education regarding the types and sources of carbohydrates can empower patients to make healthier choices, contributing to overall nutrition and diabetes control (Bentzen et al., 2016). To achieve the best health results, people with type 1 diabetes should manage their carbohydrates, since this helps them give the right amount of insulin and control their blood sugar levels (Figure 7.7).

7.2.2. Meal Planning and Carbohydrate Counting

Effective meal planning and carbohydrate counting are essential components in the management of Type 1 Diabetes (T1DM), as they facilitate better glycemic control. When people count carbs, they are encouraged to watch their daily food intake very closely. This approach provides an opportunity to achieve near-normal blood glucose levels while coordinating with insulin therapy and physical activity, as outlined in recent research (Abdelghaffar et al., 2015). Meal planning encourages a structured diet that aligns with personal preferences and lifestyle, promoting nutritional balance without sacrificing enjoyment, which is often a challenge in managing T1DM (Kubbe et al., 2019). As a result, using these approaches helps control metabolism and also improves patients' knowledge about what to eat. To summarize, using meal planning and carbohydrate counting is important for the health of people with T1DM now and in the future.

7.2.3. Importance of a Balanced Diet

Taking care of Type 1 diabetes mainly depends

on having a nutritious diet. A proper diet plan helps manage blood sugar and also prevents serious problems linked to the disease. People with Type 1 diabetes need to eat foods that are rich in nutrients and avoid those that contain a lot of refined sugar and unhealthy fat. According to (Ghazeeri et al., 2021), a balanced intake of carbohydrates, proteins, and healthy fats is vital, particularly since high glycemic index foods can worsen insulin sensitivity and increase diabetes-related risks. Furthermore, research highlights that the management of obesity, often a co-morbidity in diabetic patients, requires adherence to a hypocaloric diet emphasizing balanced macronutrient distribution to mitigate health risks (Busetto et al., 2015). For this reason, a well-planned diet is necessary for people with Type 1 diabetes to maintain their health and enjoy a better quality of life (Figure 7.8).

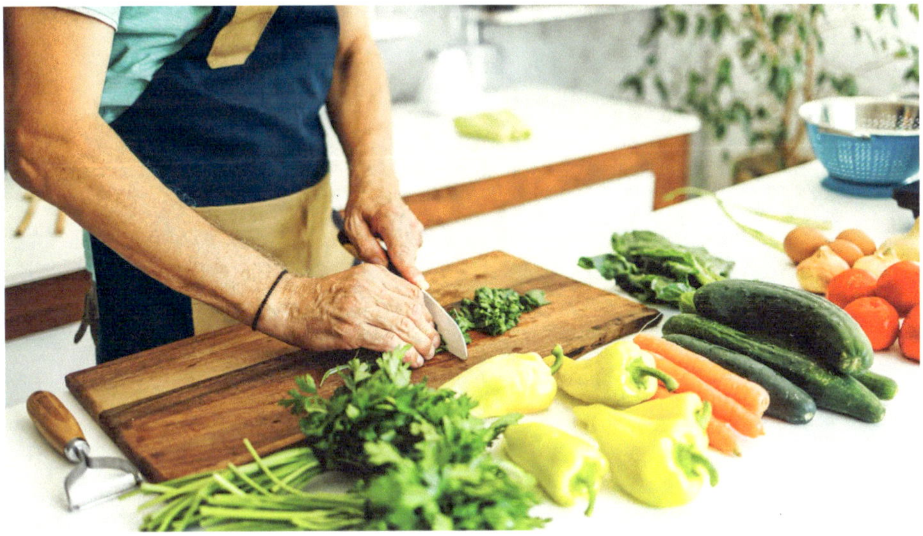

Figure 7.8. A well-structured dietary plan not only aids in controlling blood glucose levels but also plays a crucial role in preventing long-term complications associated with the condition.

Source: https://images.everydayhealth.com/images/diet-nutrition/what-to-eat-when-you-have-hiv-00-intro-alt-1440x810.jpg

7.2.4. Impact of Physical Activity on Blood Sugar

People with Type 1 diabetes should make exercise a regular habit, as it greatly affects their blood sugar. Being active improves how the body uses insulin, which may result in better control of blood sugar. The American Diabetes Association suggests that people with diabetes exercise moderately for at least 150 minutes a week to achieve good health results. Taking part in this amount of physical activity is good for your weight and also improves your heart, muscles, and bones. Furthermore, studies indicate that structured exercise regimens positively affect hemoglobin A1c (HbA1c) levels, demonstrating the long-term benefits of physical fitness in diabetes management (Petrovic et al., 2015). With regular exercise routines, like Pilates or other moderate exercises, individuals living with Type 1 diabetes gain increased autonomy and better metabolic control, ultimately leading to a healthier lifestyle (Randall et al., 2016).

7.2.5. Strategies for Healthy Eating

Taking care of Type 1 diabetes requires following healthy eating strategies, which play a big role in controlling blood sugar and a person's well-being. To follow a diabetes-friendly diet, you should eat more whole foods, fruits, vegetables, lean proteins, and whole grains and less of the processed foods that contain a lot of sugar and unhealthy fats. Tailored interventions can enhance adherence to these dietary recommendations, as evidenced by programmatic efforts aimed at postpartum populations, such as STAR MAMA, which integrates health literacy and culturally relevant strategies to promote dietary changes among women with a history of gestational diabetes (Althavale et al., 2015). Furthermore, recognizing the specific constraints of working irregular shifts, such as nights, conveys the need for tailored eating strategies that overcome specific healthy eating barriers (D'Annibale et al., 2022). They instruct Type 1 diabetes patients to choose foods suitable for them (Figure 7.9).

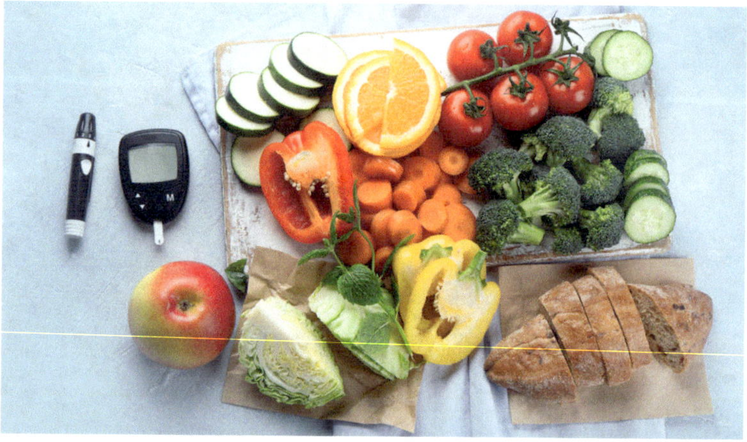

Figure 7.9. Effective management of Type 1 diabetes necessitates incorporating strategic approaches to healthy eating, which significantly influence glycemic control and overall well-being.

Source: https://makingindiaheartstrong.com/wp-content/uploads/2024/03/shutterstock_1711155652.jpg

7.2.6. Managing Diabetes During Social Events

It can be hard for people with Type 1 diabetes to manage social events, since the food served and the routine can change, which can cause their blood glucose levels to vary. When managing such occasions, it is important to prepare ahead and watch blood sugar levels to determine the right amount of insulin for the coming meal. Moreover, people can help their friends understand diabetes, which can lead to a supportive atmosphere and less pressure when eating. Participating in discussions surrounding non-severe nocturnal hypoglycemic events (NSNHEs) reveals that these instances greatly affect patients' daily functioning, suggesting that awareness and preparation can mitigate their impact during gatherings (Pohlman et al., 2012). Additionally, maintaining good glycemic control not only enhances participation in social events but also promotes overall psychological well-being, encouraging increased adherence to dietary and exercise routines in diverse social contexts (Harrison et al., 2020).

7.2.7. Importance of Hydration

Drinking enough water is vital for Type 1 diabetes patients because it helps control their body's functions and health. It is important to drink enough fluids, since diabetes may damage the body's circulatory and renal systems. Water serves as a calorie-free alternative to sugar-sweetened beverages, which are linked to weight gain and increased insulin resistance, further complicating diabetes management (Deguara et al., 2016). In addition, not drinking enough fluids can result in hyperglycemia, a situation that is harmful for blood sugar control and might make diabetic complications worse if ignored. As a result, choosing water instead of sugary drinks helps people stay hydrated and follow a healthy lifestyle that is necessary for managing diabetes. Addressing hydration in educational contexts, such as schools, can be instrumental in promoting better health outcomes for children with Type 1 diabetes, emphasizing the necessity of preventive strategies (Poldermans et al., 2009) (Figure 7.10).

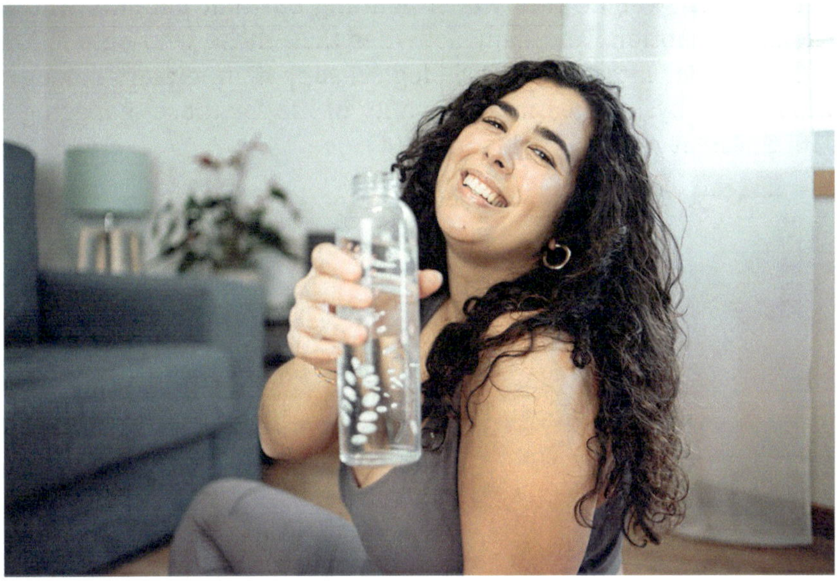

Figure 7.10. Hydration plays a critical role in the management of Type 1 diabetes, impacting both metabolic control and overall health.

Source: https://i0.wp.com/health.umms.org/wp-content/uploads/2023/02/Diabetes-Hydration_1200.jpg?fit=1100%2C733&ssl=1

7.2.8. Role of Dietary Supplements

In managing Type 1 diabetes, taking dietary supplements can be very important for controlling metabolism and promoting good health. It is shown that certain oral nutritional supplements can lead to better postprandial effects, mainly by affecting blood sugar and insulin levels. For instance, a study highlighted that oral diabetes-specific nutritional supplements demonstrated lower glycemic index values and reduced insulin area under the curve when compared to standard formula options, suggesting their potential utility in enhancing postprandial glucose regulation (Angarita Dávila et al., 2019). Furthermore, the interplay between dietary protein and fiber is essential, as both macronutrients independently modulate insulin-mediated glucose control, which is a critical aspect of Type 1 diabetes management. Although higher protein and fiber combinations did not yield significant improvements in postprandial glucose responses in some trials, enhancing dietary fiber remains a vital consideration in supplement strategies to better manage this chronic condition (Amankwaah et al., 2017).

7.2.9. Psychological Aspects of Dietary Management

Looking into the psychological side of dietary management in people with Type 1 Diabetes shows that there is a link between mental health and proper self-care. Because they must be very careful with their diet, many people feel anxious and stressed, mainly about what to eat and checking their blood sugar. Since people with diabetes face strong emotions, this can sometimes make it hard for them to stick to their treatment plan. According to studies, dealing with these psychosocial issues matters, as a large number of those severely obese had anxiety and depression, which influenced their efforts to manage their weight. It is worth pointing out that patients who had surgery had better results in terms of emotions and daily activities than those who only followed a diet. Such findings highlight the need for integrated psychological support in dietary management strategies, ultimately enhancing both physical health and quality of life for those managing Type 1 Diabetes (Kumar et al., 2010; Azran et al., 2017) (Figure 7.11).

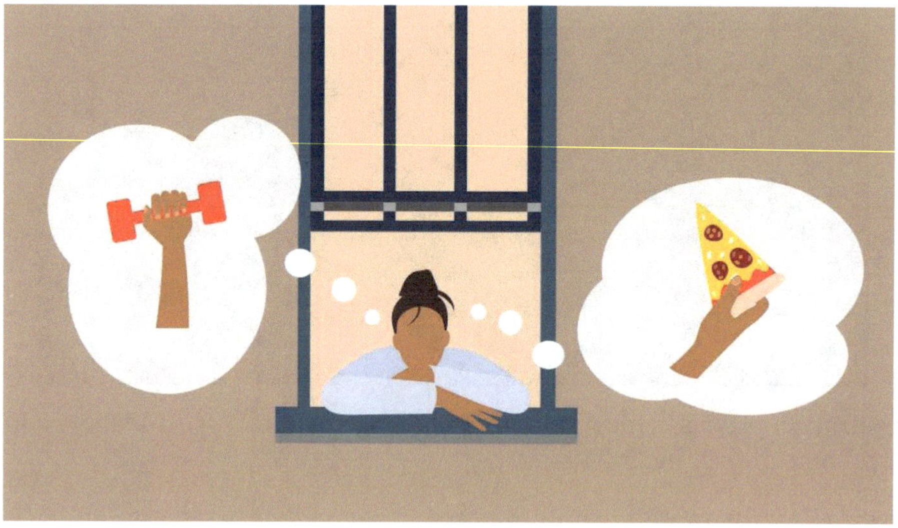

Figure 7.11. Exploring the psychological aspects of dietary management in individuals with Type 1 Diabetes reveals a complex interplay between mental well-being and effective self-care practices.

Source: https://assets.clevelandclinic.org/transform/LargeFeatureImage/e42ce2b2-3123-4158-8ff8-4a0ef3134614/bored-person-exercise-eat-1213399274

7.3. Monitoring and Technology

Since taking care of Type 1 diabetes patients is crucial, monitoring devices are important to help them achieve good outcomes. Continuous glucose monitoring (CGM) and intermittently scanned continuous glucose monitoring (isCGM) systems have transformed how individuals manage their glycemic levels, enabling real-time data tracking that informs immediate decision-making regarding insulin doses and dietary adjustments. It is good to use these technologies while exercising, since they help control diabetes and blood sugar. However, the complexity of CGM systems often poses challenges for both patients and healthcare professionals in interpreting the data effectively (Moser et al., 2020). Additionally, advancements in glucose monitoring technology contribute to improved quality of care and cost-effectiveness, addressing the broader diabetes epidemic in the United States (Ashworth et al., 2016). As a result, even though some issues remain, these new technologies make it simpler to deal with Type 1 diabetes.

7.3.1. Importance of Regular Blood Glucose Monitoring

Effective management of Type 1 diabetes depends on regular testing of blood glucose levels, which greatly affects the health outcomes of people with this condition in the long run. Regular testing of blood glucose allows patients to notice how their insulin, diet, and exercise affect them, helping them make suitable changes to their treatment plans.

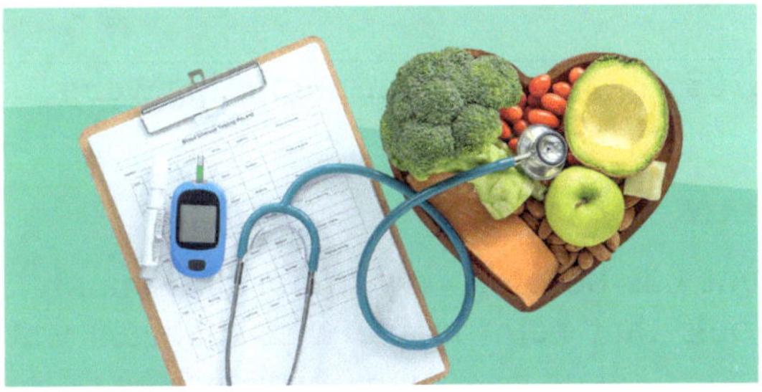

Figure 7.12. By routinely assessing blood glucose levels, patients can better understand their response to insulin therapy, dietary changes, and physical activity, enabling personalized adjustments to their management plans.

Source: https://www.singlecare.com/blog/wp-content/uploads/2020/10/Blog_110420_Living_with_diabetes.png

Thus, people can avoid sudden issues caused by blood sugar levels and lower their chances of suffering from significant diabetes-related issues. Furthermore, data indicate disparities in diabetes management across different population groups, highlighting the need for accessible monitoring resources (Diamant et al., 2003). Despite advancements in diabetes care, many individuals struggle to maintain optimal control, emphasizing the importance of tailored interventions and support systems (Anto et al., 2007). Monitoring blood sugar levels is important for diabetes patients to handle their condition and live well (Figure 7.12).

7.3.2. Continuous Glucose Monitoring Systems

In the context of managing Type 1 Diabetes, continuous glucose monitoring (CGM) systems represent a significant advancement in diabetes care, allowing for real-time glucose tracking and improved metabolic control. It is easier for patients to choose insulin and new habits because these systems constantly check blood sugar, unlike glucometers that only do it occasionally. Moreover, the integration of CGM with technologies like continuous subcutaneous insulin infusion (CSII) has shown promise in reducing hypoglycemic episodes and improving overall quality of life. Research indicates that such technological integration can provide better glycemic control, particularly for individuals with high baseline HbA1c and frequent hypoglycemia (Hovorka et al., 2015). However, it is also crucial to note that CGM accuracy can be compromised during exercise, which poses challenges for effective diabetes management during physical activity (Bondía Company et al., 2021). Therefore, although CGMs are very helpful, their weaknesses should be recognized and dealt with in medical care.

7.3.3. Use of Insulin Pumps and Smart Pens

With insulin pumps and smart pens, people living with Type 1 diabetes can now receive insulin more accurately, which leads to better health results. Insulin pumps infuse insulin under the skin all the time and make adjustments automatically, while smart insulin pens have calculators and memory to help people stick to the right doses. The integration of these devices with Continuous Glucose Monitoring (CGM) systems further amplifies their effectiveness, as evidenced by recent studies highlighting improved glycemic control and patient engagement in self-management behaviors. For instance, the transition from multiple daily injections to smart insulin pen systems has shown beneficial effects, such as decreasing mean glucose levels and increasing Time In Range, thus facilitating better overall diabetes management (Pantanetti et al., 2025; Singh et al., 2025). Thanks to this technology, patients can be more involved in looking after their diabetes (Figure 7.13).

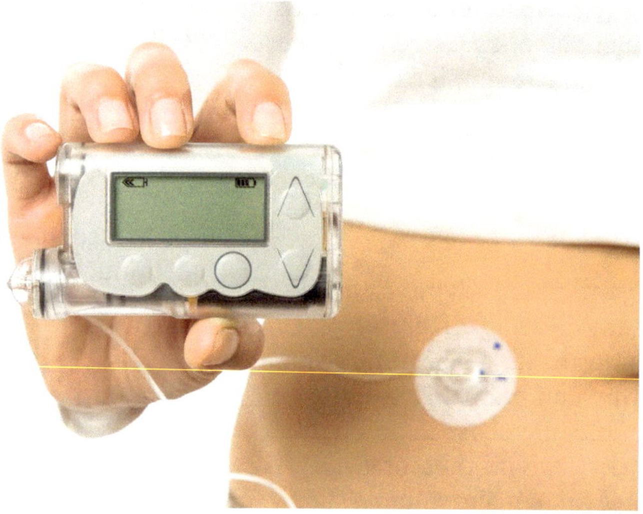

Figure 7.13. Insulin pumps offer continuous subcutaneous insulin infusion, allowing for dynamic adjustments based on real-time glucose monitoring

Source: https://gluroo.com/wp-content/uploads/2023/03/all-about-insulin-pumps.jpg.webp

7.3.4. Mobile Apps for Diabetes Management

The use of mobile applications in diabetes management has become very important, mainly for people with Type 1 diabetes. They provide various tools that help people with diabetes watch their health and keep track of their data. While systematic reviews have demonstrated the efficacy of mobile applications in improving glycemic control among Type 2 diabetes patients, there is a notable deficiency in data regarding their impact on Type 1 diabetes management (Carter et al., 2016). Even so, research is showing that mobile technology could greatly assist people with Type 1 diabetes in leading an active life and following their treatment plans. For example, some applications encourage regular physical activity, which is essential for maintaining optimal health in diabetic patients (Hewitt et al., 2016). Since mobile technology is advancing, we should look into how it can better manage diabetes and help patients.

7.3.5. Telehealth and Remote Monitoring

Telehealth and remote monitoring have made it much easier for patients with Type 1 diabetes to take care of their health. Such technologies allow patients to regularly talk to healthcare professionals and also help monitor blood sugar levels in real time, which supports better control of the disease. As highlighted in the literature, enabling technology can significantly expand primary care clinicians' capacity to coordinate complex care efficiently, allowing specialized consultations to be integrated within primary care settings (Nesbitt et al., 2017). Additionally, telehealth addresses critical accessibility issues faced by patients in rural and remote areas, where healthcare services are often limited due to geographical barriers (Bywood et al., 2013). Remote monitoring and telehealth allow people with Type 1 diabetes to handle their condition well and enjoy a better quality of life (Figure 7.14).

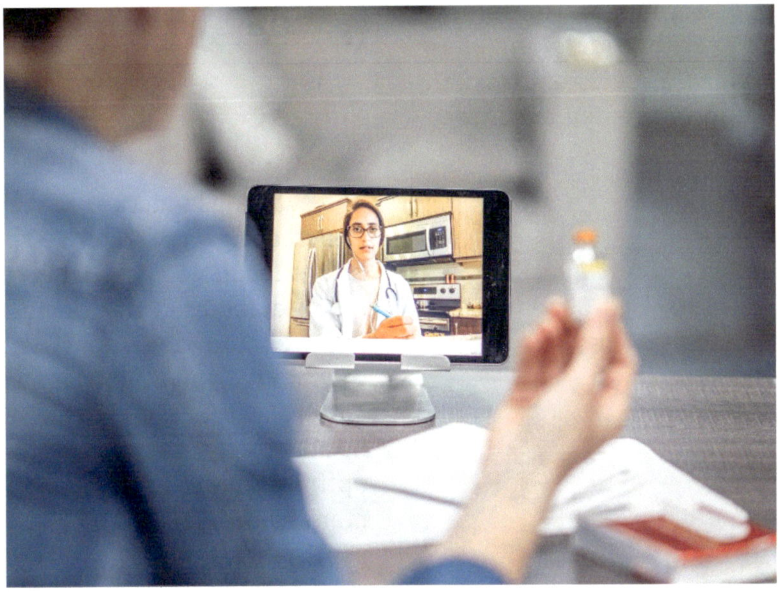

Figure 7.14. In the realm of managing Type 1 diabetes, telehealth and remote monitoring have emerged as transformative solutions, enabling patients to engage in their care with unprecedented convenience.

Source: https://www.endocrinologyadvisor.com/wp-content/uploads/sites/9/2020/04/Remote-medical-appointment_G_1219044064.jpg

7.3.6. Data Analysis for Better Management

Data analysis helps make patient care and self-management better in the management of Type 1 Diabetes. Leveraging mobile health (mHealth) technologies can provide critical insights into patients' daily glucose levels, medication adherence, and lifestyle behaviors. For instance, the use of biometric devices alongside SMS text messaging enhances communication between patients and their healthcare providers, thereby promoting active patient engagement in chronic care management (Chen et al., 2017). Additionally, self-monitoring of blood glucose has shown significant correlations to improved self-management practices; patients who engage with their data often report greater autonomy over their condition, despite facing challenges such as insufficient support from healthcare professionals (Bond et al., 2014). So, a strong data analysis framework enables patients and helps healthcare teams choose treatments that lead to better health results in those with Type 1 Diabetes.

7.3.7. Role of Wearables in Diabetes Care

Wearable technology is very useful in treating Type 1 Diabetes, helping both patients and doctors become more effective. Devices such as continuous glucose monitors (CGMs) and smart insulin pens provide real-time data, enabling users to track their glucose levels and insulin administration with unprecedented accuracy.

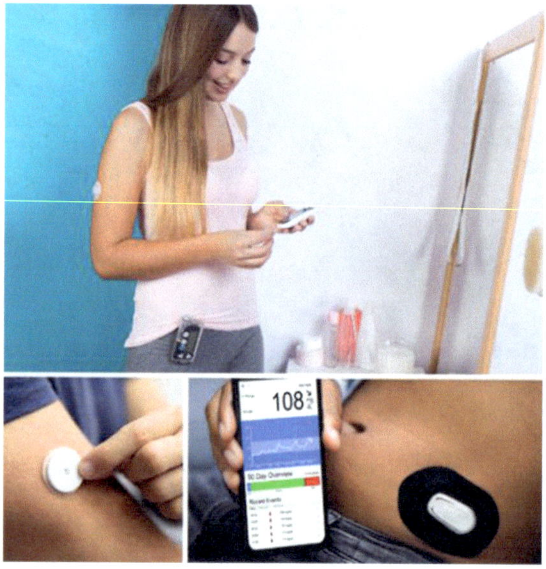

Figure 7.15. Devices such as continuous glucose monitors (CGMs) and smart insulin pens provide real-time data, enabling users to track their glucose levels and insulin administration with unprecedented accuracy.

Source: https://diabetes.org/sites/default/files/styles/large/public/2023-09/CGM-advo-L2-lady-patch-screen_0.jpg?itok=MaEStE7w.

Caring for their health makes people more aware of what they eat and how much they move each day. Furthermore, the increased transparency in health data creates opportunities for more personalized care strategies, facilitating a shift in the traditional patient-provider dynamic, wherein patients become active participants in their care journey (Gabriels et al., 2018). Despite these advantages, challenges remain, including the need for effective integration of wearable data into clinical practice and the emphasis on evidence-based content within health apps to ensure meaningful engagement (Antoniou et al., 2017). As a result, you should think ahead about using wearables to get the best outcomes (Figure 7.15).

7.3.8. Future Technologies in Diabetes Management

The evolving landscape of diabetes management is increasingly characterized by the integration of future technologies, particularly in the realm of type 1 diabetes (T1D). Using mobile applications and wearable devices in digital health is a new way to involve patients and easily monitor their blood sugar levels. These innovations are crucial in addressing the complexities of T1D, where optimal glycemic control remains elusive for many patients due to adherence issues and psychological barriers, as highlighted by recent studies (Delamater, 2017). Additionally, the gamification of diabetes management presents opportunities for patients to access personalized strategies, fostering a more proactive stance toward their health (Pancheva et al., 2024). With new technology appearing, it is important to keep researching and developing these tools so they help individuals with T1D and are easy to use.

7.3.9. Patient Engagement with Technology

The use of technology in managing Type 1 diabetes greatly improves how patients take care of themselves and stay involved. Thanks to continuous glucose monitoring systems and mobile applications, patients can monitor their blood sugar levels in real time and take part in managing their diabetes. Still, there are difficulties, mainly in making these technologies available and easy to use. Research reveals that many diabetes educators find the use of technology burdensome, indicating a fragmentation in care delivery and support (Gallagher et al., 2016). Furthermore, issues related to inadequate knowledge among healthcare providers and patients about diabetes complications often precipitate unscheduled hospital admissions, underscoring the necessity for improved patient engagement strategies (Coates et al., 2021). Doctors and nurses should improve their abilities and a good support network should be given to patients to help them make the right decisions (Figure 7.16).

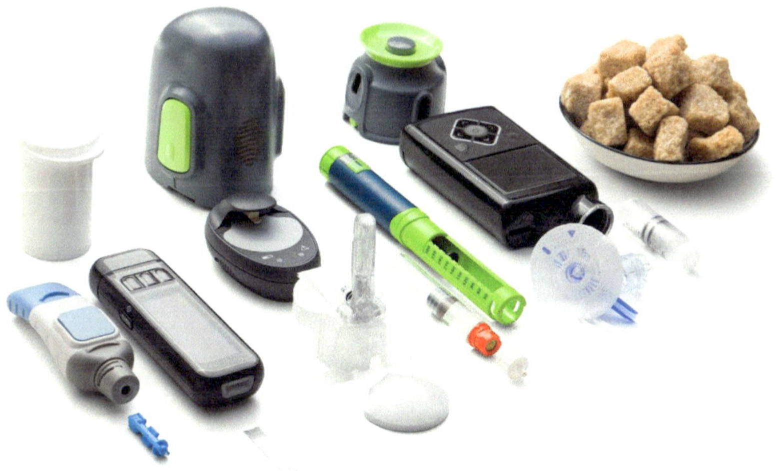

Figure 7.16. The integration of technology into the management of Type 1 diabetes represents a pivotal advancement in enhancing patient engagement and self-care.

Source: https://www.endocrine.org/-/media/endocrine/images/patient-engagement-webpage/condition-page-images/diabetes-and-glucose-metabolism/diabetes_technology_pe_1796x943.jpg

A CLOSER LOOK

POSTPRANDIAL GLUCOSE (PPG) MANAGEMENT

Postprandial glucose (PPG) management refers to controlling blood sugar levels after meals to prevent spikes that can lead to complications in people with diabetes. A person's PPG should be 180 mg/dL or less, and it usually rises 1 to 2 hours after a meal. A good way to manage diabetes is to have balanced meals, limit portion sizes, stay active, and follow the doctor's advice on taking medications or insulin. Keeping an eye on PPG is very important to avoid cardiovascular disease in people with normal fasting glucose but high glucose levels after meals.

Summary

Treating Type 1 diabetes in adolescents calls for a detailed and individualized plan that considers what they go through. Such families often deal with a lot of stress and family issues related to diabetes, which may negatively impact their health. As highlighted in recent studies, effective engagement of adolescents in their own diabetes care can lead to improved self-management and a reduction in related complications (Carroll et al., 2018). Furthermore, integrating resilience-promoting factors such as coping strategies, positive affect, and self-efficacy into nursing practice can empower these individuals, fostering a greater sense of control over their condition (Steele et al., 2019). If healthcare professionals focus on shared decision-making and psychosocial matters, they can design interventions that help patients and teens handle their new lives.

In brief, managing Type 1 Diabetes needs a mix of different strategies for proper care. This kind of management depends on giving each patient personalized insulin therapy that matches their food habits, exercise levels, and personal choices. Additionally, education and support play critical roles; for instance, support from healthcare professionals, including nurses, is crucial to help patients navigate the challenges of their condition, particularly in terms of lifestyle modifications and weight management, as evidenced by Nicky Kime's insights (Kime et al., 2013). Clinical pharmacy services can also guide patients and healthcare workers on how to control diabetes. This holistic approach not only addresses physiological aspects but also emphasizes emotional and educational support, ensuring that patients are well-equipped to handle their diabetes effectively (Biddle et al., 2014).

References

1. Abdelghaffar, S. (2015). Nutritional management of type 1 diabetes. https://core.ac.uk/download/322425193.pdf (accessed on 11th June 2025).
2. Moser, O., Riddell, M. C., Eckstein, M. L., Adolfsson, P., Rabasa-Lhoret, R., van den Boom, L., Gillard, P., Nørgaard, K., Oliver, N. S., Zaharieva, D. P., Battelino, T., de Beaufort, C., Bergenstal, R. M., Buckingham, B., Cengiz, E., Deeb, A., Heise, T., Heller, S., Kowalski, A. J., Leelarathna, L., ... Mader, J. K. (2020). Glucose management for exercise using continuous glucose monitoring (CGM) and intermittently scanned CGM (isCGM) systems in type 1 diabetes: position statement of the European Association for the Study of Diabetes (EASD) and of the International Society for Pediatric and Adolescent Diabetes (ISPAD) endorsed by JDRF and supported by the American Diabetes Association (ADA). *Diabetologia*, *63*(12), 2501–2520. https://doi.org/10.1007/s00125-020-05263-9 (accessed on 11th June 2025).
3. Aguayo, G. A., Augstein, P., Auzanneau, M., Cosson, E., et al. (2024). Sex inequalities in cardiovascular risk factors and their management in primary prevention in adults living with type 1 diabetes in Germany and France: Findings from DPV and SFDT1. https://core.ac.uk/download/652069629.pdf (accessed on 11th June 2025).
4. Aleppo, G., Fonseca, V. A., Garg, S. K., Hirsch, I. B., et al. (2019). Optimizing postprandial glucose management in adults with insulin-requiring diabetes: Report and recommendations. https://core.ac.uk/download/322802198.pdf (accessed on 11th June 2025).
5. Almeida, M., Andrade, C., da Silva Moreira, S., de Souza Teles, M., et al. (2019). Sex differences and correlates of poor glycemic control in type 2 diabetes: A cross-sectional study in Brazil and Venezuela. https://core.ac.uk/download/323081941.pdf (accessed on 11th June 2025).
6. Althavale, P., Fisher, L., Gonzalez-Mendez, E., Handley, M., et al. (2015). Applying the COM-B model to creation of an IT-enabled health coaching and resource linkage program for low-income Latina moms with recent gestational diabetes: The STAR MAMA program. https://core.ac.uk/download/323074056.pdf (accessed on 11th June 2025).
7. Amankwaah, A. F., Campbell, W. W., Chen, N., McCrory, M. A., et al. (2017). Effects of higher dietary protein and fiber intakes at breakfast on postprandial glucose, insulin, and 24-h interstitial glucose in overweight adults. https://core.ac.uk/download/215930164.pdf (accessed on 11th June 2025).
8. AMBROSIADOU, B. V.; Vadera, S.; SHANKARAMAN, Venky; Goulis, D.; and Gogou, G.. Decision Support Methods in Diabetic Patient Management by Insulin Administration Neural Network vs. Induction Methods for Knowledge Classification. (2000). *Proceedings of the ICSC Symposium on Neural Computation 2000: May 23-26, Berlin*. 852-858. **Available at:** https://ink.library.smu.edu.sg/sis_research/1147(accessed on 11th June 2025).
9. American Diabetes Association, Bailey, C. J., Banting, F., Battelino, T., Beato-Víbora, P., Beck, R. W., Bergenstal, R. M., et al. (2018). Recent updates on type 1 diabetes mellitus management for clinicians. https://core.ac.uk/download/157728573.pdf (accessed on 11th June 2025).
10. Amiel, S. A., Dawoud, D., Fenu, E., Higgins, B., et al. (2017). Basal insulin regimens for adults with type 1 diabetes mellitus: A cost-utility analysis. https://core.ac.uk/download/287580946.pdf (accessed on 11th June 2025).
11. Amiel, S., Barnard, K., Beckwith, A., Brennan, A., et al. (2017). A cluster randomized trial,

cost-effectiveness analysis and psychosocial evaluation of insulin pump therapy compared with multiple injections during flexible intensive insulin therapy for type 1 diabetes: The REPOSE trial. https://core.ac.uk/download/82893694.pdf (accessed on 11th June 2025).

12. Angarita Dávila, L. C., Aparicio, D., Bermúdez Pirela, V. J., Cisternas, A., et al. (2019). Effect of oral nutritional supplements with sucromalt and isomaltulose versus standard formula on glycemic index, entero-insular axis peptides and subjective appetite in patients with type 2 diabetes: A randomized cross-over study. https://core.ac.uk/download/222767716.pdf (accessed on 11th June 2025).

13. Anto, N., Bastiaens, H., Chow, E., Griffiths, R., et al. (2007). Understanding the diversity and dynamics of living with diabetes: A feasibility study focusing on the case. https://core.ac.uk/download/1387204.pdf (accessed on 11th June 2025).

14. Antoniou, P. E., Bamidis, P. D., Karagianni, M., Rivera Romero, O., et al. (2017). Towards evidence-based m-health application design in cancer patient healthy lifestyle interventions. https://core.ac.uk/download/187421621.pdf (accessed on 11th June 2025).

15. Ashworth, S., Coustasse, A., Paul, D. P., III, et al. (2016). Evaluation of glucose monitoring technologies for cost-effective and quality control/management of diabetes. https://core.ac.uk/download/232723891.pdf (accessed on 11th June 2025).

16. Auckland, S., Bachmann, M., Barton, G., Clark, M., et al. (2019). Recruitment, retention, and training of people with type 2 diabetes as diabetes prevention mentors (DPM) to support a healthcare professional-delivered diabetes prevention program: The Norfolk Diabetes Prevention Study (NDPS). https://core.ac.uk/download/210994844.pdf (accessed on 11th June 2025).

17. Avdal, E. Ü., Sofulu, F., Polat, G., & Düzgün, G. (2024). Effect of variables of sociodemographic on disease management skills on individuals with type 1 and type 2 diabetes receiving insulin therapy. https://core.ac.uk/download/614356998.pdf (accessed on 11th June 2025).

18. Azran, C., Batterham, R. L., Busetto, L., Dicker, D., et al. (2017). Practical recommendations of the Obesity Management Task Force of the European Association for the Study of Obesity for the post-bariatric surgery medical management. https://core.ac.uk/download/141699962.pdf (accessed on 11th June 2025).

19. Balamurugan, A. N., Alexander, G., Allen, M., Amos, A., Barber, T., Barrou, Z., Bartlett, R., et al. (2002). Pancreas and islet cell transplantation. https://core.ac.uk/download/12205582.pdf (accessed on 11th June 2025).

20. Bentzen, S. M. R., Christensen, T., Ewers, B., Knudsen, L., et al. (2016). Relative validity of a web-based food frequency questionnaire for patients with type 1 and type 2 diabetes in Denmark. https://core.ac.uk/download/84000899.pdf (accessed on 11th June 2025).

21. Bergenstal, R. M., Fleming, G. A., Heinemann, L., Holl, R. W., et al. (2017). Improving the clinical value and utility of CGM systems: Issues and recommendations: A joint statement of the European Association for the Study of Diabetes and the American Diabetes Association Diabetes Technology Working Group. https://core.ac.uk/download/132211400.pdf (accessed on 11th June 2025).

22. Biddle, M. A., & Kennedy, A. G. (2014). Practical strategies for pharmacist integration with primary care: A workbook. https://core.ac.uk/download/215154018.pdf (accessed on 11th June 2025).

23. Błaszczak, K., Dąbrowska, A., Kruszewski, A., Kucharska, A., et al. (2024). Sport and type 1 diabetes–A great value but also a challenge: Review of the literature and guidelines. https://core.ac.uk/download/620863019.pdf (accessed on 11th June 2025).

24. Bond, C. S., & Hewitt-Taylor, J. (2014). How people with diabetes integrate self-monitoring of blood glucose into their self-management strategies. https://core.ac.uk/download/20442840.pdf (accessed on 11th June 2025).

25. Bondía Company, J., Diez, J. L., Laguna Sanz, A. J., Muñoz Fabra, M., et al. (2021). A comprehensive review of continuous glucose monitoring accuracy during exercise periods. https://core.ac.uk/download/611753529.pdf (accessed on 11th June 2025).

26. Buse, J. B., Davidson, M. B., Ferrannini, E., Holman, R. R., et al. (2009). Medical management of hyperglycemia in type 2 diabetes: A consensus algorithm for the initiation and adjustment of therapy: A consensus statement of the American Diabetes Association and the European Association for the Study of Diabetes. https://core.ac.uk/download/345205928.pdf (accessed on 11th June 2025).

27. Busetto, L., Fried, M., Micic, D., Schindler, K., et al. (2015). European guidelines for obesity management in adults. https://core.ac.uk/download/53528633.pdf (accessed on 11th June 2025).

28. Bywood, P. T., & Melissa. (2013). Allied health video consultation services. https://core.ac.uk/download/43335675.pdf (accessed on 11th June 2025).

29. Cąkała, M., Grzegorzak, F., Kozioł, M., Podgórniak, M., et al. (2024). Sports and diabetes–Limitations resulting from the disease in people engaging in sports. https://core.ac.uk/download/620863245.pdf (accessed on 11th June 2025).

30. Carroll, A. E., Cheng, E. R., Claxton, G. E. M., Hannon, T. S., et al. (2018). Codesigned shared decision-making diabetes management plan tool for adolescents with type 1 diabetes mellitus and their parents: Prototype development and pilot test. https://core.ac.uk/download/188008370.pdf (accessed on 11th June 2025).

31. Carter, B. R., Francisa, T., Hewitt, J., Hou, Y., et al. (2016). Do mobile phone applications improve glycemic control (HbA1c) in the self-management of diabetes? A systematic review, meta-analysis, and GRADE of 14 randomized trials. https://core.ac.uk/download/42534392.pdf (accessed on 11th June 2025).

32. Castaneda, J., Cohen, O., Filetti, S., Glandt, M., et al. (2016). When intensive insulin therapy (MDi) fails in patients with type 2 diabetes: Switching to GLP-1 receptor agonist versus insulin pump. https://core.ac.uk/download/54537154.pdf (accessed on 11th June 2025).

33. Chen, L., Crawford, P., Dye, C. J., Edwards, M., et al. (2017). Enhancing mHealth technology in the patient-centered medical home environment to activate patients with type 2 diabetes: A multisite feasibility study protocol. https://core.ac.uk/download/237709884.pdf (accessed on 11th June 2025).

34. Coates, V., Friel, K. M., Heaton, J., MacRury, S., et al. (2021). Progression to unscheduled hospital admissions in people with diabetes: A qualitative interview study. https://core.ac.uk/download/427515929.pdf (accessed on 11th June 2025).

35. Curtis, L. H., & Schulman, K. A. (2006). Overregulation of health care: Musings on disruptive innovation theory. https://core.ac.uk/download/62553419.pdf (accessed on 11th June 2025).

36. D'Annibale, M., Gibson, R., Guess, N., Linley, J., et al. (2022). Towards targeted dietary support for shift workers with type 2 diabetes (Shift-Diabetes study): A mixed-methods case study protocol. https://core.ac.uk/download/480392875.pdf (accessed on 11th June 2025).

37. Deguara, M., & Gauci, C. (2016). Free access to drinking water in schools: Development of a survey tool. https://core.ac.uk/download/46604241.pdf (accessed on 11th June 2025).

38. Delamater, A. M. (2017). Psychological factors in evaluation and treatment of diabetes. https://core.ac.uk/download/80526620.pdf (accessed on 11th June 2025).

39. Diamant, Allison & Babey, Susan & Brown, E & Chawla, Neetu. (2003). Diabetes in California: Nearly 1.5 million diagnosed and 2 million more at risk. Policy brief (UCLA Center for Health Policy Research). 1-8. (accessed on 11th June 2025).

40. El Kubbe, A. (2019). The difference in A1C of children and adolescents with type 1 diabetes mellitus using carbohydrate counting compared to those using a structured meal plan. https://core.ac.uk/download/286340523.pdf (accessed on 11th June 2025).

41. Ellis, M. R. C., & Jayarajah, C. (2016). Adolescents' view and experiences of living with type 1 diabetes. https://core.ac.uk/download/163076629.pdf (accessed on 11th June 2025).

42. Facchinetti, A. (2016). Continuous glucose monitoring sensors: Past, present and future algorithmic challenges. https://core.ac.uk/download/84921788.pdf (accessed on 11th June 2025).

43. Gabriels, K., & Moerenhout, T. (2018). Exploring entertainment medicine and professionalization of self-care: Interview study among doctors on the potential effects of digital self-tracking. https://core.ac.uk/download/147045100.pdf (accessed on 11th June 2025).

44. Gallagher, R., James, S., Lowe, J., Perry, L., et al. (2016). Diabetes educators: Perceived experiences, supports and barriers to use of common diabetes-related technologies. https://opus.lib.uts.edu.au/bitstream/10453/91325/4/MED%2027417141%20%20%20%20PDF.pdf (accessed on 11th June 2025).

45. Ganguly, A. P. (2018). Collateral benefits of diabetes self-management associated with self-administered outpatient parenteral antimicrobial therapy. https://core.ac.uk/download/212897302.pdf (accessed on 11th June 2025).

46. Ghazeeri, G., Ghazeeri, G., Hmedeh, C., Hmedeh, M., et al. (2021). Nutritional management in polycystic ovary syndrome: Challenges and opportunities. https://core.ac.uk/download/161103740.pdf (accessed on 11th June 2025).

47. Harrison, A., Mellor, D., Lopez-Jimenez, F., Sigal, R., Riddell, M., Turner, D., et al. (2020). Acute glycemic management before, during and after exercise for cardiac rehabilitation participants with diabetes mellitus; a joint statement of the British and Canadian Associations of Cardiovascular Prevention and Rehabilitation, the International Council for Cardiovascular Prevention and Rehabilitation and the British Association of Sport and Exercise Sciences. https://core.ac.uk/download/373290978.pdf (accessed on 11th June 2025).

48. Herbst, A., Strauss, A., King, A. C., Liese, A. D., Brazeau, A. S., Trigona, B., Dee, B., et al. (2015). "Having diabetes shouldn't stop them": Healthcare professionals' perceptions of physical activity in children with type 1 diabetes. https://core.ac.uk/download/161100451.pdf (accessed on 11th June 2025).

49. Hewitt, A., Kirk, A., MacRury, S., McMillan, K., et al. (2016). A systematic and integrated

review of mobile-based technology to promote active lifestyles in people with type 2 diabetes. https://core.ac.uk/download/132205721.pdf (accessed on 11th June 2025).

50. Hood Thabit, L., & Leelarathna, L. (2016). Basal insulin delivery reduction for exercise in type 1 diabetes: Finding the sweet spot. https://core.ac.uk/download/pdf/81614876.pdf (accessed on 11th June 2025).
51. Hovorka, R., & Mohd-Thabit, H. A. (2015). Continuous subcutaneous insulin infusion therapy and multiple daily insulin injections in type 1 diabetes mellitus: A comparative overview and future horizons. https://core.ac.uk/download/83938920.pdf (accessed on 11th June 2025).
52. Iacobini, C., Menini, S., Pesce, C., Pugliese, G., et al. (2017). Dietary interventions to contrast the onset and progression of diabetic nephropathy: A critical survey of new data. https://core.ac.uk/download/80314820.pdf (accessed on 11th June 2025).
53. Kime, N. H. (2013). Weight loss in type 2 diabetes. https://core.ac.uk/download/29018374.pdf (accessed on 11th June 2025).
54. Knaak, C., Kuenz, S., Kurpanik, M., Lachmann, T., et al. (2019). Risk factors of intraoperative dysglycemia in elderly surgical patients. https://core.ac.uk/download/225124691.pdf (accessed on 11th June 2025).
55. Kosmas, P., Lei, J., & Sun, Y. (2024). Exploring biomarker relationships in both type 1 and type 2 diabetes mellitus through a Bayesian network analysis approach. http://arxiv.org/abs/2406.17090 (accessed on 11th June 2025).
56. Kumar, S., Kyrou, I., Matyka, K., Osei-Assibey, G., et al. (2010). Self-reported psychosocial health in obese patients before and after weight loss. https://core.ac.uk/download/46368.pdf (accessed on 11th June 2025).
57. Kurukulasuriya, L. R., & Sowers, J. R. (2010). Therapies for type 2 diabetes: Lowering HbA1c and associated cardiovascular risk factors. https://core.ac.uk/download/pdf/8453221.pdf (accessed on 11th June 2025).
58. Nesbitt, T. S., & Young, H. M. (2017). Increasing the capacity of primary care through enabling technology. https://core.ac.uk/download/323070127.pdf (accessed on 11th June 2025).
59. Ness, E. (2018). Telemedicine and type 2 diabetes. https://core.ac.uk/download/217656868.pdf (accessed on 11th June 2025).
60. Pancheva, R., & Stoycheva, R. (2024). Digital horizons in type 1 diabetes care: Evaluating the impact of mobile health technologies. https://core.ac.uk/download/622091488.pdf (accessed on 11th June 2025).
61. Pantanetti, P., Cangelosi, G., Morales Palomares, S., Ferrara, G., Biondini, F., Mancin, S., Caggianelli, G., et al. (2025). Real-world life analysis of a continuous glucose monitoring and smart insulin pen system in type 1 diabetes: A cohort study. *Diabetology.* https://www.semanticscholar.org/paper/c1be99ecbfc97075c9d70ecffbc3cfc87a07ed12 (accessed on 11th June 2025).
62. Petrovic, M., & Ruiz-Montero, P. J. (2015). Transformation of anthropological status in elderly with type II diabetes through exercise: Pilates and aerobic exercise. https://core.ac.uk/download/214849366.pdf (accessed on 11th June 2025).

63. Pohlman, B., Brod, M., Wolden, M., & Christensen, T. (2012). Non-severe nocturnal hypoglycemic events: Experience and impacts on patient functioning and well-being. https://core.ac.uk/download/pdf/81092439.pdf (accessed on 11th June 2025).

64. Poldermans, D., Bax, J. J., Boersma, E., De Hert, S., Eeckhout, E., Fowkes, G., Gorenek, B., et al. (2009). Guidelines for pre-operative cardiac risk assessment and perioperative cardiac management in non-cardiac surgery: The Task Force for Preoperative Cardiac Risk Assessment and Perioperative Cardiac Management in Non-cardiac Surgery of the European Society of Cardiology (ESC) and endorsed by the European Society of Anesthesiology (ESA). https://core.ac.uk/download/55798032.pdf (accessed on 11th June 2025).

65. Rajagopal, S., et al. (2023). Investigating the impact of multiple inputs on predicting glucose level in individuals with type-1 diabetes through deep learning technique. https://core.ac.uk/download/591405263.pdf (accessed on 11th June 2025).

66. Randall, A. (2016). Integrating technology to support and maintain glycemic control in people with diabetes. https://core.ac.uk/download/162578693.pdf (accessed on 11th June 2025).

67. Singh, L. G., Gothong, C., Ash, G. I., Hernandez, R., & Spanakis, E. (2025). Advancing telemedicine using smart insulin pens with continuous glucose monitoring and telecommunication systems: A case series. *Journal of Clinical Medicine, 14.* https://www.semanticscholar.org/paper/4c3b93830cf00bf1e12793e7342001c7a54b9a5e (accessed on 11th June 2025).

68. Steele, S. (2019). Effectively enhancing health resilience in adolescents with type 1 diabetes mellitus: An integrative literature review. https://core.ac.uk/download/232981914.pdf (accessed on 11th June 2025).

69. Sugihara, E., Yokokawa, H., Isonuma, H., Mitsuhashi, K., Meijyo, M., Shiga, T., Hisaoka, T., et al. (2013). Age-specific effectiveness and safety of newly initiated insulin therapy in Japanese patients with uncontrolled diabetes. https://core.ac.uk/download/pdf/81623165.pdf (accessed on 11th June 2025).

70. Zaharieva, D. P. (2019). Basal insulin adjustments and continuous glucose monitoring during exercise in type 1 diabetes. https://core.ac.uk/download/188194623.pdf (accessed on 11th June 2025).

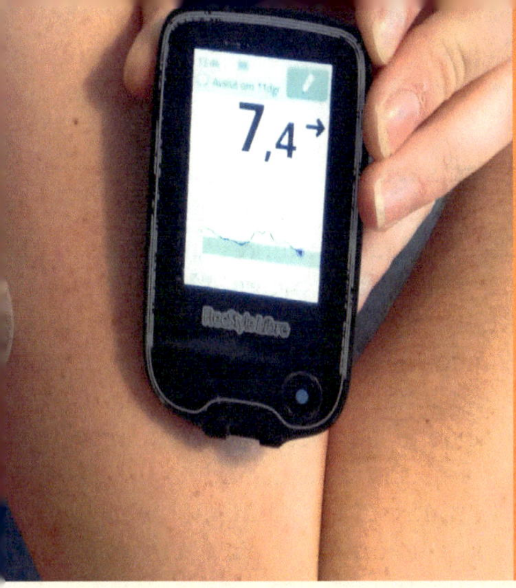

Chapter 8

MANAGEMENT OF TYPE 2 DIABETES

Contents

Introduction

Because Type 2 diabetes is becoming more common and has a major effect on health, its management is now more important in healthcare. In most cases, this condition happens when the body does not use insulin well, which causes blood glucose to rise. Recent studies have found that good management strategies should include modifying one's lifestyle, using medications, and educating patients. People with Type 2 diabetes usually need to be guided on how to check their blood sugar, choose healthy meals, and exercise to control their blood sugar well. Using several kinds of treatments at the same time is necessary for controlling diabetes and preventing serious health problems in the future. What you eat is very important for managing Type 2 diabetes, since it affects blood sugar and heart health. Studies carried out recently suggest that consuming low-glycemic index foods is useful for managing blood sugar and for lowering the risk of heart disease. As an example, one research project looked at a diet based on millet for diabetics and found that it helped control blood sugar, lowered hemoglobin A1c, and improved lipid levels in the participants. It is clear from these results that personalized diet plans help in managing diabetes, which is what the American Diabetes Association recommends. In addition, the use of educational resources helps patients and healthcare providers create diets that fit particular health needs and improve how well patients follow the diet. Psychosocial issues are important in managing Type 2 diabetes since they influence how patients follow their treatment plans and look after themselves. A person's mental and emotional state may affect their motivation, ways of coping, and overall health. The support of family, friends, or healthcare experts is very important for helping people change their lifestyle and control the disease. Educational pamphlets, such as those detailing strategies for teachers and school administrators, highlight diverse approaches to support individuals with diabetes in various settings (University of New England Applied Nutrition Program, 2020). Moreover, integrating psychological support into diabetes care can lead to improved compliance with dietary and exercise guidelines, fostering a comprehensive approach to the management of Type 2 diabetes that addresses both the physical and emotional aspects of the disease (Jali et al., 2012) (Figure 8.1).

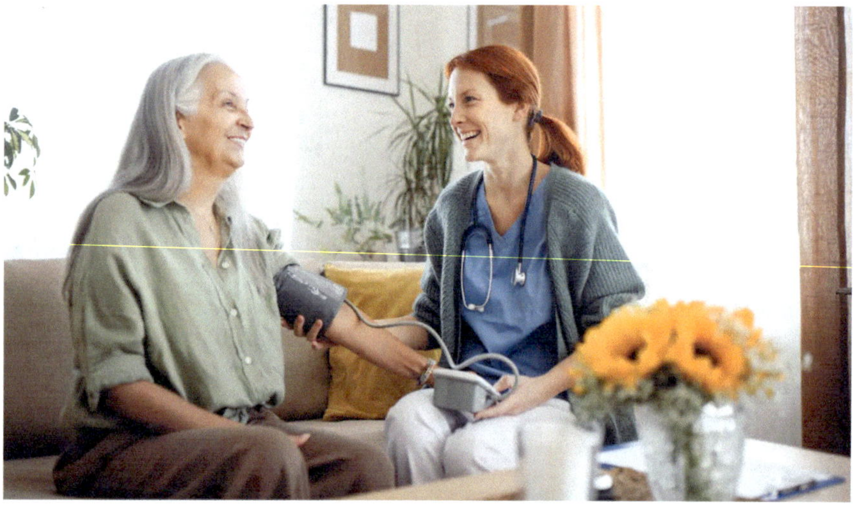

Figure 8.1. Effective management strategies encompass lifestyle modifications, pharmacological interventions, and patient education.

Source: https://drkumo.com/wp-content/uploads/2023/04/nursing-diagnosis-for-hypertension-nurse-checking-woman-blood-pressure.webp

8.1. Lifestyle Modifications

When dealing with Type 2 diabetes, changes in lifestyle are very important for better health and a better quality of life. Dietary management is a main part of these changes, and it has been proven to improve how the body handles sugar and heart disease risks linked to diabetes. Studies point out that having a customized diet is important, since it helps control blood sugar and also helps with weight control, which is crucial for many diabetic patients. Nevertheless, using these dietary strategies in clinical settings is not always easy, so people have called for simpler and more long-term approaches. The overall evidence indicates that while structured interventions can yield substantial benefits, identifying strategies that fit seamlessly into the patients' daily routines is essential for long-term adherence and success in managing diabetes effectively (Adler et al., 2018). Moving more is an important thing to do when managing Type 2 diabetes. Working out regularly helps you lose or maintain weight, makes your body respond better to insulin, and improves your health. Daily exercise can greatly help people from diverse backgrounds, like African Americans, in managing their health conditions. Among African Americans with Type 2 diabetes, changing their lifestyle, especially by being more active, helped them feel better and more confident about their health. The direct correlation between lifestyle adaptations and health outcomes illustrates the transformative potential of self-management behaviors in diabetes care, highlighting the necessity of culturally tailored programs that resonate with this demographic (Duro et al., 2017). In addition, making changes to one's lifestyle is not only up to a person but also requires community support and resources. It is important for healthcare providers to cooperate in making programs that help patients gain the skills and knowledge needed to carry out these changes, which improves their self-efficacy. In addition, projects that help people join their community and find support can encourage them to stick with healthy habits. They are very important for reducing the serious problems that often come with Type 2 diabetes, mainly for those who are more at risk. Also, when both behavioral health and physical health care are used, the effects of lifestyle changes can be better. Overall, comprehensive strategies that incorporate dietary changes and physical activity, supported by healthcare structures, are fundamental to effectively managing Type 2 diabetes and improving patients' quality of life (Duro et al., 2017; Adler et al., 2018) (Figure 8.2).

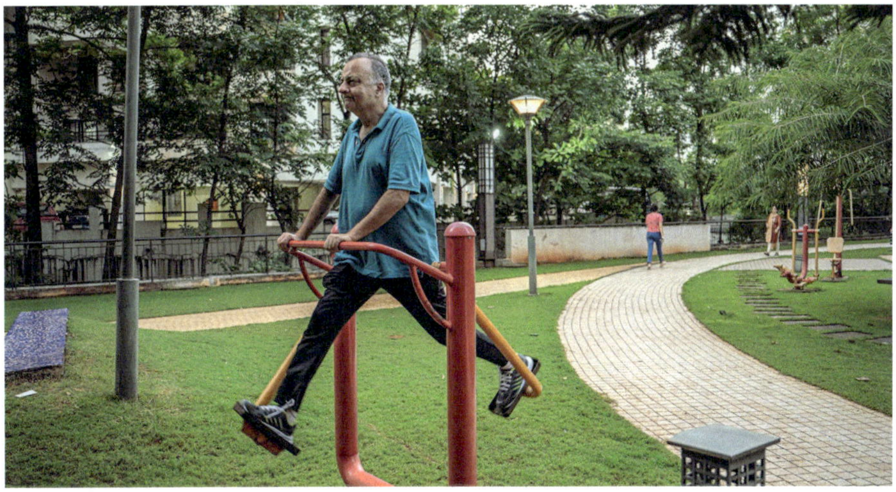

Figure 8.2. Physical activity constitutes another vital aspect of lifestyle modifications necessary for the effective management of Type 2 diabetes.

Source: https://idf.org/media/uploads/2024/08/PA-India-1700px.png

8.1.1. Dietary Changes

Changing your diet is important for managing Type 2 diabetes since it helps control blood sugar, weight, and your body's metabolism. An effective dietary plan includes lots of whole foods, such as fruits, vegetables, whole grains, lean proteins, and healthy fats, and lessens the amount of foods that are high in sugars and unhealthy fats. It is shown in studies that changing nutrition can help individuals manage their diets better and reach the best blood sugar control. For instance, a dietary and exercise self-management support program demonstrated considerable improvements in fasting blood glucose (FBG) and total cholesterol levels among participants with poorly controlled diabetes, highlighting the necessity of tailored dietary approaches in this population (Chinnawong et al., 2015). Making such changes to your diet is necessary for a complete treatment plan that helps control blood sugar and lowers the risk of diabetes complications. The purpose of changing your diet is not only to control calories; you also need to learn about macronutrients and how they affect your blood sugar levels. Many people use carbohydrate counting to help them watch their carb intake and decide on healthy foods that fit their blood sugar management. In addition, when meals people eat can affect their insulin sensitivity and blood sugar levels. According to research, using self-management programs for dietary changes can lead to meaningful improvements in clinical signs linked to diabetes. For example, individuals participating in programs that focus on dietary and physical activity guidelines exhibited marked improvements in various health parameters, including cholesterol management (Chinnawong et al., 2015). For this reason, sharing these dietary principles with people is necessary to help them control their health. Social and cultural factors should be taken into account when looking at people's food choices and Type 2 diabetes. Since people have different food customs, it might be difficult for them to make the changes suggested by doctors. If dietary education and support are culturally appropriate, it can boost a person's motivation and make it easier for them to follow a personalized plan for managing diabetes. Programs designed specifically for certain populations, such as Muslim patients in Indonesia, show promising results in enhancing dietary and exercise behaviors, which ultimately lead to improved clinical outcomes (Chinnawong et al., 2015). When we understand how culture and food habits are connected, we can make dietary changes easier for each person and help them stay healthy (Figure 8.3).

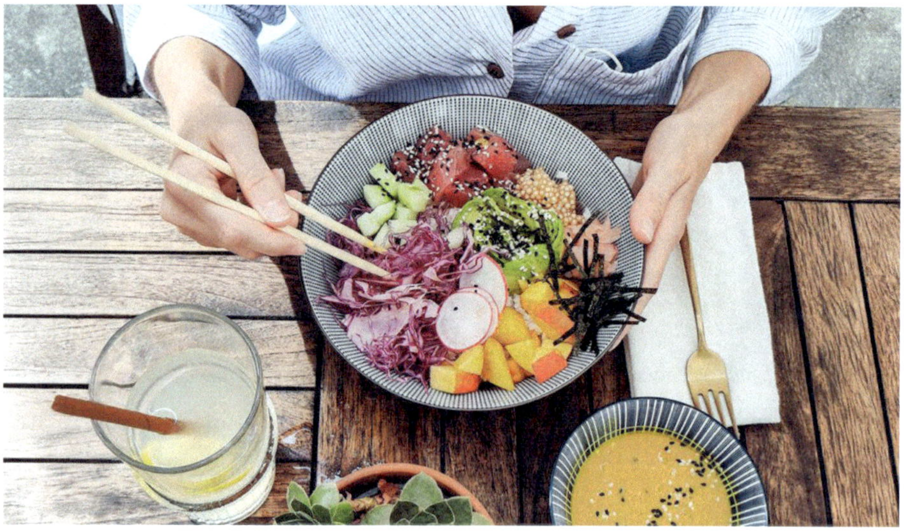

Figure 8.3. A well-structured dietary plan emphasizes the intake of whole foods, including fruits, vegetables, whole grains, lean proteins, and healthy fats, while minimizing processed foods high in sugars and unhealthy fats.

Source: https://media.post.rvohealth.io/wp-content/uploads/sites/3/2025/03/Whole-food-GettyImages-1311163305-Header-1024x575.jpg

8.1.2. Physical Activity Recommendations

The management of type 2 diabetes mellitus (T2DM) necessitates a multifaceted approach, with physical activity emerging as a cornerstone of effective treatment. It is widely accepted that exercise on a regular basis helps insulin function well, aids in losing weight, and lowers blood glucose levels, all of which are necessary for people with T2DM. The current advice for adults with diabetes is to do at least 150 minutes of moderate exercise weekly and strength-training exercises on two or more days. Despite these recommendations, research indicates that many individuals with T2DM fail to meet these activity levels, often due to a variety of barriers, including age, gender, and lack of structured support (Al-Shookri et al., 2017). Eliminating these issues is important for increasing physical activity among people with T2DM and boosting their general health. A review of studies involving older adults points out that special interventions help increase physical activity in those 65 and above who have T2DM. Evidence suggests that personalized coaching, goal setting, and the use of technology can significantly increase activity levels in this demographic (Browning et al., 2013). In addition, joining support groups with other people can encourage you and hold you accountable. Even though there are encouraging results, there is still a big gap in using effective interventions for older individuals. Most of the studies have focused on younger people, so there is a clear need for research on older adults and their special challenges with physical activity. This gap proves that it is important to provide evidence-based programs that are suitable for seniors with T2DM. For people with T2DM, doing physical activity each day is necessary to manage blood sugar levels and promote good health in the future. Strategies such as consultations, structured activity sessions, and referrals to community resources have been highlighted as effective means to encourage physical engagement (Al-Shookri et al., 2017). Health care providers help by teaching and supporting people, which encourages them to take part in regular physical activity. Since diabetes is becoming more common among older people, it is now especially important to inform people about the health benefits of exercise. Supportive systems that encourage active living can help people with T2DM go from knowing about the disease to actually managing it, which improves their quality of life (Figure 8.4).

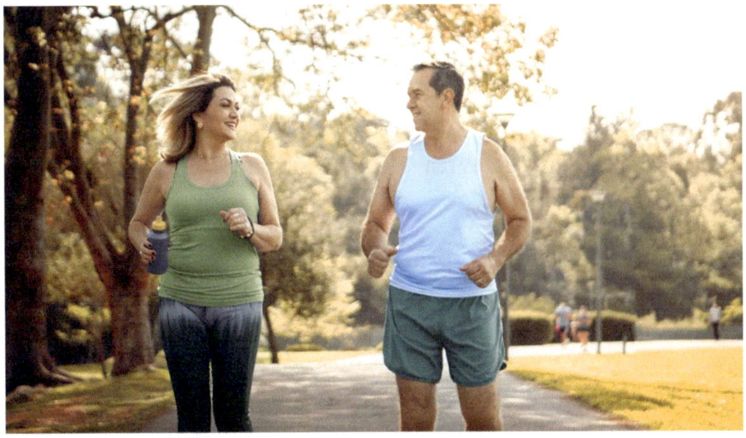

Figure 8.4. Regular physical activity has been shown to enhance insulin sensitivity, aid in weight management, and lower blood glucose levels, all vital for individuals with T2DM.

Source: https://images.everydayhealth.com/images/news/physical-activity-in-the-evening-lowers-blood-sugar-1440x810.jpg?sfvrsn=e467d573_3

8.1.3. Weight Management Strategies

Weight management is important for people with Type 2 diabetes because additional weight makes insulin resistance worse and makes it harder to keep blood sugar in check. A lot of people with Type 2 diabetes start dieting to boost their health. Looking at the findings of the Look AHEAD clinical trial gives us a better idea of how to lose weight effectively. Participants in this trial adopted a variety of intentional weight loss strategies, ranging from dietary modifications to increased physical activity, which directly correlated with their body mass index (BMI) at enrollment. This correlation highlights the necessity of tailored weight loss plans that acknowledge individual needs, preferences, and existing conditions (Ruggiero et al.). Personalized approaches are designed to help patients follow their plan and make positive lifestyle changes, which control diabetes. The use of medication to manage weight is very important for people with Type 2 diabetes. Some antidiabetes drugs, for example, glucagon-like peptide-1 receptor agonists and amylinomimetics, help patients lose weight, so they are important parts of a treatment plan.

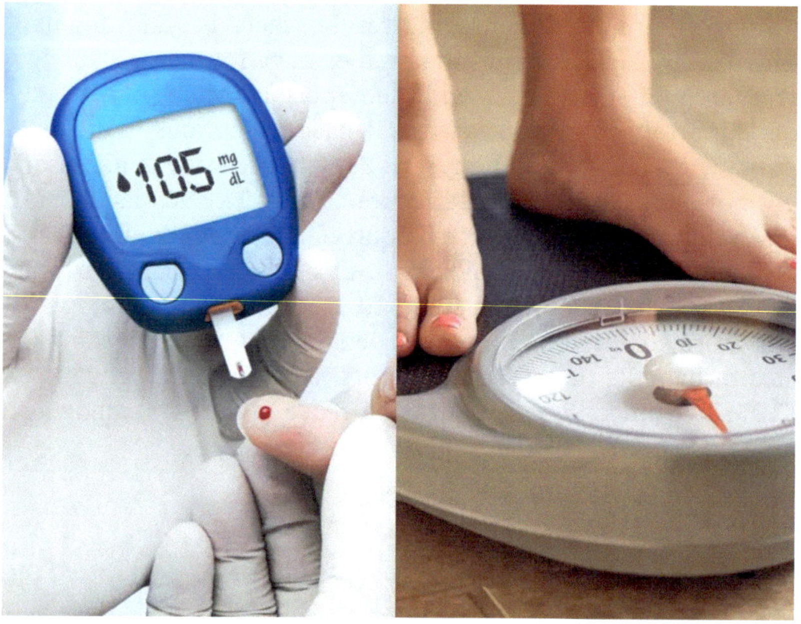

Figure 8.5. Many individuals diagnosed with Type 2 diabetes embark on weight loss journeys to improve their health outcomes.

Source: https://arogyamnutrition.com/wp-content/uploads/2021/03/weight-loss-diabetes-1-1024x768.jpg

As explained in recent studies, while insulin and sulfonylureas are usually linked to gaining weight, new medications can help people either lose or maintain their weight. The recommendation for a multidisciplinary approach emphasizes the significance of integrating lifestyle changes with pharmacological support to effectively manage diabetes and reduce cardiovascular risk factors (Kurukulasuriya & Sowers, 2010). A combination of education, using medication, and behavioral strategies helps healthcare professionals achieve the best results for patients handling their weight and glucose levels. Achieving success in weight management requires people to keep an eye on their progress and stay motivated. Frequent appointments with healthcare professionals allow patients to see how far they have come, change their strategies, and stay dedicated to their aims. Using goal setting, getting support from peers, and perhaps using mobile health applications, people can be more responsible for their weight loss. Also, joining community or group activities can help people receive social support and enjoy experiences with others. For this reason, patients are usually more encouraged when they relate to others dealing with the same problems. Managing weight by considering medical and social factors is very important for people with Type 2 diabetes to achieve lasting results (Figure 8.5).

8.2. Pharmacological Treatments

If lifestyle changes alone do not keep blood sugar under control, Type 2 diabetes management usually involves using medicines. Many types of medicines have been made to handle the different problems in the body caused by the disease. Among the drugs, metformin is the first choice because it reduces the amount of glucose made in the liver and makes insulin more effective. Additionally, newer agents such as glucagon-like peptide-1 (GLP-1) receptor agonists and sodium-glucose co-transporter 2 (SGLT2) inhibitors have emerged, offering not only glycemic benefits but also cardiovascular and renal protective effects.

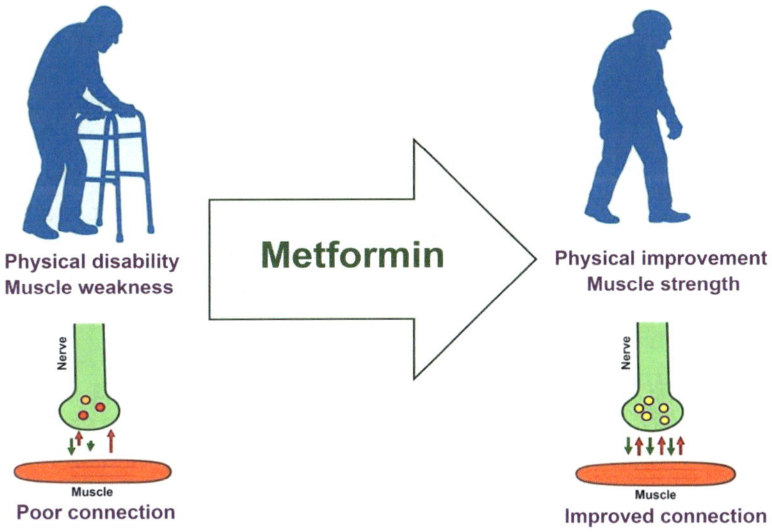

Figure 8.6. Metformin remains the first-line therapy.

Source: https://scx2.b-cdn.net/gfx/news/hires/2025/metformin-could-treat.jpg

These advancements reflect a shift towards a more comprehensive treatment paradigm that not only focuses on blood sugar control but also addresses associated risks, enhancing overall patient outcomes in managing Type 2 diabetes (Fabian et al., 2025). Both obesity and Type 2 diabetes in a person can be hard to handle and may require taking drugs. People with diabetes caused by obesity can benefit a lot from both weight loss drugs and medicines that control blood sugar. Scientists now think that using naltrexone-bupropion can help reduce appetite and improve a person's metabolic system. Emerging treatments like tirzepatide, which targets both GLP-1 and glucose-dependent insulinotropic polypeptide (GIP) receptors, have shown promise in concurrently managing diabetes and obesity, thus offering a holistic approach to treatment. Personalized pharmacological approaches are becoming increasingly important, given that responses can vary based on individual patient profiles and cultural backgrounds, underscoring the necessity of tailored therapies (Tresslor, 2008). The results of pharmacological treatments are affected by the medicines and the patients' participation in their treatment plan. How people deal with diabetes depends a lot on the cultural beliefs they have. There are cases where patients' cultural background affects how they react to their treatment. So, it is necessary to be aware of cultural differences and use sensitive ways of communicating when working with diabetes patients. As pharmacological treatments evolve, there is a pressing need for healthcare providers to ensure that patients understand the mechanisms and benefits of their medications within the framework of their personal and cultural contexts, ultimately fostering better adherence and improved health outcomes in the management of Type 2 diabetes (Tresslor, 2008) (Figure 8.6).

8.2.1. Overview of Common Medications

Doctors often use a variety of common drugs to help control blood glucose and deal with issues linked to type 2 diabetes. Because metformin helps reduce blood sugar and is unlikely to cause weight gain, it is usually the first drug recommended to people with obesity-related diabetes. It has been found that metformin improves insulin sensitivity and helps patients maintain a healthy weight, which is why it is preferred by overweight people. As obesity is linked to further complications, including cardiovascular disease and increased insulin resistance, the ability of metformin to mitigate these factors aligns with the broader treatment goals of managing type 2 diabetes effectively (Ameer et al., 2018). Consequently, metformin acts as a basic drug and also demonstrates the main idea of combining medicine with other approaches for diabetes care. Other than metformin, doctors may prescribe different medications that influence different body functions in diabetes management. Sulfonylureas are drugs that cause the pancreas to make more insulin and help lower the amount of sugar in the blood. Yet, these drugs may cause low blood sugar and weight gain, so patients should be watched closely and advised to make changes to their lifestyle. Additionally, newer agents such as glucagon-like peptide-1 (GLP-1) receptor agonists provide dual benefits of lowering blood sugars and aiding weight loss, positioning them as attractive alternatives for patients struggling with obesity (Ameer et al., 2018). Since there are many diabetes medications, healthcare providers can adjust treatment plans to suit each patient's needs and way of life. Along with drugs, experts suggest that people with type 2 diabetes also follow behavioral therapy, eat better, and exercise regularly. When medications and lifestyle changes are used together, they tend to improve the results of treatment. Those who take drugs that can make them gain weight should also be advised on nutrition and exercise to prevent this from happening. According to studies, taking care of your weight is vital for controlling blood sugar and avoiding the long-term issues that diabetes may cause. For this reason, diabetes medication is shifting to a model that includes both managing the disease with medicine and supporting the patient's general health and well-being (Figure 8.7).

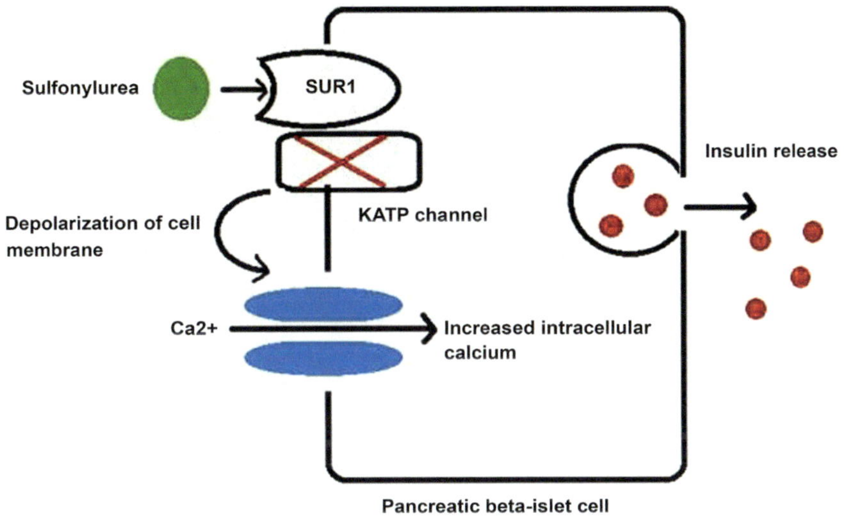

Figure 8.7. Sulfonylureas stimulate the pancreas to produce more insulin, directly lowering blood glucose levels.

Source: https://ars.els-cdn.com/content/image/3-s2.0-B9780128204726000980-f00098-03-9780128204726.jpg

8.2.2. Insulin Therapy

For those who do not control their blood sugar well enough with lifestyle and oral drugs, insulin therapy is very important. Although type 2 diabetes is mainly linked to insulin resistance, the disease can also cause a drop in the body's ability to produce insulin as time goes on. So, starting insulin helps to manage blood glucose more accurately and lessens the chances of hyperglycemia and its problems. When insulin is included in treatment, patients can reach better blood sugar levels, which helps them live healthier and happier lives. Besides, there are several ways to use insulin, and basal insulin is often given to patients with type 2 diabetes. Basal insulin is designed to give a constant supply of insulin that resembles the body's insulin release when it is not fed. According to evidence, insulin detemir given twice a day results in greater clinical benefits than other available regimens. For instance, studies have shown that this particular regimen has the highest quality-adjusted life-years (QALYs) gained compared to alternatives, underscoring its cost-effectiveness in the long term (Amiel et al., 2017). Adjusting insulin treatment to each patient's needs and wishes helps them stick with it and is therefore very important in treating diabetes. Nowadays, using insulin along with different glucose-lowering medicines is seen as an effective way to handle diabetes. Experts have studied liraglutide and similar drugs to see if they can work with insulin to help people lose weight and lower their chances of hypoglycemia. Recent studies indicate that liraglutide can significantly improve glycemic control when used as part of a regimen that includes insulin, which may provide a broader therapeutic approach for patients struggling with weight management and adherence (Cummins et al., 2011). With further progress in the field, it will be necessary to combine insulin therapy with modern drugs to give people with type 2 diabetes effective and personalized care (Figure 8.8).

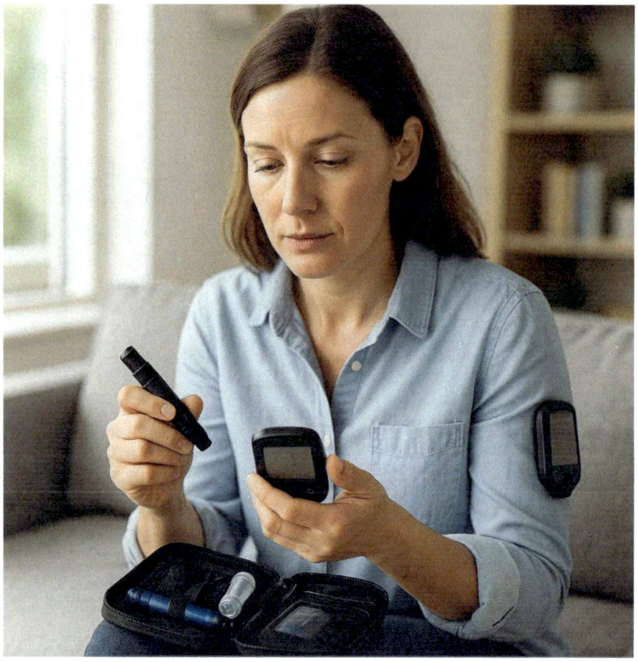

Figure 8.8. Tailoring insulin therapy to fit individual patient needs and preferences enhances adherence, making it a vital part of comprehensive diabetes care.

Source: https://www.diabetesincontrol.com/wp-content/uploads/2025/05/compressed_type1_diabetes_image.jpg

8.2.3. Monitoring and Adjusting Medications

It is very important to monitor and adjust medications in type 2 diabetes since there are many different treatments to choose from. Effective monitoring often starts with regular assessments of glycemic control through Hemoglobin A1c (HbA1c) levels. A good schedule lets healthcare professionals check blood sugar levels and assess the results of the prescribed drugs. The DiGEM study proves that using different methods of blood glucose self-monitoring can greatly impact how treatment works. By comparing different approaches to monitoring, including self-testing and conventional HbA1c measurements, the study sheds light on how tailored interventions can better support patients' long-term glycemic management and overall well-being (Farmer et al., 2005). Combining what patients say with the analysis of data helps doctors decide on medication changes. Together with regular monitoring, patients and healthcare providers should work together to adjust the patient's medication plan. Learning about proper self-monitoring gives patients the ability to be involved in their treatment. Any changes in oral glucose-lowering medication should be made based on both blood tests and the person's daily eating and exercise habits. The DiGEM trial points out that patients who use monitoring tools to check their blood glucose are more likely to take better care of their health. Such changes, in turn, may lead to improved health service cost efficiencies and enhanced clinical outcomes, bridging the gap between medication adherence and actual health improvements (Farmer et al., 2005). Besides, using standard methods for changing medications can make it easier to manage type 2 diabetes patients. The Patient-Centered Medical Home model supports carrying out complete evaluations that measure quality and costs. When healthcare systems use the data they collect, they can create specific actions that improve the quality of care. Using this process, patients and providers can communicate well, and the treatment plan is aligned with the key principles in well-known frameworks for chronic disease management. With frequent changes and updates to their medication, patients can reach better health and enjoy a higher quality of life and better outlook for the future (Figure 8.9).

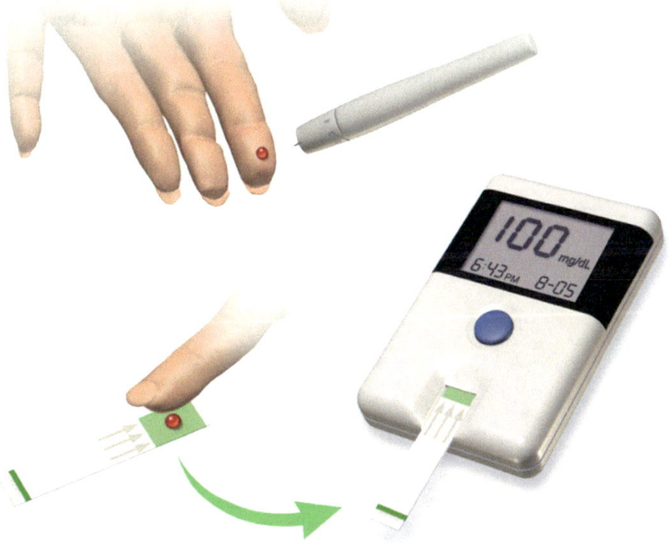

Figure 8.9. A well-structured regimen allows healthcare professionals to detect fluctuations in blood glucose levels and to evaluate the efficacy of prescribed medications.

Source: https://upload.wikimedia.org/wikipedia/commons/6/62/Blausen_0301_Diabetes_GlucoseMonitoring.png

8.3. Role of Healthcare Professionals

Caring for people with Type 2 diabetes is best done with the help of healthcare professionals who provide many different services. They are responsible for treating diabetes and also for encouraging patients to take care of their health. The way patients see their doctors' motivation can increase their own efforts to control their illnesses. Some studies show that when healthcare professionals help patients make their own decisions, it results in better control over Type 2 diabetes. Consequently, the effectiveness of mHealth and eHealth interventions has been linked to the level of engagement initiated by healthcare providers, highlighting their essential role in bridging technological tools with patient participation in healthcare management (Barello et al., 2015). The way healthcare professionals and patients interact is also highlighted by what affects the quality of diabetes care. A study carried out in the UAE revealed that several things, such as heavy workload and cultural beliefs about diabetes, can prevent healthcare workers from offering the best care. It was also found that when patients and healthcare providers communicate and cooperate well, the results of treatment can be improved. It means that healthcare professionals need to understand the organization and the culture to offer quality care. Awareness of cultural nuances and patient backgrounds is crucial in developing tailored approaches for diabetes management, reinforcing the need for culturally competent healthcare practices within the diabetes care framework (Abdulhadi et al., 2013). Besides giving treatment, healthcare professionals are responsible for creating an environment that encourages patients to stay involved. The best way to manage Type 2 diabetes is to focus on strategies that boost the motivation and teamwork of these professionals. It is necessary to help nurses strengthen their roles and also give them the tools and information to address the challenges they encounter. Thus, healthcare systems can encourage a unified way to manage diabetes, which results in better outcomes for patients. Creating a culture of collaboration among healthcare professionals and actively involving patients in their care is essential for successfully managing Type 2 diabetes and ensuring long-term adherence to treatment plans (Abdulhadi et al., 2013) (Figure 8.10).

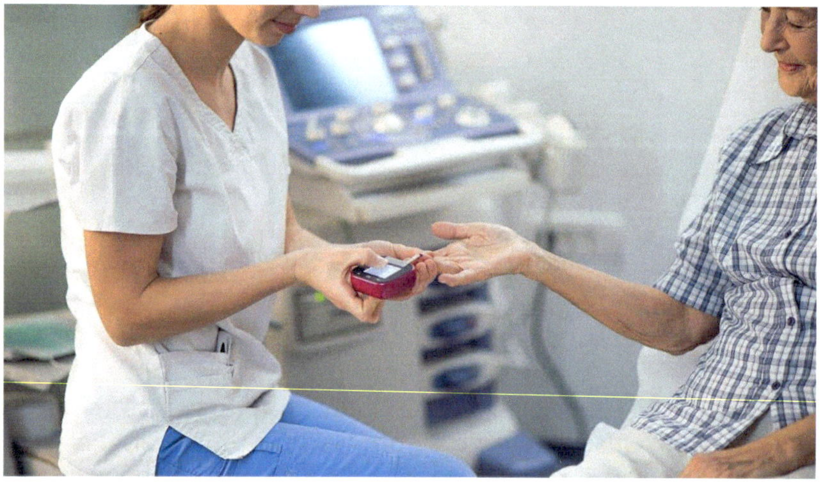

Figure 8.10. Physicians, nurses, dieticians, and health educators, are pivotal in not only diagnosing and treating diabetes but also in fostering patient engagement in self-management.

Source: https://content.jdmagicbox.com/comp/def_content_category/diabetic-educators/what-you-need-to-know-about-diab-diabetic-educators-1-icxsj.jpg

8.3.1. Importance of Regular Check-ups

Regular visits to the doctor are necessary for Type 2 diabetes because they allow problems to be found early. Those with Type 2 diabetes face a greater chance of getting cardiovascular diseases, neuropathy, and nephropathy. During routine medical visits, healthcare providers can check blood glucose, blood pressure, and lipid levels, which are necessary for handling diabetes. These visits give a chance to discuss new ways to live healthily, following medication instructions, and checking one's health regularly. Regular contact with doctors and nurses helps patients get care that changes with their health over time. Performing regular check-ups for diabetes has been helpful in lowering the number of cases and deaths caused by the disease. Healthcare practitioners can make important improvements in patient outcomes by evaluating treatments and making any needed changes. Regular checks of hemoglobin A1c are important for understanding if someone's glucose is under control, which can lead to diabetes complications. In addition, these visits usually involve checking for hypertension and dyslipidemia, which may make diabetes harder to control if they are not managed. Frequent check-ups seem to help patients stick to their prescribed treatments and follow the suggested health habits, which improves their quality of life. Besides, regular visits to the doctor encourage patients to take charge of their health. Regular consultations help people know more about their health and become responsible for their own well-being. While in these appointments, patients are encouraged to ask about anything they are unsure of and join in on making their treatment decisions. Taking part in diabetes care is important, since there is a lot of information about nutrition, exercise, and managing other diseases related to diabetes. As indicated by IDF-LFAC's commitment to providing education and support within diabetes care, regular check-ups serve to bolster patients' capacities for self-management, vital for achieving sustained health outcomes (Sigfrid et al., 2015). Such empowerment not only leads to better individual health results but also contributes to the overall efficiency of healthcare systems by reducing the incidence of emergency care and hospitalizations (Abela, 2004) (Figure 8.11).

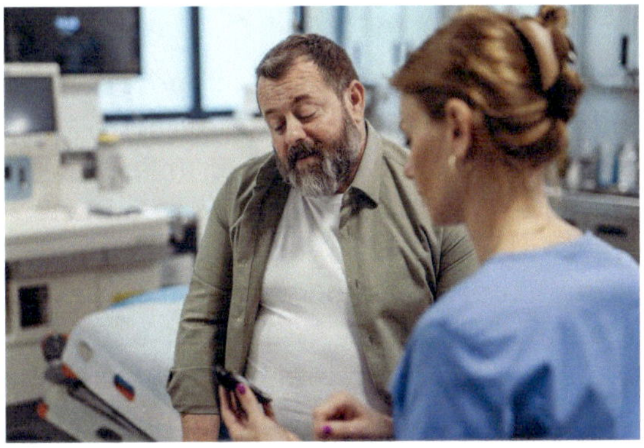

Figure 8.11. Regular check-ups are a fundamental aspect of managing Type 2 diabetes, as they facilitate the early identification of potential complications associated with the condition.

Source: https://storage.googleapis.com/treatspace-prod-media/pracimg/u-1998/shutterstock_2387615751_1.jpeg

8.3.2. Multidisciplinary Approach

The management of Type 2 diabetes (T2D) necessitates a robust multidisciplinary approach that integrates various healthcare professionals to address the complex nature of the disease. This happens because lifestyle, biology, and comorbidities affect each other in many ways. Usually, a team includes endocrinologists, dietitians, educators, nurse practitioners, and mental health professionals, who use their expertise to plan treatments for each patient. Endocrinologists pay attention to medicines, whereas dietitians help patients choose healthy meals for their metabolism. The team approach helps patients manage their blood sugar better and also stops or lessens the risk of heart problems and kidney damage, which are both essential for better health. So, having a multidisciplinary approach helps meet the many needs of people with T2D in a complete way. Moreover, as highlighted in recent literature, the complexities inherent in managing Type 2 diabetes often require targeted interventions that consider coexisting health conditions, such as chronic kidney disease (CKD) and cardiovascular issues. Since these conditions are linked to T2D, it is important to use a multidisciplinary method so that different health problems can be handled at the same time. Particularly, the Dysfunctional Adipose Tissue Approach (DATA) emphasizes weight management and lifestyle intervention as cornerstones of care, aligning with the latest insights into the metabolic challenges faced by patients. When healthcare providers focus on weight loss, they can help manage the disease and improve patients' overall health, proving that teamwork is effective in handling the many effects of T2D. (López-Martínez et al., 2024) Lastly, effective communication within a multidisciplinary team is paramount to the success of managing Type 2 diabetes. When healthcare providers talk openly, the care given is more consistent and goals are always in line. It is especially important for this coordination when treatment choices are changing rapidly and new research is being discovered. Both patients and providers gain the ability to handle T2D challenges when they continue learning and make decisions together. Besides, teaching patients about their health and how to manage themselves encourages them to stick to their treatment plans. The achievement of effective management of Type 2 diabetes and its complications is determined by the teamwork of experts, good communication, and active participation by patients (Figure 8.12).

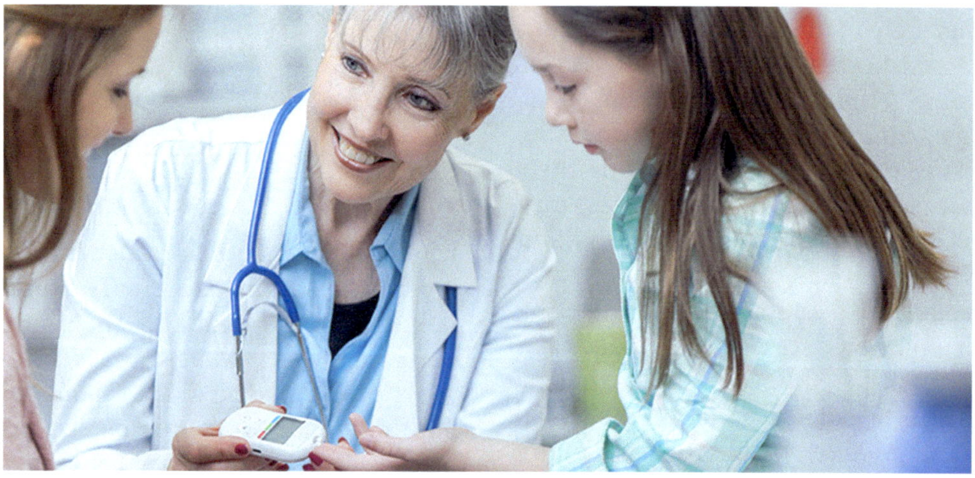

Figure 8.12. A team usually comprises endocrinologists, dietitians, educators, nurse practitioners, and mental health professionals, each contributing unique expertise to devise personalized treatment plans.

Source: https://storage.aanp.org/www/images/practice/therapeutic-areas/endo.jpg

8.3.3. Patient Education and Support

Managing type 2 diabetes requires giving patients the right information and support, as these are important for improving their self-management skills. Proper patient education helps people learn about their illness, decide on what actions to take, and take an active role in their health care. To this end, diabetes self-management education (DSME) programs have been established to bridge gaps in understanding and skills. Still, it is observed that many populations are not using these educational initiatives as much as they should. This underutilization emphasizes the need for innovative approaches, such as digital health interventions (DHI), to ensure that educational resources are accessible, available when needed, and tailored to diverse patient requirements, thereby addressing both knowledge gaps and engagement deficits in diabetes management (Michie et al., 2018). It is also important to consider the emotional and psychological aspects of diabetes management, which show why it is necessary to have more than just basic medical support. Many patients say that dealing with their condition for a long time causes stress, which often prevents them from sticking to their self-care routines. Researchers have found that traditional education programs mainly teach about medical care, but they usually miss the importance of psychological support for long-term success. When emotional and role management are part of patient education, healthcare providers help patients deal with the difficulties of diabetes. This multifaceted approach is further supported by findings indicating that enhanced emotional well-being correlates with improved self-management outcomes, highlighting the profound impact of integrating psychological support within educational frameworks (Christensen et al., 2017). Looking into the success of patient education programs shows that they help people with type 2 diabetes improve their self-care and emotional strength. For instance, studies utilizing the Health Education Impact Questionnaire (HeiQ) indicate that participants in structured educational programs exhibit improvements in various aspects of self-management shortly after the educational intervention. These advantages are improved skills, better self-observation, and better positive attitudes. Still, keeping these improvements going for a long time has proven to be tough, with results that differ from one situation to another. This underscores the importance of not only delivering patient education but also ensuring ongoing support and resources are available to patients as they adjust to their diagnosis, thereby creating a comprehensive strategy for managing type 2 diabetes effectively (Christensen et al., 2017) (Figure 8.13).

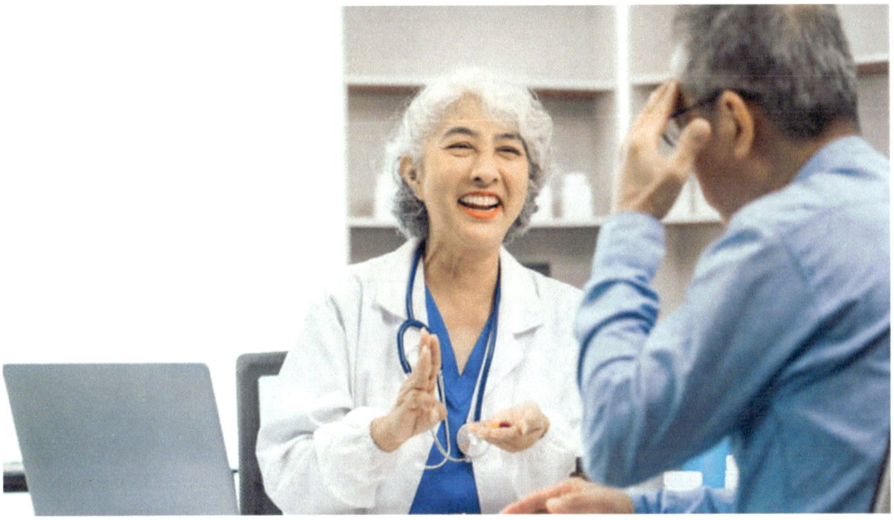

Figure 8.13. Effective patient education serves to provide individuals with critical knowledge regarding their condition, empower them to make informed choices, and encourage proactive engagement in their health care. To

Source: https://www.rightpatient.com/wp-content/uploads/2023/11/The-Future-of-Patient-Engagement-in-Medical-Practices.jpg

8.4. Psychological Aspects of Diabetes Management

How people with Type 2 diabetes manage their emotions and thoughts is very important for their health and general well-being. Living with diabetes usually requires making big lifestyle changes, which can make people feel stressed, anxious, and depressed. Such emotional issues can make it harder for patients to follow their medication and diet plans and to handle their condition on their own. Knowing the mental effects of diabetes is necessary, since people with diabetes may feel different emotions that can influence their willingness to look after themselves. Interventions that focus on mental health support, such as counseling and group therapy, have been shown to enhance coping strategies, which are critical in managing the chronic nature of diabetes effectively, illustrating the need for a holistic approach in diabetes care that integrates both physical and psychological health (Rao et al., 2015). Furthermore, learning about diabetes is very important, since it gives patients the tools to handle their condition and overcome mental challenges to treatment. Programs that use behavioral strategies and psychological help help patients follow their diabetes plan and choose healthier habits.

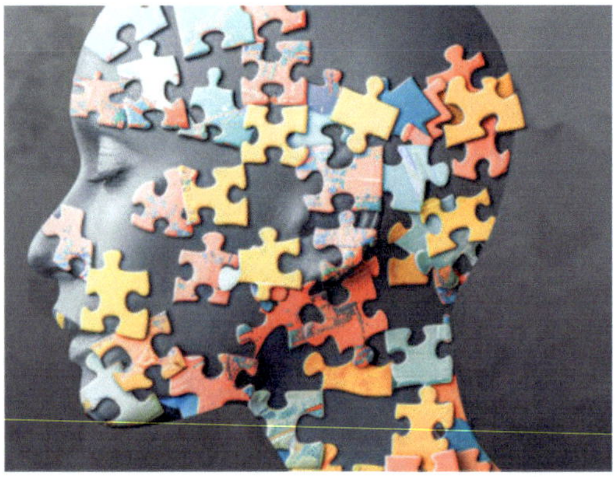

Figure 8.14. Understanding the psychological dimensions of diabetes is essential, as individuals may experience fluctuating emotions that can impact their motivation to engage in self-care behaviors.

Source: https://www.diabetologie-online.de/_storage/asset/2528502/storage/kirchheim:article-2_04-1/file/365050331/32395716.jpg

When patients are given personal advice on nutrition and blood glucose, it can help them feel more in control, so they do not feel as helpless with their condition. As people with diabetes learn more and gain helpful information, they feel more confident, become less anxious, and enjoy better health results. The integration of psychological support within educational frameworks encourages individuals to build resilience, emphasizing that managing diabetes is not solely a physical endeavor but also a psychological journey (Rao et al., 2015). Moreover, it is easy to see how psychosocial factors impact diabetes management when we look at the lives of adolescents and adults. It is clear from research that emotional problems, such as parental arguments in teenagers and stigma in adults, may strongly affect how diabetes is managed. Because they are still becoming independent, adolescents have a tough time coping with their illness, making their relationship with it more difficult. This shows that special support should be given to address these emotions, which can boost self-management and health. Health care providers should pay attention to the emotional and social effects of diabetes on their patients, as this supports the need for environments that help patients emotionally and manage their diabetes well (Figure 8.14).

8.4.1. Impact of Diabetes on Mental Health

Both the physical and mental health of a person can be seriously affected by type 2 diabetes. Living with diabetes for a long time may make people feel unsure and anxious about handling it properly. A lot of people with type 2 diabetes feel more stress handling their special diets, taking medications, and dealing with the risks of the disease. Having to deal with these psychological problems can cause more anxiety and depression, which may make it harder for people to follow their treatment plans. Studies have demonstrated that effectively addressing psychological health alongside physical health can lead to improved outcomes for patients, indicating that healthcare strategies must account for the mental wellness of individuals living with diabetes (Gao et al., 2025). It is important to understand the link between obesity and type 2 diabetes to see how it affects mental health. Because obesity often leads to metabolic issues and diabetes, people often feel stigmatized and their self-esteem decreases as a result of their extra weight and health. This stigma adds to the problems of mental health, making people feel hopeless and despairing, and also prevents them from finding good treatment and support. Because obesity and diabetes often go together, it is necessary to address society's views and give resources that help with mental health. As highlighted in recent guidelines, a holistic approach toward obesity management can improve not just physical health outcomes but also enhance the psychological well-being of patients (Barber, 2023). Recently, new approaches like precision nursing have been successful in helping people with type 2 diabetes deal with their mental health issues. Emphasizing individual plans that look after mental and physical health has led to fewer cases of anxiety and depression in patients and helped them control their blood sugar. It is important to help people with diabetes by offering mental health support, as it greatly improves their ability to manage the disease. Programs that recognize the interconnectivity between mental and physical health can lead to a better quality of life for those with type 2 diabetes, reinforcing the need for healthcare providers to adopt a comprehensive approach to management strategies (Gao et al., 2025) (Figure 8.15).

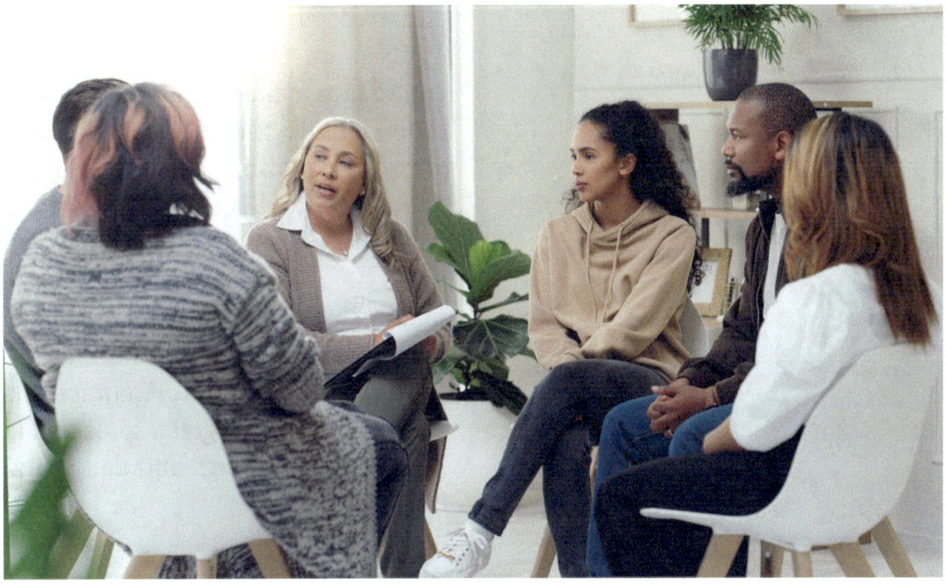

Figure 8.15. The integration of mental health support into diabetes management is vital; when patients feel supported and understood, their capacity to manage their diabetes improves significantly.

Source: https://publichealth.tulane.edu/wp-content/uploads/sites/3/2021/01/Understanding-Mental-Health-as-a-Public-Health-Issue.jpg

8.4.2. Coping Strategies

Type 2 diabetes is easier to manage when people use coping strategies that help their mental state and blood sugar levels. Using effective ways to cope can increase a person's belief in their ability to control diabetes. Research indicates that patients who engage in problem-solving and control-oriented coping strategies demonstrate higher levels of diabetes management self-efficacy compared to those employing emotion-oriented methods (Mirkohi & Rahimian-Boogar, 2016). This means that people who try to solve problems and keep control over their diabetes are more likely to have better health results. So, helping patients learn adaptive coping strategies is important in diabetes education and support programs to encourage them to look after their health. How a person manages stress is very important when looking at how diabetes is handled.

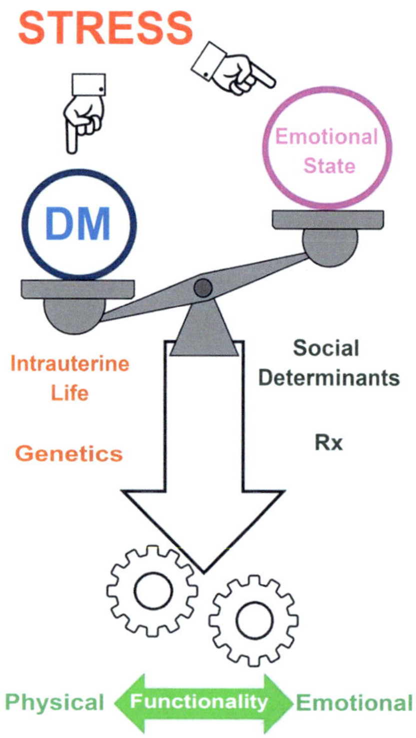

Figure 8.16. Coping strategies play a vital role in the management of Type 2 diabetes, influencing both psychological wellbeing and metabolic outcomes.

Source: Mangoulia P, Milionis C, Vlachou E, Ilias I. The Interrelationship between Diabetes Mellitus and Emotional Well-Being: Current Concepts and Future Prospects. *Healthcare*. 2024; 12(14):1457. https://doi.org/10.3390/healthcare12141457

If people with Type 2 diabetes experience a lot of stress, it can make their situation worse and may encourage them to use unhealthy coping methods that affect their diabetes care. A study investigating patients with diabetes revealed a significant association between elevated stress levels and the prevalence of maladaptive coping strategies, which can lead to poorer adherence to treatment and increased risk of diabetes complications (Mirkohi & Rahimian-Boogar, 2016). This research reveals that healthcare providers should pay attention to stress in diabetes management and include ways to reduce stress with usual treatment plans. When patients learn adaptive strategies, they may reduce their stress and manage diabetes in a more complete way. To sum up, using effective coping methods is very important for controlling Type 2 diabetes and its effects on mental health and treatment results. Encouraging people to address their problems and boosting their confidence in managing diabetes can greatly help them handle the condition. Similarly, dealing with stress and unhealthy ways of coping is necessary to avoid complications and make sure the patient follows treatment. It points out that psychological resilience and diabetes management go hand in hand, which means patients should receive all-around support when they visit a clinic. To manage diabetes well, patients should be given tools and knowledge to handle their feelings and daily routines (Figure 8.16).

8.4.3. Importance of Support Systems

The presence of support systems greatly helps patients with Type 2 diabetes to take care of themselves. Such systems include many different resources, for example, family, friends, healthcare professionals, and community organizations. Having these relationships supports individuals in making the right decisions about their health and way of life. It has been shown that learning more about diabetes and how to manage it helps people control the condition and avoid its complications. When individuals understand the necessary self-management strategies and receive encouragement from their support networks, they are better positioned to adhere to dietary guidelines, engage in regular physical activity, and monitor their health indicators effectively, thus enhancing their overall quality of life (Okeya & Brundrett, 2016). Having a structured model for chronic care that offers self-management help greatly increases patients' involvement in their diabetes care. Having full support networks encourages people to take part in making health decisions, which makes them feel responsible for their well-being. Studies reveal that people who feel well supported often improve their diet and exercise. This bond is necessary since controlling diabetes well depends on doctors' help and the patient's active involvement. Moreover, the impact of support on self-management behaviors is evident across diverse patient populations, suggesting a universal benefit of these networks in the context of healthcare treatments (Proie, 2017). It is very important to focus on social support when managing Type 2 diabetes, since it helps people feel better mentally and less alone. Since depression and anxiety are common in people with chronic illnesses, patients may have a harder time managing their health. Support networks can boost your confidence, inspire you, and offer a chance to discuss what you have gone through. So, including support systems in diabetes education and care is necessary to boost both physical and mental health. This holistic approach fosters a more supportive environment for patients, equipping them to face the daily challenges associated with their condition and promoting a more proactive stance toward their health (Proie, 2017) (Figure 8.17).

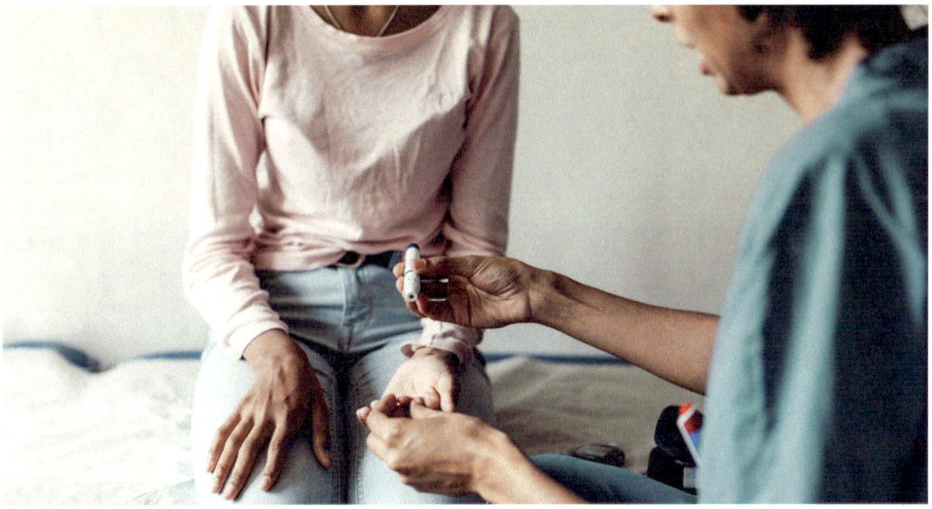

Figure 8.17. Support systems play a pivotal role in the management of Type 2 diabetes, significantly influencing patients' ability to effectively self-manage their condition.

Source: https://media.post.rvohealth.io/wp-content/uploads/2018/10/diabetes-doctor-1200x628-facebook.jpg

A CLOSER LOOK

FASTING BLOOD GLUCOSE (FBG)

Fasting Blood Glucose (FBG) is a test that measures blood sugar levels after an individual has not eaten for at least 8 hours, usually performed in the morning. It allows for checking how the body manages glucose when it has not eaten recently. Normal FBG levels range from 70 to 99 mg/dL. A blood sugar level between 100 and 125 mg/dL shows prediabetes, and two tests with a reading of 126 mg/dL or more indicate diabetes. FBG is often used to diagnose diabetes and keep an eye on glucose levels in people with the disease. Having healthy fasting glucose levels is necessary to avoid complications linked to diabetes.

Summary

To summarize, controlling Type 2 Diabetes requires both the patient's effort and the help of healthcare specialists. Patients' ability to take care of themselves is greatly affected by their self-efficacy, which is a psychological factor. It has been found that hardiness and coping strategies strongly affect a person's confidence in managing their diabetes, so health programs should aim to improve them. In particular, fostering commitment, control, and the use of effective coping mechanisms can improve self-management outcomes in patients with Type 2 Diabetes (Mirkohi & Rahimian-Boogar, 2016, 2016). For this reason, health professionals should help patients by handling these psychological issues, which results in improved health management and outcomes. The emotional aspect of having Type 2 Diabetes is very important in guiding patients' self-care routines. It has been shown in recent research that a patient's culture and emotional state play a major role in how they handle diabetes. People taking part in the study wanted to be supported by their healthcare providers, who should consider each person's individual feelings and culture. This highlights the necessity for healthcare professionals to adopt a more holistic view of patient care, where emotional support and cultural sensitivity are integral components of effective diabetes management (Furler et al., 2008). Being aware of the emotions behind patients' self-management, health experts can offer better support and achieve better health results. When these insights are applied to diabetes management, it becomes easier for patients to take part in their care and follow guidelines. As health professionals aim to form closer relationships with patients, they should pay more attention to caring for the patient's mind and feelings. When hardiness, coping strategies, and cultural factors are combined, it becomes possible to design interventions that help manage Type 2 Diabetes and also address the main health-related issues. Therefore, future practices must prioritize a comprehensive understanding of patient needs, fostering an environment in which individuals feel empowered to take control of their health narratives, thereby improving adherence and overall quality of life for those living with Type 2 Diabetes (Furler et al., 2008).

References

1. Abdulhadi, N., Al-Kaabi, J., Al-Shahib, W., Alberti, H., Alberti, H., Alhyas, L., Alhyas, L., et al. (2013). Factors affecting the motivation of healthcare professionals providing care to Emiratis with type 2 diabetes. https://core.ac.uk/download/29017990.pdf (accessed on 11th June 2025).
2. Abe, M., Norton, K., & Smith, J. (2022). The impact of a Medicare Public Health Emergency policy change for continuous glucose monitors on utilization and total cost of care for diabetes. https://core.ac.uk/download/524708748.pdf (accessed on 11th June 2025).
3. Abela, J. C. (2004). *General Practice.* https://core.ac.uk/download/46601885.pdf (accessed on 11th June 2025).
4. Adler, A. I., American Diabetes Association, Atkinson, F. S., Bansal, S., Bassler, D., Bell, K. J., Brand-Miller, J., et al. (2018). Treatment of diabetes with lifestyle changes: Diet. https://core.ac.uk/download/pdf/237685331.pdf (accessed on 11th June 2025).
5. Albright, A. L., Albright, A., Aljasem, A., American Diabetes Association, American Diabetes Association, Araiza, C., Armit, C., et al. (2010). Exercise and type 2 diabetes: The American College of Sports Medicine and the American Diabetes Association: Joint position statement. https://core.ac.uk/download/pdf/8491602.pdf (accessed on 11th June 2025).
6. Al-Shookri, A., Al Riyami, A., Brazeau, A. S., Brazeau, A. S., AlQuaiz, A., Sibai, A. M., American Diabetes Association, et al. (2017). Correlates of physical activity and sitting time in adults with type 2 diabetes attending primary health care in Oman. https://core.ac.uk/download/84592069.pdf (accessed on 11th June 2025).
7. Ameer, B., Weintraub, H., et al. (2018). Pediatric obesity: Influence on drug dosing and therapeutics. https://core.ac.uk/download/155271623.pdf (accessed on 11th June 2025).
8. Amiel, S. A., Dawoud, D., Fenu, E., Higgins, B., et al. (2017). Basal insulin regimens for adults with type 1 diabetes mellitus: A cost-utility analysis. https://core.ac.uk/download/287580946.pdf (accessed on 11th June 2025).
9. Astrup, A., Lean, M. E. J., & Roberts, S. B. (2018). Making progress on the global crisis of obesity and weight management. https://core.ac.uk/download/158368197.pdf (accessed on 11th June 2025).
10. Barber, T. (2023). How will the latest modifications to the CG189 NICE guidelines for obesity management likely impact clinical care? *Hepatobiliary Surgery and Nutrition, 12*, 413–416. https://www.semanticscholar.org/paper/b04bc821d3ec5edd2f36eb91efadc1c140a2d15c (accessed on 11th June 2025).
11. Barello, S., Bonanomi, A., Graffigna, G., Menichetti Delor, S., et al. (2015). The motivating function of healthcare professional in eHealth and mHealth interventions for type 2 diabetes patients and the mediating role of patient engagement. https://core.ac.uk/download/79150709.pdf (accessed on 11th June 2025).
12. Bartoszek, L., Kapłan, W., Lipiec, J., Olszak, M., et al. (2024). Hyperosmolar hyperglycemic syndrome: A comprehensive review of clinical presentation, diagnosis, and treatment strategies in hyperglycemic crises. https://core.ac.uk/download/597985314.pdf (accessed on 11th June 2025).

13. Furler, J., Walker, C., Blackberry, I., Dunning, T., Sulaiman, N., Dunbar, J., Best, J., & Young, D. (2008). The emotional context of self-management in chronic illness: A qualitative study of the role of health professional support in the self-management of type 2 diabetes. *BMC health services research*, *8*, 214. https://doi.org/10.1186/1472-6963-8-214(accessed on 11th June 2025).

14. Bitton, A., Abrams, M. K., & Rosenthal, M. B. (2012). Recommended core measures for evaluating the patient-centered medical home: Cost, utilization, and clinical quality. https://core.ac.uk/download/71358813.pdf (accessed on 11th June 2025).

15. Bonakdaran, S., Hezarkhani, S., Marjani, A., Rajabian, M., et al. (2013). Comparison of glycemic excursion in patients with new onset type 2 diabetes mellitus before and after treatment with repaglinide. https://core.ac.uk/download/52204666.pdf (accessed on 11th June 2025).

16. Bond, C. S. (2014). Telehealth as a tool for independent self-management by people living with long term conditions. https://core.ac.uk/download/29050943.pdf (accessed on 11th June 2025).

17. Bong, W. K., Das, J., Sneha, K., & Janszen, F. (2022). Gluco Coach—A self-management application for type 2 diabetes mellitus: User testing to understand comfort levels and sustained patient engagement. https://core.ac.uk/download/636679315.pdf (accessed on 11th June 2025).

18. Browning, C., Shariff Ghazali, S., Yasin, S., & Shajahan, Y. (2013). Interventions to promote physical activity in older with type 2 diabetes mellitus: A systematic review. https://core.ac.uk/download/153811182.pdf (accessed on 11th June 2025).

19. Okeya, E., & Brundrett, M. (2016). Knowledge of Diabetes Education Programmes and Support Systems on Type 2 Diabetes Self-Management among Black Africans in Liverpool. *Journal of Nursing and Health Science*, *5*(3), 32-38. Advance online publication. https://doi.org/10.9790/1959-0503063238(accessed on 11th June 2025).

20. Chinnawong, T. (Tippamas), Kritpracha, C. (Charuwan), & Pamungkas, R. A. (Rian). (2015). The effect of dietary and exercise self-management support program on dietary behavior, exercise behavior and clinical outcomes in Muslim patients with poorly controlled type 2 DM in a community setting in Indonesia. https://media.neliti.com/media/publications/154630-EN-the-effect-of-dietary-and-exercise-self.pdf (accessed on 11th June 2025).

21. Christensen, K. B., Christensen, U., Frøhlich, A., Hjorth Lauersen, J., et al. (2017). Assessment of short and long-term outcomes of diabetes patient education using the health education impact questionnaire (HeiQ). https://core.ac.uk/download/269293905.pdf (accessed on 11th June 2025).

22. Cummins, E. (Ewen), Royle, P., Shyangdan, D. (Deepson), Waugh, N., et al. (2011). Liraglutide for the treatment of type 2 diabetes: A single technology appraisal. https://core.ac.uk/download/9562645.pdf (accessed on 11th June 2025).

23. Dougall, R., Gillies, M., & Knifton, L. (2012). Prison health in NHS Greater Glasgow & Clyde: A health needs assessment 2012. https://core.ac.uk/download/9843474.pdf (accessed on 11th June 2025).

24. Duro, C. (2017). Effects of lifestyle changes on the health of African Americans with type 2 diabetes. https://core.ac.uk/download/147841221.pdf (accessed on 11th June 2025).

25. Eid, W., El-Gayar, O. F., Nawar, N., Timsina, P., et al. (2013). Mobile applications for diabetes

self-management: Status and potential. https://core.ac.uk/download/352610622.pdf (accessed on 11th June 2025).

26. Ellis, M. R. C., & Jayarajah, C. (2016). Adolescents' view and experiences of living with type 1 diabetes. https://core.ac.uk/download/163076629.pdf (accessed on 11th June 2025).
27. Fabian, D., Kędziora, F., Siwiec, J., Smyl, J., et al. (2025). The growing obesity epidemic: Integrating lifestyle, pharmacological, and surgical interventions for effective management. https://core.ac.uk/download/636386139.pdf (accessed on 11th June 2025).
28. Farmer, A., French, D. P., Goyder, E., Kinmonth, A. L., et al. (2005). The DiGEM trial protocol—a randomized controlled trial to determine the effect on glycemic control of different strategies of blood glucose self-monitoring in people with type 2 diabetes [ISRCTN47464659]. https://core.ac.uk/download/20330164.pdf (accessed on 11th June 2025).
29. Fisher, L., Hessler, D. M., Mullan, J., Polonsky, W. H., et al. (2012). When is diabetes distress clinically meaningful? Establishing cut points for the Diabetes Distress Scale. https://core.ac.uk/download/323073077.pdf (accessed on 11th June 2025).
30. Gao, H., Han, Y., Deng, D., & Liu, L. (2025). The intervention effect of comprehensive precision nursing in elderly patients with type 2 diabetes. *Australasian Journal on Ageing, 44*. https://www.semanticscholar.org/paper/ab934337326d1a6d59549c2571c31f745b749987 (accessed on 11th June 2025).
31. Ghodrati Mirkouhi M, Rahimian-Boogar I. Predicting diabetes management self-efficacy base on hardiness and coping strategies in patients with type 2 diabetes mellitus.J Inflamm Dis.20(4):e155981. (accessed on 11th June 2025).
32. Jali, M. V., Kamatar, M. Y., Jali, S. M., Hiremath, M. B., & Naik, R. K. (2012). Efficacy of value added foxtail millet therapeutic food in the management of diabetes and dyslipidamea in type 2 diabetic patients. *Recent Research in Science and Technology*, *4*(7). Retrieved from https://updatepublishing.com/journal/index.php/rrst/article/view/902(accessed on 11th June 2025).
33. Jacobson, A. M., Zigmond, A. S., Lai, A. Y., Chua, C. G., Eigenmann, C. A., Goh, C. S. Y., Toobert, D. J., et al. (2019). The combined diabetes and renal control trial (C-DIRECT)–a feasibility randomized controlled trial to evaluate outcomes in multi-morbid patients with diabetes and on dialysis using a mixed methods approach. https://core.ac.uk/download/163076809.pdf (accessed on 11th June 2025).
34. Kurukulasuriya, L. R., & Sowers, J. R. (2010). Therapies for type 2 diabetes: lowering HbA1c and associated cardiovascular risk factors. *Cardiovascular diabetology*, *9*, 45. https://doi.org/10.1186/1475-2840-9-45(accessed on 11th June 2025).
35. López-Martínez, M., Modrego Pardo, I., Moreno-Perez, O., Reyes-Garcia, R., et al. (2024). Are we ready for an adipocentric approach in people living with type 2 diabetes and chronic kidney disease? https://core.ac.uk/download/604467541.pdf (accessed on 11th June 2025).
36. Michie, S., Murray, E., & Pal, K. (2018). Digital health interventions for adults with type 2 diabetes: Qualitative study of patient perspectives on diabetes self-management education and support. https://core.ac.uk/download/151187935.pdf (accessed on 11th June 2025).
37. Nesbitt, T. S., & Young, H. M. (2017). Increasing the capacity of primary care through enabling technology. https://core.ac.uk/download/323070127.pdf (accessed on 11th June 2025).

38. Ness, E. (2018). Telemedicine and type 2 diabetes. https://core.ac.uk/download/217656868.pdf (accessed on 11th June 2025).

39. Proie, C. D. (2017). An Examination of Factors Affecting Hemoglobin A1c Levels and Self-Care Behaviors among Type 2 Diabetic Patients in the Primary Care Setting (Doctoral dissertation, Duquesne University). Retrieved from https://dsc.duq.edu/etd/145(accessed on 11th June 2025).

40. Rao, L. S. (2015). Redesigning treatment strategies in type 2 diabetes by treatment intensification and patient education. https://core.ac.uk/download/33562651.pdf (accessed on 11th June 2025).

41. Ruggiero, A. M., Adachi, J. D., American Diabetes Association, Bish, J. P., Bruce, R., Cho, Y., French, S. A., et al. (2025). Weight loss strategies associated with BMI in overweight adults with type 2 diabetes at entry into the Look AHEAD (Action for Health in Diabetes) trial. https://core.ac.uk/download/pdf/8113959.pdf (accessed on 11th June 2025).

42. Sigfrid, L., McKee, M., Eeles, M., Atkinson, S., & Atkinson, Z. (2015). From surviving to thriving: Evaluation of the International Diabetes Federation Life for a Child Program. https://core.ac.uk/download/80510988.pdf (accessed on 11th June 2025).

43. Tresslor, S. K. (2008). "It's a whole package": Type 2 diabetes and what it means for the body, life and self of people of Indian origin in New Zealand: A thesis presented in partial fulfillment of the requirements for the degree of Master of Arts in Psychology (with an endorsement in Health Psychology) at Massey University, Albany, New Zealand. https://core.ac.uk/download/157568844.pdf (accessed on 11th June 2025).

44. University of New England Applied Nutrition Program, "Supporting a Healthy School Environment for Students with Diabetes" (2020). *All Student-Created Educational Resources*. 163. https://dune.une.edu/an_studedres/163(accessed on 11th June 2025).

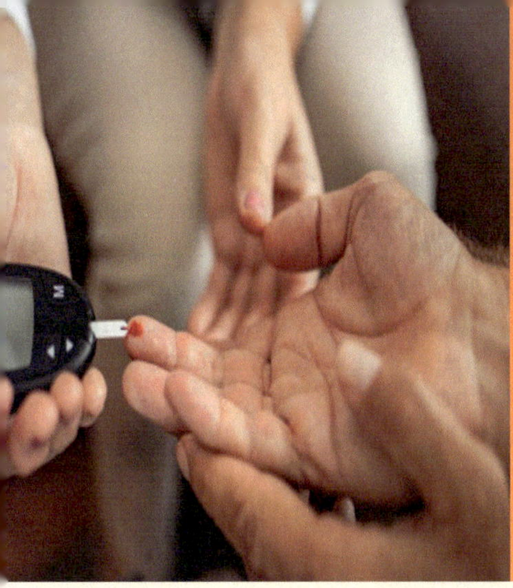

Chapter 9

DIABETIC KETOACIDOSIS, HYPERGLYCEMIC HYPEROSMOLAR STATE, AND LACTIC ACIDOSIS

Contents

Introduction

The increasing prevalence of diabetes mellitus has raised awareness about its severe complications, notably diabetic ketoacidosis (DKA), hyperglycemic hyperosmolar state (HHS), and lactic acidosis. These conditions represent critical metabolic emergencies resulting from uncontrolled hyperglycemia, which manifests when blood glucose levels exceed 15 mmol/L, or 240mg/dL (Mohajan et al., 2023). DKA mainly happens to those with type 1 diabetes, and it occurs when insulin shortage causes ketone bodies to be produced, which results in metabolic acidosis. In most cases, HHS is linked to type 2 diabetes and brings about extreme high sugar levels in the blood, and dehydration, with little or no ketoacidosis. Both conditions call for fast medical attention, since long-lasting high blood sugar can seriously harm the eyes, kidneys, heart, and immune function, which can cause severe health issues if not treated. Since these metabolic problems are linked to infections and other stresses in the body, the situation can become more difficult for doctors to manage. Recent studies have highlighted a potential link between SARS-CoV-2 infections and adverse glycemic outcomes, leading to an increased incidence of DKA and HHS among individuals with pre-existing diabetes (Al-Sa HAH'idy et al., 2022). Therefore, viral infections could make existing metabolic conditions worse or lead to diabetes in people who did not have it before. This shows that it is important to use better monitoring and management strategies to help patients with diabetes avoid these complications, especially when there are outbreaks of infectious diseases. It is important to know how hyperglycemia and external stressors are linked to prevent and treat patients who are at risk of DKA and HHS. To summarize, early detection and treatment of DKA, HHS, and lactic acidosis in people with diabetes helps prevent dangerous outcomes. Because diabetes is becoming more widespread worldwide, healthcare professionals should be knowledgeable about these metabolic emergencies to give prompt care. It is important for treatment strategies to consider each patient's other infections and health problems, as they can play a big role in the patient's outcome. By fostering an integrated approach to diabetes management, there is potential to reduce the incidence of DKA and HHS while improving overall patient outcomes in managing hyperglycemic crises (Al-Sa HAH'idy et al., 2022; Mohajan et al., 2023) (Figure 9.1).

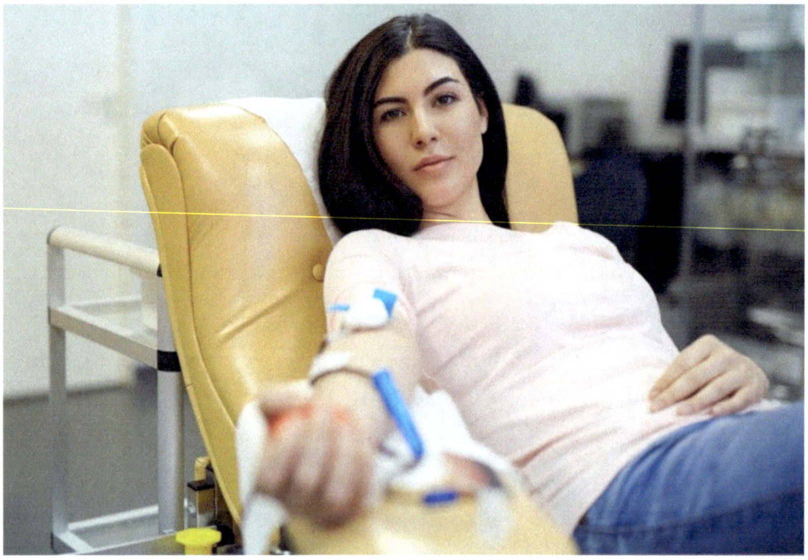

Figure 9.1. As the burden of diabetes continues to rise globally, healthcare professionals must be well-versed in the nuances of these metabolic emergencies to provide timely care.

Source: https://advinhealthcare.com/wp-content/uploads/2022/10/Blood-Donation-3-1024x683.jpg

9.1. Pathophysiology of DKA

Diabetic Ketoacidosis (DKA) is characterized by a triad of symptoms: hyperglycemia, ketonemia, and acidosis. It is triggered by a lack of insulin in sutuations of stress such as infections, emotional or physical stress such as surgeries or dehydration, or missed insulin doses. If there is not enough insulin, glucose cannot enter the peripheral tissues and this causes hyperglycemia. For this reason, the body tries to make up for the energy loss by increasing lipolysis, releasing free fatty acids that are turned into ketone bodies by the liver. Having too many ketone bodies results in metabolic acidosis, which is shown by a decreased blood pH and a high anion gap, both important signs of DKA. Effective understanding and management of these biochemical changes are essential, as failure to promptly recognize and treat DKA can lead to severe complications and even mortality (Gong et al., 2024). Electrolyte imbalances further complicate the pathophysiology of DKA. When the renal threshold is passed, too much glucose goes into the urine, causing water to be excreted as well through osmotic diuresis. As a result of diuresis, the body loses a lot of sodium and potassium. Even though the potassium levels in the blood are initially increased, the lack of insulin causes potassium to be shifted into the cells. As a result, when someone starts insulin therapy, potassium levels must be monitored, since sudden the shift of potassium into cells can result in low potassium levels in the blood, which can lead to arrhythmias. Restoration of normal electrolyte balance is equally vital during treatment to mitigate the risks associated with the electrolyte disturbances inherent in DKA (Gong et al., 2024). In addition, acidosis in DKA leads to many other effects that worsen the patient's condition. Acidosis can disrupt the functions of cells, reduce the strength of the heart's contractions, and decrease the heart's response to catecholamines, which might cause the heart to become unstable. Acidosis in the renal system reduces the kidneys' ability to remove hydrogen ions and keep bicarbonate, which makes the imbalance worse. Sometimes, DKA is shown by mental changes, which can happen because of brain swelling caused by very high blood glucose and acids. The systemic nature of DKA requires a multidisciplinary approach to manage not only the acute metabolic derangements but also to gauge and treat potential underlying precipitating factors, thereby improving patient outcomes and reducing the risk of recurrence (Modi et al., 2020) (Figure 9.2).

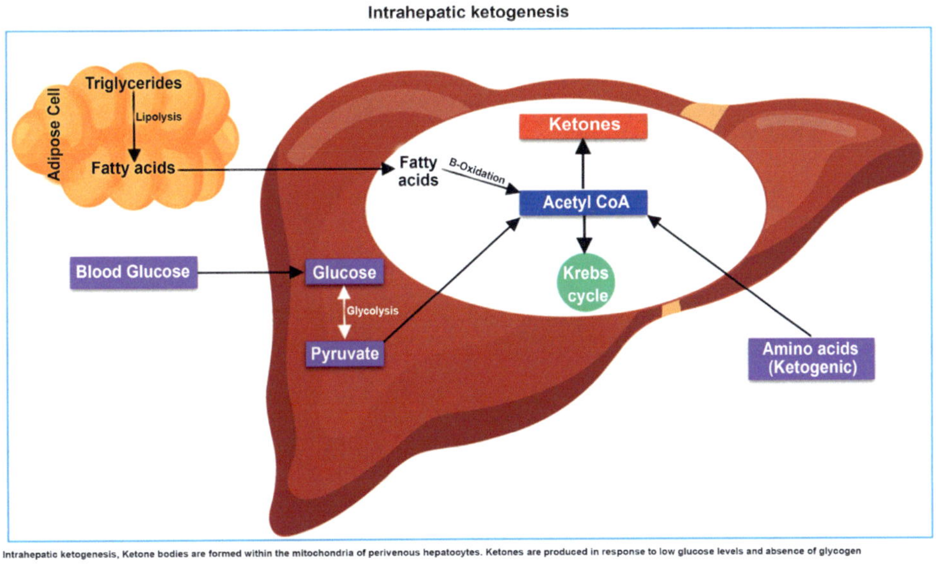

Figure 9.2. Diabetic Ketoacidosis (DKA) is characterized by a triad of symptoms: hyperglycemia, ketonemia, and acidosis.

Source: https://recapem.com/wp-content/uploads/2021/06/diabetic-ketoacidosis-intrahepatic-ketogenesis.png

9.1.1. Mechanism of Insulin Deficiency

The mechanism of insulin deficiency plays a critical role in understanding the development of acute hyperglycemic emergencies, specifically diabetic ketoacidosis (DKA) and hyperglycemic hyperosmolar state (HHS). Insulin helps the muscles and fat in the body to absorb glucose. If insulin is lacking, as it is in type 1 diabetes, glucose stays in the blood, which results in hyperglycemia. Because glucose cannot be used for energy, fat is broken down and this leads to more free fatty acids and ketone bodies in the blood. When insulin levels are low, the body goes into ketosis and this is marked by metabolic acidosis, a main feature of DKA. Thus, the mechanistic understanding of insulin deficiency is paramount for recognizing the physiological disruptions that culminate in these severe metabolic conditions, as reiterated in recent findings regarding management strategies for hyperglycemic emergencies (Anumah et al., 2007).

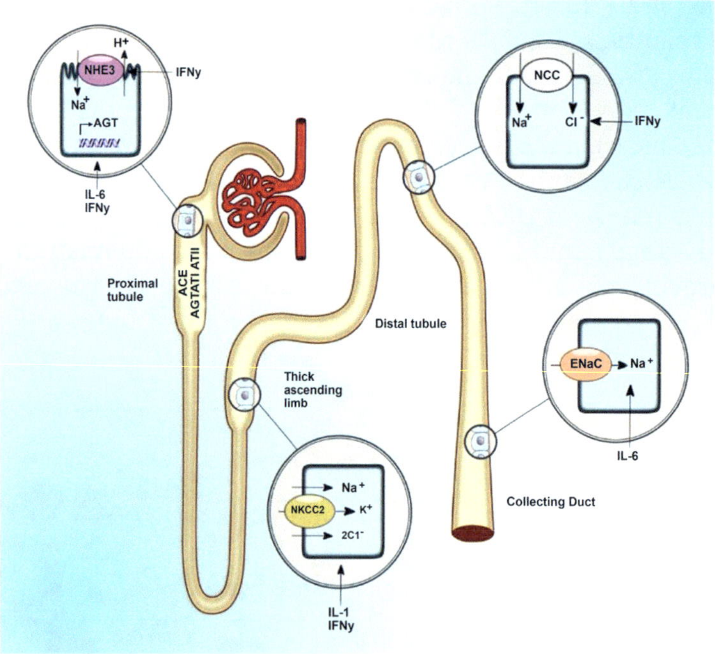

Figure 9.3. Electrolyte imbalances, particularly potassium shifts, often accompany insulin deficiency, as insulin administration in therapeutic settings is crucial for restoring normal cellular exchanges of potassium and other electrolytes.

Source: Cianciolo G, De Pascalis A, Gasperoni L, Tondolo F, Zappulo F, Capelli I, Cappuccilli M, La Manna G. The Off-Target Effects, Electrolyte and Mineral Disorders of SGLT2i. *Molecules*. 2020; 25(12):2757. https://doi.org/10.3390/molecules25122757

In addition, the effects of insulin shortage go beyond high blood sugar and play a major role in the symptoms of DKA and HHS. As insulin levels fall, glucagon, epinephrine, and cortisol are not stopped from working, which causes more glucose to be produced by the liver. Because of insulin resistance and high levels of counter-regulatory hormones, the body's metabolic state is greatly affected, and DKA appears as a rapid increase in these problems. When insulin levels are low, there are often electrolyte imbalances, mainly potassium shifts, because restoring these electrolytes with insulin is very important in therapy. Understanding these interactions is vital for clinicians tasked with managing these conditions effectively, emphasizing the need for prompt recognition and treatment (Modi et al., 2020). Finally, handling and preventing DKA is mainly based on knowing how insulin deficiency works. The purpose of intravenous insulin therapy is to correct insulin shortage and control the effects of increased glucagon and other similar hormones. This way of treating diabetes helps lower blood glucose and also stops the breakdown of fat while encouraging fat storage. That is why it is important to understand how insulin influences carbohydrate and lipid metabolism to improve the outcomes of patients with hyperglycemia. In clinical practice, the prompt restoration of insulin levels, alongside aggressive fluid and electrolyte management, is crucial to preventing the complications that arise from these metabolic derangements, underscoring the importance of swift intervention in cases of DKA and HHS (Anumah et al., 2007) (Figure 9.3).

9.1.2. Ketogenesis and Its Effects

When there are not enough carbohydrates, ketogenesis happens in the liver and results in the production of ketone bodies from fatty acids. It is important for giving extra energy, especially when people are fasting for a long time, exercising vigorously, or have diabetes and their glucose use is not well managed. In the context of diabetic ketoacidosis (DKA), the overproduction of ketone bodies results in an accumulation of acids in the bloodstream, precipitating metabolic acidosis. When ketone levels are high and blood sugar is high, it is called DKA, so it must be managed quickly to avoid serious problems.

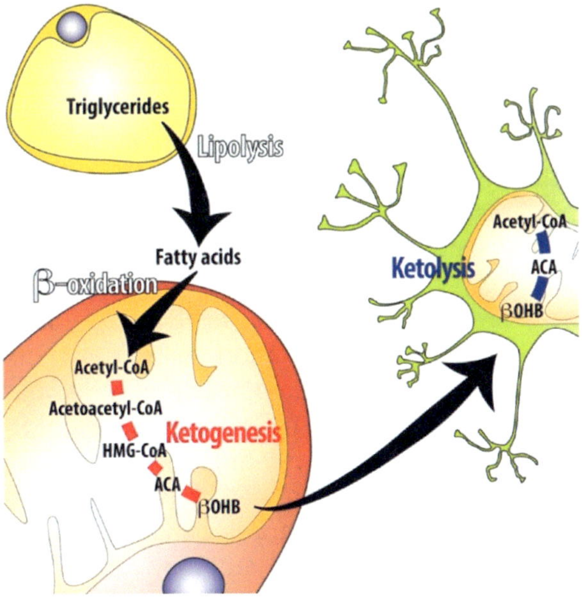

Figure 9.4. Ketogenesis is a metabolic process that occurs in the liver when there is a scarcity of carbohydrates, leading to the production of ketone bodies from fatty acids.

Source: Longo R, Peri C, Cricrì D, Coppi L, Caruso D, Mitro N, De Fabiani E, Crestani M. Ketogenic Diet: A New Light Shining on Old but Gold Biochemistry. *Nutrients*. 2019; 11(10):2497. https://doi.org/10.3390/nu11102497

The interplay between insulin deficiency and increased lipolysis leads to a pathophysiological state that exemplifies the body's shift from glucose metabolism to fat metabolism, underscoring the importance of understanding ketogenesis in clinical settings involving diabetes (Anumah et al., 2007). Because Ketogenesis increases when insulin is low, it causes serious problems with the body's metabolism. DKA causes the blood to become more acidic due to the extra ketones, which leads to the special acidosis linked to the condition. The diagnosis of DKA is confirmed through the presence of hyperglycemia, elevated ketone levels, and a significant metabolic acidosis (Modi et al., 2020). A rise in ketogenesis can upset the body's electrolyte balance, mainly affecting potassium, which may lead to various treatment difficulties. Therefore, when managing DKA, one must address the high blood sugar as well as watch and correct other metabolic problems, such as low potassium levels that can happen after insulin is given, highlighting the importance of using different treatments. Understanding the role of ketogenesis in diabetic emergencies such as DKA and hyperglycemic hyperosmolar state (HHS) is imperative for clinicians tasked with managing these acute conditions. Although ketogenesis helps us survive starvation by keeping glucose for important uses, any problems with its regulation in uncontrolled diabetes can cause major metabolic issues. Even though ketoacidosis is not as common in HHS as in DKA, both conditions are caused by a strong lack of insulin and high blood glucose levels. When health care providers understand how these metabolic pathways are linked, they can use the best interventions. The restoration of metabolic homeostasis not only alleviates acute symptoms but also aims to reduce long-term complications associated with recurrent diabetic emergencies, highlighting the importance of understanding ketogenesis and its effects in clinical practice (Anumah et al., 2007) (Figure 9.4).

9.1.3. Electrolyte Imbalances Associated with DKA

Electrolyte imbalances are a hallmark of diabetic ketoacidosis (DKA) and significantly impact the clinical outcomes in affected patients. Potassium is one of the main substances that is depleted in diabetes, due to the fact that insulin deficiency stops cells from absorbing potassium. Acidosis causes potassium to move from inside cells to the blood, which can cause a quick increase in serum potassium that is not real. Many clinicians do not pay attention to this issue, which may result in serious problems if potassium is not handled properly in treatment. When insulin therapy begins, there is a risk that potassium levels will drop fast, so it is necessary to watch and treat them carefully to avoid heart problems. The intricate relationship between insulin, electrolyte shifts, and metabolic derangements underscores the complexity of DKA management and exemplifies the necessity for interdisciplinary approaches in acute care (Hamid et al., 2010). DKA causes sodium to vary significantly, mainly because of the high blood glucose and the osmotic impact it creates. Due to dilution, the sodium level in blood may be lower than it really is, a situation called pseudohyponatremia, so it is important to measure it accurately for treatment. A disturbance in sodium levels can make the situation more difficult and may call for further actions to correct the problem. It becomes more complicated since managing fluid and electrolytes matters, as potassium and sodium are tied to kidney health and how much fluid the body has. Treatment methods should gradually improve these abnormalities and watch for any signs of renal impairment, since it is common in DKA patients. Misinterpretation of electrolyte levels might lead to inappropriate treatment, solidifying the importance of a nuanced understanding of these imbalances (Bartoszek et al., 2024). In addition, both magnesium and phosphate imbalances are common in DKA and help create the overall picture of metabolic problems. Not noticing magnesium deficiency can make muscle weakness and dysrhythmias worse, making it harder to treat the patient. As a result of insulin's effect on phosphate levels, there is a higher chance of respiratory depression and changes in how cells function. If these electrolytes are not managed well, recovery may take a long time and the patient's condition may worsen; therefore, it is important for healthcare workers to closely watch and treat these imbalances during the acute phase of DKA. Every treatment plan should involve frequent electrolyte tests and the use of supplements that are chosen for each patient to prevent the complications of these metabolic issues. Collectively, addressing the full spectrum of electrolyte imbalances is fundamental to improving outcomes for patients experiencing diabetic ketoacidosis (Hamid et al., 2010) (Figure 9.5).

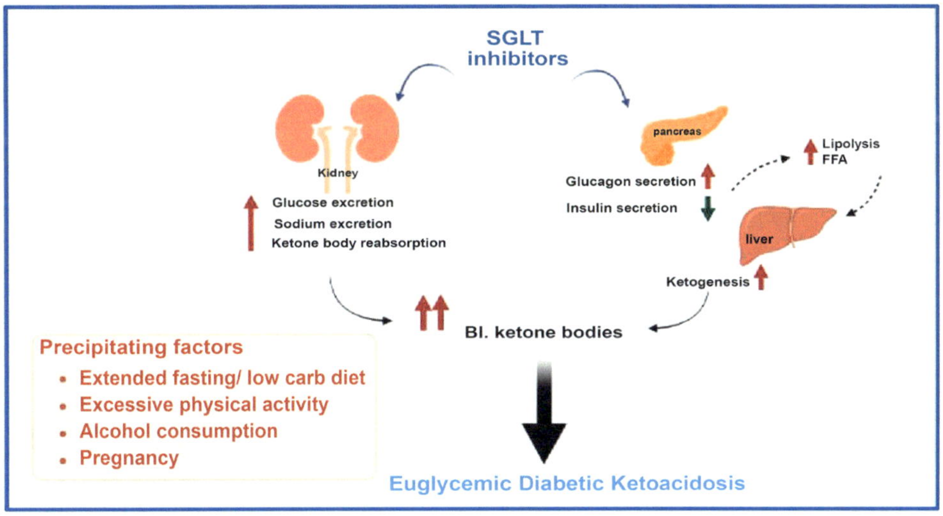

Figure 9.5. Electrolyte imbalances are a hallmark of diabetic ketoacidosis (DKA) and significantly impact the clinical outcomes in affected patients.

Source: El-Remessy AB. Diabetic Ketoacidosis Management: Updates and Challenges for Specific Patient Population. *Endocrines*. 2022; 3(4):801-812. https://doi.org/10.3390/endocrines3040066

9.2. Pathophysiology of HHS

The hyperglycemic hyperosmolar state (HHS) is a serious diabetic emergency characterized by extreme hyperglycemia, dehydration, and hyperosmolarity without significant ketoacidosis. It happens mainly in those with type 2 diabetes, often caused by infections, certain drugs, or not drinking enough water. A lack of insulin and insulin resistance in HHS prevent glucose from being used well, so blood glucose levels rise above 600 mg/dL. Having high blood glucose levels leads to osmotic diuresis, which makes dehydration and electrolyte problems worse. The symptoms that appear are mental confusion, frequent urination, and increased thirst as the body tries to get rid of extra glucose through urine. To manage and diagnose HHS well, it is important to know this pathophysiology, especially in older people and those who have other health problems. HHS affects electrolyte balance, mainly in the case of sodium and potassium. When glucose rises, it makes the body lose water from inside the cells, which increases the concentration of osmoles in the blood. Because of this change, hyponatremia may happen, which makes it more difficult to manage HHS. Moreover, as a result of dehydration, the kidneys do not function properly and are unable to remove both glucose and electrolytes from the body. When there is extra fluid in the body, the serum electrolytes might not show the true levels. HHS patients need their fluid and electrolyte levels to be closely monitored while their hearts and brains are carefully watched. Swift identification of these electrolyte changes is necessary, since they may result in significant complications such as heart rhythm problems and disturbances in the brain, proving once again why pathophysiology plays a vital role in HHS management. New studies have shown that there is a link between increased serum tumor markers and the problems caused by HHS. For instance, levels of carcinoembryonic antigen (CEA) have been found to correlate positively with osmolarity in patients with HHS, suggesting that increased CEA may serve as a predictor for the severity of the condition (Gong et al., 2024). Besides, it has been noted that serum iron levels are linked to certain tumor markers, suggesting that diabetes may be related to hidden malignancies. By knowing these connections, doctors can improve the accuracy of diagnosing HHS and its related problems. By integrating biochemical analyses into the clinical framework, healthcare providers can achieve a comprehensive understanding of an individual's metabolic dysfunction, ultimately enhancing patient outcomes in cases of hyperglycemic crises such as HHS (Palmiere, 2015) (Figure 9.6).

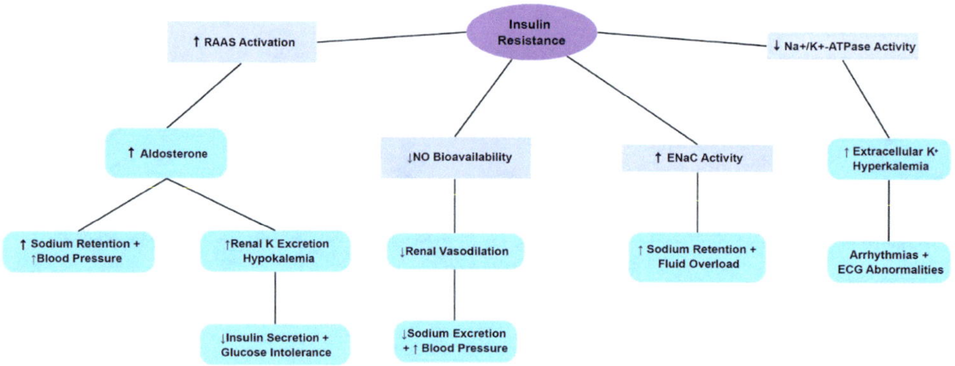

Figure 9.6. Elevated blood glucose concentrations result in osmotic diuresis, which exacerbates dehydration and electrolyte imbalances.

Source: Crintea IN, Cindrea AC, Mederle OA, Trebuian CI, Timar R. Electrolyte Imbalances and Metabolic Emergencies in Obesity: Mechanisms and Clinical Implications. *Diseases*. 2025; 13(3):69. https://doi.org/10.3390/diseases13030069

9.2.1. Mechanism of Insulin Resistance

The mechanism of insulin resistance plays a crucial role in the pathophysiology of diabetic ketoacidosis (DKA) and hyperglycemic hyperosmolar state (HHS). Insulin usually helps glucose enter into the tissues where glucose is stored, but if there are certain pro-inflammatory cytokines, insulin's action is blocked and glucose levels rise in the blood. Hyperglycemia is responsible for both DKA and HHS, and it also increases the likelihood of lactic acidosis because of insufficient glucose for cells and the related anaerobic metabolism. For this reason, learning about insulin resistance is very important to grasp the rise of these serious complications in diabetic patients, especially in terms of their physical and chemical aspects. Frequently, chronic insulin resistance leads to problems with pancreatic beta-cells, which makes it harder to manage diabetes and its sudden complications. When insulin is produced less due to continuous insulin resistance, the liver makes more glucose through gluconeogenesis, which further increases high blood sugar. This situation is especially noticeable in Type 2 diabetes, since the body's insulin needs can become so high that the beta cells cannot keep up. DKA makes the situation very serious, as more lipolysis results in the buildup of ketone bodies and leads to metabolic acidosis. The difficulty of handling these conditions is increased by the need for intensive treatment. Enhancing insulin sensitivity allows medical experts to support proper regulation of blood sugar. Apart from high blood sugar, insulin resistance can result in electrolyte problems and contribute to the disturbances related to lactic acidosis. Increased blood sugar levels often go together with changes in important electrolytes, making it harder to treat patients in emergency situations. Insulin therapy is important in treating DKA and HHS because it helps bring down glucose and also replaces potassium in cells, which is often missing in these cases. However, insulin resistance can lead to more acidosis, as the body's cells do not work efficiently, which increases the patient's risk of complications. Effective management of these metabolic derangements hinges on a thorough understanding of the mechanism of insulin resistance, which ultimately informs therapeutic strategies aimed at preventing the onset of DKA, HHS, and lactic acidosis in vulnerable populations, as noted in the literature (Palmiere, 2015) and the clinical characterization of DKA (Modi et al., 2020) (Figure 9.7).

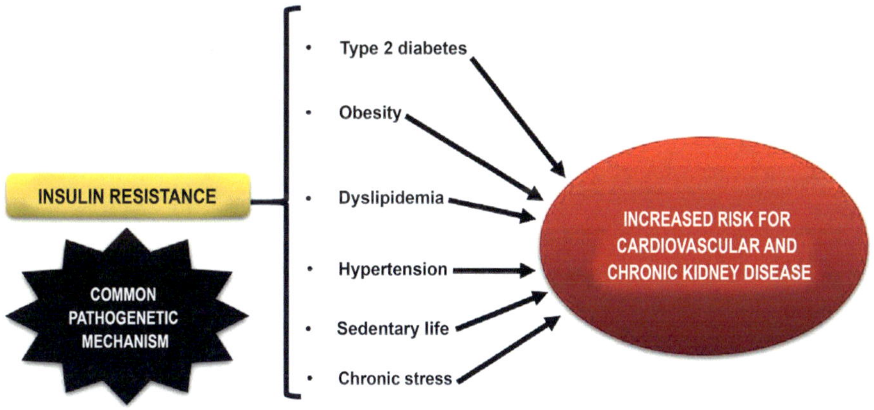

Figure 9.7. By restoring insulin sensitivity, medical professionals can mitigate emergencies and promote a better regulatory environment for glucose homeostasis.

Source: Papakonstantinou E, Oikonomou C, Nychas G, Dimitriadis GD. Effects of Diet, Lifestyle, Chrononutrition and Alternative Dietary Interventions on Postprandial Glycemia and Insulin Resistance. *Nutrients*. 2022; 14(4):823. https://doi.org/10.3390/nu14040823

9.2.2. Hyperglycemia and Osmotic Diuresis

The phenomenon of hyperglycemia is intricately linked to osmotic diuresis, a pivotal pathological process that manifests during acute hyperglycemic crises such as Diabetic Ketoacidosis (DKA) and Hyperglycemic Hyperosmolar State (HHS). If blood glucose goes above 180 mg/dL, the kidneys start to excrete extra glucose because of the osmotic effect it creates in urine. As a result of this osmotic effect, there is a lot of urine produced and the body becomes dehydrated. Therefore, patients may develop serious problems with fluids and electrolytes, which could lead to extra problems if not addressed properly. Glycosuria and the associated increase in urine output contribute significantly to the severity of the hyperglycemic crisis, marking osmotic diuresis as a critical factor in understanding the clinical implications of these metabolic disorders (Ekpebegh et al., 2011). When treating patients, it is necessary to notice how osmotic diuresis affects sodium and potassium levels, since hyperglycemia causes these electrolytes to be lost and should be corrected during treatment. In some patients with hyperglycemic crises, hypernatremia complicates the management of fluid imbalances. Research indicates that individuals admitted for hyperglycemic crises often present with altered serum sodium levels, a condition associated with older age and altered consciousness, as well as newly diagnosed diabetes (Ekpebegh et al., 2011). Because hyperosmolarity is very severe in these patients, careful monitoring and the right fluid replacement plan is necessary, since mishandling may make their electrolyte problems worse and delay their recovery. Doctors and nurses should assess patients well to guide the replacement of fluids and electrolytes needed for managing hyperglycemia and its osmotic diuresis. The main goal of the initial treatment is to calculate how much water, sodium, and potassium the patient needs to restore normal body functions. While the treatment continues, it is necessary to adjust the replacement fluids according to the patient's losses, urine output, and changes in their blood chemistry. Regularly checking a patient's health and blood tests, mainly for glucose, sodium, and potassium, is necessary to prevent metabolic acidosis and problems with electrolytes. Taking a dynamic approach to fluid management helps to reduce the harmful effects of osmotic diuresis and therefore improves outcomes for patients with high blood sugar and promotes their recovery in DKA and HHS (Figure 9.8).

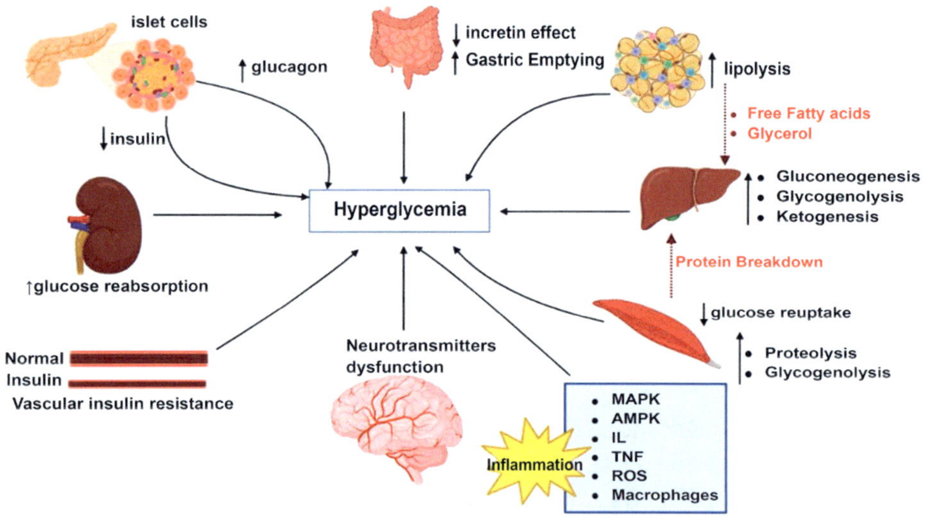

Figure 9.8. The phenomenon of hyperglycemia is intricately linked to osmotic diuresis, a pivotal pathological process that manifests during acute hyperglycemic crises such as Diabetic Ketoacidosis (DKA) and Hyperglycemic Hyperosmolar State (HHS).

Source: Naz R, Saqib F, Awadallah S, Wahid M, Latif MF, Iqbal I, Mubarak MS. Food Polyphenols and Type II Diabetes Mellitus: Pharmacology and Mechanisms. *Molecules*. 2023; 28(10):3996. https://doi.org/10.3390/molecules28103996

9.2.3. Complications Arising from HHS

The Hyperglycemic Hyperosmolar State (HHS) presents a myriad of complications that significantly contribute to patient morbidity and mortality. HHS is mainly found in patients with type 2 diabetes and may result in serious dehydration, problems with electrolytes, and disturbances in the nervous system. When blood glucose rises too high, it causes fluid to shift from the intracellular space to the extracellular space, following an osmotic gradient. This increases the risk of coma, kidney failure and shock. Often, complications are increased by the health problems that are more common in this group, for example, cardiovascular disease and chronic kidney disease. For this reason, it is crucial to notice the early signs of HHS so that proper treatment can be given as soon as possible and the patient's condition can improve. In addition, HHS may result in dangerous changes in a person's metabolism. Changes in potassium levels in the blood may cause arrhythmias or a heart attack for patients. If hyperosmolarity is present, it can affect the brain and cause changes in mental status or seizures. If a person's condition becomes very serious, they may slip into a coma, so urgent medical care is needed. It is very important to notice these signs early and use the right treatment methods. In many cases, patients are given fluids and their electrolyte levels are corrected carefully while being watched continuously to prevent complications. Mortality rates can be as high as 20%, which is 10 times more than with diabetic ketoacidosis. Early medical treatment is necessary and prevention with adequate management of diabetes lowers the risk of HHS. In addition to the physical effects, HHS causes various psychosocial problems. A slow and sneaky start to HHS may cause people to visit healthcare settings late, making their problems worse and resulting in longer hospital stays. Patients may also experience emotional challenges because of having to go to the hospital often, the effects of chronic illness on their daily lives, and the interruptions to their regular activities. Such factors may make it harder for patients to stick to their treatment plans and worsen the progress of diabetes. Consequently, a holistic approach to patient care must be adopted, encompassing not only the physical management of HHS but also addressing the psychological, social, and educational needs of patients to holistically improve outcomes in diabetic care and management (Anumah et al., 2007) (Figure 9.9).

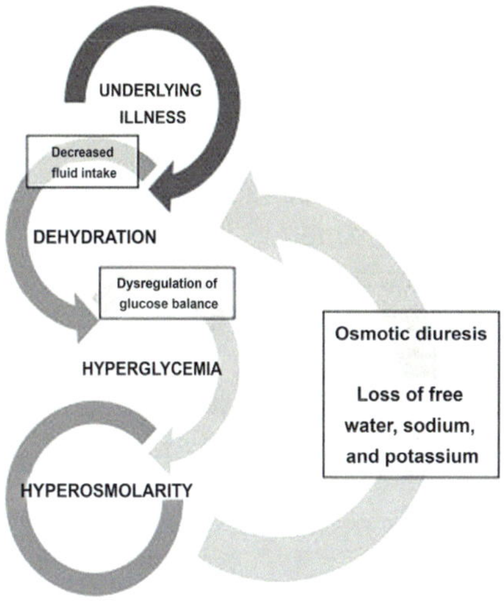

Figure 9.9. The Hyperglycemic Hyperosmolar State (HHS) presents a myriad of complications that significantly contribute to patient morbidity and mortality.

Source: https://ars.els-cdn.com/content/image/1-s2.0-S0733862723000743-gr2.jpg

9.3. Pathophysiology of Lactic Acidosis

The pathophysiology of lactic acidosis is critical to understanding its implications in pathological states such as diabetic ketoacidosis (DKA) and hyperglycemic hyperosmolar state (HHS). The main cause of lactic acidosis is an imbalance in the body between making and eliminating lactate, especially when there is not enough oxygen in the tissues and metabolism is changed. Due to insufficient insulin in diabetes, especially when it is DKA, cells are unable to use glucose properly, which results in anaerobic metabolism. Therefore, lactate production rises, which causes acidemia. In addition, reduced oxygen in the limbs of diabetic patients can make the problem worse, as lactate keeps accumulating because the liver and kidneys cannot remove it fast enough. So, the combination of these metabolic problems highlights the need to regularly check lactate levels in diabetic patients who are very ill. The link between lactate and particular diabetes complications shows how lactic acidosis develops in the body. Evidence indicates that individuals with diabetes mellitus, particularly those experiencing acute myocardial infarction (AMI), exhibit markedly elevated lactate concentrations when compared to non-diabetics. For instance, a study demonstrated that blood lactate levels in type 2 diabetes patients with AMI averaged 4.54±1.44 mmol/L, significantly higher than the 3.19±1.005 mmol/L seen in nondiabetic counterparts (Mitic et al., 2016). This finding proves that lactate is a significant marker for predicting the outcome of diabetes patients. In particular, when lactate is high, there is a greater risk of heart failure, arrhythmias, and cardiogenic shock, which suggests that elevated lactate points to poor outcomes for these patients. In the field of forensics, it can be difficult to diagnose lactic acidosis, especially when thinking about the sudden effects of diabetes as possible causes of death. Since lactic acidosis is connected to metabolic problems, a thorough examination of biochemical parameters is required to find out the exact cause. Using blood lactate levels as well as new parameters helps in the medical examination of deaths resulting from diabetes complications, such as DKA and HHS. The ability to conduct biochemical assessments postmortem may provide crucial insights, enabling medics to discern the involvement of metabolic derangements in fatalities (Palmiere, 2015). So, knowing about lactic acidosis as part of metabolic problems helps both doctors and forensic experts see its importance and why it should be better understood (Figure 9.10).

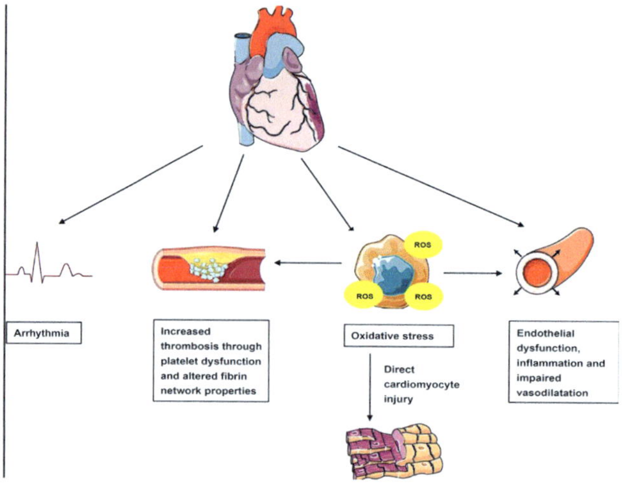

Figure 9.10. Individuals with diabetes mellitus, particularly those experiencing acute myocardial infarction (AMI), exhibit markedly elevated lactate concentrations when compared to non-diabetics.

Source: https://www.researchgate.net/publication/310467742/figure/fig2/AS:1086746599137323@1636111988398/Mean-blood-lactate-levels-in-patients-with-acute-myocardial-infarction-and-diabetes.jpg

9.3.1. Causes of Increased Lactate Production

In the context of diabetic emergencies, understanding the mechanisms leading to increased lactate production is crucial, particularly in conditions like Diabetic Ketoacidosis (DKA). Mainly, high lactate levels are caused by a lack of oxygen in tissues and an increase in anaerobic metabolism, which happen in situations of metabolic stress. A lack of insulin and an increase in glucagon and cortisol in DKA lead to glucose intolerance and cause problems in metabolism. Because of this, the body cannot use glucose properly, so lactate builds up as a result of anaerobic glycolysis. Consequently, lactate levels rise, contributing to the formation of lactic acidosis, a significant factor in DKA pathology (Modi et al., 2020).

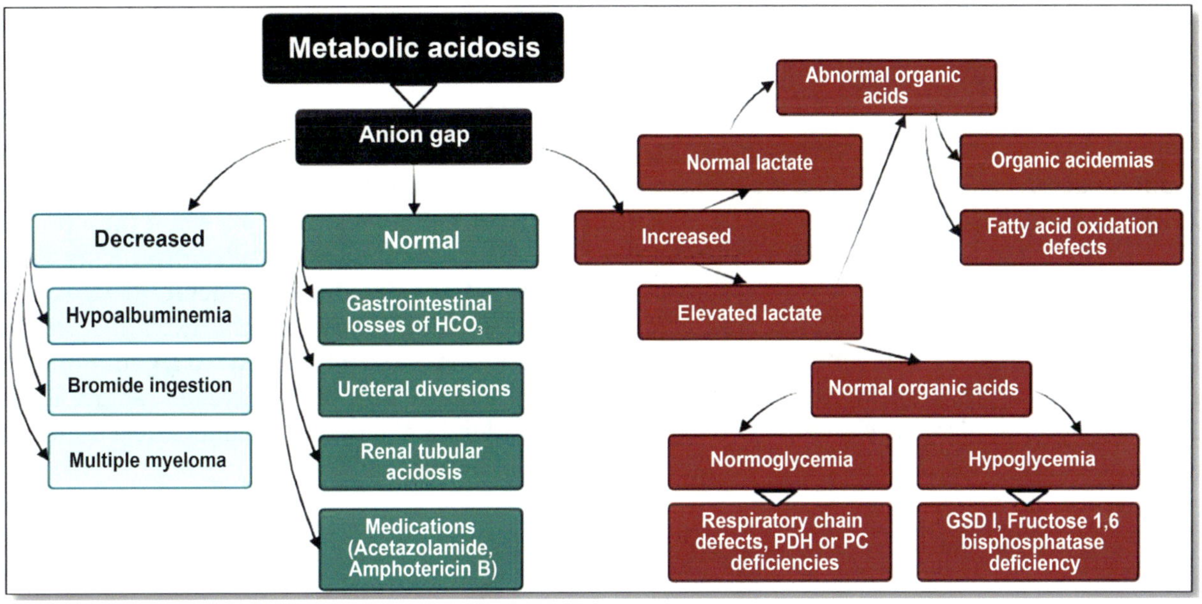

Figure 9.11. Elevated lactate levels primarily stem from tissue hypoxia and enhanced anaerobic metabolism, prevalent in states of metabolic stress.

Source: Belu A, Filip N, Trandafir LM, Spoială EL, Țarcă E, Zamosteanu D, Ghiga G, Bernic J, Jehac A, Cojocaru E. Lactate, an Essential Metabolic Marker in the Diagnosis and Management of Pediatric Conditions. *Diagnostics*. 2025; 15(7):816. https://doi.org/10.3390/diagnostics15070816

Being aware of these mechanisms matters a lot to healthcare providers, as it helps them address the risks caused by high lactate in DKA. Hyperglycemic Hyperosmolar State (HHS) also plays a critical role in lactate production, albeit through different metabolic pathways. Extreme elevations in blood sugar in HHS lead to more water being lost, which causes dehydration and reduces the supply of oxygen to the body's tissues. Lack of blood flow in the peripheral tissues leads to anaerobic respiration, which causes more lactate to be made. The changes in metabolism are very significant, since the lactic acidemia that follows makes the patient's condition even more serious. It was also found that sepsis, which is common with HHS, tends to make the metabolic issues even worse. Sepsis correlates with prolonged insulin infusion and hospital stay due to increased lactate levels, underscoring the need for vigilance in monitoring these patients

(Hamza et al., 2016). So, it is important to understand the various aspects of lactate production in HHS to manage the results well. Apart from diabetes, different medical conditions may cause lactate levels to rise, mainly in critically ill patients with DKA or HHS. When a person has severe dehydration and loses a lot of blood, it can cause the oxygen supply to be out of balance, making lactic acidosis worse. Besides, when infections like sepsis occur, the body's metabolic rate rises and causes more stress, resulting in the use of anaerobic metabolism and higher lactate levels. In pediatric populations experiencing DKA, the duration of insulin infusion has been found to be significantly linked to persistent electrolyte disturbances, emphasizing that inappropriate metabolic states can lead to lactate overproduction (Hamza et al., 2016). Having a clear idea of how these factors interact is necessary for designing effective approaches to help patients who have these acute problems (Figure 9.11).

9.3.2. Impaired Lactate Clearance Mechanisms

Impaired lactate clearance mechanisms are crucial in understanding the pathophysiology of metabolic disturbances associated with diabetic emergencies, particularly in diabetic ketoacidosis (DKA) and lactic acidosis. A rise in lactate levels in people with diabetes happens when their bodies have trouble using glucose and there is not enough oxygen in the tissues. Besides producing more lactate, the liver and kidneys are less able to get rid of it from the blood. If lactate clearance is hindered, for example in cases of acute illnesses like myocardial infarction, the extra lactate can cause severe acidosis. Clinicians must appreciate that factors like low tissue oxygenation and defective glucose metabolism in diabetic patients contribute not only to heightened lactate levels but also to poorer prognoses, emphasizing the need for vigilant monitoring and intervention in those presenting with DKA or lactic acidosis (Mitic et al., 2016).

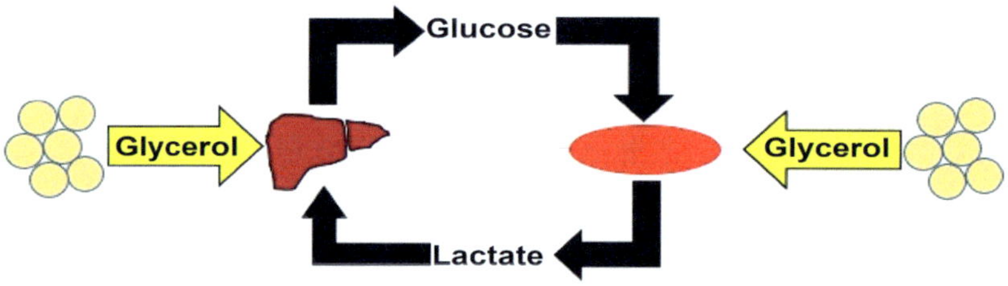

Figure 9.12. In individuals suffering from diabetes, lactate production can increase significantly due to inadequate glucose metabolism and concurrent tissue hypoxia.

Source: Shah, Ankit, Yujue Wang, and Fredric E. Wondisford. 2022. "Differential Metabolism of Glycerol Based on Oral versus Intravenous Administration in Humans" *Metabolites* 12, no. 10: 890. https://doi.org/10.3390/metabo12100890

The complexity of impaired lactate clearance is particularly pronounced in the context of hyperglycemic hyperosmolar state (HHS). When a patient has HHS, their blood glucose levels can increase a lot, resulting in too much urination and dehydration. The reason for this is that the kidneys are not working properly and are not receiving enough blood due to dehydration. The presence of lactate adds to the metabolic acidosis as well as worsens the main problem of high blood sugar. Furthermore, the risk of developing lactic acidosis in hyperglycemic states highlights the interconnected nature of these conditions, reinforcing the importance of addressing both hyperglycemia and lactate clearance mechanisms in management strategies (Modi et al., 2020). Fast and effective actions are necessary to avoid the problems that may result from poor lactate clearance. Doctors mainly use various methods to restore fluid in the blood, correct electrolyte problems, and give urgent insulin to reduce blood glucose levels in DKA and HHS. At the same time, clinicians should keep an eye on lactate levels during the entire treatment process. Knowing how lactate is produced, cleared, and linked to blood sugar helps doctors make better choices and leads to better patient results. Ultimately, recognizing and addressing impaired lactate clearance mechanisms will prove integral in the holistic management of patients suffering from DKA, HHS, and associated forms of lactic acidosis (Mitic et al., 2016) (Figure 9.12).

9.3.3. Relationship between Lactic Acidosis and Tissue Hypoxia

The relationship between lactic acidosis and tissue hypoxia is critical in understanding the pathological states associated with diabetic ketoacidosis (DKA) and hyperglycemic hyperosmolar state (HHS). When the body makes more lactic acid than it can clear, it is known as lactic acidosis, and this usually happens when tissues do not receive enough oxygen. When diabetic patients suffer from acute conditions such as myocardial infarction, insufficient oxygen and impaired glucose use in the body can worsen lactic acidosis. It was found in an important study that people with diabetes and high lactate levels were more likely to suffer from heart failure and arrhythmias. This suggests that in scenarios where oxygen availability is compromised, as seen in DKA and HHS, the resultant lactate accumulation may serve as a crucial marker for evaluating patient prognosis and the severity of metabolic derangements (Mitic et al., 2016). Also, the connection between lactic acidosis and tissue hypoxia is made more complex by the metabolic problems that occur in diabetes mellitus. Impaired glucose metabolism reduces the body's energy production and also encourages anaerobic glucose breakdown, which increases lactate levels. In diabetic patients, this phenomenon is clear since their bodies cannot deal with hypoxia as well as healthy people can. A new study has shown that high levels of lactate in DKA patients result in important changes in the heart and kidneys, pointing out the wider effects of metabolic acidosis when there is not enough oxygen. The findings illustrate that understanding lactate dynamics is essential, as elevated lactate levels not only signify increased anaerobic metabolism but also serve as an indicator of worsening hypoxia in the context of diabetic complications (Gong et al., 2024). Noticing the effects of lactic acidosis with tissue hypoxia in DKA and HHS helps medical staff take more effective actions. Lactate levels can show the current metabolic condition of a patient and how they react to different treatments. As lactate can mean both a problem with metabolism and poor blood flow, it is crucial to use it to monitor responses to treatment. If patients show high lactate levels, it may be necessary to treat them with interventions that improve oxygenation and bring metabolic processes back to normal. Since lactic acid levels in diabetic patients are tied to their health outcomes, it is necessary to address both oxygen supply to the tissues and their metabolism. This multifaceted view aids healthcare providers in delivering targeted treatments that address the root causes of lactic acidosis while simultaneously mitigating the effects of tissue hypoxia present in DKA and HHS (Mitic et al., 2016) (Figure 9.13).

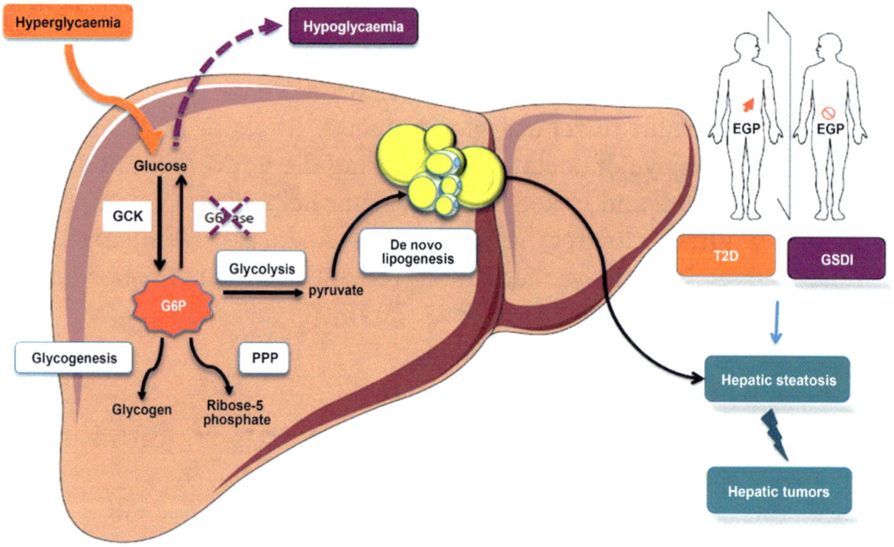

Figure 9.13. The impairment in glucose metabolism not only limits energy production but also contributes to the anaerobic breakdown of glucose, leading to increased lactate production.

Source: Rajas F, Gautier-Stein A, Mithieux G. Glucose-6 Phosphate, a Central Hub for Liver Carbohydrate Metabolism. *Metabolites*. 2019; 9(12):282. https://doi.org/10.3390/metabo9120282

9.4. Clinical Presentation of DKA

The clinical presentation of diabetic ketoacidosis (DKA) is often characterized by a triad of hyperglycemia, ketonemia, and metabolic acidosis. Patients frequently exhibit symptoms such as excessive thirst (polydipsia), frequent urination (polyuria), and abdominal pain, which can sometimes mimic an acute abdomen. As the disease continues, patients can start to feel nauseous and throw up, which may result in dehydration and problems with their electrolytes. One of the signs of DKA is that the breath has a fruity odor, which is caused by acetone made during the breakdown of fatty acids. In the case of COVID-19, the symptoms of DKA can be more noticeable, which makes the infection more severe and increases the risk of health complications. The combination of respiratory difficulties and metabolic problems is challenging for healthcare workers to handle. It is very important to recognize DKA in patients with diabetes, as its symptoms may change fast. Those who already have diabetes may experience DKA after an infection, after surgery, or when they do not follow their insulin treatment. It is becoming clear that DKA can affect patients with newly diagnosed diabetes, especially when they are facing illness or severe metabolic changes. In addition, studies show that the severity of DKA in those with COVID-19 can be increased, which may lead to poorer results. Elevated mortality rates in such cases underscore the need for prompt and aggressive management strategies, including intravenous insulin therapy and careful monitoring of electrolytes, especially potassium, which can fluctuate significantly during treatment (Hasan et al., 2020; Al-Sa HAH'idy et al., 2022). It is important to detect DKA early and act fast to control the abnormal changes in metabolism. Dehydration is corrected by giving intravenous fluids, and insulin is given to help glucose uptake and stop the formation of ketones. During treatment, it is necessary to check electrolytes, mainly potassium, since imbalances in this area can cause dangerous heart problems. With the introduction of SGLT2 inhibitors, diabetes management now includes new issues because these drugs may still cause DKA in people with normal blood sugar. The interplay between DKA and concurrent infections like COVID-19 has underscored the need for a tailored therapeutic approach to manage glycemic goals effectively while preventing adverse events (Hasan et al., 2020; Al-Sa HAH'idy et al., 2022). For this reason, it is important to recognize the signs of DKA to help patients in both regular and emergency care (Figure 9.14).

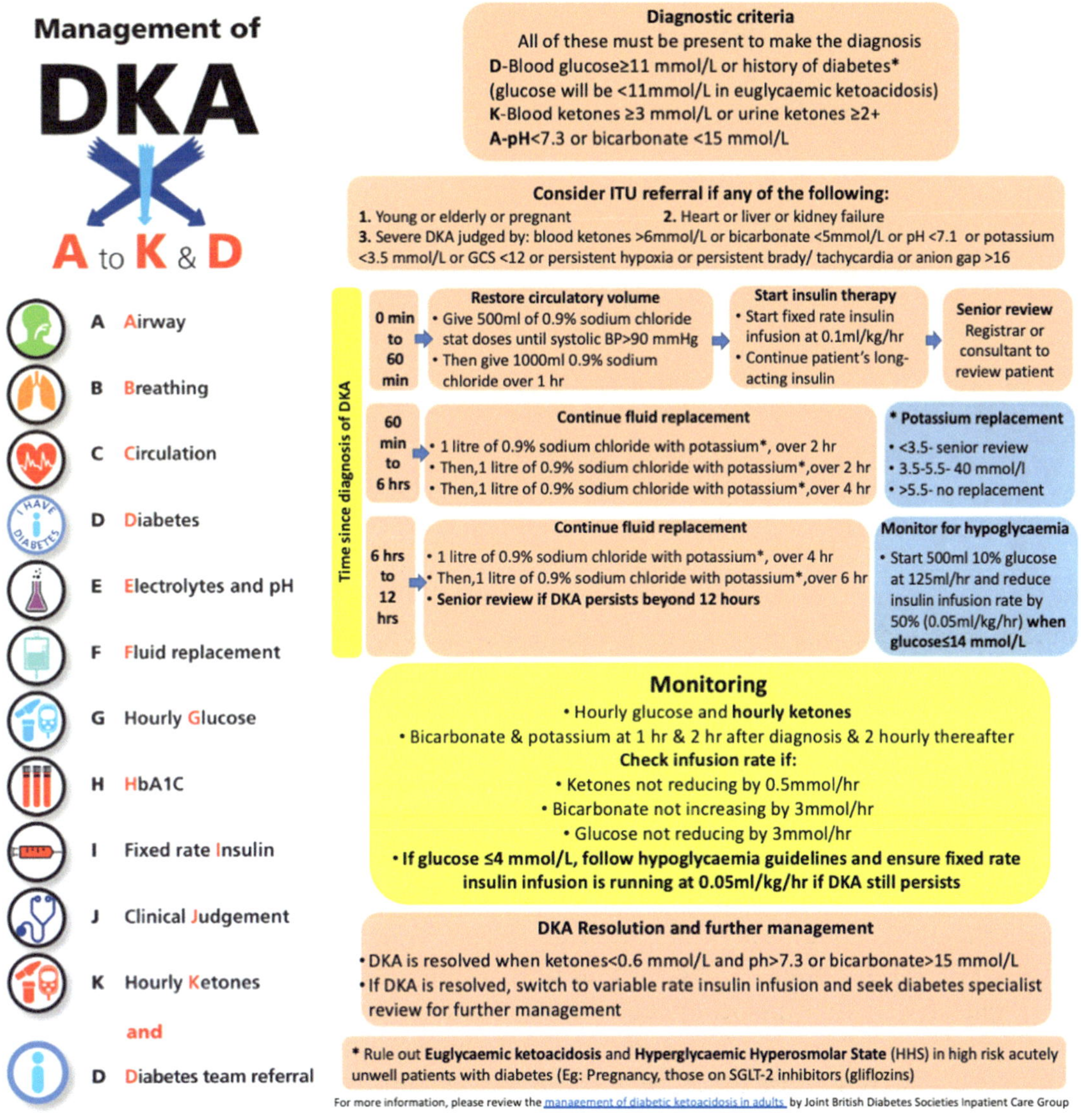

Figure 9.14. Intravenous fluids are initiated to correct dehydration and restore hemodynamic stability, while insulin is administered to facilitate the uptake of glucose and halt ketogenesis.

Source: https://onlinelibrary.wiley.com/doi/10.1111/dme.14788

9.4.1. Symptoms and Signs of DKA

The presentation of diabetic ketoacidosis (DKA) is marked by a constellation of symptoms that typically escalate rapidly, necessitating prompt recognition and intervention. At the beginning, patients can have frequent urination, increased thirst, and hunger, which happen because of high blood sugar. As the condition worsens, patients usually feel tired and weak, which reduces their ability to function normally.

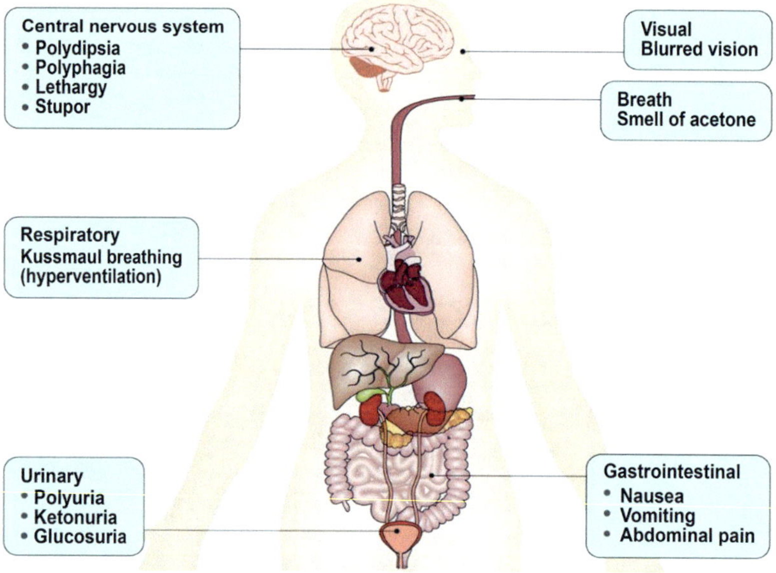

Figure 9.15. The metabolic derangements inherent in DKA also contribute to more severe manifestations such as abdominal pain, nausea, and vomiting, which can mimic gastroenteritis and complicate clinical assessments.

Source: https://media.springernature.com/lw1200/springer-static/image/art%3A10.1038%2Fs41572-020-0165-1/MediaObjects/41572_2020_165_Fig3_HTML.png

The changes in metabolism in DKA also cause abdominal pain, nausea, and vomiting, which can make DKA look similar to gastroenteritis and complicate how doctors assess the patient. Moreover, as acidosis occurs and blood flow to the brain decreases, a person may become confused or very tired. Because of these symptoms, it is clear that DKA is complicated and requires a thorough check-up to tell it apart from other medical problems, especially in urgent cases. With the worsening of the disease, patients will develop Kussmaul respirations due to the metabolic acidosis. This kind of breathing is the body's effort to let out carbon dioxide and balance its blood acid-base levels. Fruity or acetone-like breath is usually a clear sign of ketoacidosis, which happens when there are too many ketones in the blood. Besides, patients are often dehydrated, which makes their mucous membranes dry and their skin less taut, both of which may indicate how severe the disease is. Hypotension and tachycardia may occur in patients, which shows the body is losing fluids and reacting to this by increasing the heart rate. All these symptoms and signs together show the metabolic problem of DKA as well as its effect on the patient's body, which requires prompt and careful medical care. It is very important to recognize diabetic ketoacidosis since it can lead to a fast decline in a patient's condition. In most cases, the criteria are high plasma glucose, low pH, low serum bicarbonate, and the presence of ketones in blood and urine. It is essential to differentiate DKA from conditions such as hyperglycemic hyperosmolar state (HHS) and lactic acidosis, where the clinical presentations may overlap but require distinct treatment approaches (Bartoszek et al., 2024). Furthermore, there exists a variant known as Euglycemic DKA, where ketoacidosis can occur despite normal or only mildly elevated blood glucose levels, complicating diagnosis and management (Jalili et al., 2019). Promptly spotting the multiple symptoms of DKA can result in better outcomes for patients through early treatment (Figure 9.15).

9.4.2. Diagnostic Criteria for DKA

The diagnosis of diabetic ketoacidosis (DKA) is critical for timely intervention in hyperglycemic emergencies. The condition requires three things: high blood glucose, ketones in the system, and a high anion gap acidosis. When the blood glucose level is more than 250 mg/dL, it is usually a clear sign of the condition.

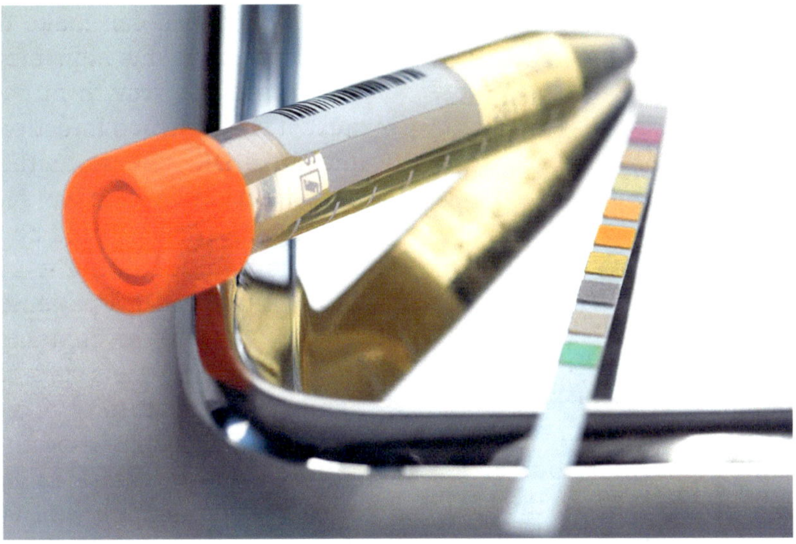

Figure 9.16. The detection of ketoacids, which may be assessed through blood tests or urinalysis, confirms the process of lipolysis contributing to increased ketone production.

Source: https://img.lb.wbmdstatic.com/vim/live/webmd/consumer_assets/site_images/article_thumbnails/BigBead/ketones_bigbead/1800x1200_ketones_bigbead.jpg

The presence of ketoacids, which can be checked through blood or urine tests, indicates that lipolysis is taking place and is the cause of more ketones. The presence of metabolic acidosis is confirmed by checking the blood pH and bicarbonate levels; a pH lower than 7.30 and less than 15 mEq/L of bicarbonate in the blood shows acidosis. This tripartite diagnostic approach ensures an accurate identification of DKA, allowing for prompt management that can significantly mitigate associated morbidity and mortality (Gong et al., 2024). It is important to understand the body's response to DKA when looking at the criteria for its diagnosis. If insulin is lacking, glucose is not used by the body's tissues, so the liver raises glucose production and begins to break down fat. As well as increasing blood glucose, this process causes a number of metabolic changes, such as the creation of ketoacids such as beta-hydroxybutyrate and acetoacetate. Ketoacids play a role in increasing the anion gap, leading to more metabolic acidosis, which is one of the main signs of DKA. Interestingly, recent studies have elucidated the relationship between various serum markers and the severity of DKA, suggesting that biomarkers such as CA199 may offer additional insights into the patients acidotic state (Gong et al., 2024). For this reason, understanding these biochemical pathways well helps doctors make accurate diagnoses. Also, it is very important to identify and manage DKA early in patients with diabetes to avoid serious consequences. Proper management consists of restoring normal blood volume, giving insulin to lower blood glucose, and filling potassium levels in the body. All of these elements are important for correcting the body's metabolic problems and dealing with infections or missed insulin intake. Moreover, the incorporation of evolving clinical guidelines and insights from contemporary research allows for an enhanced framework for managing DKA (Modi et al., 2020). If healthcare providers follow the same guidelines for diagnosis and treatment, patients can benefit a lot, so it is important to pay close attention to early detection of DKA and its related metabolic issues in diabetes-related emergencies (Figure 9.16).

9.4.3. Common Complications Associated with DKA

Diabetic Ketoacidosis (DKA) is known for its rapid onset and severe complications, primarily affecting individuals with type 1 diabetes. Some of the main risks of DKA are dehydration and imbalances in electrolytes, mainly hypokalemia, which may cause fatal heart problems if not managed swiftly. DKA causes the body to produce too many ketone bodies, which leads to acidosis and greatly affects the body's acid-base balance. Clinical symptoms such as frequent urination, thirst, and abdominal pain are seen in this condition, and if they are not handled well, they may result in serious issues such as cerebral edema. The identified need for intensive monitoring and intervention during the management of DKA emphasizes the complexity of treatment, requiring multiple therapeutic modalities, including fluid replacement and insulin therapy to stabilize the patient and mitigate further complications associated with the condition (Anumah et al., 2007). One more issue that often occurs with DKA is infections, which can make the situation even more difficult. The high blood sugar in DKA encourages the growth of bacteria, which can cause urinary tract infections or pneumonia and make DKA worse at the same time. The fact that infections can worsen DKA shows that treating infections should be a key part of DKA treatment. In addition, the possibility of acute kidney injury in DKA patients, especially when they are very dehydrated and have electrolyte problems, makes their care more difficult. This highlights the necessity of a multidisciplinary approach to care, incorporating not only insulin and fluid therapy but also vigilant monitoring for signs of infection and renal compromise (Bartoszek et al., 2024). Another problem that can happen in DKA is cerebral edema, and it is most common in children. Although the exact cause is not known, it is believed that fast changes in the amount of osmolality in the blood lead to fluid moving into the brain. Patients who experience altered consciousness because of brain issues may need fast interventions to avoid permanent damage to the brain. When this complication is noticed, doctors ensure they give fluids slowly to prevent the brain from swelling. It is important to be aware and ready to use hyperventilation or mannitol if cerebral edema happens. The implications of these complications further reinforce the need for meticulous attention to detail during the management of DKA to ensure optimal patient outcomes (Anumah et al., 2007) (Figure 9.17).

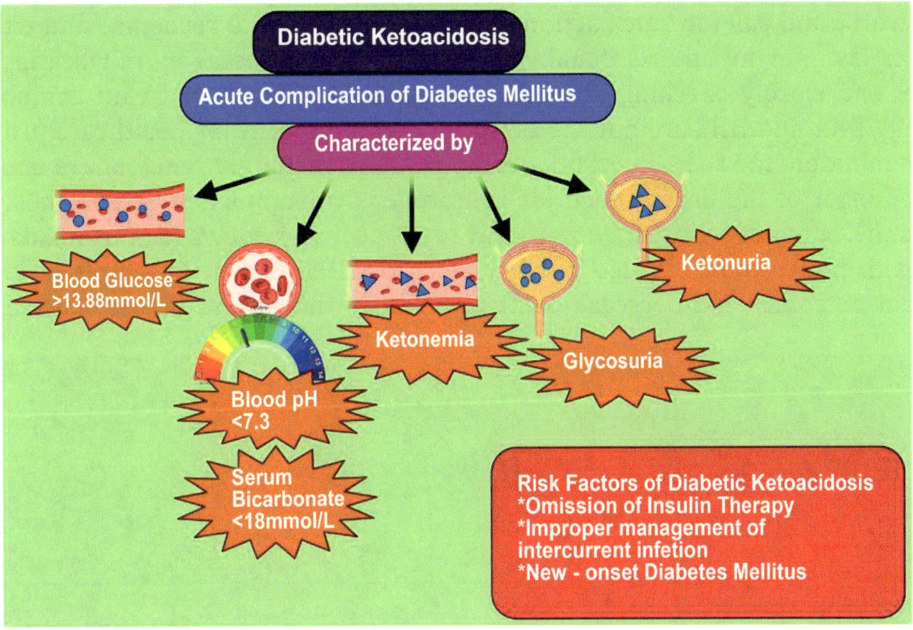

Figure 9.17. The hyperglycemic environment in DKA creates a favorable breeding ground for pathogens, often leading to urinary tract infections or pneumonia, which can simultaneously precipitate and worsen DKA.

Source: Ahmad R, Narwaria M, Singh A, Kumar S, Haque M. Detecting Diabetic Ketoacidosis with Infection: Combating a Life-Threatening Emergency with Practical Diagnostic Tools. *Diagnostics*. 2023; 13(14):2441. https://doi.org/10.3390/diagnostics13142441

9.5. Clinical Presentation of HHS

The clinical presentation of Hyperglycemic Hyperosmolar State (HHS) is distinctly characterized by severe hyperglycemia, elevated serum osmolarity, and an absence of significant ketoacidosis. Patients typically present with symptoms such as excessive thirst (polydipsia), frequent urination (polyuria), and, in some cases, altered mental status due to the dramatic shifts in osmotic balance within the central nervous system. Unlike Diabetic Ketoacidosis (DKA), where metabolic acidosis is prominent, HHS presents with a more insidious onset and often involves older populations with underlying comorbidities, such as cardiovascular diseases. Recent studies indicate that the mortality rate in HHS patients remains alarmingly high, with one analysis revealing a 31% mortality rate specifically associated with HHS, emphasizing the critical nature of recognizing this condition early to initiate appropriate clinical management (Akinrinmade et al., 2011). Apart from the usual signs, HHS may also cause neurological problems that can be seen as confusion, sleepiness, or seizures. For instance, a case study involving a 37-year-old woman detailed the emergence of involuntary movements, such as chorea, linked to her HHS diagnosis, underscoring the neurological complications that can arise from severe hyperglycemic states (Hamid et al., 2010). Most of these problems happen because HHS causes severe hyperosmolality, which may harm the blood-brain barrier and result in cerebral edema. So, as HHS continues, patients may display symptoms of metabolic issues as well as symptoms of dehydration and altered electrolytes, which can make the situation worse and call for quick action. It is very important to recognize and treat HHS right away due to its fast-moving nature. Usually, doctors manage diabetes by rehydrating the patient, giving insulin, and closely checking the patient's electrolyte levels to avoid complications. The ways to manage DKA and HHS are not the same, so it is important for healthcare providers to tell them apart. In addition, the risk of potential complications, including renal failure and thrombosis, serves as a reminder of the urgent need for comprehensive supportive care in these patients, as noted by the stark outcomes illustrated in recent retrospective reviews (Akinrinmade et al., 2011). Therefore, health professionals should be very alert for HHS, mainly in people at higher risk, to improve patient outcomes and decrease deaths caused by this severe illness (Figure 9.18).

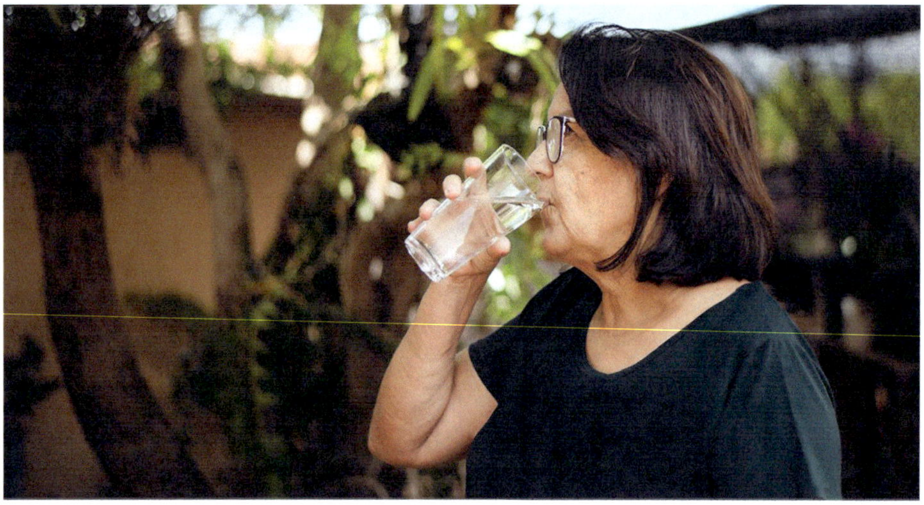

Figure 9.18. Patients typically present with symptoms such as excessive thirst (polydipsia), frequent urination (polyuria), and, in some cases, altered mental status due to the dramatic shifts in osmotic balance within the central nervous system.

Source: https://media.post.rvohealth.io/wp-content/uploads/2025/03/senior-woman-drinking-from-water-glass-outdoors-1200x628-facebook.jpg

9.5.1. Symptoms and Signs of HHS

The Hyperglycemic Hyperosmolar State (HHS) is a potentially life-threatening condition frequently observed in individuals with uncontrolled diabetes, particularly type 2 diabetes mellitus. A major sign of HHS is extremely high blood sugar, usually over 600 mg/dL, which causes a rise in osmolarity. Having a high osmolar state makes the body lose a lot of water, and this is seen as dry skin, dry mouth, and frequent urination. With the progression of the condition, people may develop neurological symptoms like confusion, tiredness, and seizures. Because insulin is not working properly in HHS, glucagon and epinephrine are released in higher amounts, which makes blood sugar levels rise further and leads to the main symptoms of fluid and electrolyte imbalance. Signs of HHS in patients are often found during physical examination, such as mental changes and symptoms of dehydration, for example, dry mucous membranes and loose skin. Tachycardia can develop in patients when they lose fluids as a way to maintain blood flow. Unlike Diabetic Ketoacidosis (DKA), HHS typically does not display significant metabolic acidosis; however, patients may present with varying degrees of electrolyte abnormalities, such as hypokalemia, stemming from both renal loss and cellular shifts. The existence of lactic acidosis may make the situation more severe; therefore, checking the arterial blood gases is very important for managing these patients. Noticing these symptoms helps diagnose the condition and shows why quick action is needed to avoid serious outcomes such as coma or death that can happen without treatment. Various biochemical markers have been found to point to various metabolic problems that can occur in HHS. Elevated levels of specific tumor markers, such as carcinoembryonic antigen (CEA), have been reported in patients with HHS, suggesting a potential linkage between hyperglycemic states and underlying pathophysiological changes in iron homeostasis and osmolarity. A study found that osmolar levels are strongly related to several markers of heart and kidney function, so it is important to thoroughly check the metabolism of these patients. Besides, understanding the mild symptoms of HHS, especially when there are other health issues, allows us to look into treatment plans that help with both urgent symptoms and the core metabolic problems. Thus, understanding the symptoms and signs of HHS is crucial for clinicians aiming to mitigate the morbidity associated with this complex condition (Hamza et al., 2016; Gong et al., 2024) (Figure 9.19).

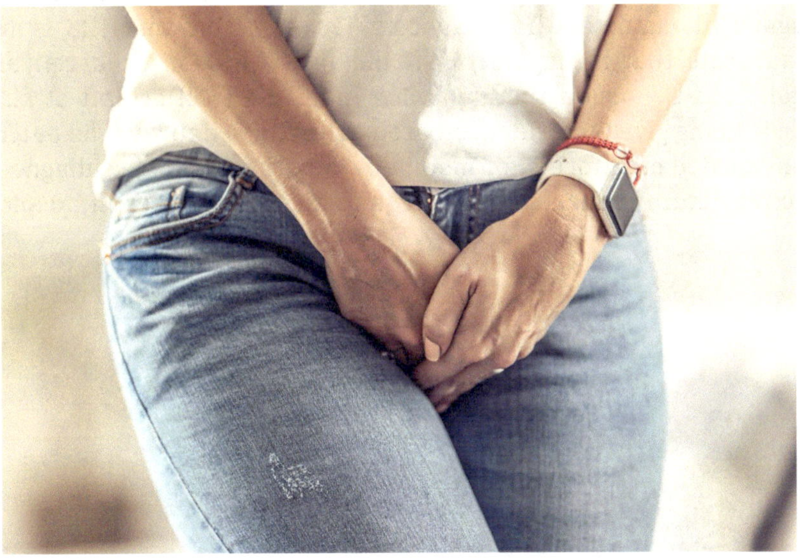

Figure 9.19. Elevated osmolar state results in significant dehydration, which in turn manifests through excessive thirst, frequent urination, and, ultimately, dry skin and mucous membranes.

Source: https://www.verywellhealth.com/thmb/NMTgZKEN7Pk36MeukkeAsWkshz0=/1500x0/filters:no_upscale():max_bytes(150000):strip_icc()/VWH-GettyImages-1364344572-80c3835603ab4c749857bcba86928bcb.jpg

9.5.2. Diagnostic Criteria for HHS

The diagnostic criteria for Hyperglycemic Hyperosmolar State (HHS) are essential for timely identification and management of this serious condition, which predominantly affects individuals with type 2 diabetes. HHS is mainly defined by very high blood sugar levels, which usually go over 600 mg/dL, and a high osmolality that is higher than 320 mOsm/kg. Unlike Diabetic Ketoacidosis (DKA), there is typically a lack of significant ketosis or acidosis in HHS, which is evident from arterial blood gas analyses showing a normal arterial pH and low ketone levels. It is very important because it affects the first steps taken and the long-term care plan for the patient. Clinicians must pay attention to electrolyte abnormalities, mainly in sodium and potassium, since they can make the patient's condition more complex and require extra care during treatment. In addition, the clinical symptoms of HHS are important and usually involve severe dehydration, a change in mental state, and very high blood sugar. Sometimes, symptoms can progress quickly and result in confusion, tiredness, and even coma in the most severe cases. When these symptoms are found, a quick biochemical check is needed to determine if the patient has hyperglycemia and related changes. It is very important to notice HHS early, as patients with this condition often have other health problems that make their condition more serious. A detailed history and physical checkup by clinicians helps them tell HHS apart from other diabetic emergencies, proving that thorough evaluation is needed for patients with hyperglycemia issues. Such diligence aligns with emerging treatment guidelines that stress the importance of accurate diagnosis for optimal intervention and management (Dhatariya et al., 2025). The latest guidelines suggest that healthcare providers must be aware of the latest changes in HHS criteria. According to detailed information on diabetes management, it is recommended that teams from different areas of medicine join forces to make sure the right diagnosis is made and misdiagnosis between DKA and HHS is avoided. Moreover, these guidelines advocate that management should focus first on fluid rehydration to combat hyperosmolality, followed by insulin therapy when indicated (McDermott et al., 2022). It means that more attention is being given to evidence-based methods to improve the outcomes for patients. Besides, using sophisticated monitoring for metabolic factors can enhance diagnosis and treatment, highlighting the active nature of managing hyperglycemic emergencies in hospitals (Figure 9.20).

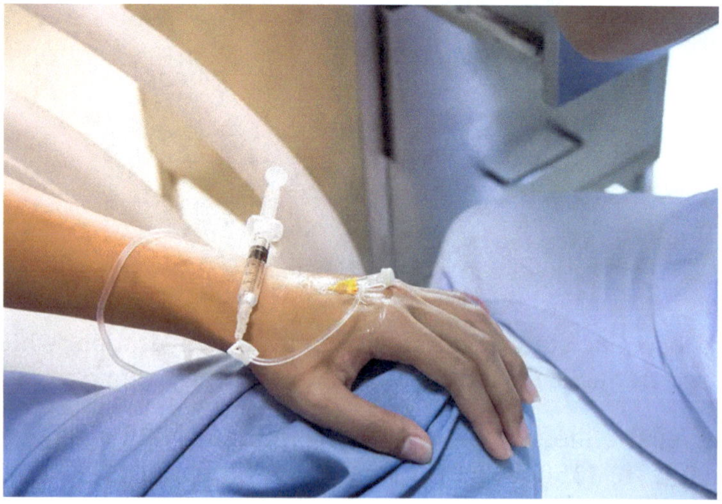

Figure 9.20. Clinicians must be vigilant for other metabolic derangements such as electrolyte imbalances, especially in sodium and potassium levels, which further complicate the clinical picture and necessitate careful monitoring and management during treatment.

Source: https://pharmaceutical-journal.com/wp-content/uploads/2022/08/electrolytes-lead.jpg

9.5.3. Common Complications Associated with HHS

Hyperglycemic Hyperosmolar State (HHS) is a serious condition that presents several common complications, reflective of its metabolic derangements. Most patients experience extremely high blood sugar, which causes them to become very dehydrated and results in electrolyte problems. Hyperglycemia-induced osmotic diuresis may cause acute kidney injury and make fluid and electrolyte loss even worse. Many times, this condition calls for giving intravenous fluids and dialysis if it is severe. Besides, HHS may cause thromboembolic events because of the increased tendency to clot caused by dehydration and electrolyte changes, which can harm blood vessels. The mortality associated with these complications highlights the necessity for early diagnosis and aggressive management, emphasizing the crucial role of healthcare professionals in detecting the warning signs of HHS in at-risk populations, particularly those with poorly controlled diabetes (Anumah et al., 2007). HHS often causes infections that play a major role in increasing the number of cases. A rise in blood glucose may weaken the immune system, which makes patients more likely to get infections in the urinary tract and lungs. These infections increase the level of sugar in the blood and may also lead to more insulin resistance, making it harder to treat HHS. It is important to identify and manage infections quickly since they may cause HHS and can greatly improve a patient's outcome. Furthermore, health care professionals need to monitor patients for signs of infection, especially as infections may be atypical in presentation in this population due to their overall metabolic state (Akms et al., 2020). The effects of HHS on patients' mental well-being should not be ignored, as they may feel very distressed about their condition and the way it is managed. The concern about diabetes-related problems, hospital stays, and lasting effects can cause anxiety and depression, which might influence a person's willingness to follow treatment and their health in general. In addition, both patients and their caregivers should learn about managing diabetes and the early signs of hyperglycemic emergencies. Having counseling and diabetes education programs can help reduce the psychosocial issues people with diabetes face. Overall, understanding the multifaceted nature of HHS, encompassing physical, mental, and social aspects—will enhance patient management and reduce the incidence of adverse outcomes associated with this severe diabetic complication (Anumah et al., 2007) (Figure 9.21).

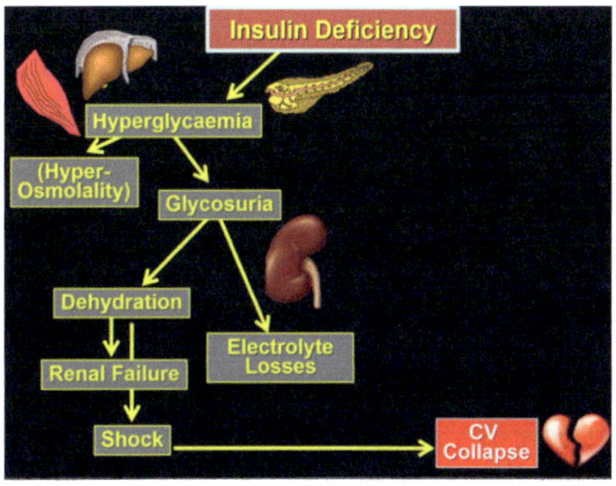

Figure 9.21. The osmotic diuresis stemming from hyperglycemia can precipitate acute kidney injury, exacerbating fluid and electrolyte depletion.

Source: https://quizlet.com/gb/262202003/t1-l16-acute-complications-of-diabetes-flash-cards/

9.6. Management and Treatment Strategies

Effective management and treatment strategies for diabetic ketoacidosis (DKA) hinge on a multifaceted approach that emphasizes rapid intervention and ongoing evaluation. The main goal in therapy is to replace fluids, helping restore the blood volume and improve the kidneys' blood supply. Usually, isotonic saline is given first so that clinicians can slowly change the rate according to the patient's blood sugar levels and hydration. Insulin therapy is also important for treating ketosis and bringing blood glucose levels back to normal, so it is usually given intravenously since DKA is very severe. Both insulin and fluid are needed for a fast response in the management of DKA. Evidence suggests that timing and dosing of interventions significantly impact patient outcomes, thereby necessitating vigilant monitoring of electrolytes, particularly potassium, which can shift dramatically during treatment (Al-Sa HAH'idy et al., 2022). In cases where hyperglycemic hyperosmolar state (HHS) is present, management strategies may differ slightly due to the specific pathophysiological underpinnings of this condition. Although fluid and insulin administration are still very important, the goal is to slowly get the serum glucose back to normal to prevent problems linked to fast changes in osmolality. It is especially important to monitor electrolytes, mainly potassium, because it can cause serious, life-threatening problems during HHS. Therapeutic strategies must be personalized, taking into consideration individual comorbidities, such as diabetes, obesity, and hypertension, noted to contribute to increased morbidity and mortality from conditions like COVID-19 (Katsiki et al., 2021). For this reason, it is important to use these factors to help patients and reduce the risks of hyperglycemic crises. Besides, recognizing lactic acidosis and using appropriate treatment strategies for its cause is very important. It is very important to deal with the main reason for lactic acidosis, such as a lack of oxygen in the tissues or metabolic issues. The first phase of treatment often includes giving fluids through a vein to boost circulation and help organs get enough blood, along with correcting any underlying problems with the patient's metabolism.

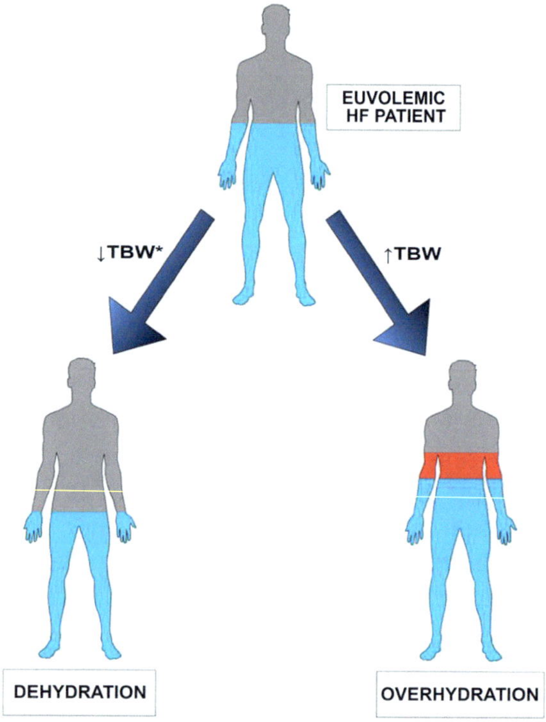

Figure 9.22. Typically, isotonic saline is administered initially, allowing clinicians to gradually adjust the rate based on the patient's glycemic trends and hydration status.

Source: Wittczak A, Ślot M, Bielecka-Dabrowa A. The Importance of Optimal Hydration in Patients with Heart Failure—Not Always Too Much Fluid. *Biomedicines.* 2023; 11(10):2684. https://doi.org/10.3390/biomedicines11102684

Lactic acidosis can indicate that the patient's condition is getting worse, which means they must be watched closely during treatment. Since these metabolic disorders are related, it is helpful for endocrinologists, intensivists, and nephrologists to work together. Understanding the connections between lactic acidosis and infections, including those related to SARS-CoV-2, may also inform management practices, representing a critical aspect of treatment in affected patients (Al-Sa HAH'idy et al., 2022) (Figure 9.22).

9.6.1. Treatment Protocols for DKA

The management of Diabetic Ketoacidosis (DKA) necessitates a structured and immediate approach to treatment, incorporating fluid rehydration, insulin therapy, and electrolyte monitoring. Giving fluids is very important, since it restores blood volume and helps reduce the level of ketones in the body, which lessens the effects of acidosis. Usually, the first step is to use isotonic saline to treat dehydration, based on the amount of fluid the patient is missing. As soon as hemodynamics are stabilized, insulin therapy must be given, since it helps bring blood glucose down and stops the production of ketones, helping the body recover. Giving regular insulin intravenously is often suggested, since it can be adjusted quickly and acts fast to treat both high blood sugar and high ketones at the same time. During DKA treatment, it is necessary to carefully watch electrolytes, especially potassium, since insulin can affect how potassium is present in the blood. Insulin causes potassium to enter the cells, which may cause hypokalemia and lead to serious heart rhythm problems and other problems. Thus, serum electrolytes need to be checked at least once every one to two hours during treatment to manage potassium and make sure its level is normal. Healthcare providers should be careful for the possibility of "refeeding syndrome" when giving fluids and electrolytes to patients who have not eaten properly for a long time. It is necessary to keep track of the patient's condition by regularly assessing clinical parameters, since there is a risk of cerebral edema and the possibility that care will need to be increased. The length of a patient's stay and their outcomes are important signs of how well the protocols work, and studies point out that hyperglycemic crises have different complication rates. According to research, DKA has shown a significantly lower mortality rate compared to Hyperosmolar Diabetic Ketoacidosis (HDKA) and Hyperglycemic Hyperosmolar State (HHS) in various clinical settings, which may reflect not only differences in treatment response but also variances in patient demographic factors and underlying conditions (Akinrinmade et al., 2010, 2011). It is very important for treatment plans to consider these differences to improve how patients are cared for and their long-term results (Figure 9.23).

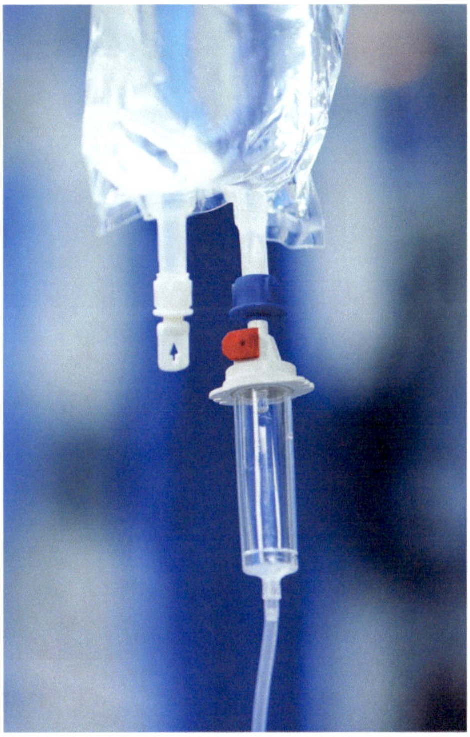

Figure 9.23. The initiation of fluid resuscitation is pivotal, as effective rehydration helps restore blood volume and dilute circulating ketone bodies, thereby lessening the severity of acidosis.

Source: https://i0.wp.com/anaesthesianews.wordpress.com/wp-content/uploads/2022/05/iv-bag-istock-peopleimages-844400642-2400.jpg?fit=1200%2C1200&ssl=1

9.6.2. Treatment Protocols for HHS

Effective treatment protocols for Hyperglycemic Hyperosmolar State (HHS) focus on addressing the severe hyperglycemia and dehydration often seen in affected patients. In the beginning, doctors give the patient a lot of intravenous fluids to increase the blood volume and improve kidney function for eliminating extra glucose. It is very important to use the right fluid; isotonic saline is given at first, and as dehydration improves, hypotonic solutions are given. The rapid correction of volume status is vital, as studies indicate that patients with HHS often face prolonged hospital admissions and elevated mortality rates, particularly when not adequately rehydrated (Akinrinmade et al., 2011). The first step is to ensure proper fluid management, since this supports the following insulin treatment and correction of electrolyte problems that are key to recovery. Along with giving fluids, insulin therapy is very important for managing HHS. After the first steps of rehydration, intravenous insulin is given to help lower blood sugar and promote the use of glucose by other tissues. The aim of insulin therapy is to slowly reduce blood glucose by 50 to 75 mg/dL per hour to prevent any problems that can result from a fast drop. Potassium levels should be checked regularly during insulin therapy since insulin may cause them to drop, which can result in hypokalemia.

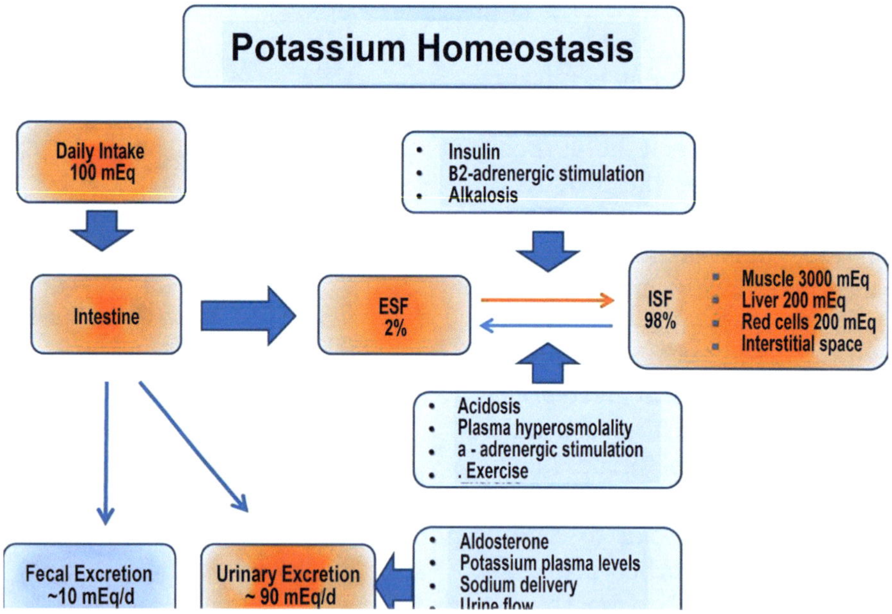

Figure 9.24. Monitoring critically important electrolytes, particularly potassium, is essential during insulin therapy, as insulin can lead to shifts in potassium levels, potentially resulting in hypokalemia.

Source: https://ec.bioscientifica.com/view/journals/ec/7/4/images/EC-18-0109fig1.jpeg

The careful titration of insulin not only aids in glycemic control but also significantly affects patient outcomes; higher mortality rates are reported in HHS cases if insulin is not initiated promptly after fluid replenishment (Akinrinmade et al., 2010). Treatment for HHS also involves fixing metabolic problems and regularly checking the patient's condition. If the levels of sodium and potassium are abnormal, they should be checked and corrected carefully to avoid dangerous outcomes. For this reason, doctors must regularly assess the patient in the lab to guide the treatment and keep the patient's condition stable. Regular observation by nurses helps to find any changes or complications as soon as they start. While mortality rates in patients with HHS remain a significant concern, effective implementation of these treatment protocols can improve outcomes drastically, underscoring the importance of timely intervention and meticulous management (Akinrinmade et al., 2011) (Figure 9.24).

9.6.3. Management of Lactic Acidosis

Handling lactic acidosis that occurs in diabetes-related problems requires different methods. High lactate levels due to either increased production or reduced clearance are the main signs of lactic acidosis, and this is usually seen in hypoxia, sepsis, or metabolic changes. The first step in clinical management is to find and solve the cause, which might require making sure the tissues receive enough blood and oxygen. For patients with diabetic complications, such as those in hyperglycemic hyperosmolar state (HHS) or diabetic ketoacidosis (DKA), timely recognition of lactic acidosis is crucial. In these situations, medical staff use fluid replacement, monitor the patient's electrolytes, and treat high blood sugar with insulin, since hyperglycemia can worsen metabolic acidosis. It is crucial to address lactate levels, which means the care team should be involved in managing the patient. Managing lactic acidosis is made more difficult by the fact that its causes can change, affecting how treatment should be done. The main concern should be to regularly check the patient's blood pressure, blood sugar, and lactate levels. If lactic acidosis lasts for a long time, doctors may also treat it by giving sodium bicarbonate to correct severe acidosis. Nevertheless, giving bicarbonate is not always accepted, and it should only be used when metabolic acidosis severely affects the patient's blood pressure and heart rate. It is important to treat any infections or other illnesses that may have led to DKA or HHS, since this can greatly improve the patient's condition. Working together across different medical fields helps healthcare providers give the best treatment and reduce the risks of lactic acidosis. It is important to carefully oversee lactic acidosis in DKA and HHS, and use a unique strategy for each patient. Since lactic acidosis may point to a serious illness, taking immediate action is important to prevent bad outcomes.

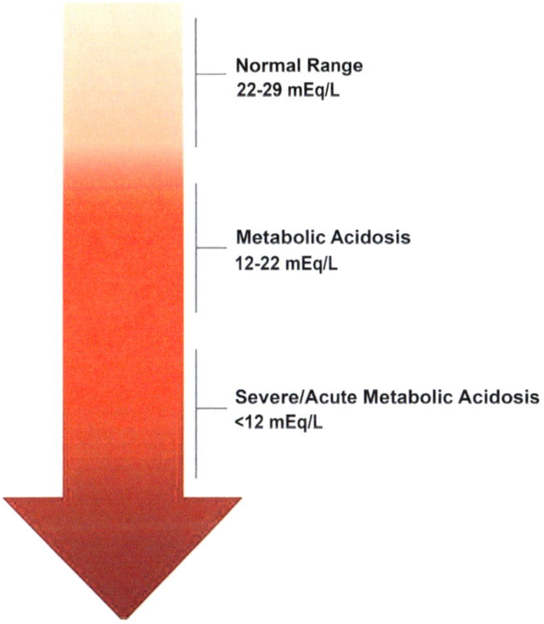

Figure 9.25. In cases where lactic acidosis is persistent, the standard therapeutic interventions may be complemented by the administration of sodium bicarbonate to correct severe acidosis. The normal range of serum bicarbonate is between 22 and 29 mEq/L. Levels below 22 mEq/L indicate metabolic acidosis.

Source: https://upload.wikimedia.org/wikipedia/commons/thumb/8/88/Bicarbonate_Levels_in_Metabolic_Acidosis.jpg/960px-Bicarbonate_Levels_in_Metabolic_Acidosis.jpg

It is necessary to regularly monitor lactate levels and check a patient's overall condition to manage their treatment well. While carrying out management plans, it is necessary for healthcare providers to address electrolyte problems and any complications in diabetic patients. The use of evidence-based guidelines ensures that care is given in the same way, which makes patients safer and aids in their recovery. As research advances and improves understanding of the interplay between these metabolic derangements, ongoing vigilance and adaptability in management strategies will remain key to successful outcomes in patients experiencing lactic acidosis (Modi et al., 2020; Bartoszek et al., 2024) (Figure 9.25).

A CLOSER LOOK

KETOACIDOSIS

Ketoacidosis, most commonly seen as diabetic ketoacidosis (DKA), is a serious and potentially life-threatening complication of diabetes, especially type 1. When the body does not have enough insulin, it uses fat for energy and creates ketones as a result. If ketones increase in the blood, the blood becomes acidic and this causes symptoms such as excessive thirst, frequent urination, nausea, vomiting, abdominal pain, rapid breathing, and confusion. If untreated, DKA can lead to coma or death. Treatment requires giving fluids, insulin, and adjusting the patient's electrolytes. Prompt medical attention is essential.

Summary

In summary, the critical examination of DKA, HHS, and lactic acidosis reveals the intricate relationship these conditions share as acute metabolic complications of diabetes mellitus. Even though each condition is different, they all result in problems caused by low insulin levels and not having enough water. Dealing with acute crises as soon as possible and in the right way is crucial; if these issues are not handled, patients may suffer serious consequences and even die. DKA is more common in people with type 1 diabetes, which shows why it is important to keep monitoring and educating them about ways to prevent it. In addition, the numbers related to these complications highlight the health challenges connected to diabetes. DKA is still a major reason for health problems and deaths, mainly among children and adolescents with type 1 diabetes, so it is important to focus on early healthcare. It is very important to use biochemical analyses in making a diagnosis for these conditions. New diagnostic techniques give important information about metabolic problems and help doctors plan appropriate treatments. The best way to manage DKA and HHS is by hospitalizing the patient on time, giving them fluids and electrolytes intravenously, and providing insulin treatment. In conclusion, the relationship between DKA, HHS, and lactic acidosis proves that diabetes care needs to keep advancing through more research. The identification and refinement of novel biomarkers, as mentioned, may facilitate earlier detection and improved prognostication in acute cases (Akms et al., 2020). It is also important to educate both patients and caregivers about these acute metabolic conditions, since knowing the early signs and symptoms helps with quick action. Since lactic acidosis may make diabetes treatment more difficult, learning about its link to metabolic changes is helpful for doctors. Collectively, addressing these issues holistically will pave the way for reducing the burden of these life-threatening complications and enhancing the quality of life for individuals living with diabetes (Palmiere, 2015).

In summary, DKA, HHS, and lactic acidosis are three distinct metabolic derangements that primarily affect individuals with diabetes or underlying metabolic disorders. DKA is usually linked to Type 1 diabetes and appears as high blood sugar, ketones in the blood, and acidic blood. The main symptoms in patients are high blood sugar, a lot of ketones, and acidosis. On the other hand, HHS is usually found in people with Type 2 diabetes and involves very high blood sugar and high blood osmolality but not much ketosis or acidosis. Since ketoacidosis is absent in HHS, the symptoms are less noticeable, such as changes in mental function and dehydration, which can complicate both diagnosis and treatment. This differentiation is crucial for emergency and long-term interventions in diabetic patients experiencing these acute conditions (Shao et al., 2021). Although lactic acidosis is not limited to diabetic patients, it has its own way of developing and showing symptoms. It is marked by a higher amount of lactic acid in the blood, which often happens due to problems that reduce oxygen supply or slow metabolism in the body. Lactic acidosis in diabetic patients may happen if sepsis, shock, or any other problem that reduces tissue oxygenation occurs. While DKA and HHS are linked to insulin problems, lactic acidosis is mainly caused by the body's need to produce energy without oxygen. In the clinic, lactic acidosis can show signs that are similar to DKA and HHS, such as quick breathing and changes in mental state, which makes it harder to tell them apart. However, the correction of lactic acidosis often focuses on addressing the underlying cause rather than the insulin therapy central to managing DKA and HHS (Shao et al., 2021). It is important to know the main differences among these three conditions for effective treatment. Treating DKA and HHS starts with giving intravenous fluids and insulin to stabilize a person's metabolism, and HHS usually requires more time in the hospital because of its severe nature. Alternatively, dealing with lactic acidosis is about finding and addressing the reasons for it, which could involve no insulin therapy. It is important to use this kind of approach, since incorrectly diagnosing these conditions may lead to ineffective treatment that worsens the patient's health. Clinicians must thus remain vigilant in distinguishing the subtle yet significant variations among DKA, HHS, and lactic acidosis, ensuring tailored interventions that reflect the unique pathophysiological mechanisms at play in each disorder.

References

1. Abd Hamid, H., Das, S., Othman, H., Umar, I., et al. (2010). A case of hyperosmolar hyperglycemic state with involuntary movements–diagnostic dilemma and clinical considerations. https://core.ac.uk/download/pdf/8696563.pdf (accessed on 11th June 2025).
2. Modi, A., Agrawal, A., & Morgan, F. (2017). Euglycemic Diabetic Ketoacidosis: A Review. *Current diabetes reviews*, *13*(3), 315–321. https://doi.org/10.2174/1573399812666160421121307(accessed on 11th June 2025).
3. Ahmed, A. M. S., Ahmed, J. U., Musa, A. K. M., Rahim, M. A., Rahman, M. R., Samad, T. G., Haque, H. F. G., et al. (2020). Clinical spectrum and management of diabetic ketoacidosis: Experience in a tertiary care hospital. https://core.ac.uk/download/357351893.pdf (accessed on 11th June 2025).
4. Akinrinmade, A., Badri, M., Blanco-Blanco, E., Ekpebegh, C. O., et al. (2010). Hyperglycemic crisis in the Eastern Cape province of South Africa: High mortality and association of hyperosmolar ketoacidosis with a new diagnosis of diabetes. https://core.ac.uk/download/230850546.pdf (accessed on 11th June 2025).
5. Al-Sa'idy, H. A. H., Al-Snafi, A. E., & Alyousif, B. T. (2022). An insight to the diabetic ketoacidosis and lactic acidosis among the SARS-CoV-2 infected individuals. *Magna Scientia Advanced Biology and Pharmacy, 6*, 036–073. https://doi.org/10.30574/msabp.2022.6.1.0071 (accessed on 11th June 2025).
6. Anumah, F. O. (2007). Management of hyperglycemic emergencies in the tropics. https://core.ac.uk/download/543362753.pdf (accessed on 11th June 2025).
7. Bartoszek, L., Kapłan, W., Lipiec, J., Olszak, M., et al. (2024). Hyperosmolar hyperglycemic syndrome: A comprehensive review of clinical presentation, diagnosis, and treatment strategies in hyperglycemic crises. https://core.ac.uk/download/597985314.pdf (accessed on 11th June 2025).
8. Bhati, V., Lala, D., Lala, K., Patil, A., et al. (2020). A study to assess the clinicopathological spectrum of acute complications of diabetes mellitus type II. https://core.ac.uk/download/552654942.pdf (accessed on 11th June 2025).
9. Dhatariya, K., Savage, M., Sampson, M., Matfin, G., & Scott, A. (2025). Severe hyperglycemia, diabetic ketoacidosis, and hyperglycemic hyperosmolar state. https://drketandhatariya.com/publications/case_reports/2014/book_chapters/DKA%20and%20HHS%20-%20Endocrine%20and%20Metabolic%20Medical%20Emergencies%20.pdf (accessed on 11th June 2025).
10. Dorin, R. I., Ing, T. S., Konstantinov, N. K., Malhorta, R., et al. (2013). Principles of quantitative fluid and cation replacement in extreme hyperglycemia. https://core.ac.uk/download/232720328.pdf (accessed on 11th June 2025).
11. Driver, C. (2016). Metformin does not prevent glucose intolerance but improves renal function and reduces oxidative stress in type 1 diabetes. https://core.ac.uk/download/196550634.pdf (accessed on 11th June 2025).
12. Ekpebegh, C. O., Longo-Mbenza, B., Nge-Okwe, A., Ogbera, A. O., et al. (2011). Advanced age,

altered level of consciousness and a new diagnosis of diabetes are independently associated with hypernatremia in hyperglycemic crisis. https://core.ac.uk/download/pdf/8571281.pdf (accessed on 11th June 2025).

13. Gong, M., Li, Y., Wen, S., Xu, D., Xu, Z., Yuan, X., Yuan, Y., et al. (2024). The effect of diabetic ketoacidosis and hyperosmolar hyperglycemic on the metabolic tumor markers: A real-world retrospective study. https://core.ac.uk/download/635262309.pdf (accessed on 11th June 2025).
14. Hamza, M. (2016). Metabolic derangements in pediatric diabetic ketoacidosis in a tertiary care hospital. https://core.ac.uk/download/235654953.pdf (accessed on 11th June 2025).
15. Hasan, S. S., Kow, C. S., Bain, A., Kavanagh, S., Merchant, H. A., & Hadi, M. A. (2020). Pharmacotherapeutic considerations for the management of diabetes mellitus among hospitalized COVID-19 patients. *Expert Opinion on Pharmacotherapy, 22*, 229–240. https://doi.org/10.1080/14656566.2020.1837114 (accessed on 11th June 2025).
16. Jalili, M., & Niroomand, M. (2019). Atypical feature of diabetic ketoacidosis with low or normal plasma glucose: A narrative review. https://core.ac.uk/download/pdf/327264238.pdf (accessed on 11th June 2025).
17. Katsiki, N., Gómez-Huelgas, R., Mikhailidis, D. P., & Pérez-Martínez, P. (2021). Narrative review on clinical considerations for patients with diabetes and COVID-19: More questions than answers. *International Journal of Clinical Practice, 75*. https://doi.org/10.1111/ijcp.14833 (accessed on 11th June 2025).
18. Keltanen, T. (2015). *Postmortem Biochemistry: Analysis of Metabolic Imbalance*. https://core.ac.uk/download/33736520.pdf (accessed on 11th June 2025).
19. Levy, D. (2017). *Diabetes Emergencies*. https://doi.org/10.1002/9781119052210.ch2 (accessed on 11th June 2025).
20. McDermott, M. T., & Trujillo, J. M. (2022). *Diabetes Secrets*. https://imp.dayawisesa.com/wp-content/uploads/2023/09/Diabetes-Secrets-2022.pdf#page=28 (accessed on 11th June 2025).
21. Mitic, J., Jovanovic, A., Peric, V., Stolic, R., Markovic-Jovanovic, S., & Smilic, T. (2016). Hyperlactatemia and the outcome of type 2 diabetic patients suffering acute myocardial infarction. https://core.ac.uk/download/193658264.pdf (accessed on 11th June 2025).
22. Mohajan, D., & Mohajan, H. (2023). Hyperglycemia among diabetes patients: A preventive approach. *Innovation in Science and Technology, 2*, 27–33. https://doi.org/10.56397/ist.2023.11.05 (accessed on 11th June 2025).
23. Palmiere C. (2015). Postmortem diagnosis of diabetes mellitus and its complications. *Croatian medical journal, 56*(3), 181–193. https://doi.org/10.3325/cmj.2015.56.181Shao, S., Yang, Q., Pan, R., Yu, X., & Chen, Y. (2021). Interaction of severe acute respiratory syndrome coronavirus 2 and diabetes. *Frontiers in Endocrinology, 12*. https://doi.org/10.3389/fendo.2021.731974 (accessed on 11th June 2025).

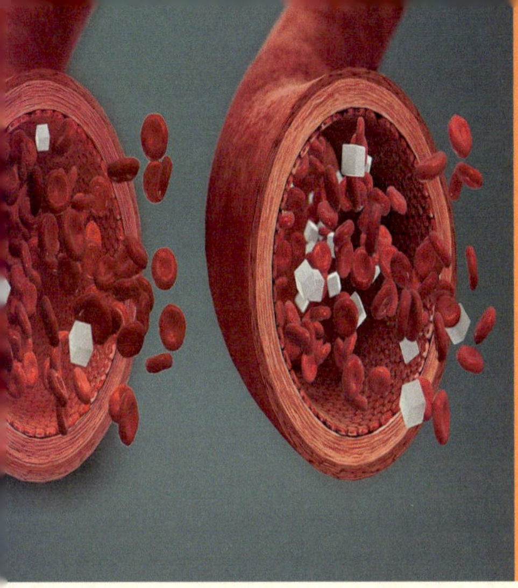

Chapter 10

HYPOGLYCEMIA

Contents

Introduction

Hypoglycemia is a serious condition for people with diabetes since it can happen when they use insulin or other blood glucose-lowering drugs. If hypoglycemia is not treated quickly, it can cause serious problems with a person's nervous system. It is important to know the ways, reasons, and strategies for handling hypoglycemia to help patients and improve their quality of life. Because of recent medical progress, doctors can now use several treatments to keep blood sugar levels under control and reduce the risk of hypoglycemia. The purpose of this chapter is to discuss these interventions and highlight the problems and successes involved in using them in clinical care. Hypoglycemia occurs more often in Type 1 diabetes patients, since they rely on insulin as a main treatment. Some people with diabetes are often worried about more episodes of low blood sugar, which may keep them from following the right treatment plan. It is clear from Cryer's findings that both education and support are important due to the many types of treatments needed for hypoglycemia. There are many approaches, from changing habits to taking medicines, that can be chosen based on a person's needs. In addition, new treatments and continuous glucose monitors are set to transform the way hypoglycemia is managed, which is why healthcare professionals must keep up with new discoveries and technology. Besides the medical difficulties involved in hypoglycemia, it is necessary to pay attention to the mental and emotional effects on those who have it. Since it is difficult to predict when hypoglycemia will occur, it is important to treat both the physical and mental effects of the condition. This chapter takes a closer examination of the interventions highlighted in recent studies, particularly those addressing Type 1 diabetes management, where numerous potential therapies have demonstrated efficacy while still requiring further validation (Heller et al., 2008). The examination of hypoglycemia will allow us to understand it better and use this knowledge to help patients manage their condition more effectively (Figure 10.1).

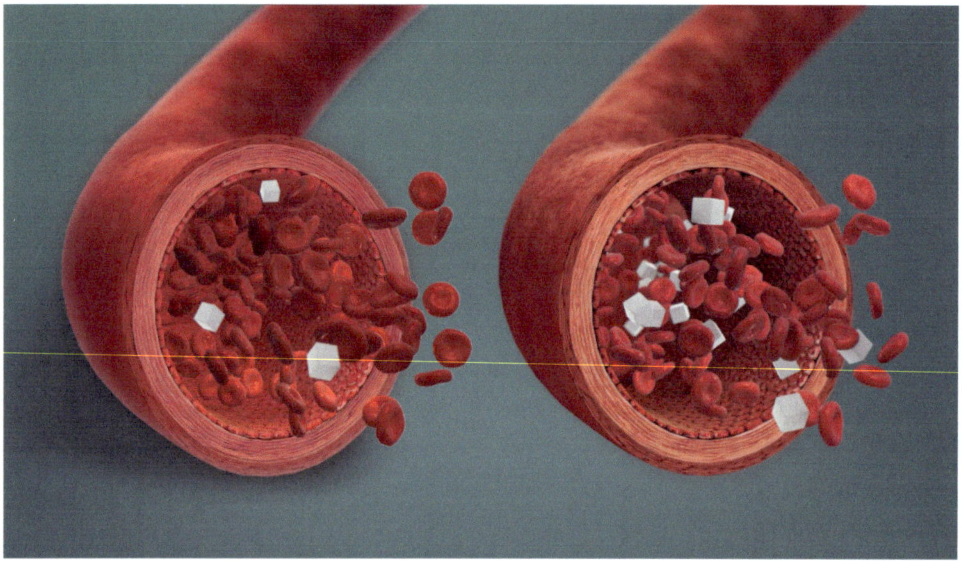

Figure 10.1. Hypoglycemia.

Source: https://upload.wikimedia.org/wikipedia/commons/e/ea/Hypoglycemia.jpg

10.1. Causes of Hypoglycemia

Many things can cause hypoglycemia, including what you eat, your medications, and your body's functions. One of the main reasons is that insulin or insulin secretagogues are given by doctors to manage diabetes. They bring down blood glucose by helping cells absorb glucose, but if the dose is wrong or if people do not eat enough carbohydrates, they may experience hypoglycemia. If someone is not active enough, but still eats the same amount, it can increase the chance of hypoglycemia. When people take part in unplanned or strenuous exercise, their blood glucose may drop quickly since they may not be eating enough carbohydrates. In some cases, hypoglycemia happens because of certain medical conditions or syndromes, not only because of drug use. Adrenal insufficiency is an important condition that weakens the body's ability to manage glucose properly. Besides, individuals with liver diseases can suffer from low blood sugar levels, as the liver's ability to make glucose from other sources is reduced. Such instances highlight that health problems in the body can make it more difficult for a person to manage their blood sugar. Notably, the understandings derived from extensive clinical trials, as highlighted in studies like Hypo-RESOLVE, emphasize the need to ascertain glucose levels that precipitate hypoglycemia, thereby addressing both physiological predispositions and medication-related risks (De Galan et al., 2020). Both mental and daily habits play a major role in causing hypoglycemia. When people are stressed, anxious, or their routine changes, it can cause low blood sugar. As an example, cortisol is a stress hormone that usually makes blood glucose levels rise, but long-term or sudden emotional stress can cause irregular glucose levels because of unpredictable eating or insulin use. In addition, not planning meals well and excessive drinking can often lead to hypoglycemia. Alcohol prevents the body from producing glucose and may result in low blood sugar, mainly for people who drink alcohol on an empty stomach. It is very important to understand all the causes, as this helps doctors treat patients and plan ways to prevent the harmful effects of hypoglycemia (Figure 10.2).

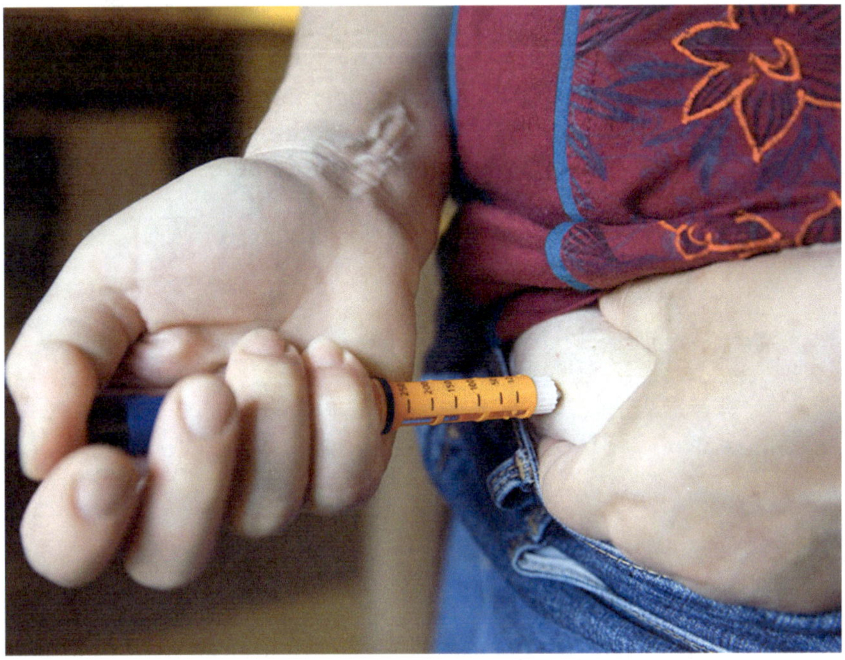

Figure 10.2. One of the primary contributors is the administration of insulin or insulin secretagogues, which are commonly prescribed to manage diabetes.

Source: https://i0.wp.com/diabetesvoice.org/wp-content/uploads/2020/03/Insulin-injection-800px.jpg?fit=800%2C600&ssl=1

10.1.1. Insulin Overdose in Diabetic Patients

Insulin overdose is a serious problem for diabetic patients, since it may result in hypoglycemia, a condition where blood sugar drops dangerously low. This side effect is usually made worse by the fact that insulin therapy must be given with great care to control blood sugar. Overdose, no matter if it is accidental or intended, can make it hard for the body to use its glucose, which may cause symptoms such as shaking, confusion, seizures, and passing out. Insulin therapy's narrow therapeutic window underscores the need for ongoing patient education regarding proper dosing and the signs of hypoglycemia, as well as the implementation of systems that facilitate monitoring and support for those at risk of overdose (Baud et al., 2007). It is important to handle an insulin overdose quickly to bring blood glucose back to a safe level. Usually, traditional methods use glucose given by mouth or through a vein to fight the effects of insulin. However, these strategies can present challenges; for instance, if the hypoglycemic episode is prolonged, there may be a risk of further hypoglycemia later due to rebound insulin secretion (Gris et al., 2005). It underlines the need to learn about the effects of insulin on the body and the possible problems caused by taking too much. Alternative therapies, for example, the use of glucagon, can be applied, but they have their own problems, mainly in people who have other health conditions that may stop glucagon from working well. Along with treating acute cases, educating people and preventing insulin overdose in the long run is very important. Providers in healthcare should encourage using personalized plans that take into account a patient's lifestyle, any other health problems, and how they react to insulin therapy. Taking part in regular check-ups and using continuous glucose monitoring tools helps patients take care of their diabetes and avoid dangerous hypoglycemia. Furthermore, public awareness campaigns can help demystify insulin therapy for both patients and caregivers, reducing stigma around its use and encouraging proactive engagement in diabetes management (Baud et al., 2007). To summarize, a combination of learning, watching, and quick action is necessary to minimize the number of insulin overdoses in people with diabetes (Figure 10.3).

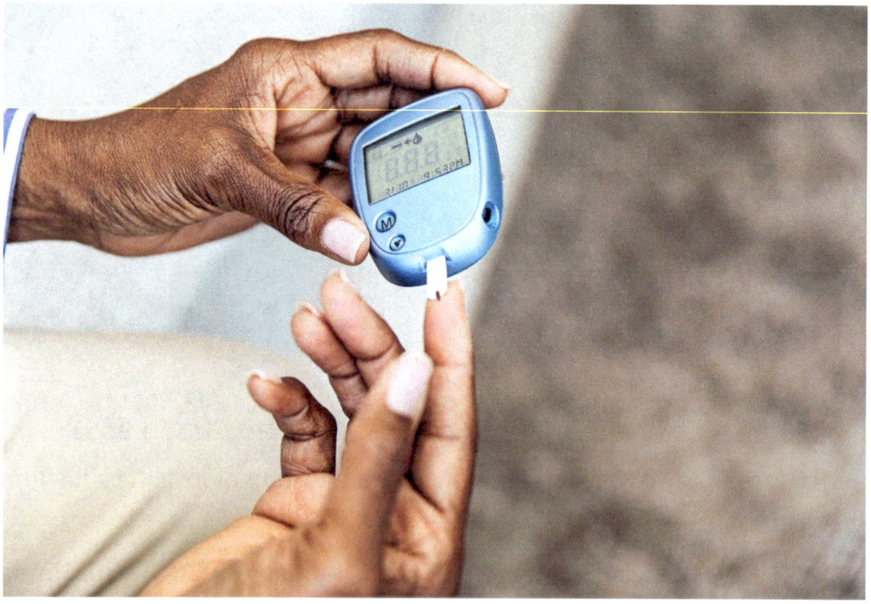

Figure 10.3. Insulin overdose represents a critical concern for diabetic patients, particularly as it can lead to severe hypoglycemia, a condition characterized by dangerously low blood sugar levels.

Source: https://www.health.com/thmb/9-gXEbNyC4g8NVHkWOc1ZZU_RII=/1500x0/filters:no_upscale():max_bytes(150000):strip_icc()/Diabetes-Insulin-GettyImages-1184019335-2000-9a522969b24d4cb3908b6e0e0f272999.jpg

10.1.2. Excessive Alcohol Consumption

Excessive alcohol consumption has significant implications for metabolic processes, particularly concerning hypoglycemia. Alcohol interferes with the liver's capacity to release glucose into the bloodstream, a function that is crucial for maintaining blood sugar levels. When large amounts of alcohol are consumed, the liver prioritizes metabolizing the alcohol over gluconeogenesis, the process of producing glucose from non-carbohydrate sources. In individuals who engage in heavy drinking, this metabolic shift can lead to dangerously low blood sugar levels, particularly when alcohol is consumed on an empty stomach or in conjunction with inadequate carbohydrate intake. The resulting hypoglycemia can manifest as confusion, weakness, and in severe cases, loss of consciousness or seizures, underscoring the need for awareness and moderation in alcohol consumption among at-risk populations.

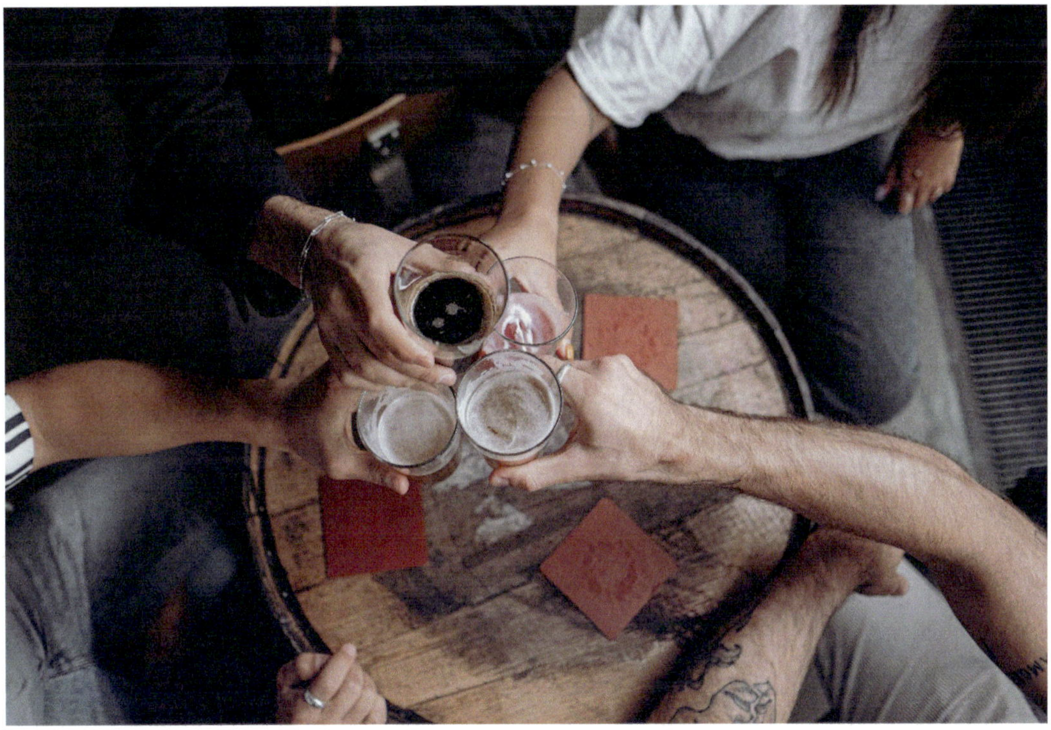

Figure 10.4. Alcohol interferes with the liver's capacity to release glucose into the bloodstream, a function that is crucial for maintaining blood sugar levels.

Source: https://cdn.prod.website-files.com/64c196f6a5062cbed770a366/65b51708b114c87c713477af_pexels-cottonbro-studio-5530171%20(1).jpg

Moreover, the relationship between hypoglycemia and excessive alcohol intake is further complicated by the type of nutrition associated with heavy drinking. Those who consume large quantities of alcohol often neglect balanced meals, which can exacerbate the risk of hypoglycemia. The failure to consume adequate macronutrients, particularly carbohydrates, can lead to insufficient glycogen stores in the liver, which are vital for glucose production during fasting states or in times of stress induced by alcohol consumption. Furthermore, the quality of dietary choices made during episodes of binge drinking tends to be poor, further contributing to nutrient deficiencies that can impair metabolic health. This cycle of neglect highlights the importance of addressing dietary habits alongside alcohol consumption to mitigate the risk of hypoglycemia and associated complications. Addressing the clinical implications of excessive alcohol consumption and its effects on hypoglycemia demands a nuanced understanding of individual health frameworks. Clinicians must consider the overall dietary patterns and lifestyle choices that can contribute to the risk of hypoglycemia. For instance, recommendations may include nutritional education focused on the importance of balanced meals containing carbohydrates, particularly for individuals who consume alcohol regularly. Additionally, interventions should provide strategies for recognizing early warning signs of hypoglycemia, emphasizing the need for immediate management, such as consuming glucose tablets or sweet beverages, to counteract low blood sugar levels. This comprehensive approach addresses not only the immediate effects of hypoglycemia but also the underlying dietary habits and metabolic factors that contribute to the risks associated with excessive alcohol consumption, ensuring a more holistic management strategy for affected individuals (Figure 10.4).

10.1.3. Hormonal Deficiencies

A lack of hormones can cause hypoglycemia and is connected to different clinical disorders. Insulin, glucagon, and similar hormones are necessary for maintaining a stable level of glucose in the blood. Because of low insulin levels in Type 1 diabetes, the body cannot manage blood glucose levels properly. If a patient injects too much insulin or does not eat enough carbohydrates, they are likely to get hypoglycemia. In the same way, if glucagon is not secreted in enough amounts, it can make hypoglycemia worse by hindering the liver from releasing glucose. Since hormones are involved in this process, understanding it well is important for handling hypoglycemia. In addition, hormonal deficiencies can cause problems besides those of insulin and glucagon. Cortisol and epinephrine are other hormones that play a big role in regulating blood glucose. During times of stress, cortisol from the adrenal glands helps maintain the right level of glucose in the body. If cortisol is not present in enough amounts, the body may have trouble managing low blood sugar, causing the problem to happen repeatedly. Likewise, epinephrine quickly stimulates the liver to release glucose that has been stored.

A lack of hormones in people with adrenal insufficiency or similar conditions may increase their risk of experiencing hypoglycemia. Because hormones play a key role in human physiology, changes in glucose levels can easily lead to health problems. More cases of obesity and the related metabolic disorders are making the situation of hormonal deficiencies and hypoglycemia more complex. Bariatric surgery has been proven to change hormone levels, which helps to improve blood sugar control. Changes in hunger and metabolism hormones are common for patients after gastric bypass or sleeve gastrectomy, resulting in better insulin sensitivity. At the same time, after surgery, patients may develop new hormone problems that need to be managed properly to avoid more hypoglycemia. A clear understanding of these hormonal adaptations is critical for healthcare providers to ensure that patients are monitored effectively post-surgery for any potential repercussions, including the risk of hypoglycemia (Miras & le Roux, 2013; Azran et al., 2017). As more is needed in obesity treatment, examining hormones and their role in hypoglycemia will continue to be very important (Figure 10.5).

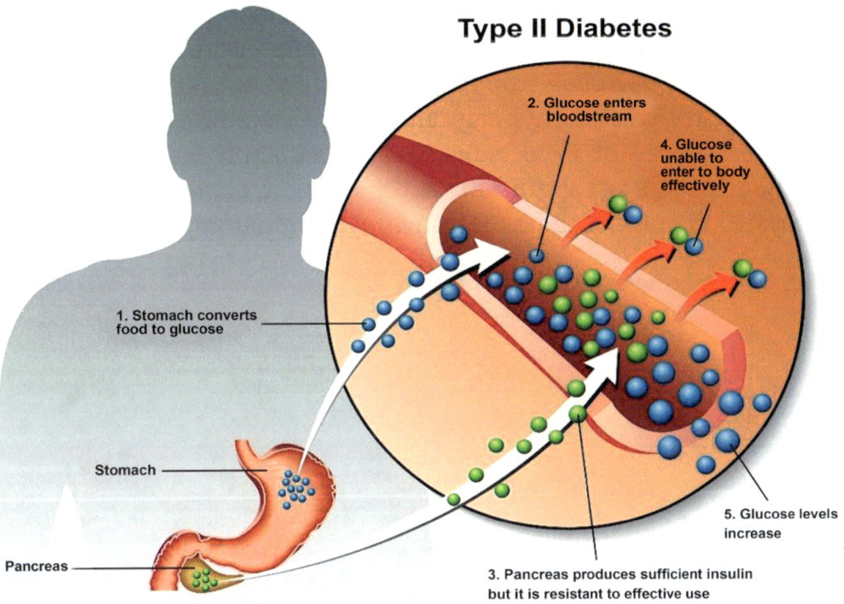

Figure 10.5. A deficiency in insulin, often seen in conditions like Type 1 diabetes, results in an inability to regulate blood glucose levels effectively.

Source: https://www.news-medical.net/images/Article_Images/ImageForArticle_1622_17155939945222654.jpg

10.2. Symptoms of Hypoglycemia

Hypoglycemia can cause different physical and mental symptoms that may seriously affect a person's well-being. Since these symptoms are easy to notice and include dizziness, trembling, irritability, and confusion, patients and their caregivers must recognize them right away. There are situations where cognitive problems appear, and these require support from others, as research on the clinical aspects of the condition shows. Besides, suffering from low blood sugar several times can make a person anxious and fearful, which can make it harder to control diabetes. Understanding the comprehensive spectrum of symptoms is vital for timely intervention, thereby mitigating the risk of severe health consequences associated with hypoglycemia, as elaborated in ongoing research efforts aimed at clarifying these issues (De Galan et al., 2020). In addition, the fact that non-severe hypoglycemia can cause several problems underlines the importance of being aware of symptoms. Although lighter symptoms can be dealt with, if hypoglycemia keeps happening, it can lead to heart problems and higher medical bills. It is also believed by psychologists that repeated episodes of migraines can increase stress and lower the quality of life, making the person's health worse. The Hypo-RESOLVE project points out that a better classification of hypoglycemia may have a major impact on how medical professionals work. If healthcare providers set clearer limits and learn the factors connected to hypoglycemia, they can handle these symptoms more effectively. Ultimately, improving symptom recognition and response can alleviate the broader psychological impact on individuals (De Galan et al., 2020). Sometimes, drugs taken for other health problems can make hypoglycemia and its symptoms worse. As an illustration, a case study reveals that a young person with a psychiatric illness experienced serious hypoglycemia because of lithium therapy. When the medication was stopped, the episodes stopped, which shows that paying attention to drug-related side effects is important for treating hypoglycemia. This situation highlights that symptoms may be caused by metabolic issues or by certain drugs, so doctors should assess patients in many ways. Integrating understanding of symptoms and possible treatments helps healthcare providers establish better ways to manage diabetes for each patient, aiming for better care (Figure 10.6).

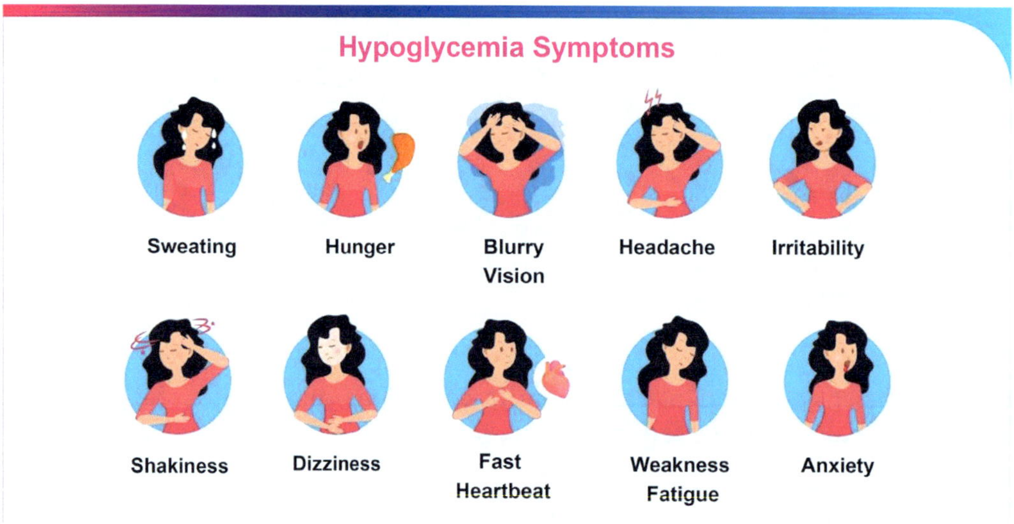

Figure 10.6. The symptoms of hypoglycemia encompass a wide range of physiological and psychological manifestations that can significantly impact an individual's well-being.

Source: https://www.fitterfly.com/blog/wp-content/uploads/2023/06/Hypoglycemia_1-02-scaled.jpg

10.2.1. Physical Symptoms (e.g., Sweating, Trembling)

When someone has hypoglycemia, their sweating and trembling are important signs that show the condition is starting and its severity. These symptoms happen when the body's systems react to low blood sugar, as the sympathetic nervous system gets activated. The release of adrenaline causes sweating, which helps the body deal with a drop in glucose levels. When we feel stress, our muscles start to tremble because the body is trying to make energy. Understanding these symptoms is imperative, especially since their presentation can vary among individuals, complicating the identification of hypoglycemia, particularly in unusual cases, such as in the elderly or pregnant women who are more vulnerable to these effects (Huda et al., 2019). If hypoglycemia is not quickly spotted and managed, it can get worse and result in serious concerns like problems with thinking and risky behavior. Those with type 1 diabetes are more likely to experience severe hypoglycemia, as it happens in about one out of three cases caused by insulin therapy. Those affected may initially exhibit noticeable physical symptoms like trembling; however, they often delay seeking intervention due to various reasons, including misjudging their situation or feeling embarrassed (Barendse et al., 2014). As a result, these symptoms can become more serious, which shows how important it is to notice and deal with them right away. If people recognize and handle sweating and trembling, they can avoid quick risks and may improve their health in the future. To manage hypoglycemia well, one must notice the symptoms and also use specific education to help people act fast. Informing people about the need to look for early symptoms can help them take quick action, since early intake of a glucose source can prevent the condition from getting worse. For example, sharing knowledge about the physical changes that happen with sweating and trembling can help people react better. When education is tailored to a person, strategies can better handle the behavioral and thinking differences that cause unique responses to low blood sugar. Ultimately, coordinating knowledge with actionable prevention plans fosters an environment where individuals can proactively manage their condition, marking a crucial step in the fight against severe hypoglycemia and its debilitating symptoms (Huda et al., 2019) (Figure 10.7).

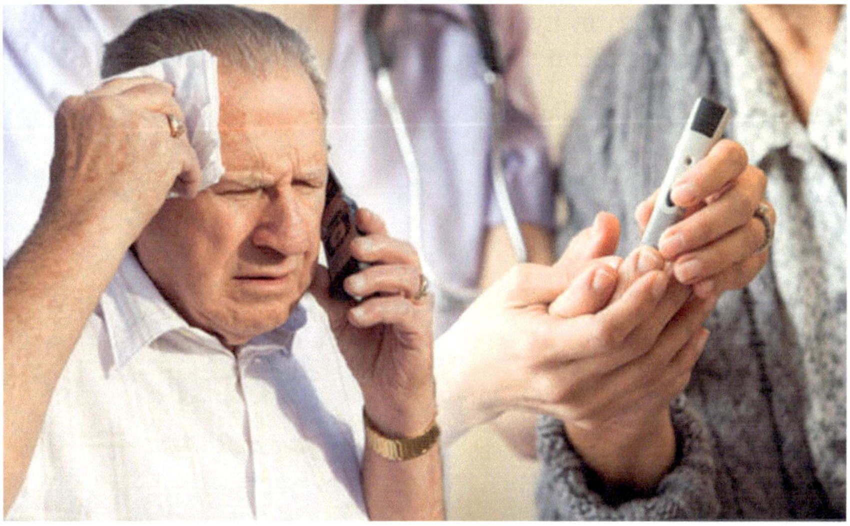

Figure 10.7. The physical symptoms associated with hypoglycemia, such as sweating and trembling, are critical indicators of this condition's onset and severity.

Source: https://cdn.images.express.co.uk/img/dynamic/11/590x/diabetes-type-2-blood-sugar-levels-sweating-hypoglycemia-985876.jpg?r=1532978390659

10.2.2. Cognitive Symptoms (e.g., Confusion, Irritability)

Cognitive changes caused by hypoglycemia are very important for understanding how glucose management affects people with diabetes. A fall in blood glucose causes the brain to show signs of not working properly. When someone has hypoglycemia, confusion, irritation, and slow thinking may appear, which means it is very important to act quickly. People may find it challenging to pay attention or use information, which makes it hard to complete daily tasks and make decisions. These symptoms can escalate the risks associated with hypoglycemia if not promptly addressed, emphasizing the importance of early recognition and treatment strategies to mitigate potential cognitive impairments during acute incidents of low blood sugar, which can have severe consequences if not handled appropriately (Paluchamy et al., 2019). In addition, the level of cognitive symptoms can change a lot based on who the person is and the surrounding circumstances. For instance, elderly patients and those with preexisting cognitive impairments may exhibit heightened sensitivity to hypoglycemia, leading to more pronounced cognitive symptoms such as severe confusion or emotional disturbances (Huda et al., 2019). Unlike older patients, younger people may not notice the effect until their blood glucose levels drop a lot. Experiencing hypoglycemia in the past can affect how someone recognizes symptoms; with time, they may not notice low blood sugar and this can make their thinking problems worse during these episodes. Because of this, healthcare workers can adjust their education and care plans to suit the particular needs of each patient group. Helping patients with their thinking problems during hypoglycemia is very important for their recovery. Some strategies are to teach people about the early symptoms of low blood sugar, encourage routine checks of blood glucose, and make treatment plans that fit each person's lifestyle. When patients learn self-management, they can react quickly to hypoglycemia and avoid serious mental issues. Additionally, research into neuroimaging studies has showcased how these cognitive symptoms manifest at the neural level, providing insights into effective methods for restoring cognitive function during episodes of hypoglycemia and highlighting the importance of constant vigilance in managing this complex condition (Huda et al., 2019) (Figure 10.8).

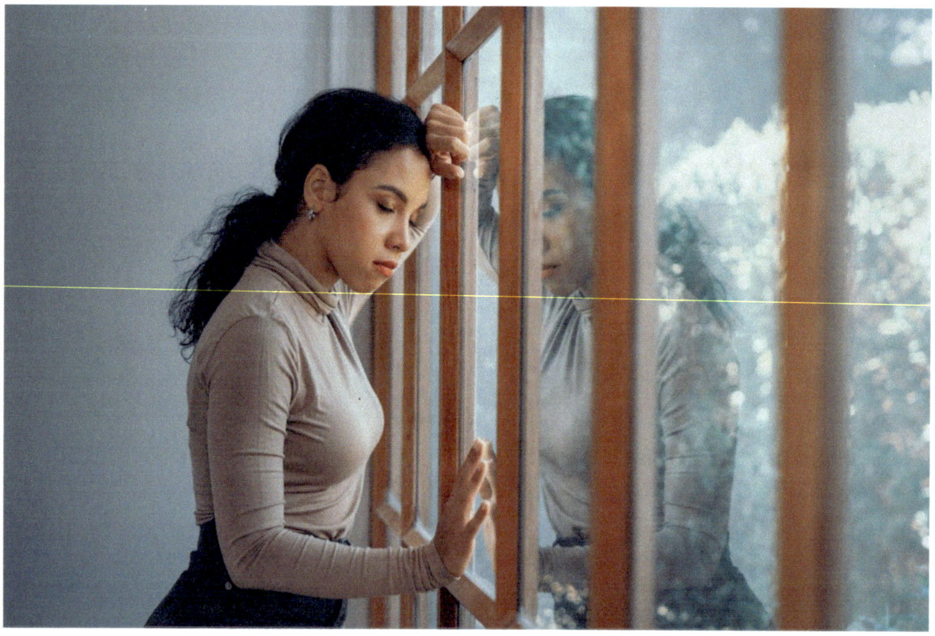

Figure 10.8. Cognitive symptoms associated with hypoglycemia are paramount in understanding the broader implications of glucose management in individuals with diabetes.

Source: https://cdn.prod.website-files.com/64eec5ed1ea74a7194cd16a3/663bbda7c016849973f1ce73_1.%20Low%20Blood%20Sugar%20Anxiety%40x2.jpg

10.2.3. Severe Symptoms (e.g., Seizures, Loss of Consciousness)

Severe hypoglycemia leads to symptoms that may seriously harm a person's brain and nervous system. Seizures and losing consciousness are the most concerning symptoms to see in a patient. If blood glucose falls below 50 mg/dL, it may lead to significant neuroglycopenia, a situation where the brain does not have enough glucose to work properly. Because of this, the brain's cells do not function properly, which can lead to mental changes, seizures, or fainting. These symptoms should be recognized right away, since they may lead to serious problems if ignored. Since the brain needs glucose to function properly, it is important to intervene right away to lessen these serious effects and return the body to normal. When horses have severe hypoglycemia, clinicians have observed seizures and changes in their mental state. A study on ninety horses with hypoglycemia showed that 42% had seizures and most of them were also obtunded and disoriented. The fact that these symptoms appear when blood glucose drops low proves that glucose is very important for brain functioning. Events such as paroxysmal discharges observed in electroencephalogram (EEG) examinations support the occurrence of seizures in affected subjects.

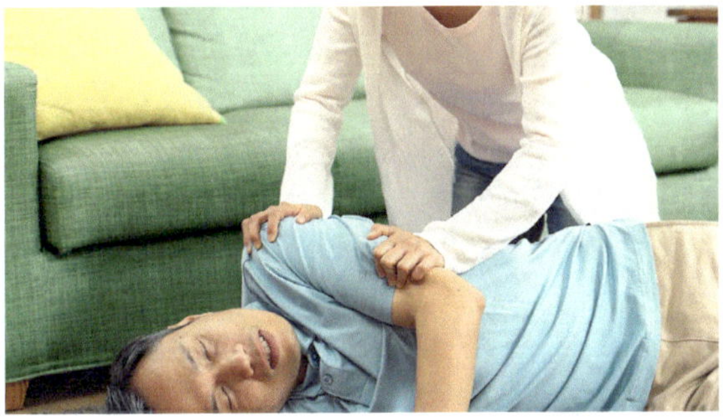

Figure 10.9. Diabetic seizures.

Source: https://images.everydayhealth.com/images/diabetes/what-is-a-diabetic-seizure-1440x810.jpg?sfvrsn=8cd24a42_3

These findings demonstrate that it is important for all animals to have enough glucose to avoid damage to the brain and nervous system. It points out that glucose is important for nutrition and also greatly affects the health of the nervous system. In addition, severe hypoglycemia has a major effect on a person's level of awareness and ability to move. If blood glucose levels are very low, for example, below 42 mg/dL, a brief period can result in severe mental problems, seizures, and unconsciousness. The connection between these symptoms and low glucose levels shows how the brain's functions, such as sensory processing and coordination, may be affected. Since fast and proper treatment is important for avoiding brain damage, caretakers and healthcare providers must learn the signs of hypoglycemia. The presence of serious neurological problems in horses and other animals as a result of hypoglycemia shows that it is important to act quickly and carefully to prevent these conditions, highlighting the global importance of normal glucose levels in health (Figure 10.9).

10.3. Diagnosis of Hypoglycemia

A person with suspected hypoglycemia is diagnosed by looking for symptoms, measuring blood glucose, and finding out the reasons behind it. Signs of hypoglycemia in the clinic may be palpitations, sweating, and anxiety, or they may be confusion, seizures, or passing out. According to the usual definition, hypoglycemia happens when blood glucose goes below 70 mg/dL, but some patients can show symptoms at levels higher than this because of their past glycemic experience. For this reason, it is important to do a complete clinical check and check blood glucose levels accurately to confirm the diagnosis. Knowing about a patient's medications and medical conditions helps healthcare providers find the reason for hypoglycemia and avoid future episodes. It is also hard to diagnose hypoglycemia because many different conditions can cause blood glucose to decrease. Insulinoma, adrenal insufficiency, and some neurogenic problems are the usual causes. Excessive insulin, not eating, or being physically inactive for a long time may cause hypoglycemia in patients with diabetes. To support a better understanding of these conditions, special clinical indicators for hypoglycemia have been developed. For instance, Black et al. (2010) highlight the development of clinical performance indicators which encompass hypoglycemia as one of the targeted areas for national assessment in prehospital care. They make it possible for emergency teams to compare their actions and find the most effective ways to help patients. In addition, how the management plan is put in place after diagnosis is very important for preventing and treating hypoglycemic episodes. When hypoglycemia is confirmed, the usual first steps are to give the patient fast-acting carbohydrates like glucose tablets or sweet drinks to raise their blood glucose levels quickly. When a patient is too weak to consume food or drink safely because of severe hypoglycemia, health professionals may need to give glucose or glucagon by injection. In the long run, strategies include teaching about diet, making changes to medications, and regularly checking blood sugar levels, mainly for those with diabetes. Additionally, recent studies indicate that short-term glycemic variability may impact health outcomes, as noted in Helleputte et al. (2020). Knowing about these factors helps clinicians handle the immediate results of hypoglycemia and also improve overall blood sugar management for patients who might develop hypoglycemia (Figure 10.10).

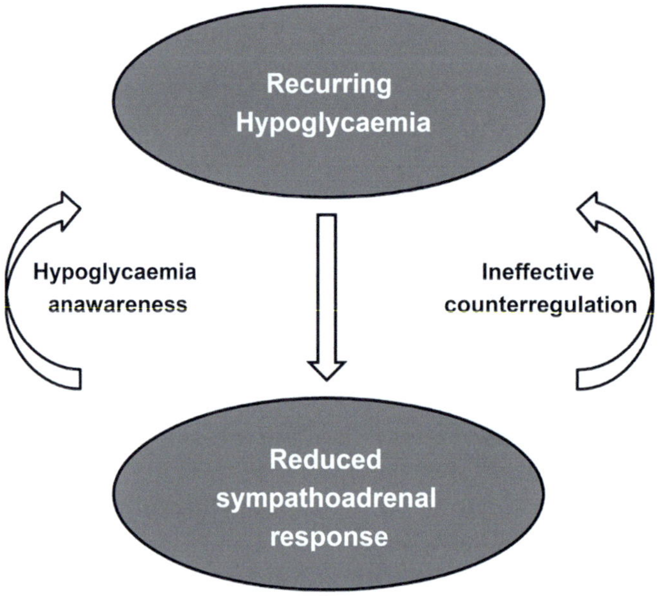

Figure 10.10. Clinically, symptoms of hypoglycemia can present as neurogenic manifestations, such as palpitations, sweating, and anxiety, or neuroglycopenic symptoms, which include confusion, seizures, or loss of consciousness.

Source: Christou MA, Christou PA, Kyriakopoulos C, Christou GA, Tigas S. Effects of Hypoglycemia on Cardiovascular Function in Patients with Diabetes. International Journal of Molecular Sciences. 2023; 24(11):9357. https://doi.org/10.3390/ijms24119357

10.3.1. Blood Glucose Testing Methods

It is very important to use blood glucose testing, especially when someone has hypoglycemia, since quick detection helps avoid serious complications. For many years, fingerstick blood samples checked with glucometers have been the main way to measure glucose. These devices give quick results and help people control their blood sugar well. Still, these devices may give unreliable results because of human mistakes and differences in devices. Since hypoglycemia can occur all of a sudden, it is essential to have better and continuous monitoring to respond quickly when glucose levels become too low. For this reason, new technological developments are changing blood glucose testing, introducing new methods that make monitoring easier and more accurate for everyone. Recent research has introduced methods utilizing continuous glucose monitoring (CGM) systems, which offer a more comprehensive view of blood glucose fluctuations throughout the day. The sensors are put under the skin and give instant readings on blood sugar, so users can be warned about both high and low blood sugar levels. Notably, the integration of personalized medicine approaches and artificial intelligence (AI) is paving the way for more sophisticated detection systems, particularly in nocturnal hypoglycemia scenarios. Studies have demonstrated that applying AI algorithms to raw electrocardiogram (ECG) signals can enhance the identification of hypoglycemic events, significantly contributing to patient safety. As the field of glucose monitoring continues to evolve, these emerging technologies not only improve the detection of dangerous glucose levels but also alleviate the burden of frequent fingersticks, ultimately enhancing the quality of life for diabetic patients (Pecchia et al., 2020). Having non-invasive ways to test blood glucose is a major progress in dealing with hypoglycemia. Some researchers are trying out optical sensing and breath analysis to help people who are reluctant to do frequent blood tests. With such approaches, patients can have their glucose levels checked without needing any invasive tests. Therefore, they make it possible to monitor blood glucose levels in real time, which helps detect hypoglycemia early. Also, bringing together these non-invasive approaches with excellent data connectivity gives healthcare providers the ability to watch patients from a distance and respond quickly if required. As technologies continue to progress, it becomes increasingly essential to evaluate their efficacy and integration into traditional care protocols, ensuring that they effectively address the complexities of hypoglycemia management while promoting patient adherence (Pecchia et al., 2020) (Figure 10.11).

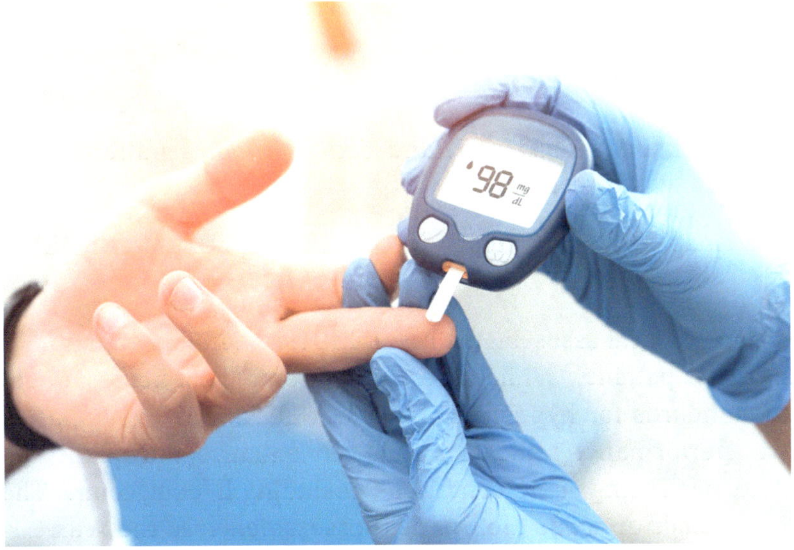

Figure 10.11. The importance of blood glucose testing methods cannot be overstated, particularly in the context of hypoglycemia, where timely detection is crucial for preventing severe complications.

Source: https://www.myamericannurse.com/wp-content/uploads/2020/04/blood-glucose-testing.jpg

10.3.2. Clinical Assessment and Patient History

A thorough review of the patient's medical history and a proper assessment by the clinician help with diagnosing and treating hypoglycemia. The assessment starts by examining the symptoms the patient has, for example, tremors, sweating, confusion, and palpitations. Noticing these symptoms helps healthcare providers tell if they are related to hypoglycemia. Alongside symptomatology, obtaining a detailed patient history is crucial. It requires finding out about the patient's medical history, such as past hypoglycemia, how they handle diabetes, what they eat, if they take their medications, and their general lifestyle. With this knowledge, doctors can diagnose the issue and choose the best ways to deal with the dangers of hypoglycemia.

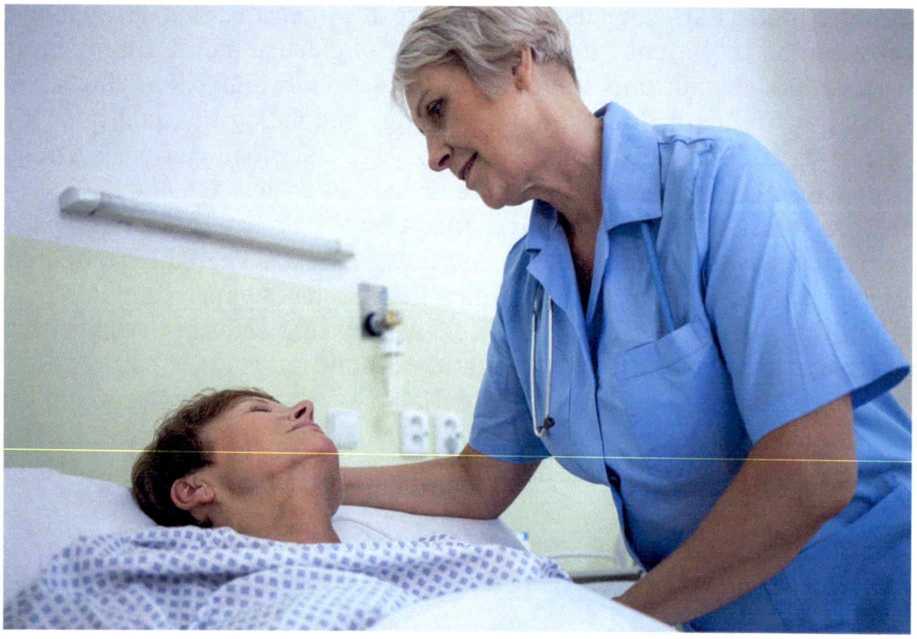

Figure 10.12. Effective clinical assessment and comprehensive patient history are pivotal in diagnosing and managing hypoglycemia.

Source: https://cdn.ps.emap.com/wp-content/uploads/sites/3/2019/12/INDEX-assessment-Alamy-HC680B.jpg

To sum up, thorough clinical assessments result in more detailed questions and a clearer view of the diseases that affect patients. While assessing patients, it is necessary to follow guidelines that match national standards for hypoglycemia. (Black et al., 2010) emphasizes the importance of structured clinical performance indicators that can enhance the quality of prehospital care provided to patients experiencing acute conditions, including hypoglycemia. These guidelines can help healthcare professionals organize their patient assessments, so they can take action promptly using evidence-based methods. Also, by using clinical indicators to standardize assessment, we can set quality care standards and stress the value of correct patient information. If practitioners assess how well these indicators work, they can keep improving their strategies and provide patient care that follows international standards. In addition, using common procedures in clinical assessments improves patient safety and results in situations of hypoglycemia. When clinicians grasp the details of a patient's case, they can create unique care plans that handle the patient's specific risk factors and other illnesses. Vekemans et al. (2011) illustrate the necessity of well-defined case definitions and assessment criteria, which not only aid in diagnosis but also support healthcare providers in delivering precise interventions swiftly. Using clinical information in treatment plans can help design individualized care plans, which may increase how well patients stick to their treatment. Focusing on both the clinical results and the patient's background allows clinicians to handle hypoglycemia more successfully, making safety, effectiveness, and patient needs the main priorities (Figure 10.12).

10.3.3. Differential Diagnosis

Since hypoglycemia may appear similar to other acute conditions, using differential diagnosis is very important in its treatment. If patients display confusion, seizures, or loss of consciousness due to low blood glucose, clinicians should tell these symptoms apart from seizure disorders, metabolic problems, or acute stroke.

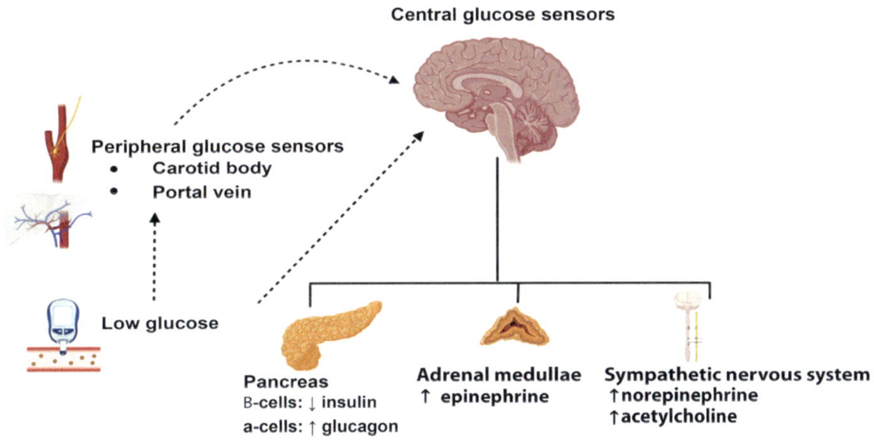

Figure 10.13. Conditions such as insulinoma, adrenal insufficiency, or glycogen storage diseases may lead to recurrent hypoglycemic episodes, complicating the clinical picture.

Source: https://www.endocrinepractice.org/cms/10.1016/j.eprac.2022.11.010/asset/52b9cd43-3c87-4cc0-b5e4-6a801d0ff8ce/main.assets/gr1_lrg.jpg

This is very important since confusing hypoglycemia with an ischemic stroke may result in serious health issues and the wrong treatment. According to medical literature, when a person has severe low blood sugar, they may experience problems similar to a stroke, so it is important to evaluate them closely. So, it is important to combine a thorough review of the patient's medical history and a physical examination to make the right diagnosis and choose the best treatment. Even though imaging studies may not always prove that hypoglycemia is present or show its effects on the brain, they can still give useful information for the differential diagnosis. Several studies, including case reports, have shown that brain imaging in hypoglycemic patients occasionally reveals abnormalities that mimic acute ischemic stroke, with specific patterns of cortical or subcortical lesions observable in approximately 20% of such cases (Iwai et al., 2012). Some of the findings may appear as reduced diffusion on MR images or as areas with low density on CT scans. So, it is important to be careful when interpreting radiological studies, since hypoglycemia may cause false results in assessing acute brain problems. To summarize, linking clinical data to imaging results can help doctors make correct diagnoses and choose better treatments. Healthcare providers should use a consistent process to identify the possible causes of hypoglycemia, since there are many possible reasons. Cases of insulinoma, adrenal insufficiency, or glycogen storage diseases can result in many episodes of low blood sugar, making the situation more difficult to manage. It is very important for these possibilities to be recognized, especially in patients who have diabetes or take drugs that may change insulin levels. A review of the literature has shown that the link between how severe and long-lasting hypoglycemia is and neurological problems is not always clear. Due to these difficulties, emergency departments ought to focus on checking blood glucose in patients who have sudden neurological problems, and make hypoglycemia a key point in their diagnosis. As a result, people affected by these conditions receive prompt and suitable care to avoid negative outcomes (Figure 10.13).

10.4. Treatment Options for Hypoglycemia

Efficient management of hypoglycemia depends on quick and suitable treatment to avoid its negative consequences. Usually, the first step is to quickly give the person carbohydrates such as glucose tablets, sugary drinks, or candy to raise their blood sugar level. In the case of severe hypoglycemia and unresponsiveness, people may need glucagon or glucose given through a vein. Recent studies underscore the importance of preparing healthcare settings with appropriate resources, such as Hypo Boxes, which contain essential supplies for treating hypoglycemia (Boyle et al., 2015).

Having such measures in hospital wards has led to better and quicker management of hypoglycemia, which has reduced the number of complications for patients in the hospital. Apart from immediate care, it is important to use long-term plans to help prevent more episodes of hypoglycemia. Those who keep having low blood sugar may find it helpful to change their insulin doses or try continuous glucose monitoring. With these technologies, people can constantly check their blood glucose and act early if their levels are dropping too low. Also, education is important in the long run, since patients must understand their diabetes, recognize the early signs of low blood sugar, and know how to act when this happens. Effective patient education can empower individuals to manage their health proactively, reducing their reliance on emergency interventions and decreasing the overall burden on healthcare services (Amiel et al., 2017).

It is important for healthcare providers to use many strategies to treat hypoglycemia, including making treatment plans that match each patient's needs and lifestyle. This approach acknowledges that different regimens, such as basal insulin therapies, may yield varying results for patients with diabetes, particularly regarding quality-adjusted life years (QALYs) and cost-effectiveness (Amiel et al., 2017). Adjusting therapies allows for better control of blood sugar with fewer chances of hypoglycemia. As studies progress, using new treatments, for example, dual hormone infusion and closed-loop insulin delivery, may help improve both the effectiveness and safety of hypoglycemia management in patients (Figure 10.14).

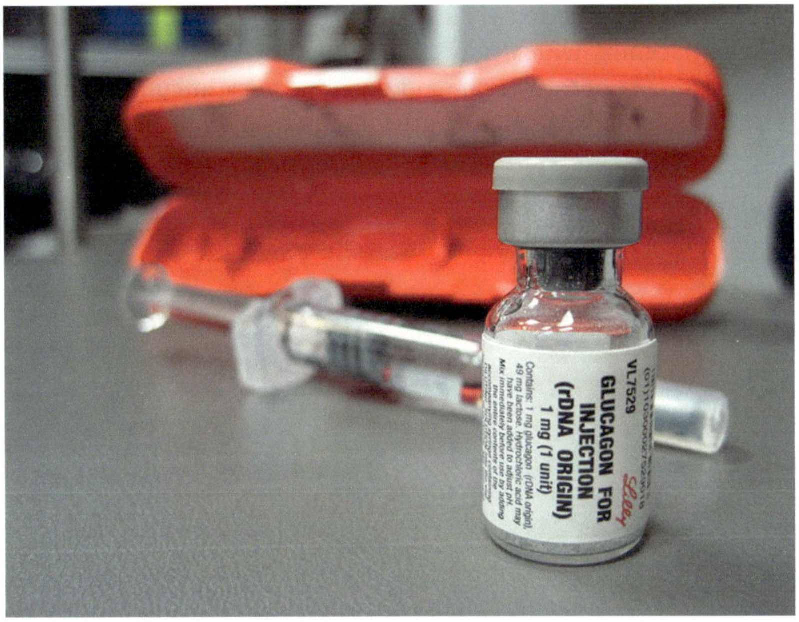

Figure 10.14. For individuals with severe hypoglycemia, particularly those who become unresponsive, glucagon injections or intravenous glucose may be necessary.

Source: https://www.collegeems.com/wp-content/uploads/2019/02/Glucagon_Image.jpg

10.4.1. Immediate Treatment (e.g., Glucose Tablets, Juice)

Treating hypoglycemia right away is necessary to avoid the worsening of symptoms and possible problems caused by low blood sugar. The quick correction of low blood glucose is very important when someone has a hypoglycemic episode. Quick remedies include glucose tablets and juice, since they are absorbed into the bloodstream very fast. A lot of people find that glucose tablets are easy to carry and always provide the right amount of glucose. On the other hand, juice is usually more enjoyable to drink, especially by people who find it hard to swallow or who need to drink more fluids. Still, what to do depends on the individual's likes and the situation surrounding the hypoglycemic episode. It is very important that individuals are ready to use these immediate treatments for managing their condition. Timely use of glucose tablets and juice is necessary to make sure they are effective in treating hypoglycemia. It is known that many people with diabetes may not seek treatment when they have mild symptoms because they either don't know or can't think clearly. This delay can exacerbate the severity of the episode, potentially leading to severe hypoglycemia, which necessitates more invasive interventions or even emergency medical assistance (Barendse et al., 2014). In addition, the availability of preferred glucose sources in the environment can make it difficult for people to follow their immediate treatment plans. Many people say they prefer some ways of treatment because they are tasty or easy to use, so healthcare providers should focus on strategies that suit patients' lives and tastes. Making sure people know the importance of treating hypoglycemia promptly also plays a big role in the outcomes. Knowing the possible problems and risks linked to late glucose administration is very important for giving glucose on time. Teaching people and caregivers about these symptoms and the quick use of glucose tablets or juice can result in improved ways to handle and prevent them. Notably, those with a history of recurrent severe hypoglycemia often exhibit unique psychological barriers, such as fear of rebound hyperglycemia, which may hinder their willingness to treat early (Laureano et al., 2018). Since hypoglycemia is both worrying and can be very uncomfortable, informing patients about quick treatment options is very important for handling diabetes well and achieving better health (Figure 10.15).

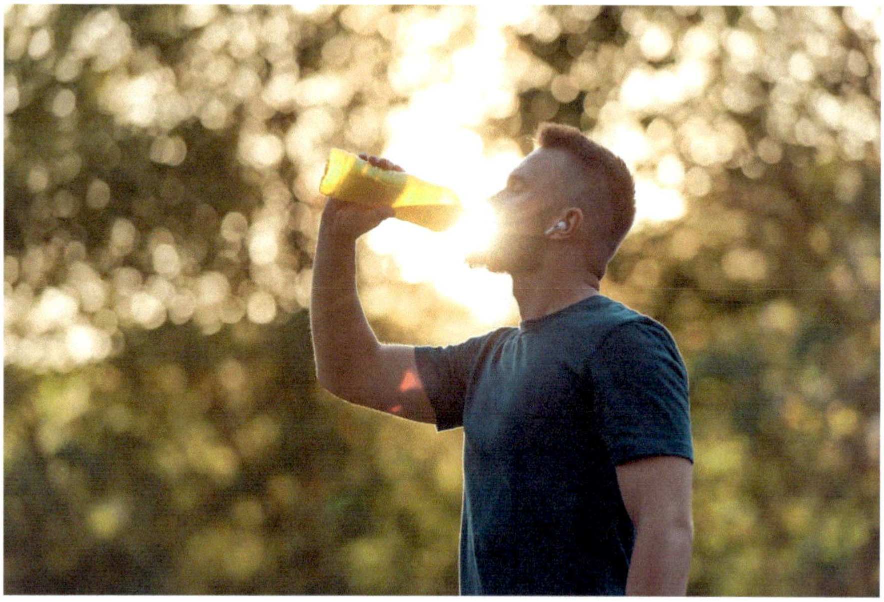

Figure 10.15. Common immediate treatments include glucose tablets and juice, which provide a quick source of carbohydrates that can be rapidly absorbed into the bloodstream.

Source: https://cdn.prod.website-files.com/64eec5ed1ea74a7194cd16a3/67e2df7f349230960e5cc50f_2.%20HEADER.jpg

10.4.2. Long-term Management Strategies

Having a good long-term strategy for hypoglycemia is vital for people with diabetes, mainly those who take insulin. They involve a complete plan that covers education, monitoring, and treatment plans that are suited to each person. Knowledge gained through education allows patients to spot hypoglycemic symptoms and realize why it is important to keep their blood glucose stable. Keeping an eye on blood glucose levels lets patients find out what affects their sugar levels, so they can make the right changes to their diet and lifestyle. Taking care of your diabetes yourself is important since it helps you become independent and lowers the chance of severe low blood sugar. Besides, having a team of healthcare professionals can assist patients in choosing the best management strategies, which helps improve their long-term results. Managing diabetes over a long period is especially important because of the difficulties linked to strict blood sugar control. Basically, achieving a low HbA1c is necessary to prevent complications, but it could result in more hypoglycemic episodes. It is important to consider the relationship between changes in blood sugar and the way diabetes is managed. Evidence indicates that fluctuations in glucose levels can impact cardiovascular health, particularly in patients with type 1 diabetes mellitus (T1DM). So, it is important for long-term strategies to assess glycemic variability well to improve treatments that help avoid risks and maintain healthy blood sugar levels. Continuous glucose monitoring (CGM) technology can be instrumental in this regard, providing real-time data that supports informed decision-making. Lastly, the use of behavioral strategies in long-term management plans is very important for patients' well-being. Making positive changes in diet and exercise can help manage blood sugar and lower the number of hypoglycemic episodes. In addition, dealing with anxiety about low blood sugar is very important for patients following their treatment plans. Some patients with hypoglycemia start to worry about it, which may cause them to overuse carbohydrates or skip their insulin. Dealing with these mental barriers with help from counseling or support groups can encourage a better approach to managing diabetes. As shown in existing research, a multifaceted approach that combines education, technology, and psychological support is vital for effective long-term management of hypoglycemia in diabetes care (Barnard et al., 2010; Helleputte et al., 2020) (Figure 10.16).

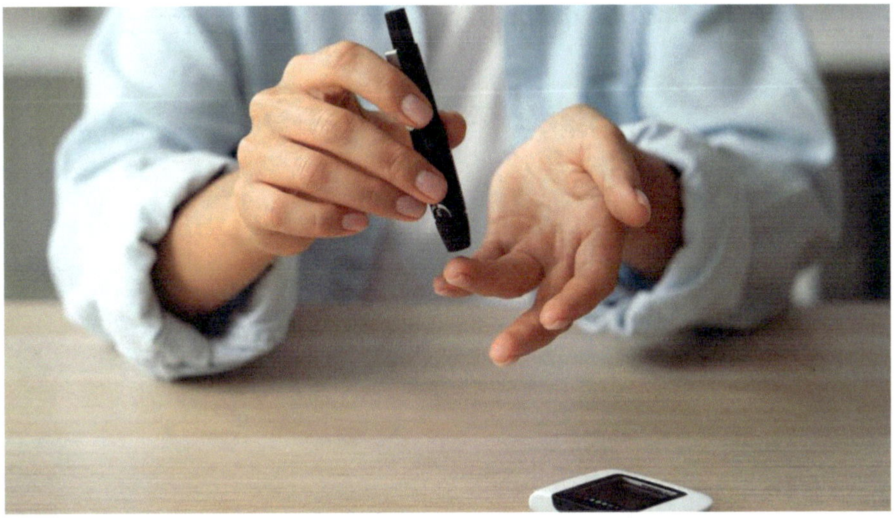

Figure 10.16. Education empowers patients with the knowledge to recognize hypoglycemic symptoms and understand the importance of maintaining stable blood glucose levels.

Source: https://ilshospitals.com/blog/wp-content/uploads/2024/04/Hypoglycemia-1038x576.jpg

10.4.3. Role of Glucagon in Severe Cases

When hypoglycemia is severe and other methods do not work, glucagon becomes very important in managing the condition. Glucagon is a hormone produced by alpha cells in the pancreas and mainly helps raise blood glucose levels by encouraging the liver to produce new glucose and break down its glycogen stores. This hormone helps control blood sugar levels when there is a major drop in blood sugar. If someone with type 1 diabetes has a serious episode of low blood sugar, glucagon can quickly help raise blood sugar. Significantly, using glucagon in emergencies may help stop a person from passing out or having a seizure, which highlights its key importance in managing hypoglycemia. Even though glucagon helps in severe hypoglycemia, there are still some difficulties with using it. The way glucagon is delivered is a problem, since it must be injected, which can be hard for those experiencing hypoglycemia in an emergency. Still, new glucagon formulations that are easy to give, such as nasal sprays, may help more people get the treatment they need in acute cases. In addition, new research is looking at glucagon's ability to help with both low blood sugar and high blood sugar in people with diabetes. Because these new therapies are being used, both diabetes care providers and patients should be well informed about how to use glucagon in hypoglycemic emergencies, as is recommended by new clinical guidelines. It has been discovered that glucagon plays a role in new diabetes treatments, not only in treating emergency low blood sugar. Lately, better methods for managing blood sugar in type 1 diabetes have highlighted the usefulness of glucagon in regular medical care. Although the UKPDS made clear the need for good glycemic control, recent diabetes drugs and insulins may not be enough to avoid hypoglycemia, so glucagon is still needed in serious cases. Knowing more about glucagons and their effects on new treatments can assist healthcare providers in controlling hypoglycemia. Consequently, integration of glucagon therapy within broader treatment paradigms can potentially lead to improved clinical outcomes, not only in preventing severe hypoglycemic events but also in addressing related complications and optimizing patient quality of life, as emphasized in studies on diabetes management and care advancements (Heller et al., 2007; DiMeglio et al., 2018) (Figure 10.17).

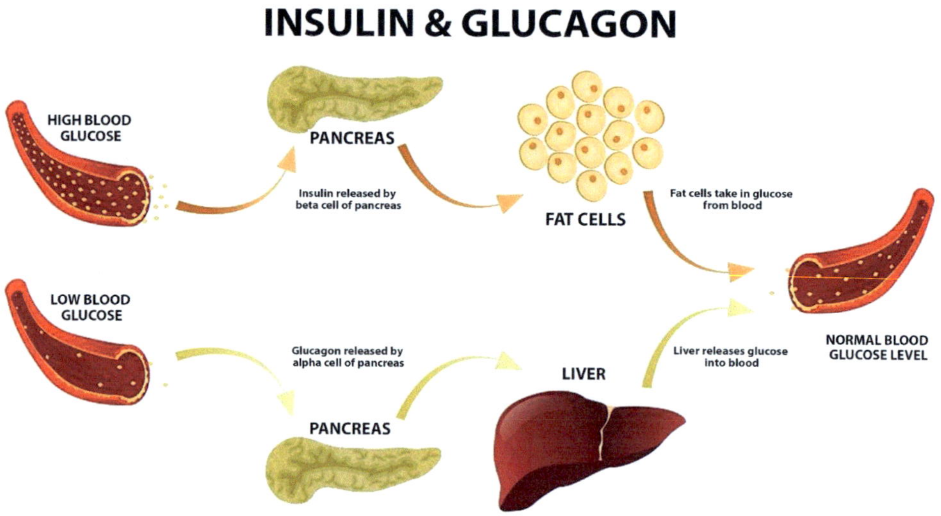

Figure 10.17. Glucagon, a hormone secreted by the alpha cells of the pancreas, functions primarily to increase blood glucose levels by stimulating hepatic gluconeogenesis and glycogenolysis.

Source: https://www.news-medical.net/images/Article_Images/ImageForArticle_25538_17322956522701880.jpg

10.5. Prevention of Hypoglycemia

Effective prevention of hypoglycemia involves a multi-faceted approach that prioritizes patient education, lifestyle adjustments, and rigorous monitoring of blood glucose levels. Education plays a pivotal role, equipping individuals with diabetes and their caregivers with the knowledge needed to recognize early signs of hypoglycemia and understand the critical importance of maintaining stable blood glucose levels. Moreover, lifestyle adjustments, such as dietary modifications that emphasize balanced carbohydrate intake, can significantly mitigate the risk of hypoglycemic episodes. Regular consultation with healthcare professionals ensures that individuals are adapting their treatment plans to their lifestyle changes and personal health conditions. In particular, comprehensive education and training deliver essential strategies that empower patients, ultimately leading to better self-management and preventing severe hypoglycemia, which can necessitate external assistance (De Galan et al., 2020). The integration of technology within diabetes management has emerged as a revolutionary strategy to prevent hypoglycemia. Continuous glucose monitoring systems allow for real-time tracking of glucose levels, providing users with immediate feedback and alerts when levels approach dangerous thresholds. This proactive approach not only aids in prevention but also fosters a sense of autonomy for patients, encouraging them to engage actively in their diabetes management. Furthermore, advancements in glucose-sensing technology, demonstrated through projects like Hypo-RESOLVE, aim to establish clearer thresholds for hypoglycemia risk while examining the diverse clinical impacts of hypoglycemic occurrences. By utilizing these advanced technologies, healthcare systems can effectively enhance patient outcomes, reducing both the frequency of hypoglycemic events and the associated psychological and economic burdens faced by individuals and families suffering from diabetes (De Galan et al., 2020). In addition to patient education and technological advancements, the establishment of clinical performance indicators plays a critical role in preventing hypoglycemia within healthcare systems.

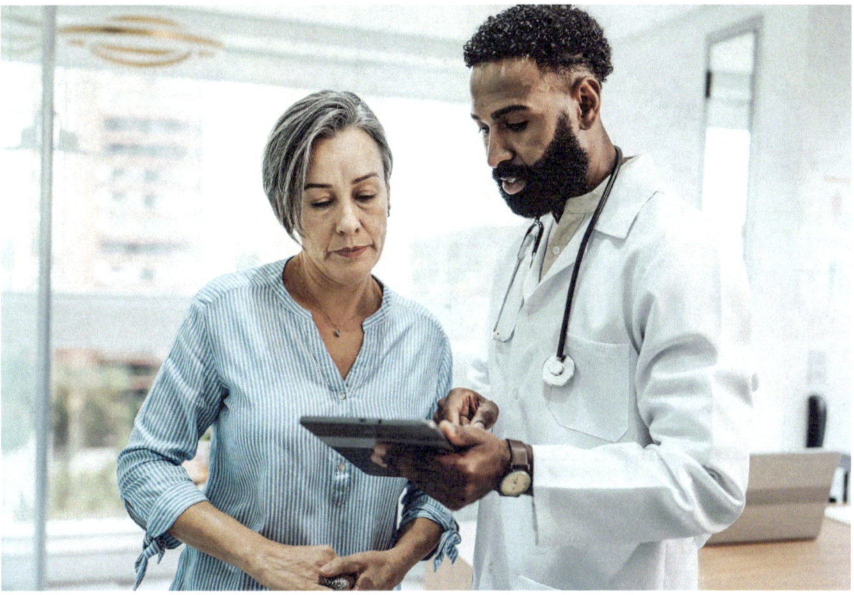

Figure 10.18. Regular consultation with healthcare professionals ensures that individuals are adapting their treatment plans to their lifestyle changes and personal health conditions.

Source: https://img.lb.wbmdstatic.com/vim/live/webmd/consumer_assets/site_images/article_thumbnails/BigBead/general_practitioners_what_to_know_bigbead/1800x1200_general_practitioners_what_to_know_bigbead.jpg

These indicators, when developed in collaboration with clinicians, service users, and health policymakers, can benchmark performance and drive improvements in patient care. They provide a framework for ensuring that prevention strategies are not only effective but also equitable and patient-centered. For instance, establishing clear metrics for monitoring blood glucose management can help to identify variations in care quality and ensure consistent implementation of best practices across different healthcare settings. This targeted approach to quality improvement is essential to reducing the incidence of hypoglycemia and enhancing overall diabetes management, ultimately addressing critical issues that matter to both patients and clinicians (Figure 10.18).

10.5.1. Dietary Management and Meal Planning

Effective management of meals and planning a diet is important for preventing and controlling hypoglycemia, mainly in people with diabetes. One important part of controlling blood glucose is to prepare meals that have the right amounts of carbohydrates, proteins, and fats. Carbohydrates are especially necessary because they influence the amount of glucose in the body. When people consume complex carbohydrates, they can avoid experiencing rapid drops in their blood sugar. To do this, one should know about the glycemic index and plan meals so that blood glucose stays stable.

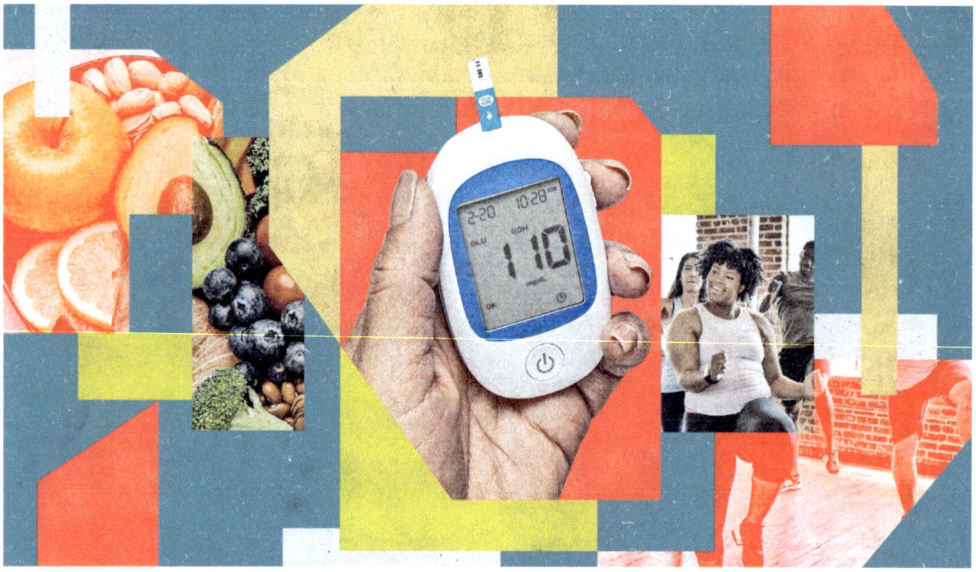

Figure 10.19. Carbohydrates, in particular, are vital since they directly affect glucose levels.

Source: https://static01.nyt.com/images/2024/10/15/well/11Well-Blood-Sugar/11Well-Blood-Sugar-videoSixteenByNineJumbo1600-v2.jpg

Besides, people should keep in mind that exercise can make insulin work better and, if they do not adjust their diet, this could lead to hypoglycemia. Besides considering the main nutrition in meal planning, people should be aware of the possible signs and symptoms of hypoglycemia to help them respond quickly. Having several small meals each day can help you keep your blood sugar levels steady. This way of eating is especially helpful for people who exercise regularly, since their blood sugar may change more easily during exercise. Snacks and meals should be planned so that people eat well before and after exercising. Managing blood glucose levels is not only about what people eat; it also requires knowing how different foods affect insulin and metabolism, which means each person should have a meal plan suited to their own needs. Besides, the results of weight management strategies, including those from bariatric surgery, are connected to diet planning and meal preparation. After bariatric surgery, patients may deal with certain nutritional issues that could lead to hypoglycemia. If sugars are quickly absorbed and meal planning is not done right, it may cause reactive hypoglycemia. As noted in the literature, adequate pre-operative and post-operative dietary education is essential in these cases to prevent complications associated with both obesity and subsequent weight loss surgery (Azran et al., 2017). This points out that a multidisciplinary way of managing diet is important, where healthcare providers guide patients on healthy meals and teach them to control their co-morbidities, so that blood glucose levels are maintained and hypoglycemic episodes are prevented (Figure 10.19).

10.5.2. Monitoring Blood Glucose Levels

Monitoring blood glucose levels is an essential component in the management of hypoglycemia, particularly for individuals with diabetes who are undergoing treatment with insulin or insulin secretagogues. Regular monitoring enables patients to track fluctuations in their glucose levels, thus allowing for timely interventions when hypoglycemia is detected. As hypoglycemia may lead to severe cognitive dysfunction, the importance of consistent monitoring cannot be overstated. Inadequate awareness of one's glucose status can result in unaddressed drops in blood sugar, which heightens the risk of severe complications, including adverse cardiovascular outcomes and increased mortality rates, as indicated by De Galan et al., (2020). Moreover, the advancement in glucose monitoring technology, including continuous glucose monitors (CGMs), facilitates real-time data collection, empowering patients to make informed decisions and maintain their blood glucose within a safe range.

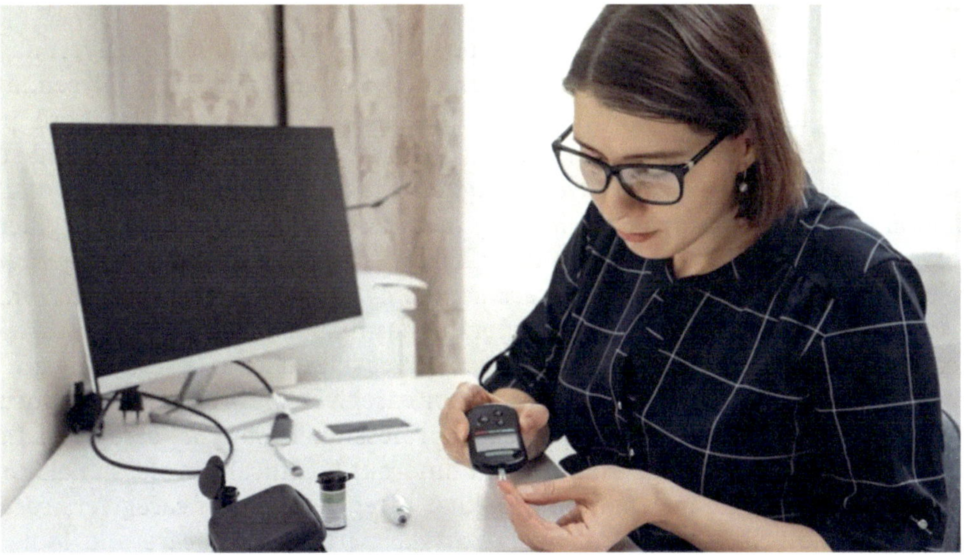

Figure 10.20. Regular monitoring enables patients to track fluctuations in their glucose levels, thus allowing for timely interventions when hypoglycemia is detected.

Source: https://drkumo.com/wp-content/uploads/2023/03/woman-checking-normal-blood-sugar-levels-by-age-1024x576.webp

The design and purpose of monitoring protocols can significantly impact the outcomes associated with hypoglycemia. The integration of evidence-based guidelines surrounding monitoring frequency and techniques is crucial for ensuring that both healthcare providers and patients are aligned in their approach to managing blood glucose levels. As highlighted in studies conducted as part of the Hypo-RESOLVE initiative, understanding predictors of hypoglycemia can aid in refining classification systems and setting appropriate thresholds for intervention, ultimately improving patient care (De Galan et al., 2020). It is not only the immediate detection of hypoglycemia that matters but also the long-term implications of monitoring strategies. By establishing effective monitoring protocols, healthcare systems can reduce the psychological and economic burdens that accompany hypoglycemia, addressing the broader impacts on both individuals and the healthcare system. Incorporating advanced technologies alongside traditional monitoring practices fosters a more comprehensive understanding of blood glucose dynamics. The utilization of glucose sensors and mobile health applications can enhance patient engagement and adherence, creating a more proactive approach to diabetes management. These technological advancements, identified in the ongoing research of the Hypo-RESOLVE initiative, illustrate the significance of monitoring beyond mere blood sugar readings, as they facilitate insights into trends and patterns over time (De Galan et al., 2020). Enhanced monitoring not only aids in preventing hypoglycemic events but also contributes to the psychological well-being of patients, alleviating anxiety around potential episodes. Therefore, a multifaceted approach to monitoring blood glucose levels serves as a robust foundation for addressing the complex challenges of hypoglycemia, promoting improved patient outcomes and reducing healthcare costs (Figure 10.20).

10.5.3. Education for Patients and Caregivers

It is very important for patients and caregivers to be well educated about hypoglycemia, mainly for those with chronic diseases such as diabetes. By teaching patients about hypoglycemia, education helps them know how to recognize it, what causes it, and how to treat it. Therefore, people with diabetes become more involved in their care and take action quickly when their blood sugar drops. Besides, when educational programs are well-designed, they can help both patients and caregivers manage common issues, for example, by showing them how to check their blood glucose, decide on good diets, and communicate well with their health team. Such support encourages patients to feel more confident and also helps caregivers handle hypoglycemia emergencies, which is good for both parties' health. It is clear that when a person has diabetes and dementia, caregivers need special education to manage the situation properly. Studies have shown that looking after someone with hypoglycemia and dementia can be very tough for caregivers. A proper training focused on the relationship between these conditions helps health professionals support caregivers in providing better care. Programs that encourage families and different healthcare professionals to work as a team are necessary to close the information gaps that caregivers face. If caregivers receive proper support and information, they are more likely to take part in healthcare and look after their patients' hypoglycemia, resulting in better overall care. Besides, educational initiatives should be able to respond to the specific needs of both patients and their caregivers. A good way to do this is to use images and demonstrations in educational materials to help students understand better. These strategies play a big role in helping people with different educational and health literacy levels understand each other. Also, keeping up with education helps both patients and caregivers know the newest ways to handle hypoglycemia. Offering support groups or workshops helps patients learn more and improves their ways of coping with their health problems. In the end, a good education framework for patients and caregivers helps people handle immediate issues and also teaches them how to manage hypoglycemia in the long run (Figure 10.21).

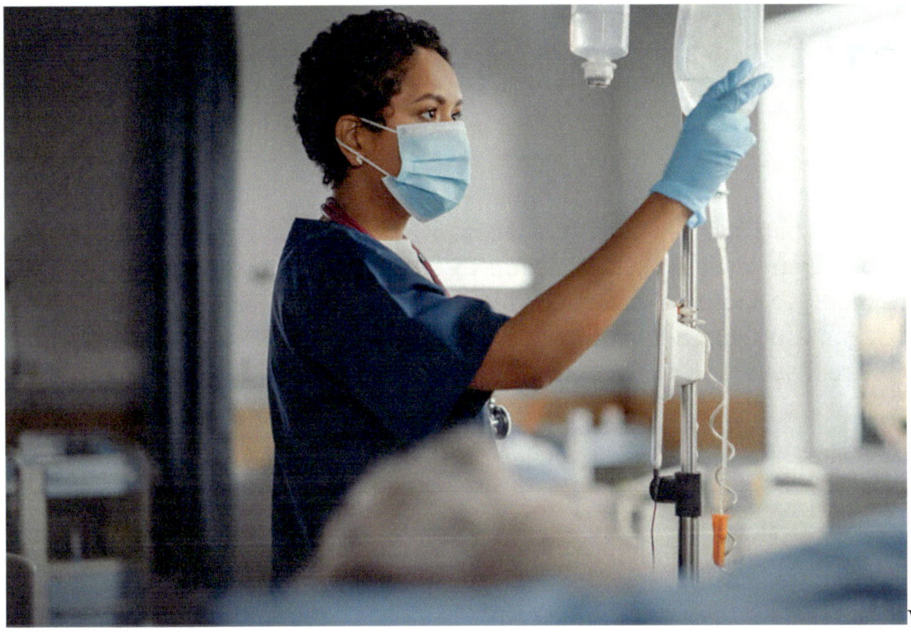

V

Figure 10.21. Education empowers patients by enhancing their understanding of hypoglycemia's symptoms, triggers, and management strategies.

Source: https://diabetesonthenet.com/wp-content/uploads/Nurse-ward-shutterstock_1985507474.jpg

A CLOSER LOOK

GLUCAGON

The alpha cells in the pancreas produce glucagon, which helps control the level of glucose in the blood. A low blood sugar level causes glucagon to tell the liver to turn glycogen into glucose and send it into the blood to increase the sugar level. It works oppositely to insulin, which helps to decrease blood sugar. Glucagon helps maintain your energy level when you are not eating. It is also used medically to treat severe hypoglycemia (dangerously low blood sugar) in people with diabetes.

Summary

Hypoglycemia creates a major issue in treating diabetes, mainly for people who use insulin or insulin secretagogues. Low blood glucose causes this condition, and it may result in symptoms ranging from slight discomfort to major brain dysfunction that requires outside help. Low blood sugar can be dangerous, leading to more heart problems and a greater chance of dying from any cause. Besides, knowing about both kinds of hypoglycemia is essential, as the non-severe version can cause harm to mental health and lead to extra costs in healthcare. The ongoing research endeavor, Hypo-RESOLVE, aims to address these gaps by examining clinical and psychological outcomes associated with various levels of hypoglycemia, ultimately refining how this multifaceted condition is classified and managed in diabetic patients (De Galan et al., 2020). It is important to look into different strategies to prevent hypoglycemia without affecting how well glycemic control is maintained. Many therapies have been proven to work differently in reducing hypoglycemia, and some have shown great benefits in actual clinical use. For example, some treatments made for Type 1 diabetes patients can help lower the number of hypoglycemic episodes without affecting the control of blood sugar. Still, some new therapies have not been completely studied, which points to the need for more research and trials. In light of the complexity of diabetes management, healthcare professionals need to remain informed about the latest interventions and guidelines to optimize patient outcomes while minimizing risks associated with hypoglycemia (Heller et al., 2008). The main purpose of Hypo-RESOLVE is to develop reliable ways of investigating hypoglycemia. The efforts will make use of large databases from many clinical trials to find the levels of glucose that may lead to negative consequences. To make sure everyone agrees on what hypoglycemia means, it is important to involve many stakeholders in the process. Looking at the various aspects of hypoglycemia is likely to highlight its complexity and may change how it is handled in medical settings. Ultimately, such progress strives to alleviate the burden faced by individuals living with diabetes, reflecting a broader commitment to enhancing quality of life (De Galan et al., 2020).

References

1. Admon, Y., Adolfsson, P., Al Khalifah, A., Arutchelvam, V., Bally, L., et al. (2017). Exercise management in type 1 diabetes: A consensus statement. https://core.ac.uk/download/77006838.pdf (accessed on 11th June 2025).
2. ADVANCE Collaborative Group, American Diabetes Association Consensus Panel, Anderson, J., Bagust, A., Billings, D., Blak, B., et al. (2018). The management of type 2 diabetes with fixed-ratio combination insulin degludec/liraglutide (IDegLira) versus basal-bolus therapy (insulin glargine U100 plus insulin aspart): A short-term cost-effectiveness analysis in the UK setting. https://core.ac.uk/download/159754627.pdf (accessed on 11th June 2025).
3. Aleman, M., Costa, L. R. R., Crowe, C., Kass, P. H., et al. (2018). Presumed neuroglycopenia caused by severe hypoglycemia in horses. https://core.ac.uk/download/323069529.pdf (accessed on 11th June 2025).
4. Almeida, M., Andrade, C., da Silva Moreira, S., de Souza Teles, M., et al. (2019). Sex differences and correlates of poor glycemic control in type 2 diabetes: A cross-sectional study in Brazil and Venezuela. https://core.ac.uk/download/323081941.pdf (accessed on 11th June 2025).
5. Amiel, S. A., Dawoud, D., Fenu, E., Higgins, B., et al. (2017). Basal insulin regimens for adults with type 1 diabetes mellitus: A cost-utility analysis. https://core.ac.uk/download/287580946.pdf (accessed on 11th June 2025).
6. Amiel, S., Barnard, K., Beckwith, A., Brennan, A., et al. (2017). A cluster randomized trial, cost-effectiveness analysis and psychosocial evaluation of insulin pump therapy compared with multiple injections during flexible intensive insulin therapy for type 1 diabetes: The REPOSE Trial. https://core.ac.uk/download/82893694.pdf (accessed on 11th June 2025).
7. Azran, C., Batterham, R. L., Busetto, L., Dicker, D., et al. (2017). Practical recommendations of the Obesity Management Task Force of the European Association for the Study of Obesity for the post-bariatric surgery medical management. https://core.ac.uk/download/141699962.pdf (accessed on 11th June 2025).
8. Barendse, S. M., Heller, S. R., Little, S. A., Rutter, M. K., et al. (2014). Cognitive, behavioral and psychological barriers to the prevention of severe hypoglycemia: A qualitative study of adults with type 1 diabetes. https://core.ac.uk/download/74233780.pdf (accessed on 11th June 2025).
9. Barnard, K., Noyes, K., Royle, P., Thomas, S., et al. (2010). Fear of hypoglycemia in parents of young children with type 1 diabetes: A systematic review. https://core.ac.uk/download/25497621.pdf (accessed on 11th June 2025).
10. Baud, F. J., Bloch, V., Collet, C., Deye, N., et al. (2007). Intentional overdose with insulin: Prognostic factors and toxicokinetic/toxicodynamic profiles. https://core.ac.uk/download/pdf/8196162.pdf (accessed on 11th June 2025).
11. Bellisle, F., Blundell, J. E., Dye, L., Fantino, M., et al. (2017). Functional food science and behavior and psychological functions. https://core.ac.uk/download/85217796.pdf (accessed on 11th June 2025).
12. Black, S., Donohoe, R., National Ambulance Clinical Audit Steering Group, Shaw, D., et al. (2010). Development and pilot of clinical performance indicators for English ambulance services. https://core.ac.uk/download/54851.pdf (accessed on 11th June 2025).

13. Boyle, J., & Livingstone, R. (2015). Improving the quality of assessment and management of hypoglycemia in hospitalized patients with diabetes mellitus by introducing 'hypo boxes' to general medical wards with a specialist interest in diabetes. https://core.ac.uk/download/42367513.pdf (accessed on 11th June 2025).

14. Helleputte, S., De Backer, T., Lapauw, B., Shadid, S., Celie, B., Van Eetvelde, B., Vanden Wyngaert, K., & Calders, P. (2020). The relationship between glycaemic variability and cardiovascular autonomic dysfunction in patients with type 1 diabetes: A systematic review. *Diabetes/metabolism research and reviews*, *36*(5), e3301. https://doi.org/10.1002/dmrr.3301(accessed on 11th June 2025).

15. de Galan, B. E., McCrimmon, R. J., Ibberson, M., Heller, S. R., Choudhary, P., Pouwer, F., Speight, J., Carlton, J., Pieber, T. R., Rosilio, M., Tack, C. J., Müllenborn, M., & Hypo-RESOLVE Consortium (2020). Reducing the burden of hypoglycaemia in people with diabetes through increased understanding: design of the Hypoglycaemia REdefining SOLutions for better liVEs (Hypo-RESOLVE) project. *Diabetic medicine : a journal of the British Diabetic Association*, *37*(6), 1066–1073. https://doi.org/10.1111/dme.14240(accessed on 11th June 2025).

16. Carral San Laureano, F., Castro Maqueda, G. R. de, Fernández Santos, J. del R., Gutiérrez Manzanedo, R. M., et al. (2018). Teachers' knowledge about type 1 diabetes in south of Spain public schools. https://core.ac.uk/download/599469941.pdf (accessed on 11th June 2025).

17. Coates, V., & Sharkey, F. (2023). Managing diabetes and dementia, a challenging duo: A scoping review. https://core.ac.uk/download/613865144.pdf (accessed on 11th June 2025).

18. DiMeglio, L. A., Evans-Molina, C., & Oram, R. A. (2018). Type 1 diabetes. https://core.ac.uk/download/228066211.pdf (accessed on 11th June 2025).

19. Farrell, C. M., Fournier, P., Hapca, S. M., Jones, T. W., et al. (2020). A randomized controlled study of high intensity exercise as a dishabituating stimulus to improve hypoglycemia awareness in people with type 1 diabetes: A proof-of-concept study. https://core.ac.uk/download/286356102.pdf (accessed on 11th June 2025).

20. Gillespie, A., Kennedy, A., Kennedy, A., Kennedy, A., Manzano, A., Reinhardt Varming, A., Sachar, A., et al. (2017). What works for whom in the management of diabetes in people living with dementia: A realist review. https://core.ac.uk/download/323306795.pdf (accessed on 11th June 2025).

21. Gris, M., Lheureux, P. E. R., Penaloza, A., Zahir, A., et al. (2005). Bench-to-bedside review: Antidotal treatment of sulfonylurea-induced hypoglycemia with octreotide. https://core.ac.uk/download/pdf/3913310.pdf (accessed on 11th June 2025).

22. Heller, S. (2007). Targeting acute hyperglycemia in clinical practice. https://core.ac.uk/download/51766.pdf (accessed on 11th June 2025).

23. Heller, S. (2008). Minimizing hypoglycemia while maintaining glycemic control in diabetes. https://core.ac.uk/download/50935.pdf (accessed on 11th June 2025).

24. Huda, M. S. B., & Loumpardia, P. (2019). Symptoms of hypoglycemia. https://core.ac.uk/download/322444894.pdf (accessed on 11th June 2025).

25. Iwai, A., Meer, A., Wain Yong, A., Megarbane, B., Boeve, B. F., Koppel, B. S., Cordonnier, C., et al. (2012). Acute symptomatic hypoglycemia mimicking ischemic stroke on imaging: A systemic review. https://core.ac.uk/download/28970070.pdf (accessed on 11th June 2025).

26. Miras, A. D., & le Roux, C. W. (2014). Can medical therapy mimic the clinical efficacy or physiological effects of bariatric surgery?. *International journal of obesity (2005)*, *38*(3), 325–333. https://doi.org/10.1038/ijo.2013.205(accessed on 11th June 2025).

27. Vekemans, J., Marsh, K., Greenwood, B., Leach, A., Kabore, W., Soulanoudjingar, S., Asante, K. P., Ansong, D., Evans, J., Sacarlal, J., Bejon, P., Kamthunzi, P., Salim, N., Njuguna, P., Hamel, M. J., Otieno, W., Gesase, S., Schellenberg, D., & Clinical Trials Partnership Committee (2011). Assessment of severe malaria in a multicenter, phase III, RTS, S/AS01 malaria candidate vaccine trial: case definition, standardization of data collection and patient care. *Malaria journal*, *10*, 221. https://doi.org/10.1186/1475-2875-10-221(accessed on 11th June 2025).

28. Paluchamy, T. (2019). Hypoglycemia: Essential clinical guidelines. https://core.ac.uk/download/322444630.pdf (accessed on 11th June 2025).

29. Pecchia, L., Pescapè, A., Porumb, M., Stranges, S., et al. (2020). Precision medicine and artificial intelligence: A pilot study on deep learning for hypoglycemic events detection based on ECG. https://core.ac.uk/download/287605709.pdf (accessed on 11th June 2025).

30. Sciberras, R. (2010). A rare cause of hypoglycemia. https://core.ac.uk/download/46602267.pdf (accessed on 11th June 2025).

31. Siriwardena, A. N. (2007). Development and use of clinical performance indicators for ambulance services and prehospital care: A discussion paper for a clinical quality improvement framework for ambulance services. https://core.ac.uk/download/16498419.pdf (accessed on 11th June 2025).

32. Szladovits, B., Glanemann, B., Darcy, H., Gajanayake, I., Simpson, K., Seth, M., McLornan, D., et al. (2018). Feline primary erythrocytosis: A multicenter case series of 18 cats. https://core.ac.uk/download/151173647.pdf (accessed on 11th June 2025).

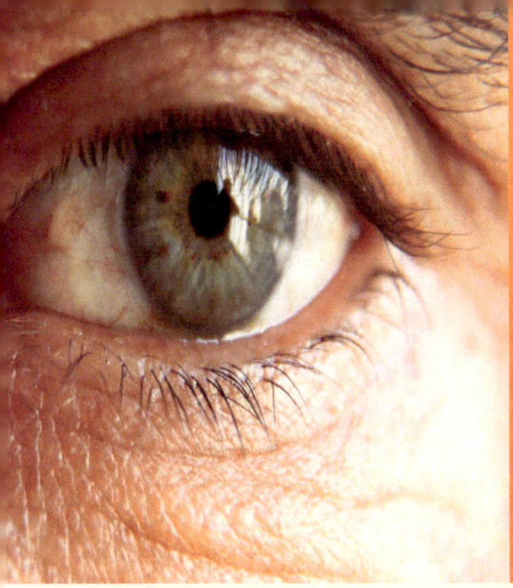

Chapter 11

DIABETIC EYE DISEASE

Contents

Introduction

Diabetic eye disease is a serious health issue because diabetes is becoming more common around the world. This issue involves different eye problems that develop due to long-term high blood sugar, and diabetic retinopathy is the most frequent case. When the disease is not treated, it may result in major vision loss and can cause blindness. It is important to know how these retinal changes happen, especially the role played by microvascular problems caused by diabetes affecting blood vessels. Therefore, this damage to the retina causes both fluid and cell growth, proving why it is important to identify and treat those at risk as soon as possible. It is important to deal with these issues for both personal patient results and for public health efforts to lower the number of diabetic complications. Diabetic eye disease costs people, their families, and the healthcare system a lot in terms of money and emotions. Patients may lose their vision and also have to deal with the mental effects of this disease. Moreover, since eye conditions require regular check-ups and treatments, patients may need laser therapy, vitrectomy, or surgery. The difficulty of treating diabetic eye disease is increased by diabetes working together with other diseases, such as high blood pressure and high cholesterol, which can worsen retinal damage. Since these factors are complex, a team of experts from different fields is needed to address all the problems related to diabetic eye disease and help patients. With the help of new technology and medical studies, it is now possible to better control diabetic eye disease. Because of telemedicine, patients who cannot easily go to an eye clinic can now be screened for retinal diseases remotely. In addition, new drugs that address the causes of diabetic retinopathy are expected to greatly change the course of the disease. For example, using neuroprotective agents is being examined to help repair neurons in the retina, and some new therapies are being developed to increase angiogenesis and strengthen blood vessels. This suggests that doctors may start using more active and coordinated care plans that focus on early treatment and regular education for diabetes patients about their eye health (Figure 11.1).

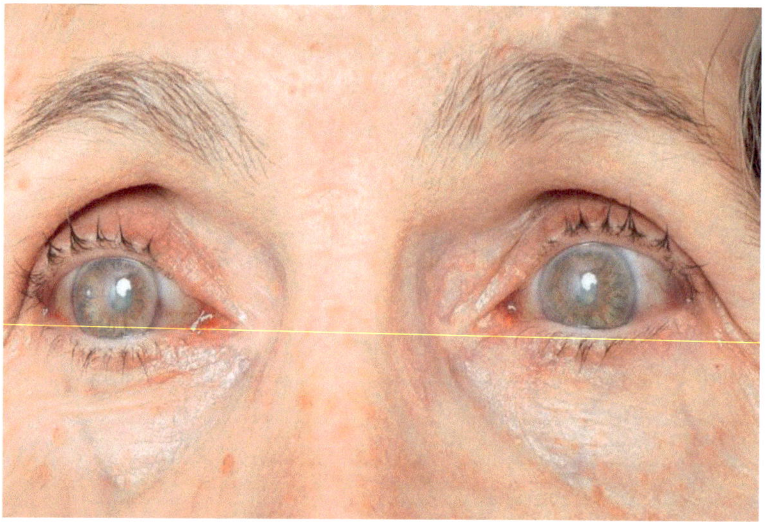

Figure 11.1. Diabetic eye disease.

Source: https://media.allaboutvision.com/cms/caas/v1/media/425468/data/f0f9a198a4fb802f620b2f52a061198e/hero-article-diabetic-retinopathy-compressor.jpg

11.1. Types of Diabetic Eye Disease

The main eye problems in diabetes are diabetic retinopathy, diabetic macular edema, and cataracts. Diabetic retinopathy happens most often and occurs when high blood sugar harms the blood vessels in the retina, leading to eye problems. Usually, it develops in stages from a mild form called non-proliferative retinopathy to a severe form called proliferative retinopathy, where new, weak blood vessels appear on the retina and can cause major vision loss. Since the condition is usually found late, it is important to have regular check-ups to catch it early. Recent advancements in prognostic technologies have facilitated the non-invasive identification of retinal damage due to prolonged hyperglycemia, potentially transforming patients' approaches to management and prevention of further disease progression, ultimately enhancing outcomes in diabetic retinopathy

(Martin et al., 2025). As well as retinopathy, diabetic macular edema is a serious problem for people with diabetes. When fluid builds up in the macula, the main part of the retina, it causes the vision to look blurry or distorted. Many times, it happens because of diabetic retinopathy and can happen at any point during the disease. Controlling blood sugar and using anti-VEGF injections, corticosteroids, or laser therapy are important in treating diabetic macular edema. The economic implications of diabetes management are significant, underscoring the necessity for integrated care that encompasses regular screening and innovative treatment options, which ultimately affect healthcare costs and quality of life for affected individuals (Middleton et al., 2007). By knowing how these eye diseases are related, we can provide patients with the right care and timely help. Cataracts are a frequent diabetic eye disease that greatly increases the chances for people with diabetes. Blurred vision is the result of these lens opacifications, and if not treated, they might cause blindness. Experts have found that diabetes may lead to cataracts earlier and more severely than in people who do not have the disease. Cataract treatment usually includes surgery, which can help a person see much better and enjoy a better quality of life. Even so, it is important to deal with diabetes-related problems like stable blood glucose and lowering hypertension to avoid cataracts. By focusing on comprehensive eye care and the interplay between diabetes management and cataract development, healthcare providers can significantly reduce the burden of diabetic eye diseases on patients, thereby enhancing their health outcomes and life satisfaction (Middleton et al., 2007; Martin et al., 2025) (Figure 11.1).

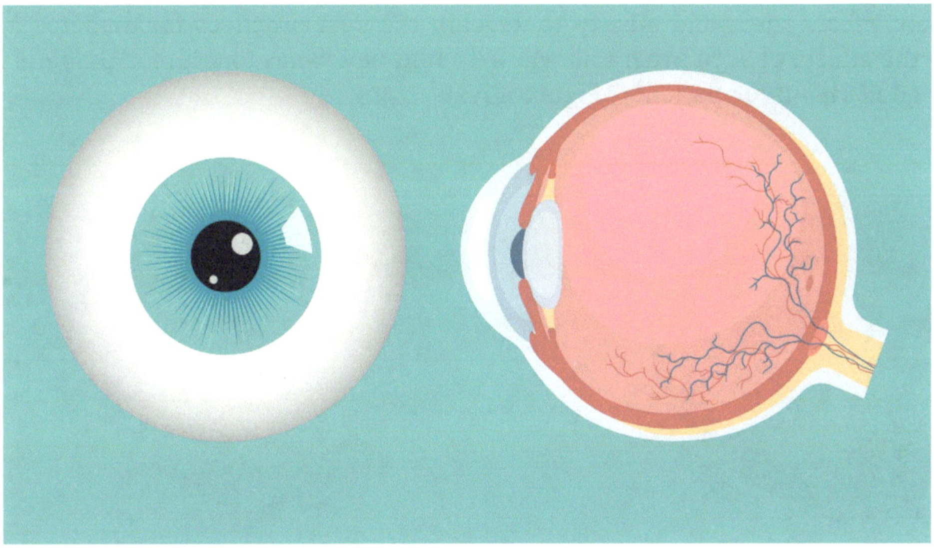

Figure 11.2. Diabetic retinopathy is the most common and occurs when high blood sugar levels damage the blood vessels in the retina, leading to vision problems.

Source: https://burjeel.com/wp-content/uploads/2022/05/shutterstock_1156809016-Converted-scaled.jpg

11.1.1. Diabetic Retinopathy

Diabetic Retinopathy (DR) represents a significant complication related to diabetes, manifesting as damage to the retinal blood vessels due to prolonged exposure to high blood glucose levels.

The stages of DR usually go from mild non-proliferative retinopathy to proliferative retinopathy, which can make vision very impaired. Unfortunately, many people are found to have eye diseases when their vision has already been affected, which proves the importance of early detection. New ways of predicting outcomes may make it possible to detect retinal changes linked to high glucose levels before they cause any clinical signs. This proactive approach not only allows for timely medical interventions but also encourages patients to implement necessary lifestyle modifications to mitigate the progression of the disease (Martin et al., 2025). Diabetic Retinopathy has a major effect on the economy because it leads to high medical bills and a loss of people's ability to work. Such models can give healthcare providers important information about how DR will develop over time and what the related expenses will be. In this way, a Markov model helps healthcare professionals to see the long-term costs of the disease and understand how changing the outlook can affect the management of DR. Such evaluations are necessary since they point out the financial burden that DR causes for both patients and healthcare providers. Economic assessments can inform policy decisions surrounding resource allocation for screening and treatment initiatives, ultimately improving patient outcomes and reducing overall expenses related to diabetes care (Martin et al., 2025). Also, technology is playing a bigger role in diabetes management, mainly for Diabetic Retinopathy. Many technology-based diabetes management programs have shown that they can check blood glucose well and motivate patients to stick to their treatment plans. These developments are necessary for both regulating blood sugar and for spotting eye diseases linked to diabetes, for example, DR. Since digital health tools are improving, it will be important to review their effectiveness and quality to develop the best practices for diabetes management. Looking into the effects of such programs will help find new ways to address Diabetic Retinopathy and support good vision for patients (Figure 11.3).

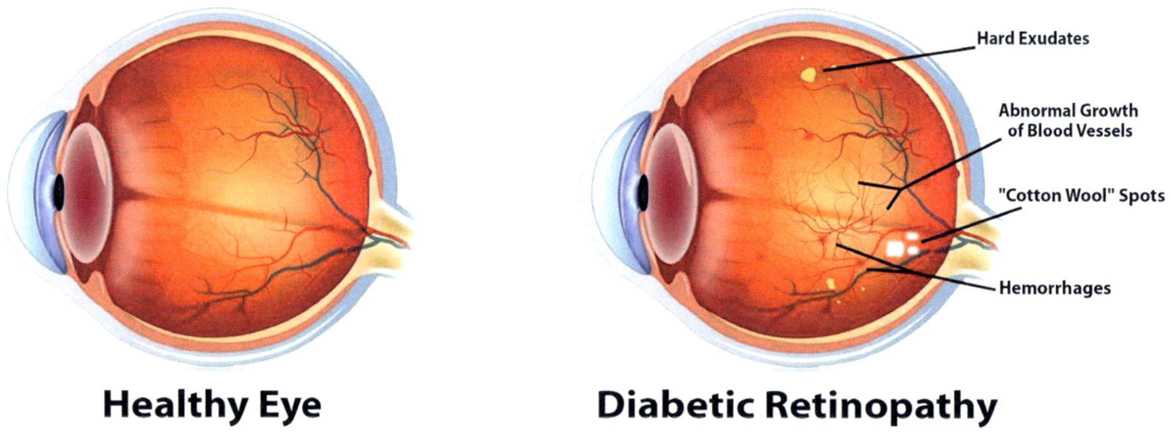

Figure 11.3. Diabetic Retinopathy (DR) represents a significant complication related to diabetes, manifesting as damage to the retinal blood vessels due to prolonged exposure to high blood glucose levels.

Source: https://specsmart.ng/cdn/shop/articles/Eyeball-Side-View-Diabetic_IMGCentury_IMGCentury.jpg?v=1737408436

11.1.2. Diabetic Macular Edema

The phenomenon of Diabetic Macular Edema (DME) is a critical consequence of diabetic eye disease, affecting a significant number of individuals diagnosed with diabetes. When fluid builds up in the macula, the main part of the retina for clear vision, it causes DME and results in blurred or distorted eyesight. If blood sugar levels stay high for a long time in diabetes, serum can leak into the retina due to increased permeability of the blood vessels. At first, this condition causes a slight vision change, but if left untreated, it can result in major visual problems. As evidence suggests, the main causes of visual impairment in individuals with diabetes include proliferative diabetic retinopathy and macular edema, indicative of the urgent need for early diagnosis and prompt intervention to mitigate the risk of vision loss, which is paramount for maintaining quality of life (Berco et al., 2015).

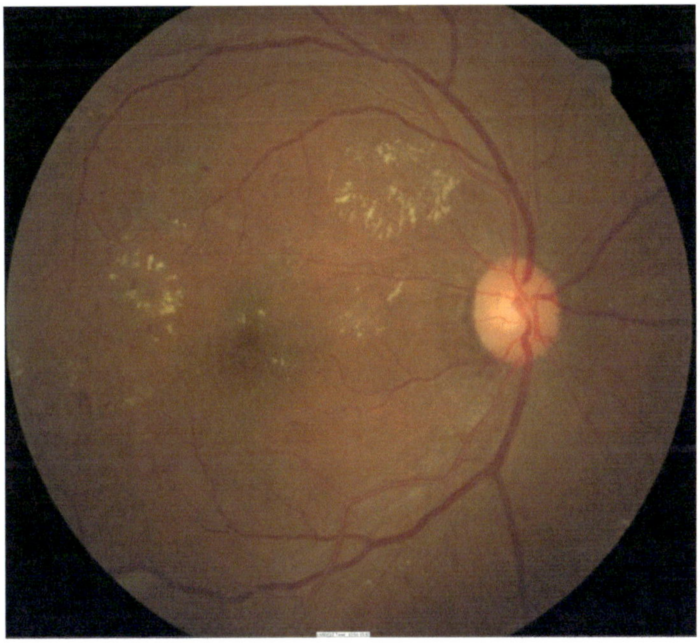

Figure 11.4. Diabetic macular edema.

Source: https://decisionmakerplus.net/wp-content/uploads/DG3620704.jpg

The treatment of Diabetic Macular Edema has advanced a lot, mainly because laser therapy was not always successful in saving vision. Recent advances in treatment modalities have introduced options such as intraocular steroid injections and antivascular endothelial growth factor (anti-VEGF) therapies. They focus on the main causes of DME by treating the inflammation and extra blood vessels found in the disease. As an example, using dexamethasone implants has led to a decrease in central macular thickness and better visual acuity in patients during the six-month follow-up, making them feel much better. As treatments continue to evolve, ongoing research is crucial for developing more effective interventions, ultimately aiming to halt the progression of DME and preserve sight for affected individuals (Bottone et al., 2016). Moreover, using various medical disciplines is necessary to handle Diabetic Macular Edema as part of diabetic eye disease. When primary care doctors and ophthalmologists cooperate, it becomes easier to detect and treat DME early, so serious complications can be avoided. Those with diabetes for a long time and those whose blood glucose is not well managed should have their eyes checked regularly. Learning how to control blood sugar, blood pressure, and modify your lifestyle is very important to reduce the risk of DME. As our understanding of diabetic eye disease continues to expand, comprehensive strategies that integrate medical, educational, and technological advancements will be pivotal in improving visual outcomes for patients suffering from this debilitating condition (Berco et al., 2015) (Figure 11.4).

11.1.3. Cataracts and Glaucoma

Visual impairment in people with diabetes is often caused by cataracts, which are a common problem of diabetic eye disease. Diabetics may experience eye conditions faster than people without diabetes. It has been found that diabetes increases the risk of cataracts, mainly because of the metabolic changes in the body, including higher sorbitol levels in the lens, which cause stress. For this reason, cataracts present a double problem, since they are related to other diabetic eye diseases like diabetic retinopathy and diabetic macular edema. For this reason, it is important for people with diabetes to have routine eye exams, since early detection and quick treatment of cataracts can help prevent vision loss and improve their lives. Glaucoma is another major issue in diabetic eye disease because it is caused by increased pressure in the eye, which may result in permanent optic nerve damage. Because of diabetes, patients are more likely to get open-angle glaucoma, and this risk can be increased by age and other eye diseases. It is especially worrying that glaucoma can develop silently, causing major vision problems before anyone notices. It has also been found that diabetes can cause changes in intraocular pressure, which makes it harder to diagnose and treat glaucoma. Healthcare providers should make sure that diabetic patients know about the risk of glaucoma and its symptoms. As the population ages, the prevalence of both cataracts and glaucoma is likely to rise, placing additional demands on healthcare systems to address these interconnected conditions effectively (Al-Namaeh et al., 2022). Taking care of cataracts and glaucoma in diabetic patients is very important since these conditions can strongly influence their daily life and wellbeing. Ocular drug delivery systems have become very important for treating these conditions. There are now technologies that help drugs enter the eye and work for a longer time, making it easier to handle glaucoma and cataract-related issues. They could increase how well patients take their medicines, reduce the number of side effects, and improve their medical results. Besides, it is evident that diabetes, cataracts, and glaucoma are all connected, so a full approach to eye care is important for this group. This integration of innovative treatments and preventive strategies is vital not only for preserving vision but also for enhancing the quality of life for individuals living with diabetic eye disease (Budhori et al., 2021) (Figure 11.5).

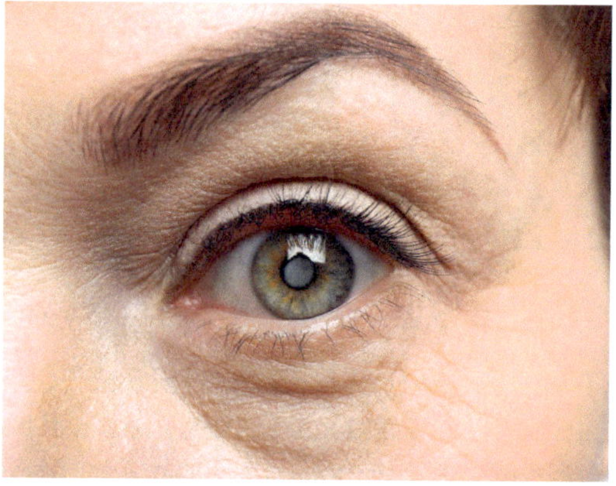

Figure 11.5. Cataracts are a significant complication arising from diabetic eye disease, often contributing to visual impairment among individuals with diabetes.

Source: https://iconeyecare.com/wp-content/uploads/sites/2/2020/11/Cataract-Condition-From-Diabetes.jpg

11.2. Causes and Risk Factors

The main cause of diabetic eye disease, mainly diabetic retinopathy, is chronic hyperglycemia, which damages the blood vessels in the retina. If blood glucose remains high for a long time, it causes many problems, including retinal capillary leakage, which creates microaneurysms and hemorrhages. When the disease worsens, retinal ischemia and neovascularization take place, affecting a person's vision. Besides, diabetic retinopathy usually starts without obvious signs, so diabetic patients need to have regular eye check-ups. Because many things can make this condition more severe, clinicians need to spot these factors in pregnant women and other high-risk patients. As reported, pregnancy can further complicate the management of diabetic retinopathy due to physiological changes that affect metabolic control and vascular health (Błaszczak et al., 2024). Being older is a major risk for diabetic eye disease, which proves that aging and diabetes-related problems are related. It is found that as people grow older, they are more likely to develop diabetic retinopathy due to their long-term diabetes and other health problems. As synthesized from recent studies, both age and diabetes duration consistently correlate with the onset of vision-threatening conditions like diabetic retinopathy (Tong et al., 2022). Moreover, having access to healthcare, the education level, and the way someone lives, such as their diet and exercise, can make risks for diseases even greater. As an example, obesity and lack of exercise increase a person's chances of developing diabetes-related eye problems, which demonstrates that there are many factors involved in the development of diabetic eye disease. Besides watching blood sugar levels, managing diabetic eye disease requires handling other risk factors that can be controlled. Smoking is known to directly cause diabetic retinopathy and also worsen diabetes. In addition, a diet that includes a lot of sugar and little nutrition can make insulin resistance worse and lead to poor glycemic control. Interventions that promote healthy lifestyle choices, such as increased physical activity and balanced nutrition, have shown potential in mitigating diabetes progression and its ocular complications (Tong et al., 2022). Given the shared risk factors between diabetic eye disease and other non-communicable diseases (NCDs), increased awareness and preventive strategies targeting modifiable lifestyles could significantly enhance patient outcomes and reduce the burden of vision impairment associated with diabetes (Figure 11.6).

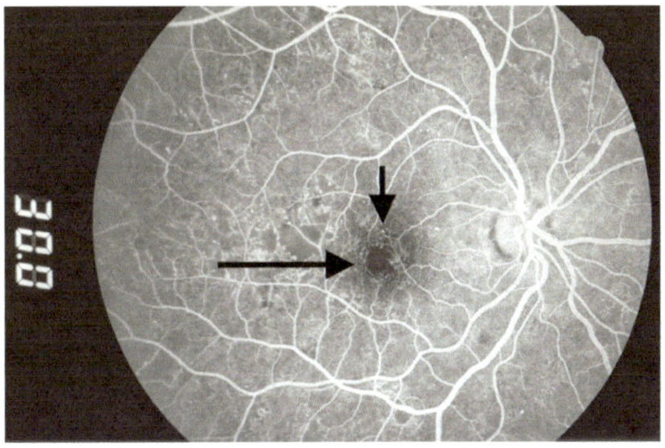

Figure 11.6. Diabetic eye disease, particularly diabetic retinopathy, arises primarily from chronic hyperglycemia, which significantly damages the blood vessels in the retina.

Source: https://www.ncbi.nlm.nih.gov/books/NBK278967/bin/diab-retinopathy-Image002.jpg

11.2.1. High Blood Sugar Levels

The relationship between high blood sugar levels and diabetic eye disease is a critical area of study within diabetes management. Chronic hyperglycemia, or sustained high blood sugar, can lead to significant vascular complications, particularly affecting the eyes. Patients with poorly managed diabetes are at an increased risk for diabetic retinopathy, which involves damage to the blood vessels in the retina. Over time, elevated glucose levels can cause the formation of new, fragile blood vessels that can leak fluid and bleed into the eye, producing vision impairment and, in severe cases, blindness. Given the silent progression of diabetic eye conditions, regular monitoring and management of blood sugar levels become essential to reduce the risk of such outcomes, emphasizing the importance of comprehensive diabetes care strategies. Effective diabetes management strategies often involve technology-enabled programs designed to help individuals maintain healthy blood sugar levels. These programs can range from continuous glucose monitoring systems to mobile applications that assist in tracking dietary habits and medication adherence. A review of various technologies used in diabetes disease management highlights the cost-effectiveness and quality implications of these interventions in the United States (Middleton et al., 2007).

When patients utilize these tools to monitor their blood sugar levels consistently, they may experience a lower incidence of diabetic eye disease. Technology not only facilitates real-time data collection but also enhances communication between patients and healthcare providers, allowing for timely interventions should blood sugar levels become dangerously high. Despite the promising nature of digital interventions, evidence shows mixed results regarding their effectiveness. A randomized study in Uruguay involving an Internet-based intervention for type 2 diabetes patients found no significant improvements in participants' knowledge, behaviors, or health outcomes, indicative of potential barriers to engagement in digital health resources (Balsa and Gandelman, 2025). This highlights that while technology offers innovative routes for managing diabetes, actual patient participation is critical for success. Factors such as demographic characteristics and personal motivation significantly affect engagement levels. Thus, to effectively combat high blood sugar levels and related complications like diabetic eye disease, a multifaceted approach integrating technology, education, and personalized support is vital for achieving better health outcomes (Figure 11.7).

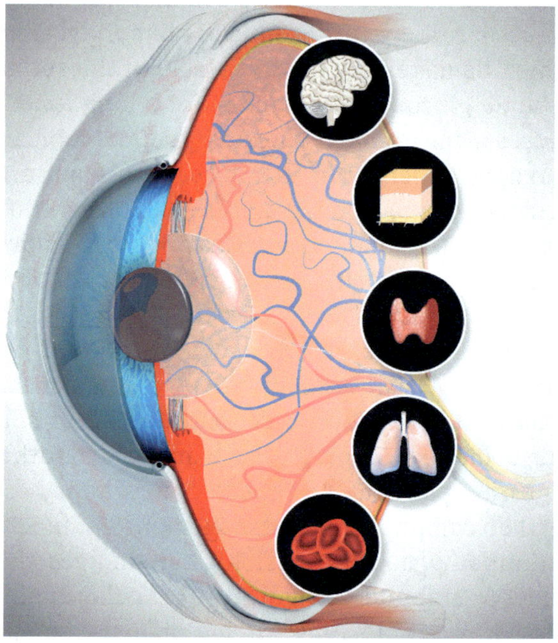

Figure 11.7. Chronic hyperglycemia, or sustained high blood sugar, can lead to significant vascular complications, particularly affecting the eyes.

Source: https://www.reviewofoptometry.com/CMSImagesContent/2022/10/RO/Screen%20Shot%202022-10-10%20at%203.27.28%20PM.png

11.2.2. Duration of Diabetes

The length of time someone has had diabetes matters a lot in the development of several complications, especially diabetic eye disease. If diabetes is not treated for a long time, the eyes of affected people may be damaged, which can result in diabetic retinopathy. It has been found that the chance of diabetic retinopathy rises a lot after five years of having diabetes, and after twenty years, almost all people with poorly managed blood sugar will get it. It shows that acting fast and managing diabetes well can help prevent eye health problems caused by diabetes.

Consequently, understanding the length of diabetes can guide clinicians in identifying patients at higher risk of developing ocular complications and implementing appropriate preventive measures (Morris et al., 2014). It is very important to understand how long someone has had diabetes and how much they follow eye care guidelines for diabetic eye disease. When patients have diabetes for a longer time, the chance of eye problems goes up and some patients may not stick to their eye check-ups. For instance, those with severe diabetic retinopathy tend to demonstrate higher adherence to follow-up eye care compared to patients with milder forms, as evidenced in studies indicating that individuals with visual impairments are more likely to prioritize such visits (Dai et al., 2017). Since their visual problems are often very noticeable, people may feel a strong urge to get medical help. As a result, knowing the length of diabetes helps doctors focus on interventions that improve eye care follow-up, mainly for those who may not pay attention to their eyes due to having few or no symptoms. These studies also point out that diabetes duration and the severity of its complications are closely linked to a person's overall health. As diabetes lasts for a longer period in patients, they are more likely to develop diabetic retinopathy and also deal with the combined effects of other health problems. When glycemic control is poor, patients smoke, or they have a low socioeconomic status, following treatment plans becomes difficult and may lead to vision loss. Many patients with minor forms of the disease are not aware of the importance of routine eye exams, so they often do not follow the treatment plan, which can cause negative results. It becomes clear that to combat the risks associated with extended durations of diabetes and mitigate the prevalence of diabetic eye disease, comprehensive strategies that address both medical and social determinants of health are essential (Dai et al., 2017) (Figure 11.8).

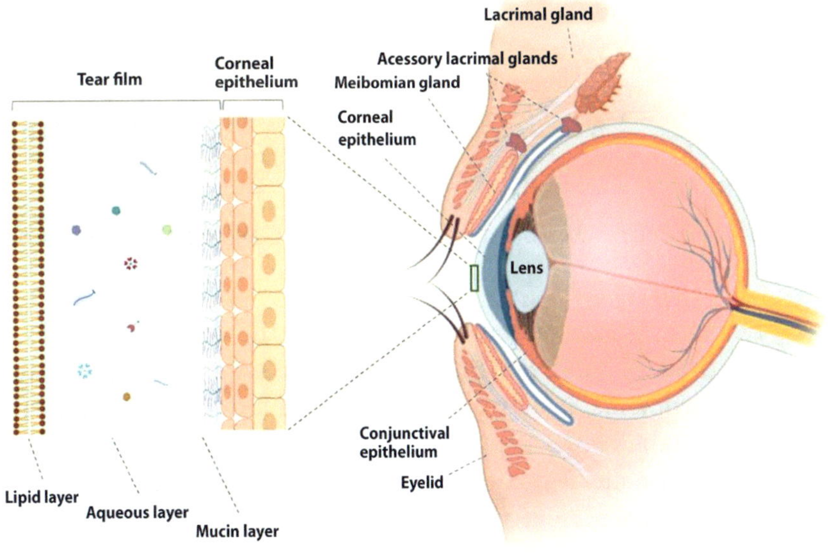

Figure 11.8. As the disease persists over time, the ocular health of individuals with diabetes is increasingly jeopardized, resulting in conditions such as diabetic retinopathy.

Source: Amorim M, Martins B, Fernandes R. Immune Fingerprint in Diabetes: Ocular Surface and Retinal Inflammation. *International Journal of Molecular Sciences*. 2023; 24(12):9821. https://doi.org/10.3390/ijms24129821

11.2.3. Other Health Conditions

When diabetes is linked to other health problems, it makes diabetic eye disease much more severe and dangerous. Having hypertension and heart disease along with diabetes can cause negative results for patients. Because of these two health issues, it becomes harder to treat diabetic patients, which can result in diabetic retinopathy and macular edema. Various studies have shown that older adults and people from the non-Hispanic Black and Hispanic populations are more likely to have complications from diabetes. These trends not only reflect a greater prevalence of diabetes but also highlight the need for targeted healthcare interventions aimed at addressing both diabetes and its associated conditions, which can lead to increased healthcare expenditures and burden on patients, as demonstrated in findings regarding diabetic complications (Kumar et al., 2019).

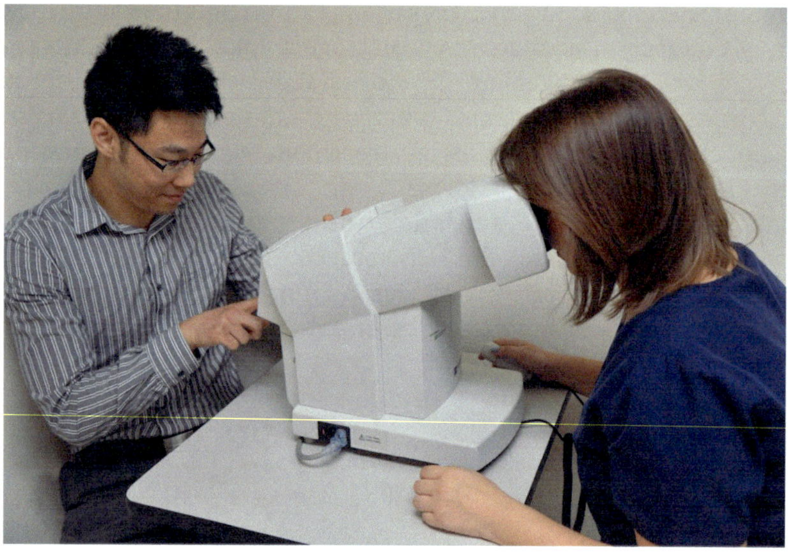

Figure 11.9. Frequency doubling technology (FDT) perimetry.

Source: https://sclerallens.com/wp-content/uploads/2014/09/Zeiss-Frequency-Doubling-Technology.jpg

When diabetic eye disease occurs with other conditions, the cost of care goes up because more health resources are required. It has been found that those with diabetes-related complications, especially eye and kidney problems, have to pay much more for their medical care each year. It is clear from data that having diabetic eye complications leads to a 33% rise in the total amount spent on healthcare each year. This financial strain not only affects individual patients but also places an immense burden on the healthcare system at large, necessitating a reevaluation of resource allocation and intervention strategies (Kumar et al., 2019). It is important to create detailed care plans that deal with eye problems in diabetes as well as other common diseases, all while keeping costs in mind. Moreover, early detection of eye diseases in diabetics is still very important for lowering the risks linked to these health problems. Conducting a variety of easy-to-use screening tests helps find and treat diabetic retinopathy early, which is vital for saving vision. A recent study suggests that employing structured screening methodologies, such as frequency doubling technology (FDT) perimetry and optical coherence tomography, can substantially improve diagnostic accuracy among elderly populations at risk for sight-threatening eye conditions. These actions may lessen the number of advanced diabetic eye diseases, proving the need for active management and regular assessment of people with diabetes, along with other health problems. If healthcare providers focus on early diagnosis and linking care, they can handle both the eye and overall health problems linked to diabetes (Figure 11.9).

11.3. Symptoms and Diagnosis

How diabetic eye disease appears can be very different from person to person, mostly based on the disease's stage. Sometimes, the first signs are very mild and people often attribute them to being tired or old. As the condition worsens, people may notice more floaters, dark spots in their eyes, and may eventually lose a lot of their vision. Since many people do not realize these symptoms at first, diabetic patients need to have regular screenings. Early detection through meticulous monitoring can facilitate timely intervention. That is why it is vital for people at risk to be aware of the possible symptoms, so they can get help before their condition becomes untreatable. Most cases of diabetic eye disease start with a complete eye examination done by an ophthalmologist or optometrist. During the examination, doctors may use visual acuity tests to check a person's ability to see at various distances. Additionally, advanced imaging techniques such as optical coherence tomography (OCT) or fluorescein angiography are frequently employed to visualize the retina in greater detail. Such methodologies help experts find out if a person has diabetic retinopathy and what complications may be present, such as macular edema or retinal detachment. Also, the use of tear fluid investigations is becoming more common as a new way to diagnose diseases. By examining the proteomic and lipidomic composition of tear fluid, researchers are uncovering potential biomarkers that could revolutionize diagnostic precision in diabetic eye disease, thus underscoring developments in diagnostic technology (Acera et al., 2016). When a disease is diagnosed promptly, it becomes easier to develop the best treatment plan. For example, recent studies have demonstrated that early intervention through treatments like intravitreal dexamethasone implants can yield significant improvements in visual outcomes for patients with central retinal vein occlusion or branch retinal vein occlusion, conditions often associated with diabetic eye disease (Autolitano et al., 2017). Although the therapy worked the same for both early and late starts, the study results showed that early diagnosis is important to achieve the best results and prevent serious problems like losing sight. For this reason, clinicians should pay close attention to monitoring and diagnosing diabetic eye disease so patients can get proper treatment as soon as possible (Figure 11.10).

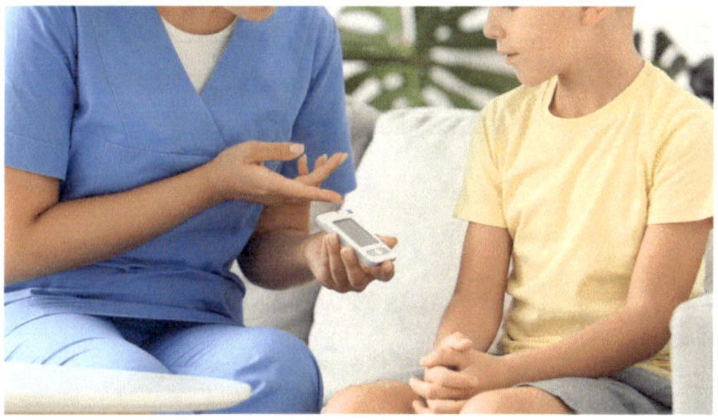

Figure 11.10. The lack of initial awareness surrounding symptoms underscores the necessity for regular screenings among diabetic patients.

Source: https://www.circufiber.com/cdn/shop/articles/Circufiber_Understanding_Diabetes_in_Children_and_Teens.png?v=1708714648

11.3.1. Early Symptoms of Diabetic Eye Disease

The early symptoms of diabetic eye disease, particularly Diabetic Retinopathy (DR), often manifest without noticeable discomfort for the patient, leading to delayed recognition and diagnosis. As the condition gets worse, people may notice that their vision is blurry, which could be the first sign that requires further examination. Such changes may not be noticed until the disease has advanced a lot. Consequently, patients with diabetes should engage in regular eye examinations, as the standard recommendation suggests annual dilated fundus examinations (DFEs) to monitor any retinal changes. Early detection is crucial because, according to research, patients with symptoms or visual impairment are more likely to follow through with timely DFEs, emphasizing the importance of recognizing these symptoms early in a patient's experience with diabetes (Dai et al., 2017). Unfortunately, most people do not know about the risk of DR until it affects their eyesight. In the early stages, people with DR may not feel the need to see a doctor since the condition is usually symptomless. With these new techniques, clinicians can spot the effects of high blood glucose before they cause any symptoms, which allows them to use interventions that could stop the disease from getting worse. This situation points out that many patients are not informed enough about diabetic eye disease and the need to manage their diabetes actively. Encouraging glycemic control and regular eye exams not only aids in symptom recognition but also enhances long-term health outcomes for those at risk of diabetic complications, reinforcing the necessity for early detection tools (Martin et al., 2025). Furthermore, following eye care advice is very important for handling the first signs of diabetic eye disease. People with more serious eye diseases are more likely to follow up on their care, probably because they start to notice their symptoms and realize how important it is to take care of their eyes. The data also reveals that demographic factors, such as smoking status and socioeconomic conditions, significantly impact adherence rates, suggesting that those with modifiable health behaviors are more likely to prioritize their vision health (Dai et al., 2017). Realizing these points encourages healthcare providers to treat the disease and the factors that may impact how patients deal with it. When patients are educated well and supported in the right way, practitioners can help them stick to their treatment and reduce the risks of diabetic eye disease (Figure 11.11).

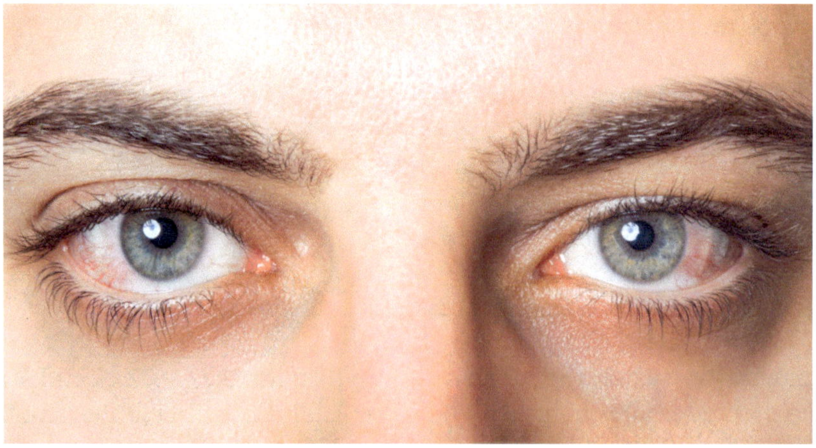

Figure 11.11. The early symptoms of diabetic eye disease, particularly Diabetic Retinopathy (DR), often manifest without noticeable discomfort for the patient, leading to delayed recognition and diagnosis.

Source: https://irp.cdn-website.com/77106691/dms3rep/multi/Urban_Optiks_Optometry_San-Diego-bloodshot+eyes.png

11.3.2. Diagnostic Tests and Procedures

Eye specialists depend on timely and correct diagnoses, which are made possible by using various tests and procedures. Teleretinal screening has become very important, especially in places where getting complete eye care is not always possible. Using advanced imaging tools, this method finds early signs of diabetic retinopathy, so healthcare providers can refer patients for more tests when necessary. A review of the program showed that the initial teleretinal referrals were in line with the final ophthalmic diagnoses, which proves how important such initiatives are in spotting sight-threatening conditions early. Additionally, with a reported mean cost of around $1000 per patient per year, it is evident that these screenings not only enhance patient outcomes but also necessitate careful resource planning in ophthalmic settings (Kroenke, 2015). Advanced optical non-invasive methods have added more value to the care of patients with diabetic eye disease. Using laser Doppler flowmetry and fluorescence spectroscopy can give more precise information about microcirculatory problems that are important for managing diabetic patients. They have been found to be effective in both rheumatology and endocrinology, mainly for problems linked to diabetes mellitus.

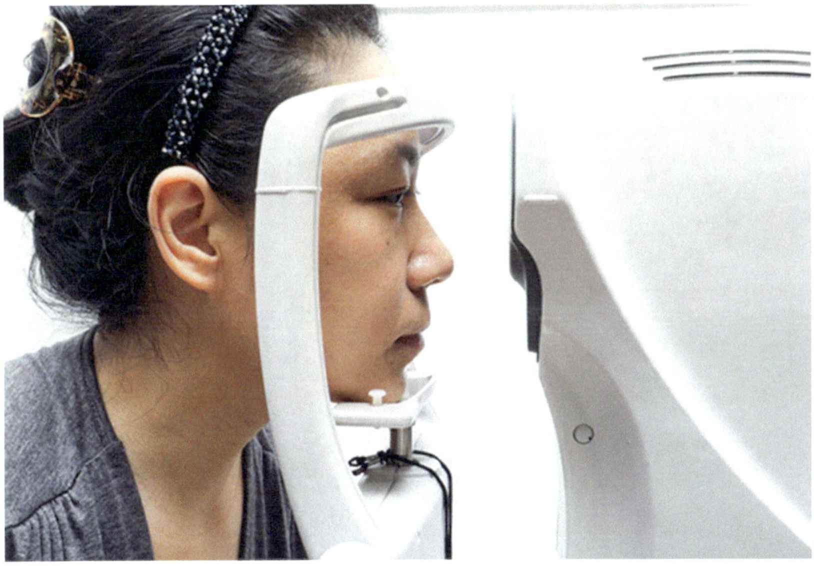

Figure 11.12. Teleretinal screening has emerged as a significant method in this regard, particularly in community settings where access to comprehensive eye care may be limited.

Source: https://clf1.medpagetoday.com/assets/images/resource-center/cs-future-telerential-imaging-60892.jpg

By using both functional tests and optical diagnostics, it is possible to learn a lot about the severity of microcirculatory disorders that are often missed but key for proper patient care. The sensitivity and specificity of these diagnostic procedures have established their value in clinical settings, allowing for earlier interventions that may prevent the progression of diabetic complications (Dremin et al., 2019). Using different diagnostic techniques is important not only for finding diabetic eye diseases but also for handling all aspects of diabetes care. Anyone with diabetes should get regular eye exams, detailed eye tests, and advanced eye scans because they are more likely to face eye problems. When teleretinal screenings are added to regular care, they help catch health problems early and show patients how important it is to stay involved in their health. With the use of these new techniques in healthcare, patients with diabetic eye disease can experience much better results. As a result, using these technologies and related infrastructure could help a lot in reducing the effects of vision loss caused by diabetes among the general population (Figure 11.12).

11.3.3. Importance of Regular Eye Examinations

Regular check-ups for the eyes are necessary for people with diabetes, mainly because they are more likely to develop diabetic eye diseases. These tests make it possible to discover conditions such as diabetic retinopathy, which, if not treated, may result in serious vision loss eventually. It has been found that getting eye care on time can help prevent or control these outcomes. For instance, a study noted that 78% of individuals with diabetes who were regularly examined followed established guidelines, demonstrating the improvement in disease management through routine check-ups (Muller et al., 2008).

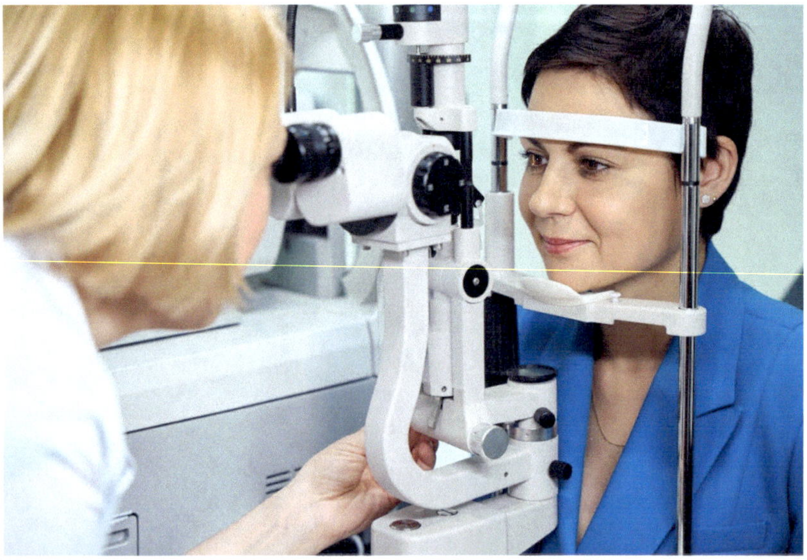

Figure 11.13. Regular eye examinations are pivotal for individuals with diabetes, primarily due to the increased risk of diabetic eye diseases.

Source: https://www.eyecareofdelaware.com/wp-content/uploads/2023/11/annual-eye-exam-diabetic-neuropathy.jpg

Evidence shows that people with diabetes for a longer time are more likely to have regular eye exams, indicating that regular care is necessary as diabetes worsens. The level of diabetic retinopathy and whether someone has vision problems are important reasons why patients may or may not keep up with eye care follow-up. Those diagnosed with moderate to severe retinopathy are more likely to comply with scheduled follow-ups, perhaps due to symptomatic experiences prompting greater awareness of their ocular health (Dai et al., 2017). Also, the study points out that controlling blood glucose levels is vital not only for the patient's overall health but also for their eye health. Because of this link, doctors advise that eye exams should be part of a diabetes patient's regular care. In addition, having regular eye exams is important because most patients say they learn about the dangers of vision loss linked to diabetes. When healthcare providers inform people about eye health, it leads them to take care of their eyes, which is very important for avoiding serious problems. In the aforementioned study, an impressive 87% of respondents acknowledged having received information about the importance of eye examinations, which correlates with their examination patterns (Muller et al., 2008). Hence, regular visits to healthcare providers help patients find out about their existing eye conditions and also learn how important it is to take preventive measures for their vision when dealing with chronic health issues (Figure 11.13).

11.4. Treatment Options

Treatment for diabetic eye disease includes different methods aimed at reducing the problems related to the condition. Since early detection of diabetic retinopathy can greatly affect the outcome, everyone should have their eyes checked regularly. When microaneurysms or hemorrhages are noticed, clinicians might advise patients to follow a monitoring plan or have laser photocoagulation to help prevent vision loss. Also, explaining to patients the value of regular check-ups encourages them to follow the right treatment steps.

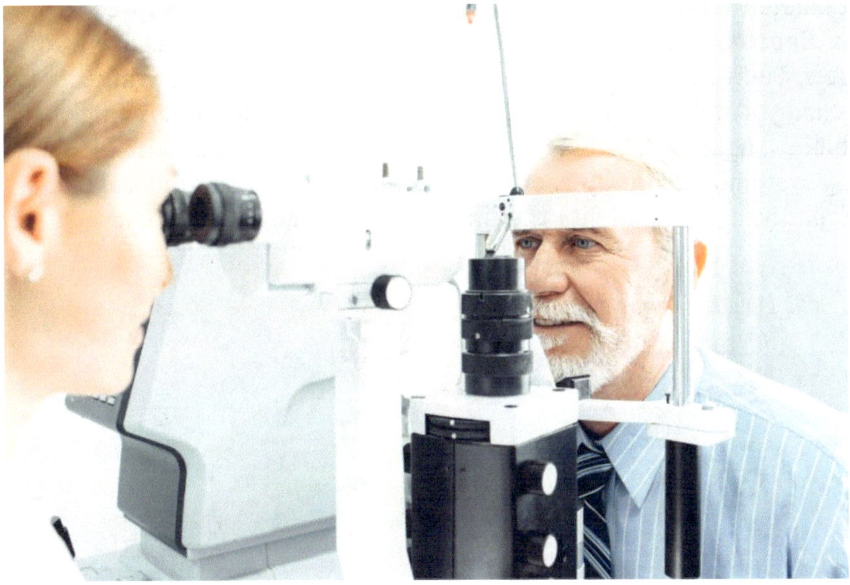

Figure 11.14. Regular monitoring through comprehensive eye examinations is fundamental, as early detection of conditions like diabetic retinopathy can significantly alter outcomes.

Source: https://www.retinaconsultantsofamerica.com/media/pages/blog/why-the-retina-matters-in-comprehensive-eye-exams/6e58c39ca7-1743384818/rca-rctx-why-retina-matters.webp

Novel technologies for diabetes management also play a crucial role in enhancing patient awareness and engagement, thereby contributing to improved overall outcomes in diabetic eye disease management (Middleton et al., 2007). When regular monitoring does not stop vision loss, it is important to use advanced treatment methods. Anti-VEGF (vascular endothelial growth factor) therapy represents a significant advancement in the pharmacological management of diabetic macular edema. They are designed to stop unusual blood vessel growth and reduce fluid leaking, which helps improve patients' vision in diabetic eye disease. Sometimes, vitrectomy is used to manage serious complications like vitreous hemorrhage. Treatment choices for diabetes are best made with the input of endocrinologists, ophthalmologists, and diabetes education specialists, so patients get the best results and face fewer issues from treatment. With the advancement of technology, the role it plays in managing diabetic eye disease is more noticeable. With digital tools, healthcare providers can offer quick care to patients who live in rural or underserved regions. By using these models, patients are more involved and healthcare providers can easily communicate, which encourages everyone to cooperate in managing diseases. Emerging research highlights the efficacy and cost-effectiveness of technology-enabled diabetes management programs, underscoring their potential to improve adherence to treatment protocols, thereby reducing the economic burden associated with diabetic eye disease (Middleton et al., 2007). The use of these new approaches will play a key role in developing future treatments and guaranteeing that patients maintain their sight (Figure 11.14).

11.4.1. Medical Management and Medications

Taking care of diabetes with proper treatment and medicine can help control the risks linked to eye disease in diabetes. If left untreated, diabetic retinopathy can cause a lot of vision loss in those with diabetes. Tight control of blood sugar is the main approach, which is usually reached by making lifestyle changes and using medications. Taking insulin and oral hypoglycemics is important for controlling blood sugar, which plays a big role in the development of diabetic eye disease. Properly handling systemic health by checking and altering medications regularly is important for preventing retinopathy, as it highlights the link between diabetes and eye health.

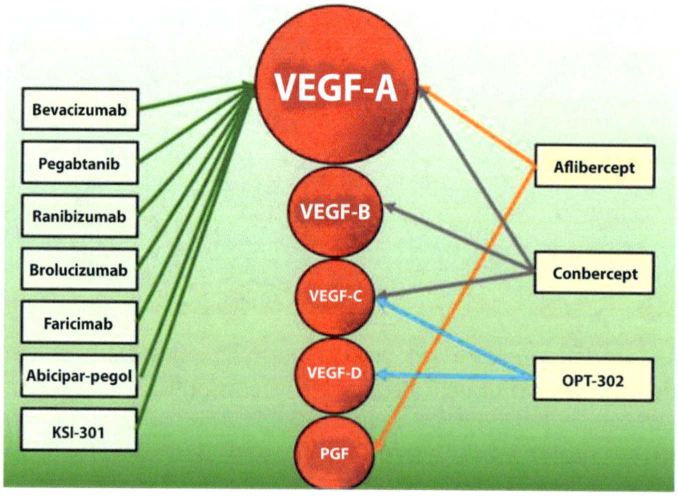

Figure 11.15. The use of anti-VEGF (vascular endothelial growth factor) drugs has revolutionized the treatment landscape for diabetic macular edema, a severe manifestation of diabetic eye disease.

Source: https://www.tandfonline.com/cms/asset/8b137a19-ceba-47c1-afb8-e030bac71030/iann_a_2064541_f0002_c.jpg

As well as controlling their glucose, patients with diabetes should have regular eye examinations. As a result, these tests can find diabetic retinopathy and other eye problems early, so treatment can start right away. The use of anti-VEGF (vascular endothelial growth factor) drugs has revolutionized the treatment landscape for diabetic macular edema, a severe manifestation of diabetic eye disease. They stop the unusual blood vessel growth seen in the condition, so patients can keep their vision and enjoy a better life. When advanced treatments are combined with information and lessons on self-management and regular eye exams, patients are more involved in their health. Furthermore, if people do not have equal access to healthcare, it can be difficult to manage diabetes and the problems it causes, for example, diabetic eye disease. It has been found through studies that people's income and ethnicity are often linked to differences in diabetes treatment and outcomes. Diamant et al. (2003) emphasize the importance of addressing these disparities to improve healthcare access and outcomes for at-risk populations. If patients know the importance of regular eye checks and medical care, they can better control diabetic eye disease. In this regard, making medications and preventive care more available to people with diabetes can help lower the number of vision problems, which improves public health and the quality of life for patients (Figure 11.15).

11.4.2. Surgical Interventions

Surgery is a key approach in managing diabetic eye disease, especially when conditions such as diabetic retinopathy and diabetic macular edema get worse. For many years, laser photocoagulation has been the main method doctors use to treat these problems and protect vision. Yet, newer methods such as vitrectomy give patients with major vision loss due to vitreous hemorrhage or retinal detachment extra treatment choices. By following these steps, surgeons can take out the cloudy vitreous gel and fix retinal detachments, which raises the chances of restoring vision. With new findings and clinical results, it is now obvious that surgery should be designed for each patient, considering how much diabetes has affected them and their general health. Surgical procedures are especially important to note when examining how bariatric surgery affects the outcomes of diabetic eye disease. Although bariatric surgery is mainly used for weight loss, it has been found to help people with type 2 diabetes and the complications that come with it, such as diabetic retinopathy. It is found that while some patients' diabetic retinopathy does not get worse after surgery, there is still a possibility of it getting worse or new cases appearing. Therefore, people who have bariatric surgery and advanced diabetic eye disease should be carefully watched and followed up. Learning about the overall results of these surgeries can give useful ideas for treating obesity and its eye-related consequences, thus improving the lives and care of these patients. Also, new surgical approaches have made it possible to address the problems related to diabetic eye disease. As an example, eye drops that contain nerve growth factor are being developed to promote better healing of the cornea. Such therapies are used for neurotrophic keratitis, a problem where the cornea loses sensitivity and can be worsened in diabetics. Using these methods, the corneal nerves are stimulated and the healing process is promoted, which benefits vision and lowers the risk of corneal ulceration. Therefore, integrating these novel surgical interventions into the management of diabetic eye disease can significantly improve patient outcomes, demonstrating the importance of evolving therapeutic strategies in response to the unique challenges posed by this complex condition (Docherty et al., 2016; Sacchetti & Lambiase, 2017) (Figure 11.16).

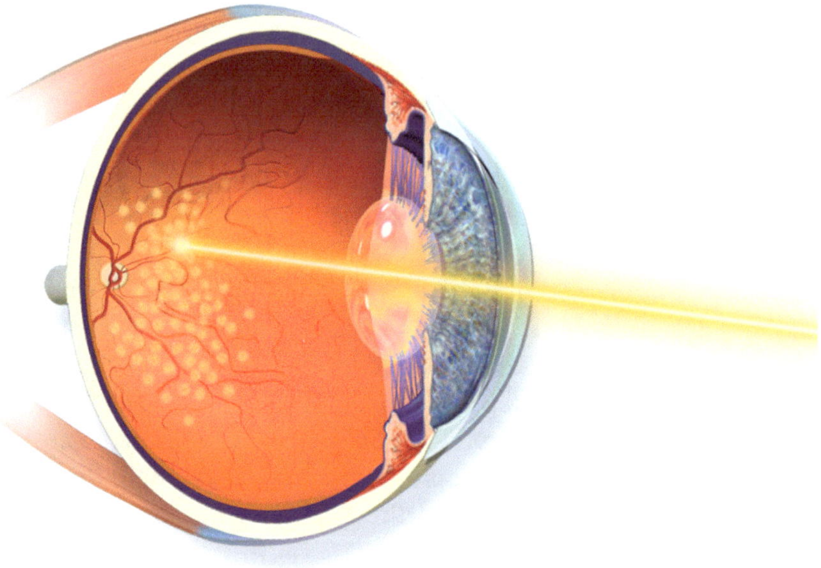

Figure 11.16. Traditional approaches, including laser photocoagulation, have long been the standard for treating these complications, aimed at preserving vision and preventing further retinal damage.

Source: https://www.texasretina.com/wp-content/uploads/2019/06/Screen-Shot-2019-06-25-at-1.11.32-PM-1200x792.png

11.4.3. Lifestyle Modifications

Changing your lifestyle is very important for controlling diabetes and avoiding diabetic eye disease, which often occurs in people with high blood sugar for a long time. Eating a healthy diet with plenty of nutrients can help control blood sugar, which reduces the chances of eye problems. A diet that includes whole grains, lean proteins, and different kinds of fruits and vegetables is good for your health. Also, it is important to cut down on processed sugars and unhealthy fats, as they may cause problems with metabolism. Keeping an eye on what patients with diabetes eat helps them control their blood sugar and decide on nutritious meals that are important for their health and vision. Taking part in regular exercise is another important change that helps with diabetes and reduces the risks of diabetic eye disease. Doing moderate activities such as walking, swimming, or cycling improves how your body uses insulin and assists in losing weight. Exercise regularly may help to lower blood sugar, which reduces the risk of developing diabetic retinopathy. Exercise is also helpful for diabetes patients since it can improve their heart health, which is important since they are more likely to develop heart problems. Doing regular exercise not only helps control diabetes but also protects the eyesight of individuals in the future. Psychosocial factors are important in helping people change their lifestyle to manage diabetes well. Problems such as anxiety and depression in a person's mental health can make it difficult for them to follow diet and exercise plans, which can lead to more eye diseases in diabetics. Assistance from doctors and community groups can motivate patients to follow their treatment plans and make better choices. Moreover, addressing barriers like low socioeconomic status is crucial, as those with inadequate access to quality care may struggle more with self-management of their diabetes (Goode et al.,

2018). Paying attention to both physical and mental health will help people prevent diabetic eye disease by making lasting changes in their lifestyles (Figure 11.17).

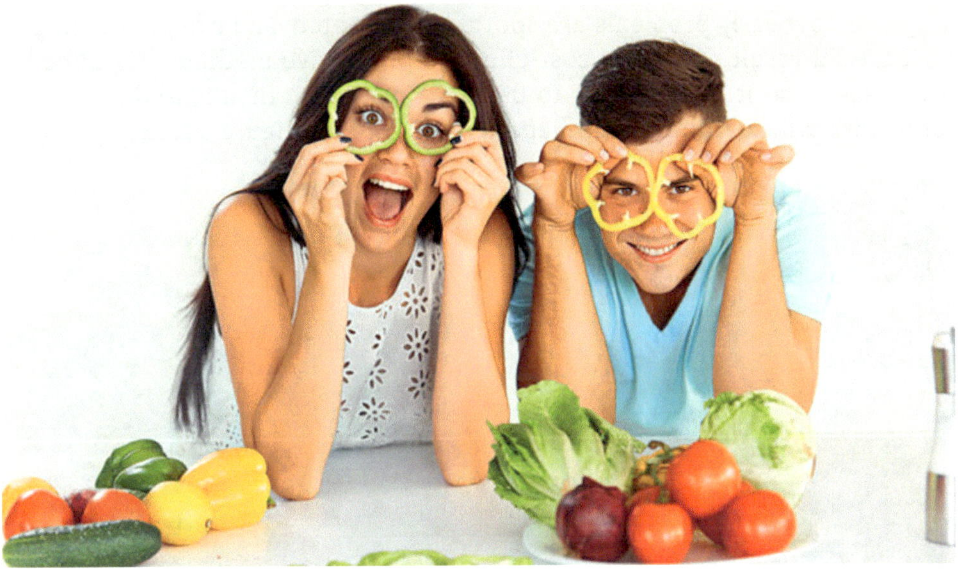

Figure 11.17. Adopting a balanced diet rich in nutrients can effectively regulate blood glucose levels, thereby minimizing the risk of eye damage.

Source: https://i0.wp.com/drvaidyaeyehospital.com/wp-content/uploads/2022/12/role-of-nutrition-in-maintaining-healthy-eyesight.jpg?fit=700%2C400&ssl=1

11.5. Impact on Quality of Life

It is important to look at how diabetic eye disease affects a person's quality of life to understand the disease better. Because of diabetes, diabetic retinopathy can cause major problems with vision and, in the worst cases, lead to blindness. Losing vision can have a major impact on a person's mental and social well-being, since it makes it hard for them to read, drive, and carry out their jobs. Such changes mean individuals have less ability to do things by themselves and need help from caregivers, which can result in them feeling even more isolated and helpless. The results are seen in the family and community as well, because the quality of life goes down for patients and those who care for them, leading to changes in daily life and emotions. There is strong proof that diabetic eye disease negatively affects a person's quality of life. Studies reveal that people with pre-symptomatic diabetic retinopathy have a lower quality of life than those who do not have the disease. Specifically, a study showed that EQ-5D-5L index values averaged 0.733 for those with pre-symptomatic conditions, compared to 0.787 for individuals free from such disease (Sampson et al., 2020). This decrease points out that diabetic eye disease can have a big impact, since even the first signs can reduce a person's well-being. It is also shown by a meta-analysis that health state utility values decrease among people with diabetic eye disease, proving that their quality of life suffers even at early stages. It is necessary to look at healthcare strategies, especially screening, to handle the effects of diabetic eye disease on people's lives. Risk-based screening can be a useful method for dealing with the negative effects of diabetic eye disease. By tailoring screening initiatives according to individual risk factors, healthcare systems can prioritize interventions for those at the highest likelihood of disease progression, as outlined in recent evaluations of health-related quality of life associated with diabetic retinopathy (Sampson et al., 2020). Taking these actions can improve how early problems are spotted and treated, and can greatly improve the lives of those involved. As a result, including cost-effective preventive methods in public health efforts may help society more, so it is necessary to use a strategy that highlights health economics and patient-centered care when dealing with diabetic eye disease (Figure 11.18).

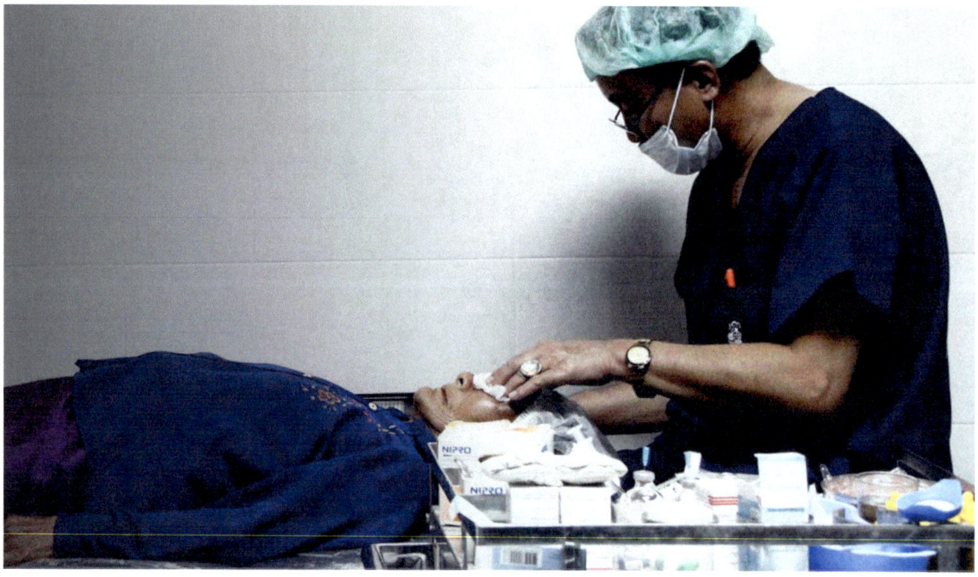

Figure 11.18. Diabetic retinopathy, a prevalent complication of diabetes, can result in substantial visual impairment and, in severe cases, blindness.

Source: https://www.hollows.org/siteassets/shared-media/au/images/laos-operation_her-banner_diabetic-retinopathy_1920x1080px.png

11.5.1. Visual Impairment and Daily Activities

Visual impairment due to diabetic eye disease has a major impact on a person's daily activities. With the progression of the condition, patients may find that their vision is not clear enough to do regular tasks. It might involve problems with reading and doing household tasks, as well as moving around public areas. A decline in vision often leads to more difficulties in everyday tasks, so it is closely tied to losing some functions. Therefore, people may end up depending more on others, which can make them feel isolated and irritated, lowering their quality of life. It proves that both the eye problems and the emotions of people with diabetes should be handled with effective interventions. A lot of older adults with vision problems are more likely to feel depressed and have mobility issues, which makes it harder for them to handle daily chores. In a study examining the relationship between dementia and age-related vision disorders, it was found that individuals displaying both cognitive decline and visual impairment were more likely to struggle with fundamental tasks of daily living than those without such impairments (Caminiti et al., 2014). It means that visual impairment can cause daily difficulties and may also bring about more significant cognitive challenges for seniors. Taking care of these two issues points out that comprehensive care should focus on helping vision and mental health, which is important for people with diabetic eye disease to keep their independence and improve their quality of life. Besides, the common fear of falling among elderly adults with visual impairment affects their movement and ability to function well. Challenges in visual perception can lead to a heightened "fear of falling" (FOF), which in turn can inhibit mobility performance and instigate avoidance behaviors (Andrew et al., 2017). Because of this avoidance, people may stop taking part in activities they once enjoyed, which only adds to their isolation and makes them less active. When people cannot see well, the danger of falling increases and their physical health also declines over the years. It is therefore necessary to focus on visual impairment in diabetic eye disease, since it can change both the physical and emotional aspects of a person's life. This way of working helps people become stronger and continue to do things on their own (Figure 11.19).

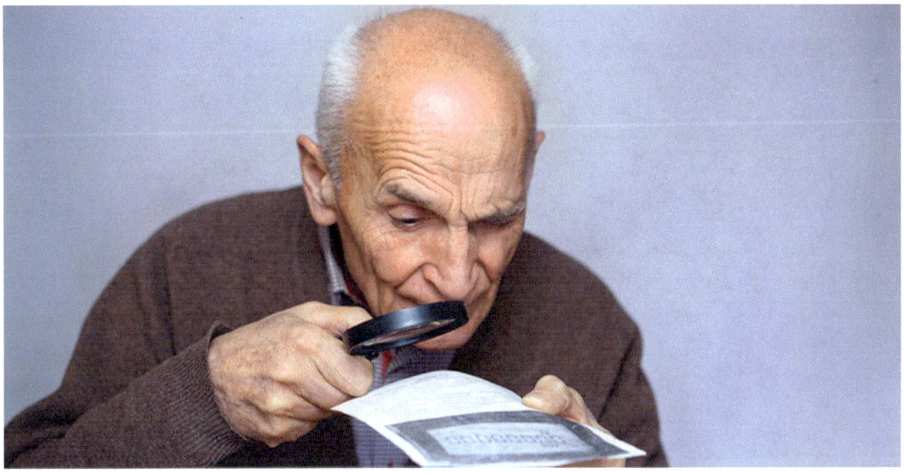

Figure 11.19. The impact of visual impairment on daily activities is profoundly significant, particularly in individuals suffering from diabetic eye disease.

Source: https://www.aoa.org/AOA/Images/Patients/Low-vision-senior.jpg

11.5.2. Psychological Effects of Vision Loss

Vision loss caused by diabetic eye disease can greatly affect a person's mental health in many ways. Those with vision impairment are likely to feel more anxious and depressed, which may negatively affect their everyday lives. When diabetic retinopathy starts, people may slowly notice the risk of blindness, which can cause them to feel emotional distress. It has been found that people with visual impairment often experience less mental health, social life, and happiness than others. As vision deteriorates, many individuals may struggle with feelings of helplessness and despair due to an inability to perform routine tasks, exacerbating their psychological challenges (Casten et al., 2019). Since poor mental health and declining vision often go together in diabetic eye disease, it is important to treat both conditions together to help patients. Besides, the combination of cultural and financial factors has a major impact on the mental reactions of diabetic patients to vision loss. If someone from a minority group does not trust the medical system, it may stop them from getting the care they need and add to their mental pressure. Research has revealed that African American patients with diabetic retinopathy exhibit higher levels of treatment mistrust, which consequently affects their glycemic control and overall health (Casten et al., 2019). Because of these gaps, it is important to provide interventions that are culturally sensitive and help both the physical and mental health of patients by encouraging trust between them and their caregivers. If healthcare systems identify and deal with these psychosocial factors, they can greatly improve the outcomes for patients. Improving the mental and social health of people with vision loss through interventions is very important. A systematic review indicated that various strategies, including counseling, peer support, and tailored employment programs, can effectively enhance mental health outcomes for those grappling with visual impairment (Gosney et al., 2009). Strong support allows patients to handle their condition better and deal with the mental effects of losing their sight. Having psychological support in addition to medical care can help patients with diabetic eye disease live better and healthier lives. Focusing on mental health and eye care at the same time shows a complete approach to patient health, pointing out the importance of managing the emotional effects of vision loss (Figure 11.20).

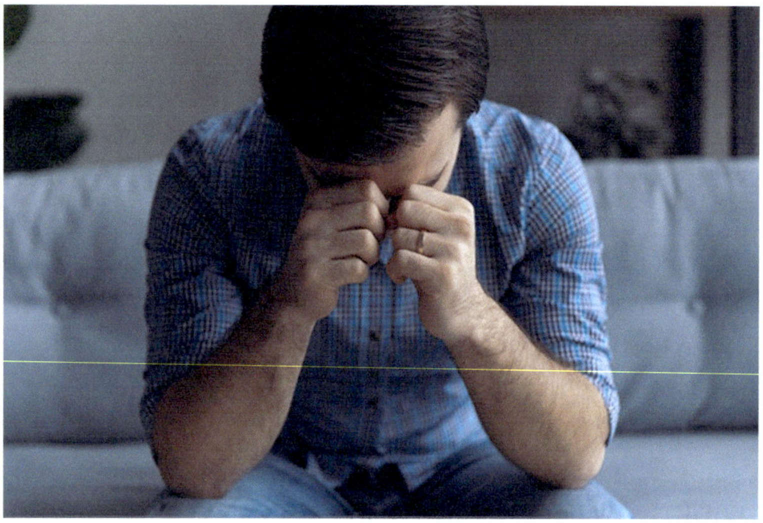

Figure 11.20. Individuals facing vision impairment often experience increased levels of anxiety and depression, which can significantly impact their quality of life.

Source: https://media.allaboutvision.com/cms/caas/v1/media/414114/data/picture/dd4b81c072a65d4831f8d498c9300f40.gif

11.5.3. Economic Burden of Diabetic Eye Disease

The costs of diabetic eye disease are an urgent issue because they go beyond the expenses for treatment and management. As more people develop diabetes worldwide, the number of related issues, such as diabetic retinopathy and macular edema, also increases, which places more demands on healthcare systems. The costs involved can have major effects on both patients and their families and communities. Since diabetes can cause blindness and low vision, the healthcare system must spend a lot on surgery, medicine, and managing the condition for life. These economic factors become even more critical when considering the impact on workforce productivity as individuals unable to work lose their income, thus further complicating their economic stability and healthcare access, highlighting the urgent need for comprehensive preventive measures and early intervention strategies (Pandova et al., 2019). Besides, the way a person's economic and cultural contexts interact is very important for accessing treatment for diabetic eye diseases. Because of differences in healthcare access, people in various economies may not get proper treatment for eye diseases in time. In some regions where people have low incomes, important screening tools and prompt clinics for intervention are often not available. The findings of a study involving elderly populations indicated that specific screening tests can identify sight-threatening diseases with reasonable accuracy, yet such testing is seldom uniformly available, especially in economically disadvantaged areas (Ctori et al., 2019). As a result of this inequality, more people become blind, and healthcare systems must handle more expenses, so it is important to improve healthcare models and make sure every group is well served. The effects of diabetic eye disease on the economy are felt by society as a whole. When more people are unable to see well, society pays for lost work and the need for additional social support. Taking care of an affected person often puts a strain on families, using up their money and changing the way they interact. In addition, if no proper preventive steps and community support are in place, the number of diabetic eye disease cases will only make the situation worse. Making sure that people can afford medicines, screening, and treatment is very important for reducing the increasing costs. The economic landscape concerning diabetic eye disease demonstrates the necessity for multi-faceted approaches that encompass preventative healthcare, patient education, and community outreach to ultimately alleviate the financial strain on both individuals and society as a whole (Pandova et al., 2019) (Figure 11.21).

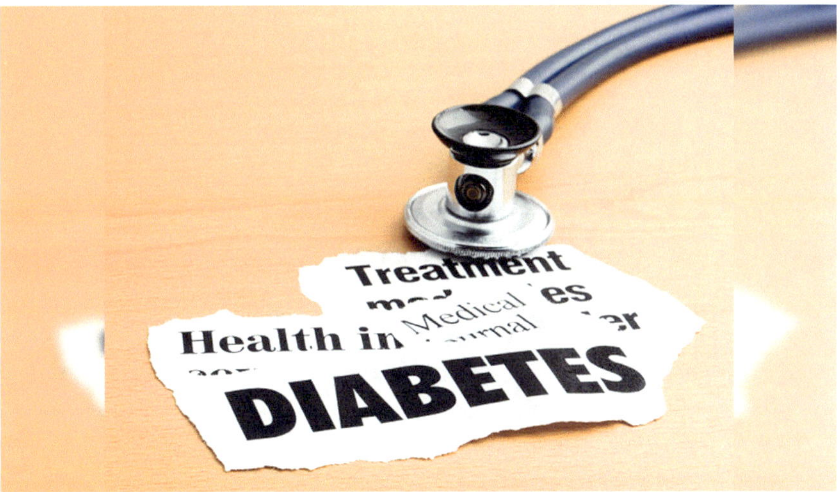

Figure 11.21. The economic burden of diabetic eye disease is a pressing concern that extends beyond the direct costs associated with treatment and management.

Source: https://img.etimg.com/thumb/width-1600,height-900,imgsize-230710,resizemode-75,msid-58120127/magazines/panache/are-you-a-diabetes-patient-who-is-often-behind-the-wheel-know-the-sugar-rules-for-safety.jpg

A CLOSER LOOK

HYPERLIPIDEMIA

Hyperlipidemia happens when there are high levels of cholesterol and triglycerides in the blood. A high intake of these fats may increase your chances of getting cardiovascular diseases such as atherosclerosis, heart attacks, and strokes. Hyperlipidemia can result from genetics, a poor diet, being overweight, not being active, or medical problems such as diabetes. Most of the time, management requires changes in lifestyle, such as eating right, exercising, and using statins to help lower the risk of heart disease.

Summary

To summarize, diabetic eye disease is a major and complicated issue in healthcare today, so it is important to know its causes and how to treat it. Diabetic retinopathy and other eye problems in diabetics are mainly caused by chronic hyperglycemia. Knowing about oxidative stress and inflammation has been very important for creating specific treatments. For instance, the role of coenzyme Q10 (CoQ10) as a potent antioxidant highlights the significance of managing oxidative stress to mitigate retinal damage associated with diabetic eye disease. The potential of CoQ10 supplementation to slow the progression of retinal degeneration underscores the need for further investigations into its therapeutic applications in managing ocular complications related to diabetes (Marcheggiani et al., 2017). Also, recent research has proven that early treatment for retinal vein occlusion can change the course of the disease for patients. Patients who get intravitreal dexamethasone injections, no matter when they receive them, tend to improve their visual acuity. Still, the way each retinal disease responds to treatment can vary a lot, so it is important for doctors to manage each patient differently. Clinicians must remain vigilant in diagnosing diabetic eye disease early and employing appropriate treatment regimens to mitigate the risk of vision loss, emphasizing the continual necessity for education and awareness within the healthcare community (Autolitano et al., 2017). It is important to use more than just medicines to manage diabetic eye disease; patients also need to be educated, change their lifestyle, and see the eye doctor regularly. Since diabetes is becoming more common around the world, the growing problem of diabetic eye disease stresses the importance of preventive care in healthcare. When eye problems are found and treated early, it can improve a patient's life and lower the chance of serious eye problems. Future research should focus on novel therapeutic modalities, including the potential of antioxidant supplementation like CoQ10 and the exploration of innovative treatment protocols to enhance patient outcomes while minimizing the overarching impact of this debilitating condition (Marcheggiani et al., 2017).

Various important points make it clear that diabetic eye disease is both complex and affects people in many ways. There is a key concern about the mechanisms that result in diabetic retinopathy, a serious problem for people with diabetes. The cause of this condition is damage to the retina's blood vessels from high blood sugar, which leads to both non-proliferative and proliferative stages. The development of diabetic retinopathy shows why it is crucial to detect the disease early and manage its symptoms, as well as use reliable screening methods. Having regular eye exams helps to prevent serious problems, such as vision loss, which can negatively affect a patient's life. This research proves that it is important to watch and treat this condition so that healthcare providers can prevent it. In addition to prevention, knowing how diabetic eye disease affects the broader healthcare system is very important. It seems that problems related to diabetic eye disease are made worse by socioeconomic factors, mainly for minority and underprivileged groups. Such differences could be caused by difficulties in getting healthcare, not having enough knowledge about diabetes, and certain cultural beliefs about it. Also, the fact that diabetes-related complications are more common among those with lower socioeconomic status shows that healthcare approaches should be customized. A solution to these problems should include good communication, culturally appropriate care, and evenly sharing resources to manage diabetic eye disease in all populations. The goal of this approach is to boost public health and reduce the health inequalities that mainly affect those who are vulnerable. The recent progress in medical research should be considered when it comes to diabetic eye disease. For example, exploring new treatments, gene therapy and improved drug delivery, may help reduce vision loss in diabetic retinopathy. New studies may find interventions that help patients and save more retinal cells. The combined work of researchers and clinicians on understanding the causes and possible treatments of diabetic eye disease is very important in dealing with this serious problem. Investing in research and using good screening methods will play a key role in improving treatment and lessening the effects of this condition on everyone. Such developments make it clearer how research, policy, and patient care are related in the fight against diabetic eye disease.

References

1. Abdelrahim, M. S. N., Abozaid, L., Abu Elgasim, M. A. E., Ahmed, M., et al. (2021). Knowledge and awareness of diabetic retinopathy among diabetic Sudanese patients, Khartoum State, Sudan, 2018. https://core.ac.uk/download/492740440.pdf (accessed on 11th June 2025).
2. Acera, A., Alonso, A., Enríquez-de-Salamanca, A., Ghaffariyeh, A., Jemal, A., et al. (2016). Tear fluid biomarkers in ocular and systemic disease: Potential use for predictive, preventive and personalized medicine. https://core.ac.uk/download/293884791.pdf (accessed on 11th June 2025).
3. Ah Tong, B., Burton, M., D'Esposito, F., Dillon, H., et al. (2022). Risk factors common to leading eye health conditions and major non-communicable diseases: A rapid review and commentary. https://core.ac.uk/download/548256039.pdf (accessed on 11th June 2025).
4. Al-Namaeh, M. (2022). Common causes of visual impairment in the elderly. https://core.ac.uk/download/524635246.pdf (accessed on 11th June 2025).
5. Andrew, L., Davis, T., & Johnson, C. (2017). The impact of visual impairments on mobility performance in community-dwelling older adults. https://digitalscholarship.unlv.edu/cgi/viewcontent.cgi?article=3923&context=thesesdissertations (accessed on 11th June 2025).
6. Autolitano, M., Basili, S., La Torre, G., Lenzi, A., et al. (2017). Comparison between "early" or "late" intravitreal injection of dexamethasone implant in branch (BRVO) or central (CRVO) retinal vein occlusion: Six months follow-up. https://core.ac.uk/download/74321801.pdf (accessed on 11th June 2025).
7. Ayares, D., & Cooper, D. K. C. (2012). Potential benefits and risks of clinical xenotransplantation. https://core.ac.uk/download/12213803.pdf (accessed on 11th June 2025).
8. Balsa, A., & Gandelman, N. (2025). The impact of ICT on health promotion: A randomized experiment with diabetic patients. https://core.ac.uk/download/pdf/6313436.pdf (accessed on 11th June 2025).
9. Berco, E., Greenwald, Y., Kleinmann, G., Pollack, A., et al. (2015). Management of diabetic retinopathy and other ocular complications in type 1 diabetes. https://core.ac.uk/download/322425431.pdf (accessed on 11th June 2025).
10. Bharti, A., Raina, B., & Sharma, P. (2020). Knowledge, attitude and practice of diabetic retinopathy amongst diabetic patients in a tertiary care hospital of Jammu. https://core.ac.uk/download/539913005.pdf (accessed on 11th June 2025).
11. Błaszczak, E., Dydyk, M., Dyrek, M., Gurdak, K., et al. (2024). Pregnancy as an important risk factor for the progression of diabetic retinopathy. https://core.ac.uk/download/636385964.pdf (accessed on 11th June 2025).
12. Borg, D., Camilleri, F., Cuschieri, S., Pace, A., et al. (2016). A review of diabetic patients' knowledge in a high prevalent European country: Malta. https://core.ac.uk/download/46604043.pdf (accessed on 11th June 2025).
13. Bottone, A., Fameli, V., Ferraresi, A. F., Giustolisi, R., et al. (2016). Intravitreal injection of Ozurdex® implant in patients with persistent diabetic macular edema, with six-month follow-up. https://core.ac.uk/download/98344485.pdf (accessed on 11th June 2025).

14. Budhori, R., Kaushik, A., Manorma, Mazumder, R., et al. (2021). Current measures against ophthalmic complications of diabetes mellitus–A short review. https://core.ac.uk/download/482244030.pdf (accessed on 11th June 2025).

15. Bulpitt, C. J., Fletcher, A. E., Hewitt, J., Smeeth, L., et al. (2005). Respiratory symptoms in older people and their association with mortality.

16. Busetto, L. (2015). Timing of bariatric surgery in people with obesity and diabetes. https://core.ac.uk/download/53528626.pdf (accessed on 11th June 2025).

17. Caminiti, G., Casu, M., Catte, O., Costaggiu, D., Dessí, S., Fossarello, M., Manconi, P. E., et al. (2014). Cognitive impairment and age-related vision disorders: Their possible relationship and the evaluation of the use of aspirin and statins in a 65 years-and-over Sardinian population. https://core.ac.uk/download/pdf/54603310.pdf (accessed on 11th June 2025).

18. Casten, R. J., & Rovner, B. W. (2019). Trust and glycemic control in Black patients with diabetic retinopathy: A pilot study. https://core.ac.uk/download/213449812.pdf (accessed on 11th June 2025).

19. Clark, M. D., Johnson, M. R. D., Owen, D., Szczepura, A., et al. (1999). The unavoidable costs of ethnicity: A review of evidence on health costs. https://core.ac.uk/download/16664278.pdf (accessed on 11th June 2025).

20. Ctori, I., Dabasia, P., Edgar, D. F., Fidalgo, D., et al. (2019). Role of advanced technology in the detection of sight-threatening eye disease in a UK community setting. https://core.ac.uk/download/288395620.pdf (accessed on 11th June 2025).

21. Dai, Y., Haller, J. A., Hark, L. A., Leiby, B. E., et al. (2017). Non-adherence to eye care in people with diabetes. https://core.ac.uk/download/129191555.pdf (accessed on 11th June 2025).

22. Diamant, Allison & Babey, Susan & Brown, E & Chawla, Neetu. (2003). Diabetes in California: Nearly 1.5 million diagnosed and 2 million more at risk. Policy brief (UCLA Center for Health Policy Research). 1-8. (accessed on 11th June 2025).

23. Docherty, N. G., Gorman, D. M., Le Roux, C. W. (2016). The effect of bariatric surgery on diabetic retinopathy: Good, bad, or both? https://core.ac.uk/download/77020446.pdf (accessed on 11th June 2025).

24. Dremin, V. V., Dunaev, A. V., Goltsov, A., Makovik, A., et al. (2019). Multimodal optical diagnostics of the microhemodynamics in upper and lower limbs. https://core.ac.uk/download/228178569.pdf (accessed on 11th June 2025).

25. Goode, P. (2018). Diabetes disparities in African Americans: A cry for help to primary care providers. https://digitalscholarship.unlv.edu/cgi/viewcontent.cgi?article=1671&context=jhdrp (accessed on 11th June 2025).

26. Gosney, M. A., Nyman, S. R., & Victor, C. R. (2009). Psychosocial impact of visual impairment in working age adults. https://core.ac.uk/download/337412.pdf (accessed on 11th June 2025).

27. Kroenke, K. (2015). Telemedicine screening for eye disease. https://core.ac.uk/download/46961457.pdf (accessed on 11th June 2025).

28. Kumar, A. (2019). Influence of diabetic kidney and eye complications on annual health expenditures using the Medical Expenditures Panel Survey 2012–2016. https://core.ac.uk/download/270046162.pdf (accessed on 11th June 2025).

29. Sacchetti, M., & Lambiase, A. (2017). Neurotrophic factors and corneal nerve regeneration. *Neural regeneration research, 12*(8), 1220–1224. https://doi.org/10.4103/1673-5374.213534(accessed on 11th June 2025).

30. Marcheggiani, F., Reilly, J., Shu, X., Tiano, L., et al. (2017). Therapeutic potential of co-enzyme Q10 in retinal diseases. https://core.ac.uk/download/293883638.pdf (accessed on 11th June 2025).

31. Martin, D., Ting, J., & Haas, M. (2025). *A Markov Model of Diabetic Retinopathy Progression for the Economic Evaluation of a Novel DR Prognostic Device, CHERE Working Paper 2007/14*. https://core.ac.uk/download/pdf/7070858.pdf (accessed on 11th June 2025).

32. Middleton, B., Cusack, C. M., Kendrick, D., Bates, D. W., Bu, D., Johnston, D., Pan, E., et al. (2007). The value of information technology-enabled diabetes management. https://core.ac.uk/download/71355637.pdf (accessed on 11th June 2025).

33. Morris, A. D., Cheng, D. T., Cromie, D. W. M., Pearson, E., Elman, G. P., Leese, G. P., Ghafour, A., et al. (2014). Rates of referable eye disease in the Scottish National Diabetic Retinopathy Screening Programmed. https://core.ac.uk/download/30660889.pdf (accessed on 11th June 2025).

34. Muller, A., Wilson, A., Bunce, C., Kelliher, C., Stefansson, E., Joner, G., et al. (2008). Care of vision and ocular health in diabetic members of a national diabetes organization: A cross-sectional study. https://core.ac.uk/download/pdf/8170329.pdf (accessed on 11th June 2025).

35. Pandova, M. G. (2019). Diabetic retinopathy and blindness: An epidemiological overview. https://core.ac.uk/download/322444061.pdf (accessed on 11th June 2025).

36. Sampson, C. J. (2020). Optimizing the cost-effectiveness of risk-based screening for diabetic retinopathy. https://core.ac.uk/download/552442742.pdf (accessed on 11th June 2025).

37. Tonna, A. (2001). Diabetes mellitus and its management: An introductory overview. https://core.ac.uk/download/46604533.pdf (accessed on 11th June 2025).

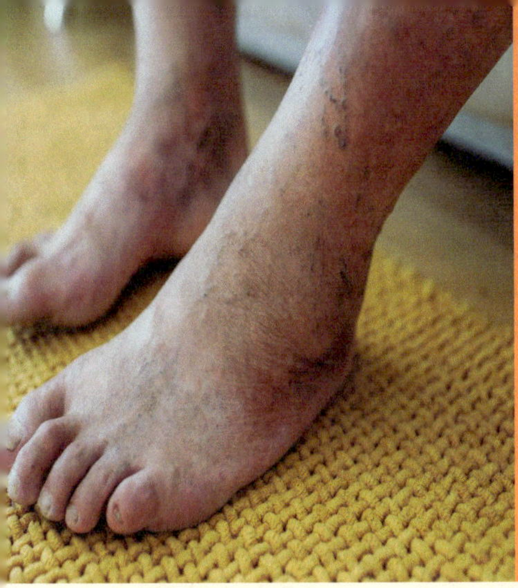

Chapter 12

DIABETIC NEUROPATHY

Contents

Introduction

Diabetic neuropathy is a major and complicated problem that affects many people with diabetes mellitus worldwide. Because of this, it is a kind of peripheral neuropathy that develops when high blood sugar causes damage to nerves in the arms and legs. There are many disorders in this condition that affect peripheral nerves and cause both sensory and motor problems. Since more people are developing type 2 diabetes, it is important to learn about diabetic neuropathy, what causes it, and what symptoms it brings. Experts say that between 60% and 70% of diabetics experience neuropathy, which demonstrates how it is a major diabetes-related issue that can greatly reduce quality of life. We will look at the different aspects of diabetic neuropathy, including its signs and symptoms, difficulties in diagnosing it, and available treatments. The symptoms of diabetic neuropathy can be as simple as a little numbness or as serious as intense pain and full paralysis. Many patients complain of numbness, tingling, and burning pain in the hands and feet. If left untreated, these symptoms may get worse and cause foot ulcers and infections, which could end in amputation. For example, John, a 62-year-old man with type 2 Diabetes Mellitus for seven years, got a dry ulcer on his foot after putting on new shoes. This example underscores the importance of recognizing early signs of neuropathy and understanding its direct implications for patient health and daily functioning(Gabriele et al., 2008). In addition, when diabetic neuropathy is of the autonomic type, it can cause problems with organs such as the heart and bladder, which makes diabetes harder to control and leads to more health complications. Since diabetic neuropathy has many different and complex symptoms, it must be investigated in a step-by-step manner. While guidelines exist for the treatment of neuropathy, the avenues for investigation lack standardization, making diagnosis challenging for clinicians (Aquilina et al., 2015). The doctor often uses clinical examination, nerve tests, and information about the patient's history to find out the extent of nerve damage and what caused it. Learning about the causes of diabetic neuropathy helps doctors provide better care and improve the results for patients. Since the condition affects many diabetics and has serious outcomes, more research and better ways to diagnose it are needed right away. When we have a clear idea about the condition, we can handle diabetic neuropathy better and reduce its effects on patients (Figure 12.1).

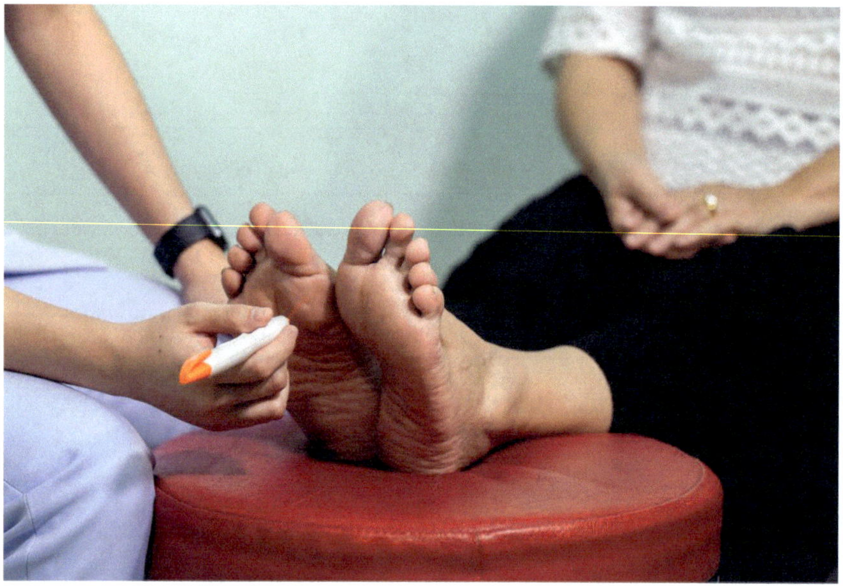

Figure 12.1. Diabetic neuropathy.

Source: https://cdn-prod.medicalnewstoday.com/content/images/articles/245/245310/foot-test-for-peripheral-neuropathy.jpg

12.1. Causes of Diabetic Neuropathy

Diabetic neuropathy is most likely to develop when diabetic patients have high blood sugar levels for a long time. Continued high blood sugar levels may result in changes in the body that harm the nerves outside the brain and spinal cord. Higher levels of glucose in the body lead to the formation of toxic substances that injure nerves. Additionally, over time, the accumulation of advanced glycation end-products (AGEs) causes oxidative stress and inflammation, which exacerbate the degeneration of nerve fibers. This connection between blood glucose and neuropathy is not accidental; studies prove that better control of blood sugar reduces the likelihood of neuropathy in people with diabetes. Having other conditions, especially heart problems, is another important reason for the development of diabetic neuropathy. People with diabetes are likely to develop hypertension, dyslipidemia, and other heart problems that make their nerve pain worse. The interaction between these risk factors and diabetic neuropathy is profound, as studies show that conditions such as high cholesterol and increased body mass index (BMI) are significantly associated with the cumulative incidence of diabetic neuropathy (Abdillah et al., 2017). Also, people with cardiovascular disease at the start of treatment are twice as likely to develop neuropathy, so treating these problems may slow down nerve damage in diabetic patients. Because of this, diabetes care should pay close attention to cardiovascular health and be managed regularly. What we eat and do has a big effect on the development of diabetic neuropathy. Smoking and being inactive are important factors that can be changed and lead to neuropathic problems. Smoking leads to more insulin resistance and poor blood circulation, which makes nerve damage worse. Consequently, patients who smoke are at a higher risk for developing more severe forms of diabetic neuropathy (Abdillah et al., 2017). A sedentary lifestyle can also cause a person's BMI to rise and result in metabolic problems that make neuropathic symptoms worse. It is very important to help people quit smoking and exercise more to lower their risk of neuropathy. If people with diabetes exercise more, they can enhance their health and reduce the risk of diabetic neuropathy (Figure 12.2).

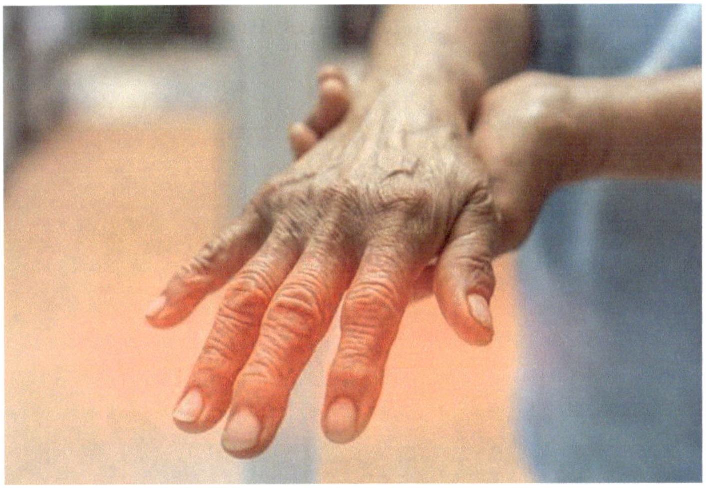

Figure 12.2. Elevated glucose concentrations initiate the conversion into various toxic metabolites, which contribute to nerve injury.

Source: https://content.health.harvard.edu/wp-content/uploads/2024/08/gettyimages-1319694149.jpg

12.1.1. High Blood Sugar Levels

Having high blood sugar, which is called hyperglycemia, is a main sign of diabetes and helps lead to diabetic neuropathy. Continued high levels of glucose may result in serious damage to nerves, mainly in the peripheral nervous system. Excess glucose in the body leads to the formation of harmful substances, which cause oxidative stress and inflammation that negatively affect the nerves. When these pathogenic processes take place, people who have high blood sugar for a long time may feel tingling, pain, and numbness in their extremities. Consequently, managing blood glucose effectively becomes paramount not only in preventing the emergence of neuropathic symptoms but also in mitigating the long-term complications associated with diabetes, which include not only sensory deficits but also the risk of amputations due to unnoticed injuries (Iqbal et al., 2019). Also, diabetic neuropathy is common among people who have had diabetes for a long time. It is estimated that almost half of the people with diabetes can experience neuropathy during their lives. Since high blood sugar can cause nerve problems, it is important to regularly check blood sugar and control it well. To lower the risk of neuropathy, people with diabetes should follow strategies that keep their blood sugar within the right range. It is also necessary to teach patients about the symptoms of nerve damage, as many people may not notice them until the condition becomes very serious. Thus, comprehensive care strategies must incorporate both preventive measures and therapeutic interventions aimed at controlling hyperglycemia (Arent et al., 2001). In addition, dealing with high blood sugar as a cause of diabetic neuropathy requires a plan that involves both patients and healthcare professionals. It requires testing hemoglobin A1c regularly and developing plans that help avoid sudden increases in blood sugar. Also, healthcare workers should encourage their patients to eat a healthy diet, be physically active, and stick to their medication to control their blood glucose. As it becomes clear that hyperglycemia can lead to diabetic neuropathy, encouraging patients to manage their diabetes well can help them live better and stop nerve damage from getting worse. Ultimately, by prioritizing the prevention and management of high blood sugar levels, we can mitigate the severe consequences of diabetic neuropathy and improve overall patient outcomes (Iqbal et al., 2019) (Figure 12.3).

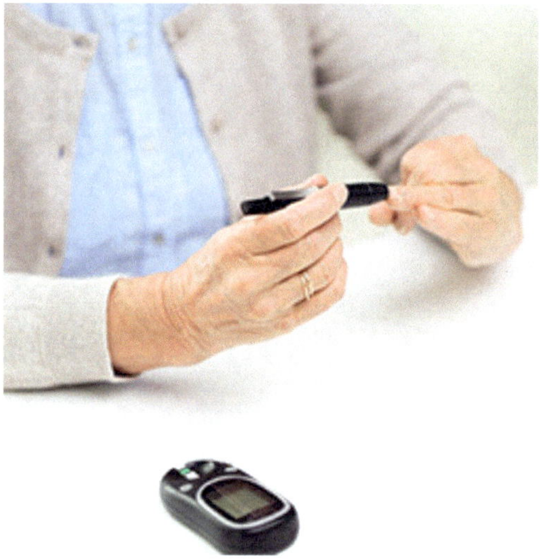

Figure 12.3. High blood sugar levels, also known as hyperglycemia, are a hallmark of diabetes and play a crucial role in the development of diabetic neuropathy.

Source: https://www.niddk.nih.gov/-/media/Images/Health-Information/Featured-Images/Diabetic_Neuropathy_square.jpg

12.1.2. Genetic Predisposition

A person's genetic background is very important in the development of diabetic neuropathy, a frequent complication of diabetes that leads to nerve damage. Both the environment and the individual's genes can make some people more prone to neuropathic damage. Genetic variations in the genes responsible for glucose metabolism may make it more likely for a person to get diabetic neuropathy. For instance, when ATP-dependent potassium channels vary, it can cause coronary blood flow problems and negatively affect the peripheral nerves of patients with diabetes. It is important to know how genes and the environment interact to guide the creation of effective prevention and treatment plans. Through research on glucose and nerve tissues, it is further shown that genetic background plays a key role in diabetic neuropathy. It has been found that high glucose levels alter the behavior of spinal roots, which can increase the nerves' resistance to hypoxia, but also negatively affect other nerves. In particular, the ventral roots were able to function well, but the dorsal roots suffered a lot of electrophysiological damage during hyperglycemia. The results imply that variations in genes might determine how nerves respond to stresses, especially when there is a high level of glucose as in diabetes.

So, genetic aspects should be taken into account when assessing the risk of diabetic neuropathy in a person. Overall, the relationship between genes and the environment gives a complete explanation of diabetic neuropathy. They are responsible for the structure and function of the brain as well as how people react to metabolic problems, for example, hyperglycemia. Besides, the role of increased anaerobic glycolysis in peripheral nerves may help reveal how the body defends itself from extreme hypoxia caused by high glucose. Every one of these factors highlights the different aspects of diabetic neuropathy and shows why it is important to treat patients according to their genetic backgrounds (Figure 12.4).

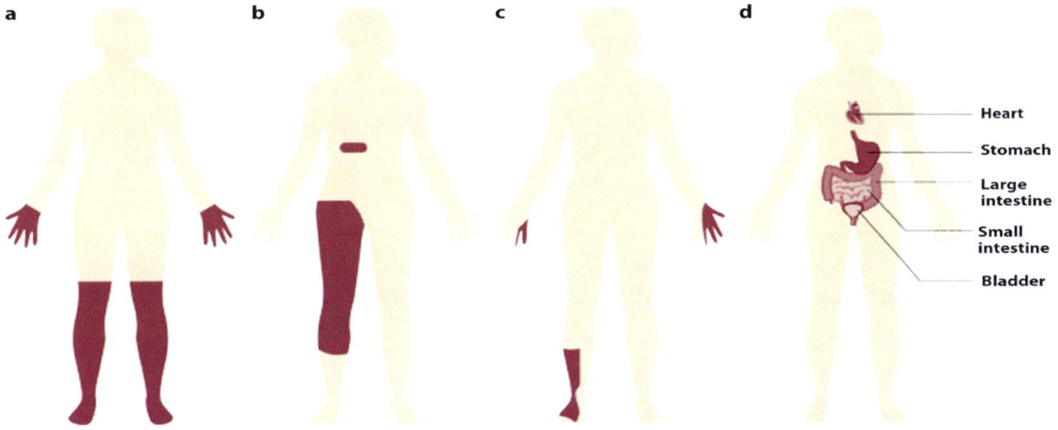

Figure 12.4. Genetic predisposition plays a critical role in the development of diabetic neuropathy, a common complication of diabetes characterized by nerve damage.

Source: https://media.springernature.com/m685/springer-static/image/art%3A10.1038%2Fs41572-019-0092-1/MediaObjects/41572_2019_92_Fig1_HTML.png

12.1.3. Lifestyle Factors

Lifestyle plays a major role in diabetic neuropathy since it can directly impact when and how fast the condition develops. It is important to pay attention to diet, exercise, and weight control since they help maintain normal blood glucose levels and protect against diabetes complications. Eating foods high in whole grains, lean proteins, and healthy fats can help control blood sugar levels and thus lower the chance of neuropathy. Furthermore, being physically active regularly helps keep your weight healthy and makes your body respond better to insulin. Such interventions can mitigate the adverse effects of chronic hyperglycemia, ultimately lowering the risk of developing diabetic neuropathy as well as other related complications described in the literature (Defeudis et al., 2015). Also, smoking and drinking alcohol can greatly increase a person's chances of developing diabetic neuropathy. In particular, smoking makes insulin resistance worse and increases the risk of heart diseases that often occur together with diabetes and its complications. It has been demonstrated that people who smoke and have diabetes are more likely to suffer from neuropathy. Although drinking alcohol is sometimes accepted in society, it may result in unstable blood sugar levels and make neuropathic symptoms worse.

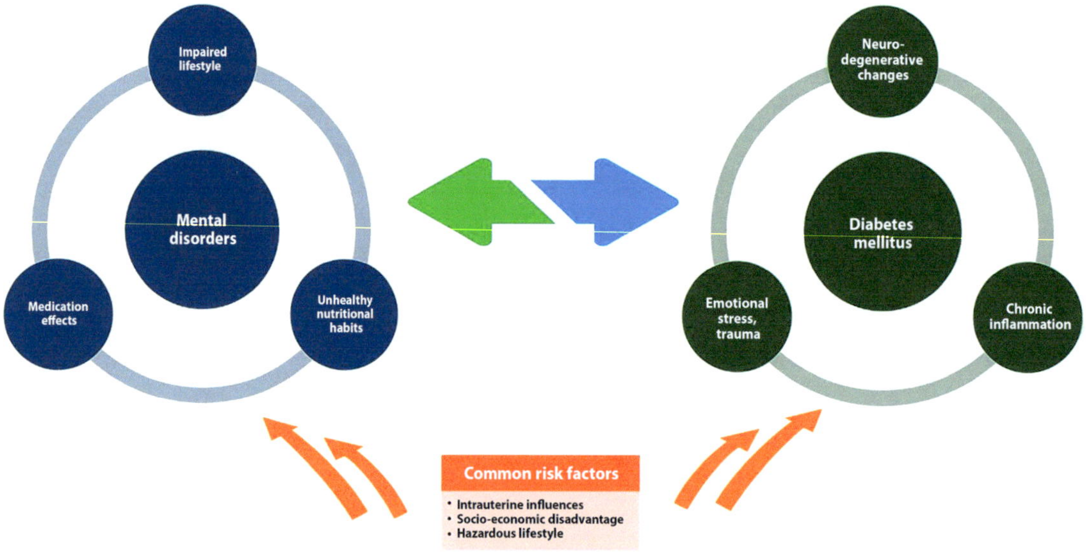

Figure 12.5. The interplay between lifestyle factors and diabetic neuropathy is significant, as these factors can directly influence the onset and progression of the condition.

Source: Mangoulia P, Milionis C, Vlachou E, Ilias I. The Interrelationship between Diabetes Mellitus and Emotional Well-Being: Current Concepts and Future Prospects. *Healthcare*. 2024; 12(14):1457. https://doi.org/10.3390/healthcare12141457

The moderation of these lifestyle choices is crucial, as they can greatly influence disease outcomes, particularly considering how additional factors, such as obesity and hypertension, interact within the diabetic population to compound the risk of complications (Kautzky-Willeret al., 2013). It is also important to pay attention to psychosocial factors in lifestyle, such as handling stress and following medication schedules, for diabetic neuropathy. Stress that continues for a long time can upset hormones, which can make blood sugar hard to control and worsen symptoms of nerve damage. If you practice mindfulness and exercise often, you can manage stress much better and improve your health. It is also necessary to follow the suggested diabetes management plans, but research has shown that women tend to be less likely to stick to these guidelines than men. This discrepancy underscores the need for tailored interventions that account for lifestyle factors, particularly in populations at risk for neuropathy, ensuring comprehensive management of diabetic complications (Kautzky-Willer et al., 2013) (Figure 12.5).

12.2. Types of Diabetic Neuropathy

A variety of nerve problems called diabetic neuropathy can happen to people with diabetes due to high blood sugar for a long period. Doctors usually divide diabetic neuropathy into four main types: peripheral neuropathy, autonomic neuropathy, proximal neuropathy, and focal neuropathy. Most of the time, peripheral neuropathy is diagnosed, and it usually leads to pain, tingling, or a loss of sensation in the hands and feet. This condition can greatly interfere with everyday activities and make it hard for a person to move around. It is important to understand these classifications to manage patients well and give them the right treatment for their symptoms. Moreover, problems related to peripheral neuropathy may lead to serious injuries such as foot ulcers, making it clear that awareness and active management are very important. In addition, autonomic neuropathy is a serious problem in diabetic neuropathy, since it affects the nerves that control involuntary body functions. Such a condition can upset the body's important functions, including how the heart beats, blood pressure is managed, and food moves through the intestines. Symptoms of this condition can be as simple as postural hypotension and as complicated as gastroparesis, showing how it can affect many parts of the body. It is often hard to notice these symptoms at first, which might result in a late diagnosis and treatment. Furthermore, when complications occur, they can worsen other health problems, so it becomes necessary to treat the neuropathy and the effects it has on the patient's overall health and diabetes control. Proximal and focal neuropathies are not common, but they should be noticed because they have different symptoms and call for special treatment. Proximal neuropathy usually causes the muscles of the thighs and hips to waste and become weak, making it hard for people to move around. In this case, focal neuropathy means that damage to specific nerves happens suddenly and affects cranial or peripheral nerves. These conditions may lead to sudden pain, weak muscles, or vision problems, which are serious for the people who have them. Since diabetic neuropathy has many aspects, it is important to know about each type and use personalized care strategies. Since doctors and researchers are always looking for better ways to treat and study neuropathies, it is still important to increase awareness and education to help patients (Figure 12.6).

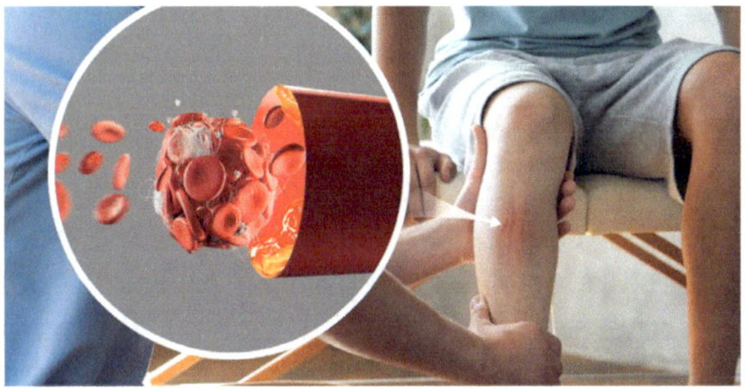

Figure 12.6. Diabetic neuropathy encompasses a range of nerve disorders stemming from prolonged elevated blood glucose levels, impacting millions of individuals with diabetes.

Source: https://longlivelives.com/wp-content/uploads/2024/03/Image-1-1.webp

12.2.1. Peripheral Neuropathy

Since peripheral neuropathy is complex, it creates many difficulties for patients with diabetes, as it is linked to a wide variety of disorders brought on by different causes. Because of high blood glucose levels, type 2 diabetes mellitus is a major reason for nerve damage in the arms and legs, known as peripheral neuropathy. It is significant that peripheral neuropathy is common globally, as studies suggest that it affects 2.4% of people, and the incidence goes up to 8% in older age groups. This underscores the importance of early detection and management, as untreated peripheral neuropathy can severely compromise an individual's quality of life, leading to complications such as ulcers or infections, further exacerbated by the underlying diabetic condition (Aquilina et al., 2015). Diabetic peripheral neuropathy may show up in many ways, but often it starts with mild symptoms like numbness, tingling, or pain in the arms or legs. When neuropathy worsens, patients may feel less sensation, which increases the chances of injuries or ulcers in the feet. For instance, a case study illustrates a 62-year-old patient with type 2 diabetes who presented with a small ulcer on his foot that developed after a change in footwear, highlighting how peripheral neuropathy can lead to serious complications from seemingly minimal trauma (Gabriele et al., 2008). For this reason, patients should be taught about foot care and checked regularly, which can greatly reduce the risks of this condition. In addition, examining peripheral neuropathy in people with diabetes is not simple and often requires a detailed, stepwise process, which may take a lot of time and money. The main focus of current clinical guidelines is on treating peripheral neuropathy, while there is a clear lack of standard ways to investigate it. It can be difficult for clinicians to find out exactly what causes neuropathy, since it can be caused by several factors, such as metabolic, vascular, and inflammatory issues. Because diabetes cases are increasing worldwide, it is now more important than ever to have efficient ways to diagnose the condition. Ultimately, addressing both the diagnosis and management of diabetic peripheral neuropathy is crucial to improving patient outcomes and preserving quality of life (Aquilina et al., 2015) (Figure 12.7).

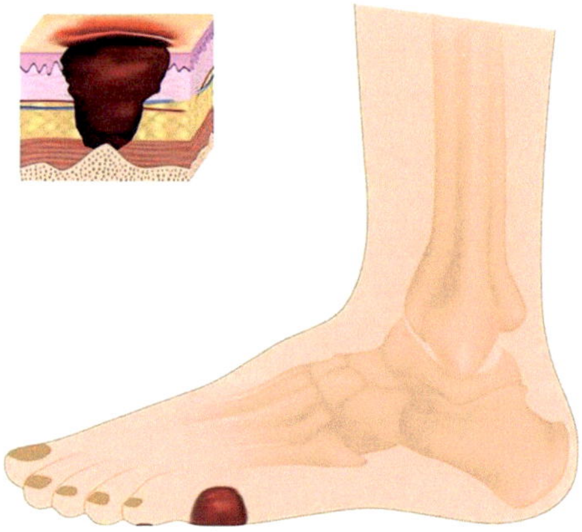

Figure 12.7. Diabetes mellitus, especially type 2, is a prominent contributor to peripheral neuropathy, which manifests as nerve damage over time due to persistently high blood glucose levels.

Source: https://novusspinecenter.com/wp-content/uploads/2017/06/Diabetic-Peripheral-Neuropathy_1200x1150.jpg

12.2.2. Autonomic Neuropathy

Because of prolonged hyperglycemia, autonomic neuropathy causes various problems in the autonomic nervous system in people with diabetes. As a result of this condition, heart rate, digestion, and sweat production are affected, which can be very harmful to a patient's health. One of the primary manifestations of autonomic neuropathy in diabetic patients is cardiovascular autonomic neuropathy (CAN), which is marked by diminished heart rate variability and impaired cardiovascular reflex mechanisms. Studies have shown that excessive glycemic variability can exacerbate the risk of developing CAN, pointing to the importance of maintaining stable blood glucose levels as part of an effective management strategy for type 1 diabetes mellitus (Helleputte et al., 2020). As a result, taking care of blood sugar levels may reduce the negative consequences linked to autonomic neuropathy. There are many factors involved in autonomic neuropathy, and hyperglycemia and oxidative stress are the main ones that lead to its development. When glucose levels remain high for a long period, it leads to problems in the mitochondria and increases oxidative stress. As a result, nerves are damaged and the functioning of the autonomic system is altered. Additionally, the presence of cardiovascular disease (CVD) in individuals with type 1 diabetes significantly impairs overall life expectancy, underscoring the critical need for intervention (Cappuccio et al., 2013). Applying intensive insulin therapy in treatment plans has been proven to lower the rate and severity of autonomic issues. The Diabetes Control and Complications Trial (DCCT) highlighted this significant association, asserting that aggressive management of blood glucose can prolong neuronal health and reduce the risk of diabetic autonomic neuropathy. In addition, the effects of autonomic neuropathy can be very serious for the heart. Altered heart function and poor blood circulation in patients with CAN may cause harmful cardiovascular events. Hypoglycemic episodes in diabetes can also affect the heart and make the condition of autonomic neuropathy more complicated. New therapeutic approaches, including glucagon-like peptide (GLP)-based treatments, are under investigation and may prove beneficial in alleviating insulin requirements while concurrently addressing neuropathic complications (Cappuccio et al., 2013). As studies progress, it is important to understand how glycemic control, autonomic function, and heart health are related to help people with diabetic neuropathy (Figure 12.8).

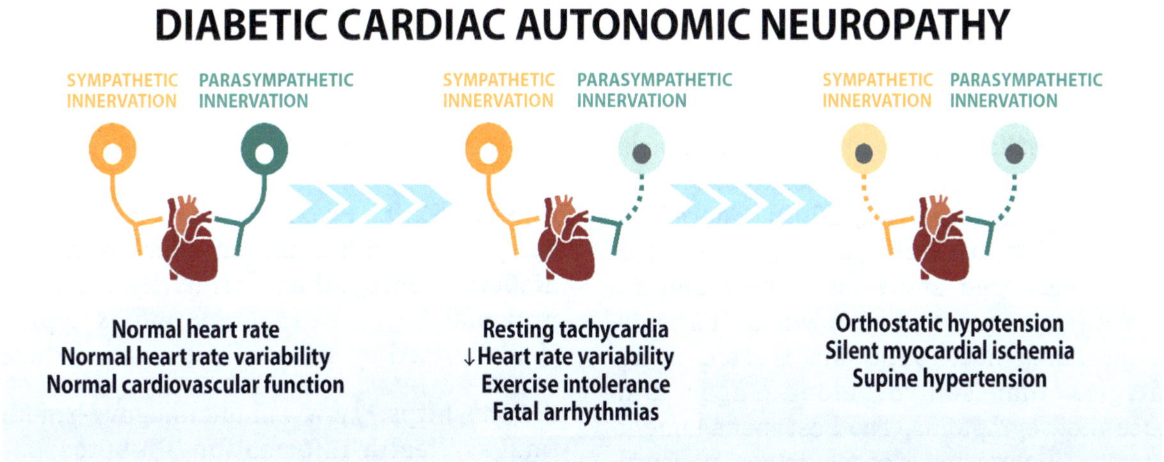

Figure 12.8. As a significant complication of diabetes, autonomic neuropathy encompasses a range of dysfunctions in the autonomic nervous system that occur in response to prolonged hyperglycemia.

Source: Sudo SZ, Montagnoli TL, Rocha BdS, Santos AD, de Sá MPL, Zapata-Sudo G. Diabetes-Induced Cardiac Autonomic Neuropathy: Impact on Heart Function and Prognosis. *Biomedicines.* 2022; 10(12):3258. https://doi.org/10.3390/biomedicines10123258

12.2.3. Proximal Neuropathy

Proximal neuropathy belongs to diabetic neuropathies and usually affects the lower extremities, causing both sensory loss and weakness. Long-term diabetes and poor control over blood sugar are the main factors that cause this condition. The first symptoms are usually a sudden pain in the hip or thigh and weakness in the legs, both of which make it difficult to move and lower the patient's quality of life. Proximal neuropathy can bring a lot of pain, and this may stop people from moving, which can weaken their muscles and worsen their daily living. As a result, understanding proximal neuropathy's implications on patient quality of life is essential as this connection lays the groundwork for appropriate therapeutic strategies aimed at managing diabetic complications (Drury et al., 2012). Many different factors, such as ischemic, metabolic, and inflammatory ones, can lead to the pathophysiology of proximal neuropathy. High blood glucose in diabetes causes changes in metabolism that may damage the nerves over the years. In addition, arterial steal can take place because of vascular problems caused by diabetes, which causes blood to be diverted away from the nerves. Such hemodynamic alterations can contribute to both diabetic neuropathy and other complications, complicating the clinical picture and challenging healthcare professionals in diagnosing and treating these conditions effectively (Calligaro et al., 2008). Therefore, it is important to investigate symptoms, the patient's past, and any existing problems to deal with the condition as a whole. Patients with proximal neuropathy are treated using strategies that control blood sugar and reduce their symptoms. The best management strategies might consist of medicines, physical therapy, and lifestyle changes that help people with the condition live better lives. Researchers believe that exercising on a regular basis can help patients by reducing neuropathy symptoms and making them stronger. Additionally, taking care of cardiovascular complications in a comprehensive way can be very helpful. By implementing these practices systematically, healthcare professionals can mitigate the impact of proximal neuropathy on individuals suffering from diabetes and facilitate a path toward better health outcomes (Drury et al., 2012). It is very important to understand how these interventions work to improve the way diabetic neuropathy is treated (Figure 12.9).

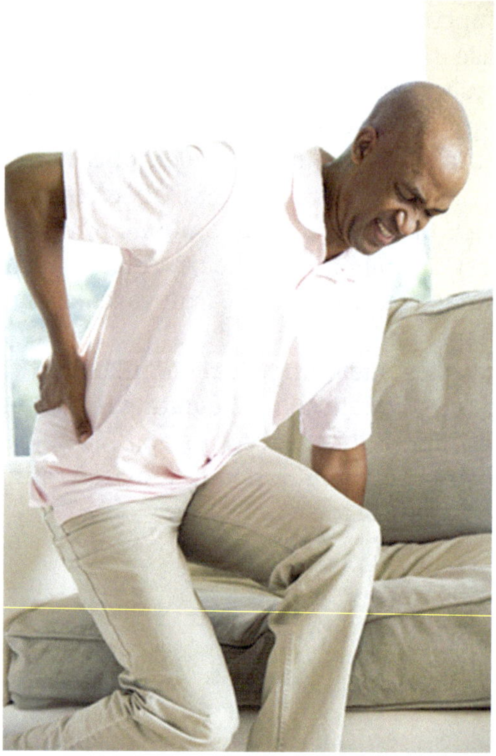

Figure 12.9. Proximal neuropathy, often categorized within the broader spectrum of diabetic neuropathies, primarily affects the proximal lower extremities and is typically characterized by sensory loss and weakness.

Source: https://www.niddk.nih.gov/-/media/Images/Health-Information/Diabetes/back_pain_330x495.png

12.3. Symptoms of Diabetic Neuropathy

Diabetic neuropathy is a frequent diabetes complication that can lead to many symptoms that greatly impact the patient's life. Often, people notice tingling, burning, or numbness, especially in their arms or legs, at the start of the disease. Most of the time, these symptoms start in the toes and move up the limbs, making the feet and hands feel like they are wearing gloves and socks. Since symptoms can gradually get worse, patients might not realize what is going on and put off getting the right diagnosis and treatment. With time, a lack of sensation may result in more injuries, infections, and conditions such as ulcers or gangrene. The interplay of prolonged hyperglycemia and oxidative stress further exacerbates nerve damage, illustrating the critical need for early identification and management of diabetic neuropathy symptoms (Aquilina et al., 2015). Diabetic people may also develop motor neuropathy, which brings its own set of problems. Signs of motor neuropathy are weakness, muscle shrinkage, and movement problems, mostly in the legs and feet. This condition can make it hard for people to move, which leads to problems with daily tasks and raises the chance of falls and more injuries. When muscles are very weak, it can cause Charcot foot, which makes the joints weak and misaligned and may cause major issues. Such physical limitations not only hinder an individual's independence but also contribute to an overall decline in mental health, emphasizing the profound impact of motor symptoms associated with diabetic neuropathy on both physical and emotional well-being (Drury et al., 2012).

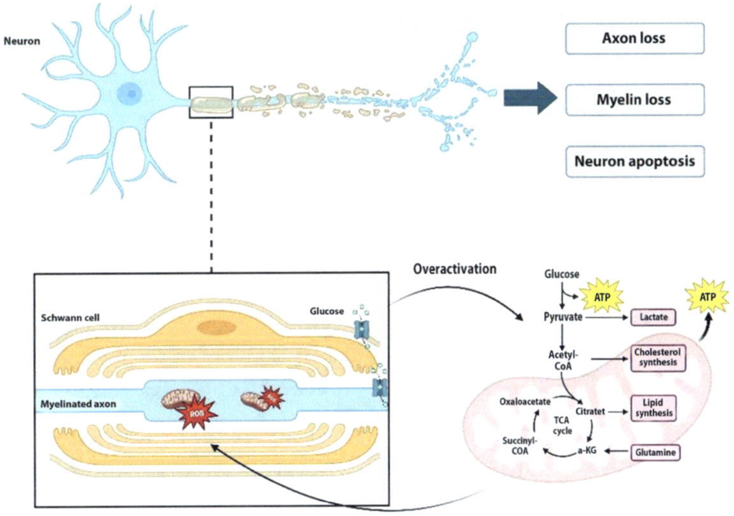

Figure 12.10. The interplay of prolonged hyperglycemia and oxidative stress further exacerbates nerve damage, illustrating the critical need for early identification and management of diabetic neuropathy symptoms

Source: Zhu J, Hu Z, Luo Y, Liu Y, Luo W, Du X, Luo Z, Hu J and Peng S (2024) Diabetic peripheral neuropathy: pathogenetic mechanisms and treatment. Front. Endocrinol. 14:1265372. doi: 10.3389/fendo.2023.1265372

Also, autonomic neuropathy can make it more difficult to control diabetes because it affects functions that the body does not control. Some symptoms are gastroparesis in the digestive system, irregular heartbeat, and changes in sweating, which makes it hard to keep body temperature under control. Dizziness when standing up may occur for some people because of orthostatic hypotension, and they may also have problems with their bladder. Since autonomic neuropathy can show in many ways, it is important to carefully watch and treat each patient with specific strategies. Given the wide-ranging symptoms associated with diabetic neuropathy, healthcare providers need to take a multifaceted approach to assessment and treatment, ensuring that patients receive comprehensive care that addresses both the physiological and psychological aspects of their condition (Aquilina et al., 2015) (Figure 12.10).

12.3.1. Numbness and Tingling

Numbness and tingling are the main signs of diabetic neuropathy, which happens when high blood sugar for a long period causes damage to nerves. When blood glucose is too high, it disrupts the nerves, which stops the nervous system from communicating properly with the body. Therefore, people may notice that their feet and hands have reduced sensitivity or feel different than before. Such symptoms can greatly lower a person's quality of life, since they may make it harder to carry out daily tasks and may raise the risk of falls and injuries. It is important to deal with these symptoms early, according to research, to prevent more damage to nerves and to help manage diabetes-related complications, which improves the patient's overall health and satisfaction.

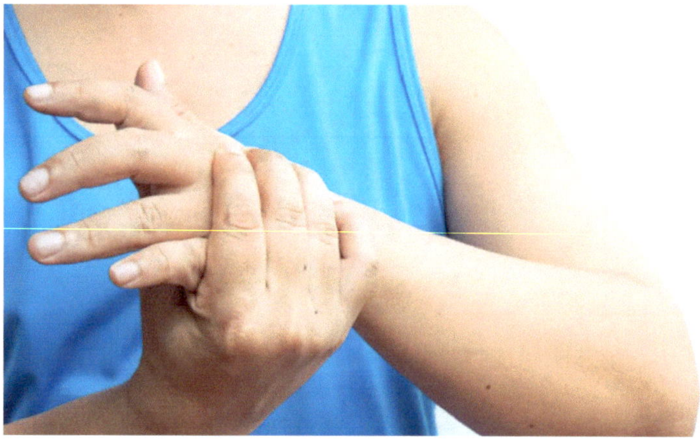

Figure 12.11. The sensations of numbness and tingling are hallmark symptoms of diabetic neuropathy, resulting from nerve damage often associated with prolonged hyperglycemia.

Source: https://images.apollo247.in/pd-cms/cms/2023-06/Shutterstock_2012022242_0.jpg?tr=q-80,f-webp,w-400,dpr-2.5,c-at_max%201000w

Doctors usually manage numbness and tingling in diabetic neuropathy with multiple treatments that help ease symptoms and promote nerve healing. Studies done in recent times have pointed out that vitamins B1, B6, and B12 are effective in reducing the symptoms of diabetic neuropathy. Among patients who received these vitamins, it was found that tingling and numbness decreased, which suggests a possible way for nerves to recover and heal. As a result, it is important to treat these conditions with methods that ease symptoms and address the main changes in the nerves. For this reason, healthcare providers should think about adding vitamin supplements to the overall care plan for people with diabetic neuropathy. Besides, Ayurveda and other traditional medicine viewpoints provide further understanding of how to handle diabetic neuropathy symptoms. The Ayurvedic framework identifies the pivotal role of the doshas—particularly Vata and Pitta, in the development and exacerbation of these symptoms (Surve et al., 2019). Practitioners try to restore balance and relieve the discomforts of neuropathy by using herbal remedies and formulas that address the doshas. The approach involves managing symptoms and, at the same time, fixing the internal issues that cause neuropathic problems. As new studies prove the benefits of both types of treatments, using them together may be more effective for handling numbness and tingling in diabetic neuropathy (Figure 12.11).

12.3.2. Pain and Sensitivity

There are both physical and mental elements that come together to create pain in people with diabetic neuropathy. Neuropathic pain, defined as pain arising from damage to the somatosensory system, affects a significant portion of the diabetic population, with estimates suggesting that around one in four diabetic patients encounter this distressing symptom (Drury et al., 2012). Apart from physical discomfort, this condition also means feeling more pain from things that do not usually hurt healthy people. As a result, some patients say that even a light touch causes them a lot of discomfort. It is important to understand the reasons behind this increased sensitivity, since it helps choose treatments that can make life better for people with diabetic neuropathy. Usually, pain from diabetic neuropathy is managed using drugs together with alternative therapies. Some pharmacological treatments are antidepressants, anticonvulsants, and topical medications meant to change the way pain is processed in the body. However, research suggests that while these medications can provide relief, they frequently come with adverse side effects that can further diminish the overall well-being of patients (Drury et al., 2012). As a result, more people are interested in complementary approaches, such as doing physical exercise and cognitive behavioral therapy, since they can ease pain and sensitivity and cause fewer severe side effects compared to drugs. When people are more active, these interventions hope to ease pain and also help with their mood and social life, making it easier to manage diabetic neuropathy. In addition, recent research stresses the role of genetics in diabetic neuropathic pain, revealing parts of the chromosomes that increase a person's chances of getting this condition. Research indicates that there may be sex-specific genetic factors that contribute to the manifestation of neuropathic pain among diabetic patients, as seen in the associations with variants on chromosome 1p35.1 and 8p23.1 (Abbott et al., 2015). They point out that treating pain and sensitivity should consider the symptoms and also the genetic background of each patient. Further research on the genetics of diabetic neuropathy can result in new treatments that are better suited to each patient (Figure 12.12).

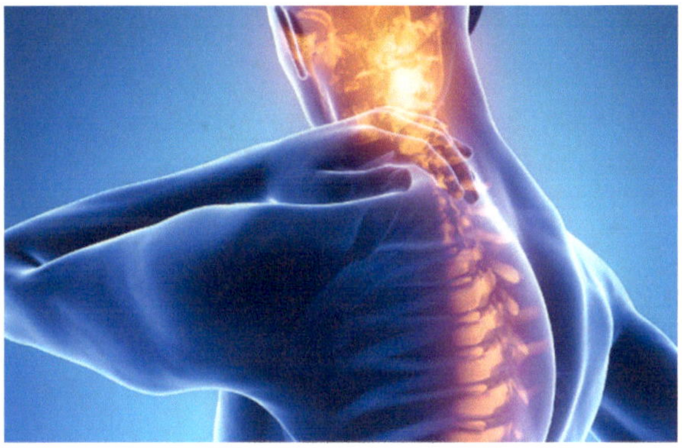

Figure 12.12. Neuropathic pain, defined as pain arising from damage to the somatosensory system, affects a significant portion of the diabetic population, with estimates suggesting that around one in four diabetic patients encounter this distressing symptom

Source: https://neuronpainclinic.com/blogs/wp-content/uploads/2023/02/Know-All-About-the-Treatment-Options-for-Neuropathic-Pain.jpg

12.3.3. Muscle Weakness

Muscle weakness is a major and disabling symptom found in people with diabetic neuropathy, which happens when high blood sugar levels affect the nerves for a long period. Changes in the peripheral nervous system result in many implications for the strength and activity of muscles. When diabetic neuropathy gets more serious, patients find it hard to maintain their strength and coordination, which makes simple daily tasks tough. Besides causing physical problems, this condition can seriously lower someone's quality of life because muscle weakness may lead to a loss of independence and movement. Thus, the relationship between muscle weakness and diabetic neuropathy proves that this disease requires both neurological and muscular care. Muscle weakness in diabetic neuropathy occurs because of direct nerve damage and also because of secondary factors such as not using the muscles enough.

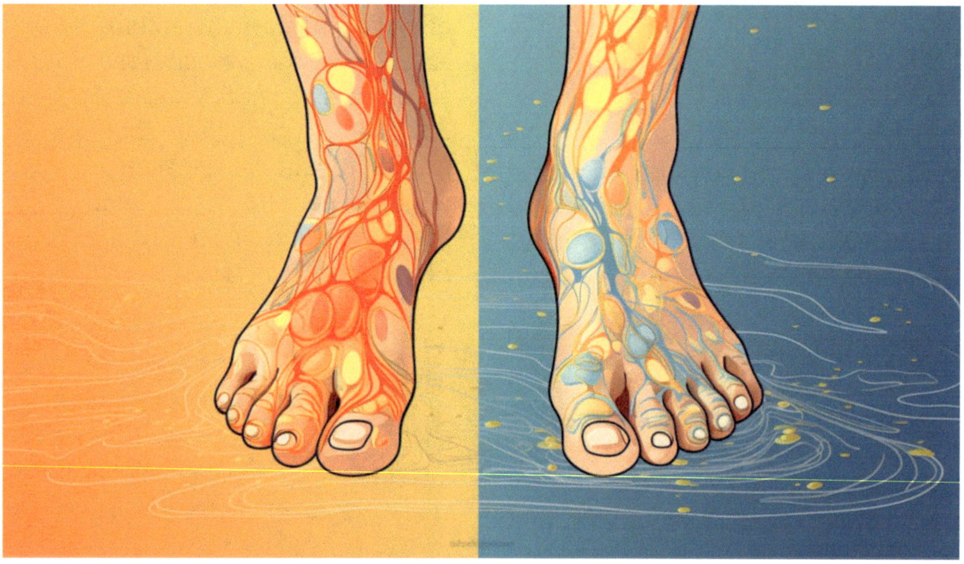

Figure 12.13. Muscle weakness is a prominent and debilitating symptom experienced by individuals suffering from diabetic neuropathy, a condition resulting from prolonged high blood sugar levels that affect nerve function.

Source: https://www.mountain-ice.com/cdn/shop/articles/00-what-causes-neuropathy-in-feet_1024x1024.jpg?v=1690892056

Dysregulation of nerve signaling can impede motor functions, leading to diminished muscle activation and strength, a concept evident in findings related to chemotherapeutic neuropathy, which also emphasizes the role of exercise rehabilitation to counteract such detrimental effects (Drury et al., 2012). Thus, it appears that similar approaches might help people suffering from diabetic neuropathy. A regular exercise routine is meant to keep muscles strong and also to assist the brain and nervous system in adapting to, fixing, or coping with the damage caused by the condition. That's why a combination of physical activity and other measures could help people with neuromuscular diseases avoid muscle weakness and improve their daily living. Even though exercise can help, dealing with muscle weakness in diabetic neuropathy is often difficult due to the patient's unique situation. Coexisting diseases, reactions to drugs, and not being aware of the right exercises often prevent people from being active. Moreover, neuropathic pain combined with weak muscles makes it challenging to treat patients, since they may be reluctant to take part in exercises that worsen their pain. An understanding of these challenges is critical for tailoring interventions that not only consider the physiological aspects of muscle weakness but also the psychological and social dimensions impacting patient compliance and motivation (Bratu et al., 2020). Since research is always advancing, it is more important than ever to create strategies that help patients fight muscle weakness and improve their lives and health with diabetic neuropathy (Figure 12.13).

12.4. Diagnosis of Diabetic Neuropathy

When diagnosing diabetic neuropathy, doctors must review the patient's health history, note the symptoms, and perform the required tests. Mostly, healthcare providers begin the process by looking at a patient's medical history, concentrating on how long diabetes has been present, how well blood sugar is controlled, and if the patient has any neuropathic symptoms in their extremities. Following this, a detailed clinical exam is done, which usually involves checking reflexes, strength of muscles, and sensory abilities.

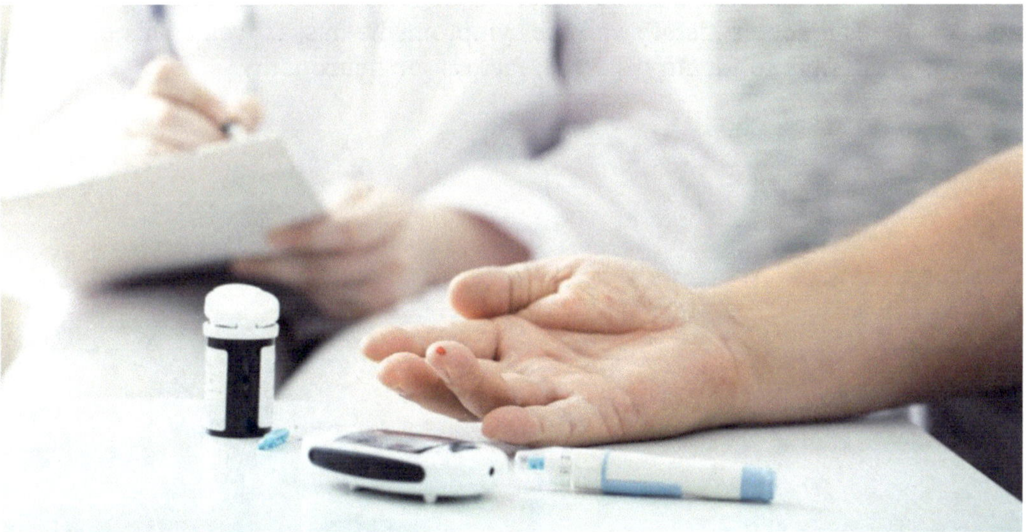

Figure 12.14. Primarily, healthcare providers initiate the diagnostic process by assessing patients' medical histories, focusing on the duration of diabetes, glycemic control, and the presence of neuropathic symptoms such as pain, tingling, or numbness in the extremities.

Source: https://lonestarneurology.net/wp-content/uploads/2022/05/5-Treatment-of-diabetic-neuropathy.jpg

These steps are vital since they make it possible to identify neuropathy correctly and tell it apart from similar conditions. Electrophysiological tests are very important for improving the diagnosis of diabetic neuropathy. They measure how well nerves carry electrical signals and can show the levels of both sensory and motor functions. Techniques like nerve conduction studies (NCS) and electromyography (EMG) help clinicians determine the extent and type of nerve damage, providing valuable information on whether the condition is primarily peripheral or autonomic. Such tools are especially useful for telling diabetic neuropathy apart from other neuropathies, including carpal tunnel syndrome, which is widespread among diabetics. (Zimmerman et al., 2022) highlights how a careful evaluation can reveal specific nerve compression issues that may coexist with diabetic neuropathy, underscoring the need for comprehensive diagnostic approaches. It is also necessary to link symptoms, diagnostic results, and what the patient says to plan the best treatment. Pain or numbness in the body usually leads to more tests to find out how much neuropathy is affecting the patient's life. As indicated in Ziegler et al. (2021), understanding the complications and mechanisms of diabetic neuropathy aids in tailoring interventions that can significantly enhance patient outcomes. It is necessary to keep an eye on patients and review their treatment plan as they go through therapy. By using this approach, it is clear that accurate diagnosis forms the base for successful management of diabetic neuropathy (Figure 12.14).

12.4.1. Medical History and Physical Examination

The medical history is necessary for diagnosing diabetic neuropathy because it gives important information about the patient's diabetes and its development. It is very important to review the duration and treatment of diabetes mellitus in the patient's medical history. For instance, John is a 62-year-old man who has had type 2 diabetes for seven years and has recently gotten a foot ulcer. Taking into account his diabetes history and the symptoms he has, as well as his use of metformin and gliclazide, it is possible to identify the risk factors for neuropathy.

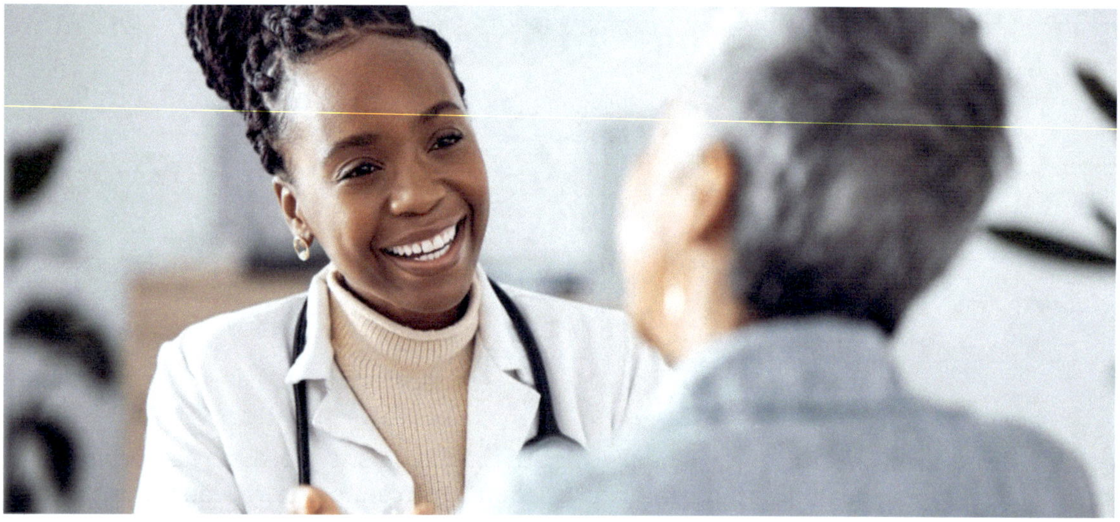

Figure 12.15. The medical history is a critical component in diagnosing diabetic neuropathy, as it provides insights into the patient's background and progression of diabetes.

Source: https://painandspinespecialists.com/wp-content/uploads/What-Is-the-Best-Treatment-for-Diabetic-Neuropathy.jpeg

Accurately gathering data about dietary habits, physical activity, previous neurological symptoms, and comorbidities allows healthcare professionals to construct a comprehensive picture that is crucial for evaluating the likelihood of neuropathy and guiding management decisions, leading to improved patient outcomes (Gabriele et al., 2008). Besides the medical history, carefully examining the patient's body is crucial for checking diabetic neuropathy. Usually, this assessment focuses on the patient's feelings, movements, and reflexes. Testing with monofilaments and tuning forks helps to measure how much sensory loss a person has. The use of standardized measures like the VA Neuropathy Scale (VANS) also significantly enhances the reliability of the assessment process. A study that discusses telemedicine protocols reveals that the VANS can assess patients' neuropathic status using both in-person and remote examinations, so it can be used in many different medical settings. By integrating these examination techniques, clinicians can better detect subtle changes in nerve function, ultimately leading to timely interventions that can prevent further complications (Jamal et al., 2019). It is important to combine a patient's medical history with a physical examination to develop a good management plan for diabetic neuropathy. If healthcare providers know the patient's history and check their current condition, they can plan the best treatment strategies. It may be necessary to keep checking for neuropathic symptoms and adjust the treatment plan according to the results of the first assessments. When this information is combined, it encourages healthcare teams to discuss the case with dietitians, endocrinologists, and podiatrists. When doctors and specialists join forces, it helps patients stick to their treatment plans. A complete medical history and thorough physical examination help in identifying the condition and managing diabetic neuropathy well, so patients face less risk of serious complications and enjoy a better quality of life (Figure 12.15).

12.4.2. Nerve Conduction Studies

Nerve conduction studies (NCS) serve as a pivotal diagnostic tool in the evaluation of diabetic neuropathy, a common complication resulting from prolonged hyperglycemia. They look at the health and performance of peripheral nerves by measuring the rate and effectiveness of electrical signals in them. In those with diabetes, the presence of neuropathy is usually linked to slower nerve conduction, which may mean there is demyelination or degeneration of nerves. When motor and sensory nerves are systematically checked, doctors can find out the type of neuropathy and decide on the right treatment. Also, when NCS is used along with clinical assessments, it helps clinicians make a correct diagnosis and manage patients' symptoms to avoid complications from nerve damage. NCS is useful not only for diagnosis but also for checking how the disease develops and how a patient responds to treatment.

NCS is especially important for learning how severe the nerve damage is and for checking if different treatments are effective. In obese Zucker rats, for example, research has proven that AVE7688 can greatly enhance nerve conduction and blood vessel function, which shows that these two systems are connected. These findings point out that NCS is crucial for both understanding the neuropathy and assessing whether medications can help improve the condition and enhance patients' lives. Thanks to new developments in NCS and a better understanding of how diabetic neuropathy works, doctors can now use personalized treatments. Studies on the vasa nervorum are making it clearer that nerve blood supply is important for the health of neurons. The fact that blood vessels near nerves are innervated by nitrergic fibers shows that more attention is being given to the relationship between nerves and blood vessels. Clinical use of these findings could help NCS work better and encourage new treatments for diabetic neuropathy, which is important for improving patient outcomes (Figure 12.16).

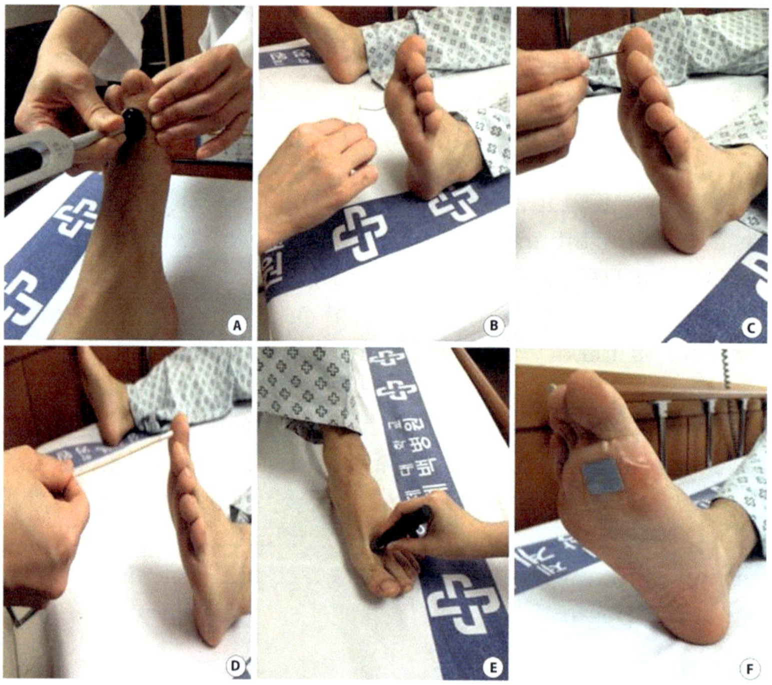

Figure 12.16. Nerve conduction studies (NCS) serve as a pivotal diagnostic tool in the evaluation of diabetic neuropathy, a common complication resulting from prolonged hyperglycemia.

Source: https://www.e-enm.org/upload/thumbnails/enm-31-230-g001.jpg

12.4.3. Blood Tests

It is very important to set up effective ways to monitor diabetic neuropathy, since detecting it early can improve treatment results. Blood tests are essential because they give important details about blood sugar levels that are necessary for preventing and dealing with diabetic problems. Specifically, hemoglobin A1c (HbA1c) levels serve as a benchmark for assessing long-term blood glucose concentrations. Having elevated HbA1c values is often linked to the advancement of neuropathy, showing that good management of blood sugar is very important. In addition to HbA1c, measuring fasting plasma glucose and postprandial levels aids in evaluating short-term glycemic variability, which has garnered attention for its potential role in the onset and acceleration of diabetic complications, including neuropathy and cardiovascular autonomic dysfunction (Helleputte et al., 2020). In addition, detailed blood tests can show other factors that increase the risk of diabetic neuropathy. These tests can be lipid profiles, renal function assessments, and inflammatory markers, and all of them can provide more information about a patient's health in relation to diabetes. In fact, dyslipidemia is common in people with diabetes and is thought to increase the risk of neuropathy, probably because it causes vascular issues. It is also important to check blood urea nitrogen and creatinine levels, since diabetic nephropathy usually occurs with diabetic neuropathy. Assessing these parameters helps healthcare providers develop a more nuanced treatment plan, targeting not only blood glucose but also other metabolic disruptions that may exacerbate neuropathic conditions (Scheen et al., 2011). Since diabetes can be very different from one person to another, interpreting blood test results for diabetic patients is not simple. For example, type 1 diabetes mellitus (T1DM) can show distinct patterns in glycemic variability and its relationship to neuropathic progression, particularly cardiovascular autonomic neuropathy (Helleputte et al., 2020). Researchers believe that T1DM patients can experience big changes in blood glucose, which may lead to autonomic dysfunction and make their condition more complex. Checking blood tests regularly can help spot trends that point out people who may be at risk. Furthermore, as patient management strategies evolve, incorporating continuous glucose monitoring can enhance the precision of glycemic assessments, fostering a more proactive approach to preventing and managing diabetic neuropathy and its cardiovascular implications (Scheen et al., 2011) (Figure 12.17).

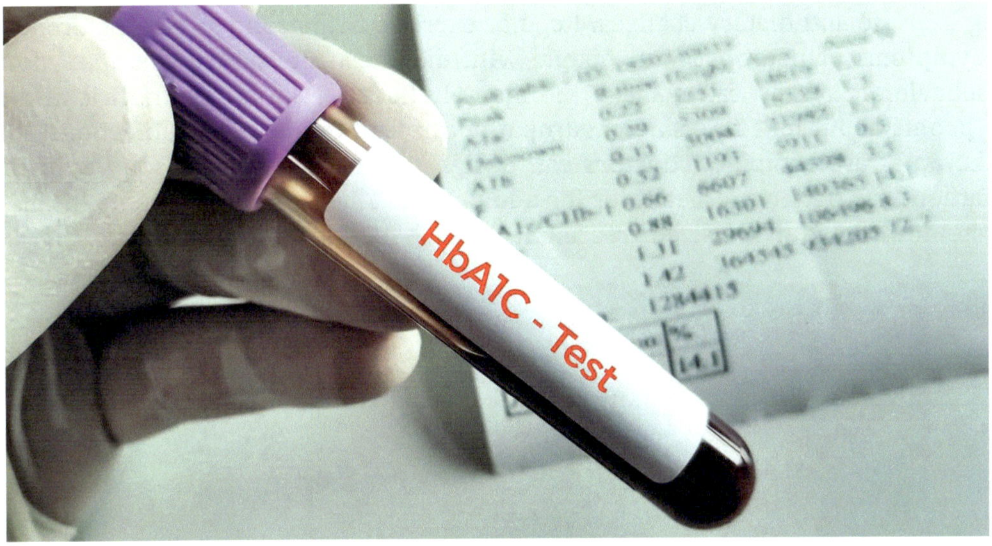

Figure 12.17. Blood tests are integral to this strategy as they provide vital information regarding glycemic control, which is paramount in preventing and managing diabetic complications.

Source: https://www.apexhospitals.com/_next/image?url=https%3A%2F%2Fbed.apexhospitals.com%2Fuploads%2FHb_A1_C2_89628bd108.jpg&w=1920&q=75

12.5. Treatment Options

Managing diabetic neuropathy requires using several approaches to relieve symptoms and improve the patient's life. Both medicine and non-medication methods are used in treatment, depending on the person's condition and how they react to therapy. Sometimes, the first step is to give patients oral drugs such as antidepressants and anticonvulsants, which have been proven to help relieve neuropathic pain. Even so, a lot of patients do not get full relief from these initial therapies, which is why extra treatment options are needed. With the progress of medical technology, new ways to handle diabetes have appeared, making traditional methods better. The integration of technology in treatment regimens offers promising benefits, as highlighted by current evaluations on cost, quality implications, and effectiveness in managing diabetic complications, thereby extending care beyond conventional methods (Middleton et al., 2007). Topical treatments, which are usually thought of as second choices, are now recognized as useful in treating diabetic neuropathy. New findings indicate that these drugs, once used only after other options, may be effective as the first treatment. Such a change in approach comes from their local use, which often causes less harm to the whole system than oral medicines. Using topical treatments for peripheral neuropathic pain is effective and safer than other options, which is why they are a good choice. With the development of new pain management strategies, it is now clear that these agents are useful for certain groups, so they can serve as alternatives to medicines taken by mouth or through an IV. As noted in recent pharmacologic treatment algorithms, increased awareness around the use of topical treatments may improve treatment adherence and overall patient outcomes in managing diabetic neuropathy (Sommer & Cruccu, 2017). Also, non-medication approaches are important parts of treating diabetic neuropathy. Some of these approaches are physical therapy, acupuncture, and making exercise and dietary changes. Regular exercise helps control blood glucose levels and eases the symptoms of neuropathy in people with diabetes. Alternative therapies, for example, cognitive-behavioral therapy, can manage the mental effects of chronic pain. It is also necessary to educate people about foot care since neuropathy can lead to ulcers and infections. When these different therapies are combined, doctors can design a custom plan that soothes pain and also helps the patient live better and healthier for a long time. The different elements in this approach point out the need for individualized treatment for diabetic neuropathy (Figure 12.18).

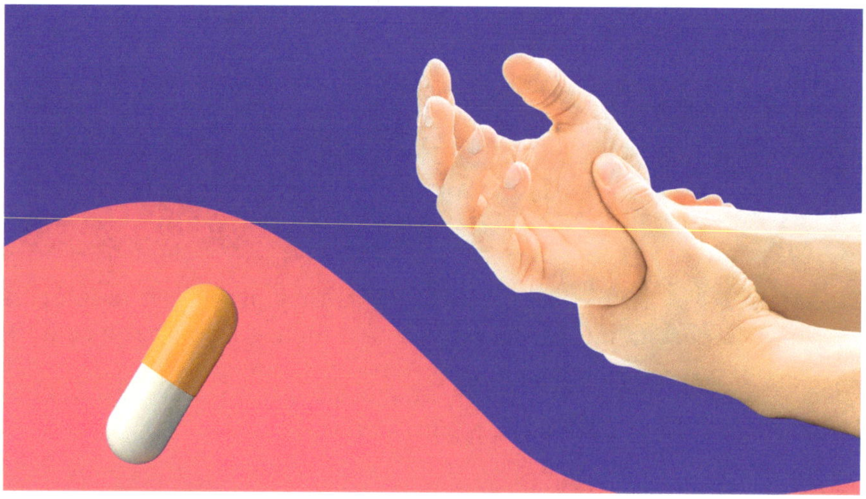

Figure 12.18. Initial management may include oral medications such as antidepressants and anticonvulsants, which have shown efficacy in reducing neuropathic pain.

Source: https://www.singlecare.com/blog/wp-content/uploads/2024/01/Blog_011624_TK_Medication_for_Nerve_Pain_2w.webp

12.5.1. Blood Sugar Management

Taking care of blood sugar is essential to avoid complications of diabetes, especially diabetic neuropathy. Higher blood glucose levels may cause nerve damage because of oxidative stress and inflammation, both of which are mainly due to problems with mitochondria. Diabetes increases the production of reactive oxygen species (ROS) in cellular mitochondria, promoting neurodegeneration over time. So, when blood sugar is maintained within the target range, it reduces the person's symptoms and the risk of nerve damage. This way of treating diabetes includes making healthy changes to diet and exercise, as well as using medications that are right for each patient. These strategies help improve the lives of diabetics and prevent future complications, for example, diabetic neuropathy. Improvements in diabetes technology have highlighted the need to always check and monitor blood glucose levels so that proper actions can be taken quickly. Automation in diabetes care has helped monitor blood sugar levels and ensure insulin is given in the best way. Because of these strategies, patients are encouraged to participate in their care, which helps them stay healthier and avoid serious issues. In addition, research shows that these programs boost diabetes care by supplying patients with personal advice and learning materials. When these tools are used in regular care, doctors can help patients control their blood sugar and, as a result, reduce the chances of painful diabetic neuropathy. As a result, the merging of technology and traditional management practices may lead to better patient results. Besides, learning about the biochemical changes caused by long-term high blood sugar gives important advice for managing diabetic neuropathy. High blood sugar for a long time can worsen problems in the mitochondria, which is considered a factor in nerve disorders linked to diabetes. Problems with mitochondria can result in too much oxidative stress, which may damage the nervous system. Hence, plans for blood sugar management should also pay attention to the impact on mitochondria for a more effective treatment approach. There are not many drugs that address these pathways, which shows why further research is necessary. As such, emphasizing holistic approaches that incorporate both glycemic control and mitochondrial health may yield significant benefits in the management of diabetic neuropathy, promoting nerve repair and regeneration alongside improved blood sugar stabilization, as discussed in the literature (Kasinathan et al., 2013) (Figure 12.19).

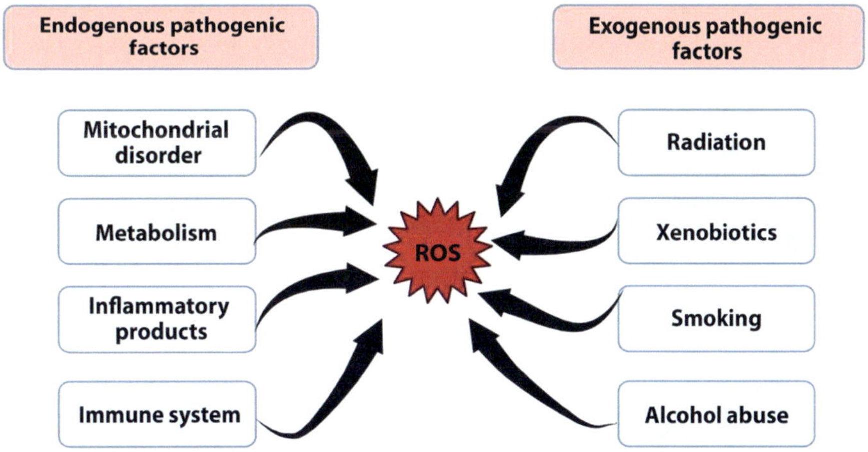

Figure 12.19. Diabetes increases the production of reactive oxygen species (ROS) in cellular mitochondria, promoting neurodegeneration over time.

Source: Zhang Z, Huang Q, Zhao D, Lian F, Li X and Qi W (2023) The impact of oxidative stress-induced mitochondrial dysfunction on diabetic microvascular complications. Front. Endocrinol. 14:1112363. doi: 10.3389/fendo.2023.1112363

12.5.2. Medications for Pain Relief

It is very hard to manage pain caused by diabetic neuropathy since neuropathic pain is so complex. Many patients do not get enough pain relief from common painkillers, so it becomes necessary to try medicines that work on neuropathic pathways. Many types of drugs have been found to help deal with this type of pain. Tricyclic antidepressants affect the levels of neurotransmitters in the brain and are proven to help by stopping pain signals. Moreover, gabapentin and pregabalin are anticonvulsants that work on calcium channels to limit the activity of pain-carrying nerves. However, the nuanced pathophysiology of neuropathic pain complicates treatment strategies, rendering complete symptom relief an elusive goal for many patients, as indicated in the literature about the limitations of current therapeutic approaches (Mutiawati et al., 2015). More people are starting to recognize topical treatments as a type of therapy that could help people with diabetic neuropathy. In the past, these drugs were used after others, but now, experts suggest using them first because they act locally and have few side effects on the body. Capsaicin and lidocaine patches are applied to the affected area to treat pain, so the drugs are delivered only to the injured nerves and not to the whole body. Such treatments are appealing to patients who react badly to standard medicines because they have a lower risk of affecting the whole body. Furthermore, the evolving pharmacologic treatment algorithms underscore the necessity of adapting pain management strategies to incorporate topical agents, which could lead to enhanced therapeutic outcomes for those suffering from diabetic neuropathic pain (Sommer & Cruccu, 2017). To summarize, managing pain in diabetic neuropathy requires knowing about both oral and topical medicines. Even though traditional analgesics can help, they are not always very effective, which is why using different methods is important. The addition of anticonvulsants and topical treatments to the treatment plan offers a better way to control pain in diabetic neuropathy patients. In the end, using a personalized method that matches treatments to each patient's needs will increase the success of pain management. Recognizing the variety in neuropathic pain treatment allows doctors to come up with personalized approaches that greatly improve the lives of their patients (Figure 12.20).

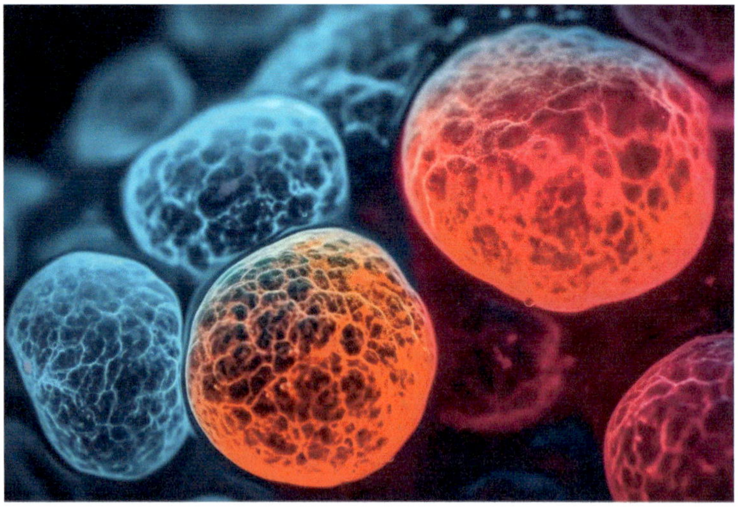

Figure 12.20. Patients often experience inadequate relief from conventional analgesics, necessitating the exploration of medications specifically targeting neuropathic pathways.

Source: https://cdn.prod.website-files.com/5d9667bad4a41e222995e15b/650afdcba859044500d6deb9_a.webp

12.5.3. Lifestyle Modifications

Managing diabetic neuropathy well involves making changes to lifestyle and using other approaches at the same time. There is no doubt that lifestyle has a major effect on diabetic complications, especially since hyperglycemia can damage nerves. Eating a balanced diet with mostly whole foods helps people control their blood sugar levels, which lowers the risk of developing and worsening neuropathy. A diet low in processed sugars and saturated fats supports stable blood glucose levels and minimizes oxidative stress, an essential factor in nerve damage, as indicated by Prabhakar (2024). Also, by regularly checking how much carbohydrate is eaten, dietary results can be improved, which benefits both the body and the quality of life for people with diabetes. Being physically active is another important change that helps control diabetes and lessen neuropathy. Doing aerobics and resistance exercises regularly can make your blood flow better, make your body more responsive to insulin, and support your metabolism. Studies have shown that consistent exercise not only aids in weight management but also reduces the severity of peripheral nerve damage, as outlined in Prabhakar (2024). Additionally, exercise helps reduce stress and lifts the mood, which matters a lot for diabetes patients, who may face mental health problems. Therefore, having a suitable exercise routine that fits each person's abilities tackles the problems of diabetic neuropathy and encourages overall diabetes management. It is also very important for patients to understand how to manage their condition on their own. Those who are informed about their health issue and its possible problems are more likely to take care of their health. It is important to have regular foot care to avoid problems caused by neuropathy. According to studies, wearing the right shoes and checking them each day helps prevent injuries that people with less feeling may miss. Moreover, ongoing communication with healthcare providers ensures personalized care planning and ongoing support, which is vital in addressing the complex nature of diabetic neuropathy, as emphasized in Hajduk-Maślak et al. (2024). All of these changes together help people with diabetes become healthier and happier (Figure 12.21).

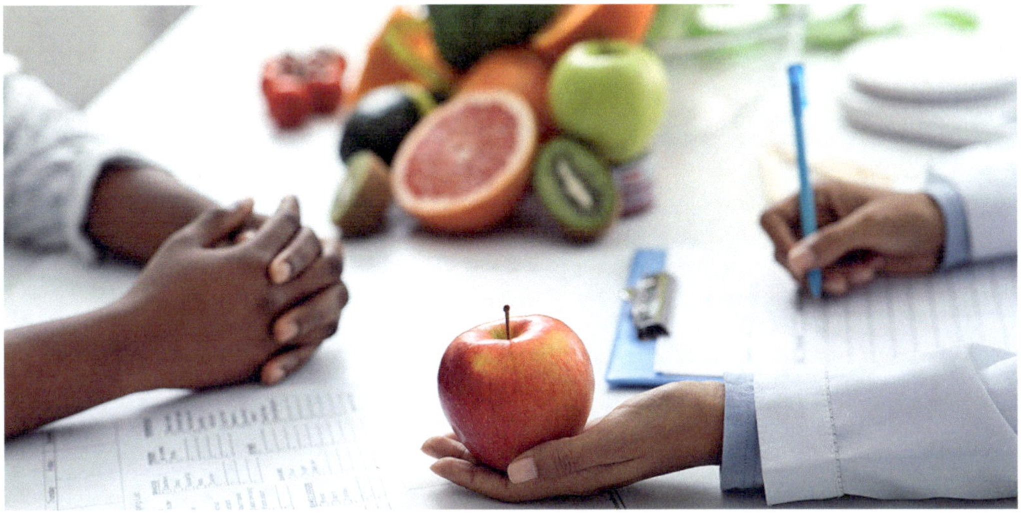

Figure 12.21. By adopting a balanced diet rich in whole foods, individuals can achieve better glycemic control, thereby reducing the risk of neuropathy onset and progression.

Source: https://irp.cdn-website.com/056e16c2/dms3rep/multi/Nutrition-Counseling.png

A CLOSER LOOK

CHARCOT FOOT

Charcot foot is a condition that damages the bones, joints, and soft tissues of the foot and usually affects people with peripheral neuropathy, especially those with diabetes. Since they cannot sense pain, patients with nerve damage often suffer from repeated injuries to their feet. With time, this results in inflammation, weak bones, and changes in the foot's shape, which can cause it to swell, redden, and become warm, and the structure of the foot may collapse. If treatment and immobilization start early, it is much less likely that the patient will develop severe deformity, ulcers, or face the risk of amputation.

Summary

Since diabetic neuropathy can be very complicated, it is important to use comprehensive methods to control and prevent it. Since neuropathy is a serious complication of diabetes, it requires paying attention to blood sugar levels and also to changes in blood sugar. Research indicates that maintaining rigorous glycemic control is paramount for patients, particularly those with type 1 diabetes mellitus (T1DM), to prevent the onset of diabetic complications, including neuropathy (Helleputte et al., 2020). As it becomes clear that glycemic variability can affect the heart's nervous system, more research is needed to find out if such changes in blood sugar can worsen nerve damage. Such knowledge can guide clinicians in designing treatment plans that control blood sugar and handle all the complications of diabetes. In addition, managing diabetes and mental health is important when considering diabetic neuropathy. Studies reveal a concerning link between depression in individuals with type 2 diabetes and poor glycemic control, which subsequently aggravates neuropathic symptoms and related complications (Chan et al., 2015). This relationship points out that taking care of mental health is necessary in diabetes care since it influences both self-management and the development of the disease. If practitioners help patients with depression and teach them about diabetes care and healthy habits, the results for patients can be better. Taking care of emotional, psychological, and physical health at the same time is likely to help more in dealing with diabetic neuropathy. To sum up, educating people about preventing and managing diabetic neuropathy helps improve the health of the public. If health workers encourage screening and inform patients about the benefits of controlling their blood sugar levels, individuals will be able to care for their health better. When healthcare professionals such as endocrinologists, psychologists, and educators team up, they can manage diabetic neuropathy more effectively due to its many causes. Since our knowledge of this condition grows, it is important to keep researching and advocating for successful intervention methods. As a result, the healthcare community can lessen the effects of diabetic neuropathy and raise the standard of living for those who have it.

To know about diabetic neuropathy, it is essential to see how many aspects it has and what effects it has on patients and healthcare providers. Diabetic neuropathy is a major problem in diabetes mellitus, involving nerve damage that can be seen as peripheral neuropathy and other forms. As a result of this form, people experience pain, tingling, and numbness in their limbs. Keeping glycemic levels under control is very important since it is necessary for avoiding diabetes complications, including neuropathy and heart problems caused by autonomic dysfunction. Research indicates that not only are stable glycemic levels vital, but also managing fluctuations in blood glucose, as excessive glucose variability may worsen the onset and progression of complications, including diabetic neuropathy and cardiovascular autonomic neuropathy, thus highlighting a broader approach to treatment strategies (Helleputte et al., 2020). Another key point in the discussion of diabetic neuropathy is the rising concern surrounding comorbid conditions, such as Charcot neuroarthropathy (CN). Even though this complication is less frequent than peripheral neuropathy, it causes joint degeneration mainly in the foot and is closely related to neuropathy, weak bones, and inflammation. Many times, CN is not recognized at first because it looks like other common problems in diabetics. Since the disease can appear in many ways, thorough examinations by doctors are important to catch it early. The main goal of traditional care is to take pressure off the affected limb to stop further changes and improve the results. Nonetheless, emerging research into potential therapies, such as bisphosphonates and calcitonin, opens the door to more effective management approaches for CN as a related complication of diabetic neuropathy (Vella & Cachia, 2008). The fact that diabetic neuropathy is quite complex points to the need for a team approach in its treatment. It is important for health care providers to control blood sugar, teach patients, identify complications early, and help with lifestyle changes. It is important for patients to realize how important it is to have regular foot exams and look after their feet to avoid neuropathy risks. Specialists like endocrinologists, podiatrists, and pain management doctors need to cooperate to handle the many complications caused by diabetic neuropathy. A complete approach to treatment by healthcare providers can improve the life of a patient, lower the chance of major complications, and help people with diabetes manage their condition better.

References

1. Abbott, C. A., Attal, N., Barrett, A. M., Barrett, D. A., Berghöfer, B., Bettoni, L., Callaghan, B. C., et al. (2015). A genome-wide association study provides evidence of sex-specific involvement of Chr1p35.1 (*ZSCAN20-TLR12P*) and Chr8p23.1 (*HMGB1P46*) with diabetic neuropathic pain. https://core.ac.uk/download/30664462.pdf (accessed on 11th June 2025).
2. Abdillah, S., Keban, S. A., & Najuah, N. (2017). The role of pharmacists in evaluating and intervening the patients with diabetic neuropathy. https://core.ac.uk/download/477852369.pdf (accessed on 11th June 2025).
3. Alessi, E., Balducci, S., Bollanti, L., Conti, L., et al. (2017). Correlates of calcaneal quantitative ultrasound parameters in patients with diabetes: The study on the assessment of determinants of muscle and bone strength abnormalities in diabetes. https://core.ac.uk/download/141696868.pdf (accessed on 11th June 2025).
4. Alsaad, S., Binmoammar, T., Hassounah, S. O. A., Majeed, R., et al. (2015). The impact of poor glycemic control on the prevalence of erectile dysfunction in men with type 2 diabetes mellitus: A systematic review. https://core.ac.uk/download/77006748.pdf (accessed on 11th June 2025).
5. Ames, J. P., Andersson, H., Appenzeller, B. M. R., Asif Muneer, A., Benesova, M., Cameron, N. E., et al. (2013). Vasa nervorum in rat major pelvic ganglion are innervated by nitrergic nerve fibers. https://core.ac.uk/download/74409974.pdf (accessed on 11th June 2025).
6. Aquilina, J., Cefai, E., & Mallia, M. (2015). A review on the investigation of peripheral neuropathy at Mater Dei Hospital. https://core.ac.uk/download/46603552.pdf (accessed on 11th June 2025).
7. Arent, S., Bruyere, S. M., & Dickson, M. B. (2001). Employment considerations for people who have diabetes. https://core.ac.uk/download/5124470.pdf (accessed on 11th June 2025).
8. Barn, R., Bus, S. A., Nollet, F., Waaijman, R., et al. (2015). Predictors of barefoot plantar pressure during walking in patients with diabetes, peripheral neuropathy and a history of ulceration. https://core.ac.uk/download/293883531.pdf (accessed on 11th June 2025).
9. Bratu, O. G., Bungau, S., Spinu Arsenie, D., Gherghiceanu, M., et al. (2020). Underactive bladder – an underestimated entity. https://core.ac.uk/download/304672906.pdf (accessed on 11th June 2025).
10. Bullen, B. (2020). Understanding what it means to be "Charcot foot health literate." https://core.ac.uk/download/287586292.pdf (accessed on 11th June 2025).
11. Vella, S. & Cachia, M. J., (2008). Charcot neuroarthropathy: Pathogenesis, diagnosis and medical management. Malta Medical Journal Volume 20 Issue 03 September 2008. https://core.ac.uk/download/46602192.pdf (accessed on 11th June 2025).
12. Helleputte, S., De Backer, T., Lapauw, B., Shadid, S., Celie, B., Van Eetvelde, B., Vanden Wyngaert, K., & Calders, P. (2020). The relationship between glycaemic variability and cardiovascular autonomic dysfunction in patients with type 1 diabetes: A systematic review. *Diabetes/metabolism research and reviews*, *36*(5), e3301. https://doi.org/10.1002/dmrr.3301(accessed on 11th June 2025).

13. Calligaro, K. D., Padberg, F. T., & Sidawy, A. N. (2008). Complications of arteriovenous hemodialysis access: Recognition and management. https://core.ac.uk/download/pdf/82369420.pdf (accessed on 11th June 2025).
14. Cappuccio, F., Ceriello, A., Genovese, S., Schnell, O., et al. (2013). Type 1 diabetes and cardiovascular disease. https://core.ac.uk/download/19553374.pdf (accessed on 11th June 2025).
15. Chan, J. C. N., China Depression in Chinese Patients with Type 2 Diabetes (DD2) Study Group, Guo, X., Ji, L., et al. (2015). Depression in Chinese patients with type 2 diabetes: Associations with hyperglycemia, hypoglycemia, and poor treatment adherence. https://core.ac.uk/download/323079139.pdf (accessed on 11th June 2025).
16. Chaturvedi, N., Eaton, S. E. M., Fuller, J. H., Ionescu-Tirgoviste, C., et al. (2005). Vascular risk factors and diabetic neuropathy. https://core.ac.uk/download/1674684.pdf (accessed on 11th June 2025).
17. Coppey, L. J., Davidson, E. P., Kleinschmidt, T. L., Oltman, C. L., et al. (2009). Vascular and neural dysfunctions in obese Zucker rats: Effect of AVE7688. https://core.ac.uk/download/pdf/8296669.pdf (accessed on 11th June 2025).
18. Cox, A. (2015). Thermal burns and smoke inhalation injuries. https://core.ac.uk/download/58826490.pdf (accessed on 11th June 2025).
19. Sommer, C., & Cruccu, G. (2017). Topical Treatment of Peripheral Neuropathic Pain: Applying the Evidence. *Journal of pain and symptom management*, *53*(3), 614–629. https://doi.org/10.1016/j.jpainsymman.2016.09.015(accessed on 11th June 2025).
20. De Gabriele, R. (2008). Assessment and management of diabetic ulcers in the primary health care setting. https://core.ac.uk/download/46602206.pdf (accessed on 11th June 2025).
21. De Marchis, M., D'Amato, A., Fedele, F., Mancone, M., et al. (2018). Diabetes mellitus and ischemic heart disease: The role of ion channels. https://core.ac.uk/download/159269109.pdf (accessed on 11th June 2025).
22. Defeudis, G., Di Emidio, C., Gianfrilli, D., Lenzi, A., et al. (2015). Erectile dysfunction and its management in patients with diabetes mellitus. https://core.ac.uk/download/54528262.pdf (accessed on 11th June 2025).
23. Derakhshanpour, F., Farsinia, M., Mirkarimi, K., Vakili, R., et al. (2015). Depression and quality of life in patients with type 2 diabetes. https://core.ac.uk/download/52205715.pdf (accessed on 11th June 2025).
24. Drury, D. G., & Wonders, K. Y. (2012). Current exercise behaviors of breast cancer patients diagnosed with chemotherapy-induced peripheral neuropathy. https://cupola.gettysburg.edu/cgi/viewcontent.cgi?article=1016&context=healthfac (accessed on 11th June 2025).
25. Hajduk-Maślak, K., Skóra, A., Galasińska, I., Michalik, B., Szypuła, A., & Sęk, M. (2024). Comprehensive Approach to Diabetic Neuropathy - A Review of the Latest Reports. *Journal of Education, Health and Sport, 62*, 107–128. https://doi.org/10.12775/JEHS.2024.62.007(accessed on 11th June 2025).
26. Grafe, P., Niedermeier, W., & Schneider, U. (1993). The paradox between resistance to hypoxia and liability to hypoxic damage in hyperglycemic peripheral nerves: Evidence for glycolysis involvement. https://core.ac.uk/download/12166407.pdf (accessed on 11th June 2025).

27. Kautzky-Willer, A., Stich, K., Hintersteiner, J., Kautzky, A., Kamyar, M. R., Saukel, J., Johnson, J., & Lemmens-Gruber, R. (2013). Sex-specific-differences in cardiometabolic risk in type 1 diabetes: a cross-sectional study. *Cardiovascular diabetology, 12*, 78. https://doi.org/10.1186/1475-2840-12-78(accessed on 11th June 2025).

28. Ho, T. K., Leigh, R. D., & Tsui, J. (2013). Diabetic foot disease and oedema. https://core.ac.uk/download/16219516.pdf (accessed on 11th June 2025).

29. Mutiawati, Endang, et al. "Pharmacologic Aspect of Neuropathic Pain." *5th Syiah Kuala University Annual International Conference 2015, Banda Aceh, Indonesia, October 2015*. Syiah Kuala University, 2015.(accessed on 11th June 2025).

30. Iqbal, N., Naz, L., Qadir, A., Sohail, S., et al. (2019). Prevalence of risk factors promoting diabetic neuropathy. https://core.ac.uk/download/227035138.pdf (accessed on 11th June 2025).

31. Jamal, N. I., Ong, M. K., Saliba, D., Wilson, C., et al. (2019). The Veterans Affairs Neuropathy Scale: A reliable, remote polyneuropathy exam. https://core.ac.uk/download/323076264.pdf (accessed on 11th June 2025).

32. Kasinathan, D., Marimuthu, P. N., & Ramar, M. (2013). Type 2 diabetic neuropathy with special reference to mitochondrial role and its effective management. https://core.ac.uk/download/236012234.pdf (accessed on 11th June 2025).

33. McIntosh, C., & Newton, V. (2008). Neuropathy—Gait changes in the diabetic foot. https://core.ac.uk/download/1652029.pdf (accessed on 11th June 2025).

34. Middleton, B., Cusack, C. M., Kendrick, D., Bates, D. W., Bu, D., Johnston, D., Pan, E., et al. (2007). The value of information technology-enabled diabetes management. https://core.ac.uk/download/71355637.pdf (accessed on 11th June 2025).

35. P. K. Prabhakar. Glucose to Complications: Understanding Secondary Effects in Diabetes Mellitus. Sumat. Med. J. [Internet]. 2024May1 [cited 2025Jul.23];7(2):87-95. Available from: https://talenta.usu.ac.id/smj/article/view/15998 (accessed on 11th June 2025).

36. Scheen, A. J., Gaede, P., Giugliano, D., Group, E., Hanson, U., Imholz, B., Philips, J. C., et al. (2011). Squatting, a posture test for studying cardiovascular autonomic neuropathy in diabetes. http://orbi.ulg.ac.be/bitstream/2268/107366/1/Squatting%2c%20a%20posture%20test%20for%20studying%20cardiovascular%20autonomic%20neuropathy%5bOCR%5d.pdf (accessed on 11th June 2025).

37. Surve, P. P. R., Shinde, R. B., Rathod, S., & Kadu, V. P. (2019). Concept of diabetic neuropathy and its management in Ayurveda. https://core.ac.uk/download/478521450.pdf (accessed on 11th June 2025).

38. Ziegler, D., Keller, J., Maier, C., & Pannek, J. (2021). Diabetic Neuropathy. *Experimental and clinical endocrinology & diabetes : official journal, German Society of Endocrinology [and] German Diabetes Association, 129*(S 01), S70–S81. https://doi.org/10.1055/a-1284-6245(accessed on 11th June 2025).

39. Zimmerman, M., Gottsäter, A., & Dahlin, L. (2022). Carpal tunnel syndrome and diabetes—A comprehensive review. *Journal of Clinical Medicine, 11*. https://www.semanticscholar.org/paper/b3ee929311ba4a7da306c28b4e40f562679993f7 (accessed on 11th June 2025).

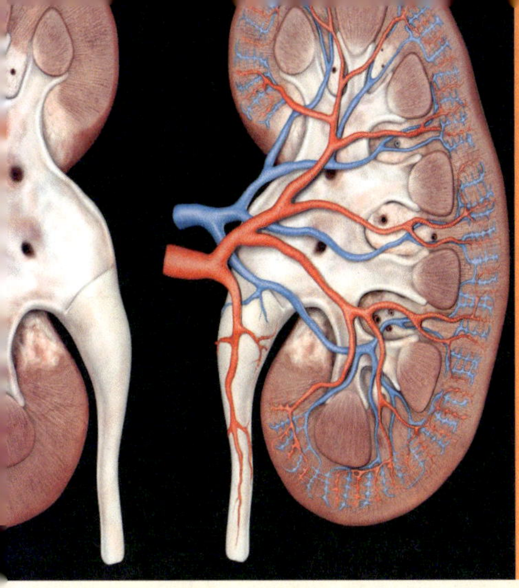

Chapter 13

DIABETIC NEPHROPATHY

Contents

Introduction

Diabetic nephropathy is a major concern for global health because it causes a continuous decline in renal function. When blood sugar remains high over a long time, this condition appears and affects the kidneys' blood flow and metabolism. The kidneys' job in removing waste and keeping fluids balanced makes it clear that these alterations are very serious, because the problems can go beyond the kidneys. The high number of diabetic nephropathy cases shows that it is very important to detect, diagnose, and treat the condition as soon as possible. Current studies point out that knowing the causes of these diseases and developing better ways to diagnose them can improve the care given to those who have them. To summarize, it is very important to study diabetic nephropathy deeply, as this helps both individuals and the public health system, as diabetes keeps increasing worldwide. The latest progress in urinary proteomics has opened up new possibilities for spotting biomarkers related to diabetic nephropathy. Combining capillary electrophoresis with mass spectrometry, researchers are now able to identify urinary protein patterns that show the development of kidney disease. Studies suggest that collagen fragments and serum albumin as biomarkers may be more accurate and sensitive compared to the current ways of detecting diseases. Because of these new techniques, urinary proteomics is very useful for finding diabetic nephropathy, following its progress, and judging the success of treatments. Also, introducing these biomarkers into clinical settings could make decisions more accurate, improving the outcomes for patients. New ways of diagnosing diseases show that precision medicine is becoming more important in treating chronic conditions such as diabetes and its complications such as nephropathy. The relationship between diabetes and diabetic nephropathy shows that many systemic problems are involved and should be studied in detail. Having high blood sugar levels for a long time is closely related to problems such as nerve damage, vascular disease, and a higher chance of heart disease, which adds to the complexity of the patient's health. It is worth noting that erectile dysfunction and diabetes are connected, since they both involve similar processes such as inflammation and problems with the blood vessels. Because of this relationship, it is important to use a variety of treatments and consider any other health problems that may affect the patient's progress. Scientists are still exploring these relations, showing how various diabetic complications are linked and why it's necessary to use a comprehensive approach to treatment. When we learn more about the causes of diabetic nephropathy and similar conditions, we can design treatment plans that address each patient's needs (Figure 13.1).

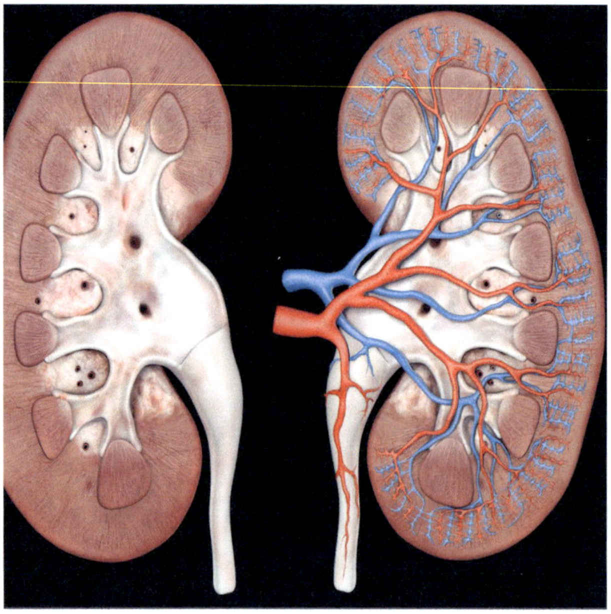

Figure 13.1. Diabetic nephropathy.

Source: https://www.yourcareeverywhere.com/health-research/health-insights/type-2-diabetes/what-is-diabetic-nephropathy-/_jcr_content/content-par/image.coreimg.jpeg/1702994800631/1295842197-.jpeg

13.1. Pathophysiology of Diabetic Nephropathy

Diabetic nephropathy (DN) is a complex disorder primarily arising from chronic hyperglycemia, leading to structural and functional alterations in the kidneys. One of the first signs of DN is that the glomerular filtration barrier becomes more permeable, which causes albuminuria, a main feature of the disease. When there is high blood sugar and changes in blood flow in the kidneys, it helps cause inflammation and oxidative stress, which leads to renal impairment. High amounts of advanced glycation end products and nitric oxide play a big role in damaging the endothelium, which makes renal damage worse. When matrix proteins build up outside the cells, mesangial cells expand and this eventually leads to scarring of the glomeruli. As the kidneys are damaged over time, diabetes causes serious health problems and shows why early treatment and detection are necessary to slow DN. As diabetic nephropathy progresses, tubulointerstitial injury becomes increasingly apparent. In particular, there is less expression of megalin and cubilin, which are necessary for reabsorbing proteins in the renal proximal tubules. It has been found that as DN progresses, the reabsorption of tubular proteins lowers, while more fibrosis and thickening of the tubular basement membrane occur, making the kidney deteriorate further. When a cell is injured, metalloproteases are activated and autophagy markers are changed, which helps in the development of fibrosis and causes cellular apoptosis. The answer indicates that the body's healing process is not normal and causes the gradual loss of nephrons. The implications of these findings point toward the necessity of developing therapeutic approaches that target both glycemic control and tubulointerstitial health in patients at risk for DN, highlighting the multifaceted nature of its pathophysiology (Bahamonde et al., 2017). A crucial aspect of the pathophysiology of diabetic nephropathy is the role of serum and glucocorticoid-regulated kinase-1 (SGK1), which is increasingly recognized for its involvement in renal sodium handling and hypertension associated with diabetes. It has been noted that increased SGK1 expression occurs in various models of diabetes, suggesting it may disturb the movement of sodium in different parts of the kidney. This protein controls the work of important sodium channels and transporters, such as NHE3 and NCC, which help maintain the right balance of sodium and blood pressure. Since SGK1 plays a key role in the development of DN, figuring out how it is regulated by different stimuli might help find new treatments for hypertension and kidney damage in diabetics. This exploration of SGK1s emphasizes the interconnectedness of diabetes-related mechanisms and renal pathophysiology, warranting further investigation to illuminate novel interventions that can alter disease outcomes (Bland et al., 2009) (Figure 13.2).

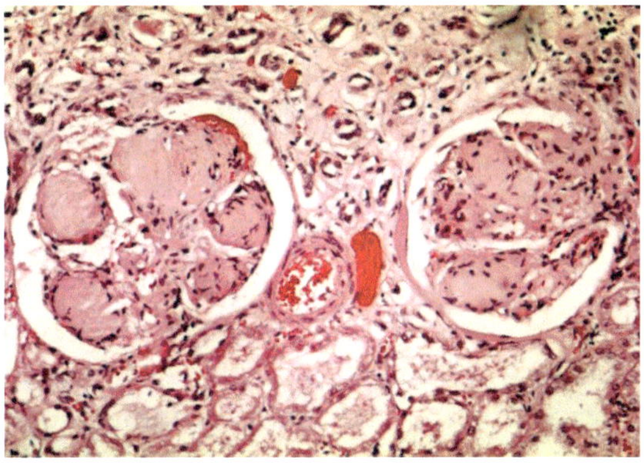

Figure 13.2. Diabetic nephropathy (DN) is a complex disorder primarily arising from chronic hyperglycemia, leading to structural and functional alterations in the kidneys.

Source: https://upload.wikimedia.org/wikipedia/commons/b/b9/Nodular_glomerulosclerosis.jpeg

13.1.1. Mechanisms of Kidney Damage in Diabetes

The development of diabetic nephropathy (DN) is intricately linked to the dysregulation of several cellular mechanisms within the kidneys. An important reason for kidney damage in diabetes is the way protein reabsorption is changed in the renal tubules. A recent study has found that the levels of megalin and cubilin have fallen, since these proteins are important for endocytosis of albumin and other proteins. Because of this, tubulointerstitial injury increases, which causes fibrosis and reduces kidney function. When these transporters decline, it interferes with protein handling and causes more proteins to build up in the tubules, which may cause more harm and inflammation. This underscores how early changes in tubular function can have deleterious implications for overall renal health, establishing a vicious cycle that propels the progression of DN (Bahamonde et al., 2017). Besides, when there is too much sugar in the blood and oxidative stress occurs together, it can lead to kidney damage in people with diabetes.

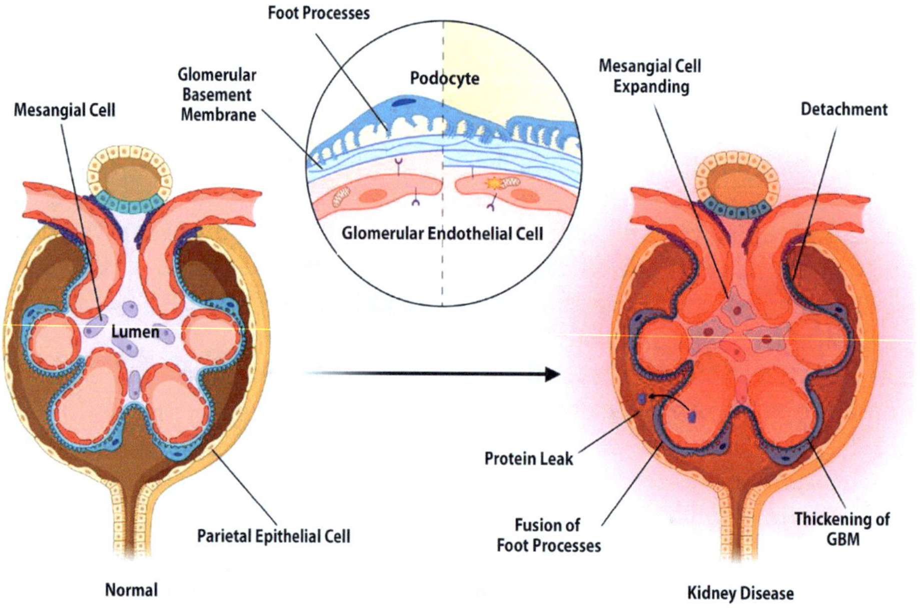

Figure 13.3. The development of diabetic nephropathy (DN) is intricately linked to the dysregulation of several cellular mechanisms within the kidneys.

Source: Deng B, Song A, Zhang C. Cell-Cycle Dysregulation in the Pathogenesis of Diabetic Kidney Disease: An Update. *International Journal of Molecular Sciences.* 2023; 24(3):2133. https://doi.org/10.3390/ijms24032133

Elevated blood glucose levels accelerate the formation of advanced glycation end products (AGEs), which subsequently enhance oxidative damage through the activation of inflammatory pathways. Because of oxidative stress, the podocytes are damaged and the glomerular filtration barrier does not work properly, which causes proteinuria in DN. Moreover, inflammation and the release of cytokines in the kidney worsen the functioning of the glomeruli. Addressing the oxidative stress through dietary interventions and pharmacological agents may offer therapeutic avenues worth exploring to mitigate the detrimental effects of hyperglycemia on kidney tissues, potentially delaying the progression of DN (Iacobini et al., 2017). Besides metabolic problems, what we eat greatly affects the health of our kidneys. New studies point out that changing your diet and the types of protein you eat can help avoid or delay diabetic nephropathy. More people are paying attention to changes such as calorie restriction and choosing which proteins to eat, mainly because eating too much protein may contribute to the worsening of kidney function. Moreover, people are becoming interested in how certain micronutrients could help reduce the kidney problems linked to diabetes. Such dietary approaches, combined with established glucose and blood pressure management strategies, highlight the potential for a holistic management plan that encompasses both metabolic control and nutritional intervention, ultimately contributing to better outcomes in patients with diabetic nephropathy (Iacobini et al., 2017) (Figure 13.3).

13.1.2. Role of Hyperglycemia in Nephropathy Development

It is clear that hyperglycemia, which means high blood sugar, plays a key role in the development of diabetic nephropathy. When hyperglycemia lasts, it causes biochemical changes that eventually harm the kidneys. The main way hyperglycemia leads to nephropathy is by activating the polyol pathway, which changes extra glucose into sorbitol with the help of the enzyme aldose reductase. The conversion of myo-inositol leads to a drop in its levels inside the cells, causing stress in the glomerulus's cells. As a result of stress, the kidneys change, become more permeable, and filter too much blood, which worsens the damage to the kidneys. Furthermore, hyperglycemia is also associated with the formation of advanced glycation end-products (AGEs) that provoke inflammatory responses and fibrosis, further compromising kidney function, a hallmark observed in diabetic nephropathy progression. Furthermore, hyperglycemia causes problems with renal blood flow, which raises the pressure in the kidneys' filtering units. High levels of glucose lead to widening of afferent arterioles and narrowing of efferent arterioles, which causes an increase in glomerular filtration rates. As a result of constant hyperfiltration, the glomeruli get damaged, which causes glomerulosclerosis and more nephron loss.

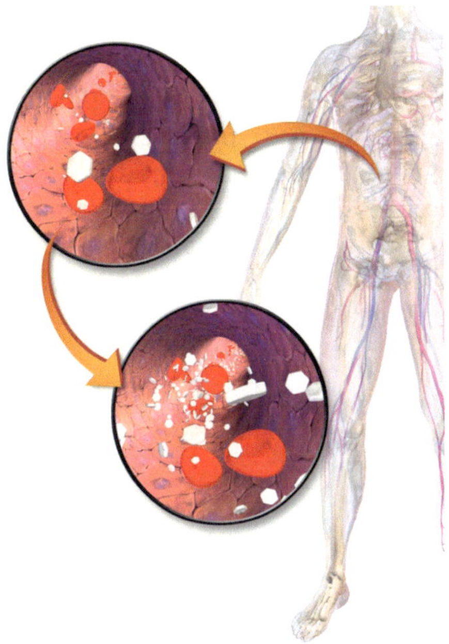

Figure 13.4. Persistent hyperglycemia triggers a series of biochemical reactions that lead to renal damage.

Source: https://upload.wikimedia.org/wikipedia/commons/c/ca/Hyperglycemia.png

It is suggested that hyperglycemia can team up with dyslipidemia to cause more damage to the kidneys. For instance, hyperlipidemic conditions characterized by elevated low-density lipoprotein (LDL) levels have been shown to exacerbate the renal impact of hyperglycemia, leading to lipid deposits and foam cell formation in the renal tissue, which is critical in the deterioration of kidney architecture and function (Alpers et al., 2004). In children, hyperglycemia can result in problems that last for a long time and affect their general health. Given the alarming rise in childhood Type II Diabetes, the manifestation of hyperglycemia during critical developmental years poses a risk for early onset of nephropathy and other complicating comorbidities, such as cardiovascular diseases and vision impairment (Kapke, 2015). Because hyperglycemia is a long-term problem, it can cause permanent kidney damage in people at a young age, so it's important to act quickly by changing habits and doing early kidney checks. If healthcare professionals know how hyperglycemia can lead to nephropathy, they can better treat diabetes and help reduce the risk of worsening kidney problems, which improves the lives of affected individuals (Figure 13.4).

13.1.3. Impact of Hypertension on Kidney Function

The connection between hypertension and kidney function is very important when it comes to diabetic nephropathy. Having high blood pressure can lead to kidney disease, causing harm to the kidneys' structure. Hypertension may harm the glomeruli in the kidneys, which results in increased proteinuria, a common symptom of nephropathy. Diabetes causes more and more problems for the kidneys, often making high blood pressure even worse. Understanding these mechanisms is crucial for addressing the overall management of diabetic patients, as controlling blood pressure can significantly impact renal outcomes, underscoring the importance of rigorous monitoring (Bland et al., 2009).

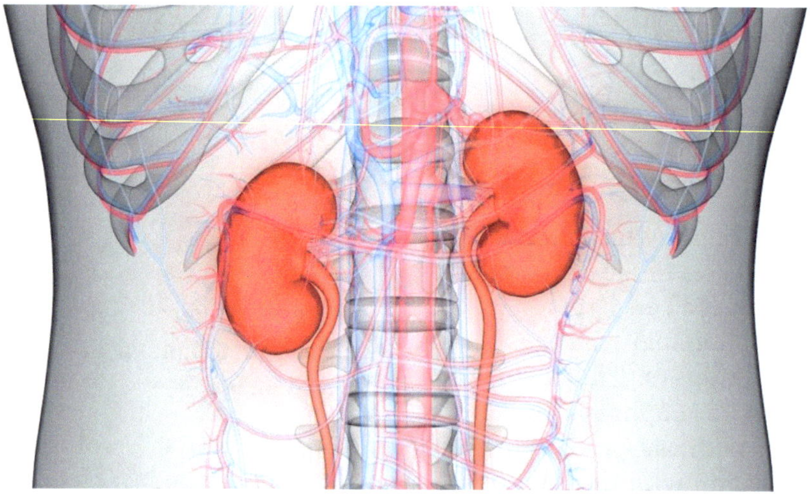

Figure 13.5. Hypertension can cause damage to the glomeruli, the tiny filtering units within the kidneys, leading to increased proteinuria, which is characteristic of nephropathy.

Source: https://sa1s3optim.patientpop.com/assets/images/provider/photos/2635335.jpg

Also, sodium transporters in the kidneys show that there is a lot of detail in how hypertension affects kidney function. Dysregulation of sodium reabsorption, particularly through pathways involving SGK1 (serum and glucocorticoid-induced kinase 1), plays a pivotal role in modulating blood pressure and, consequently, hypertensive damage to the kidneys. Many cases of diabetic nephropathy are linked to problems with sodium, which may result in extra fluid and high blood pressure. For this reason, therapies that work on sodium transport could help control blood pressure and also protect the kidneys. The evolving understanding of SGK1 functions in these processes provides a critical framework for developing specific interventions that can disrupt the harmful feedback loop between hypertensive nephropathy and diabetic complications (Iacobini et al., 2017). Taking care of one's diet may help protect kidney function in people with diabetic nephropathy. Changes in the amount of protein people eat as part of their diet have been found to help slow the progression of the disease. Eating less protein can take some stress off the kidneys, lower the pressure in the kidneys' filters, and decrease the damage to the kidney cells. Taking care of the protein source and avoiding glycotoxins can also play a key role in handling diabetic nephropathy. This approach to nutrition underlines that micronutrients and functional foods may postpone the development of kidney disease. By integrating dietary strategies aimed at hypertension control, healthcare professionals can significantly improve patient outcomes, thereby addressing both hypertension and its ramifications on kidney function more effectively (Iacobini et al., 2017) (Figure 13.5).

13.2. Risk Factors

It is very important to understand what increases the risk of diabetic nephropathy to prevent and manage it early. One of the most important issues is hyperglycemia and how it continuously affects the kidneys. When blood sugar rises to 126 mg/dl or more in diabetics, it is known to increase the risk of developing nephropathy. Besides, the length of time a person has had diabetes matters, as it can make the damage to the kidneys worse. In addition, studies have found that age and sex are important aspects for understanding these risks; for example, there is a strong link between age, the time it takes for nephropathy to develop, and the patient's sex. These interconnected variables highlight the multifaceted nature of diabetic nephropathy, making tailored interventions vital for at-risk populations (Buja et al., 2010).

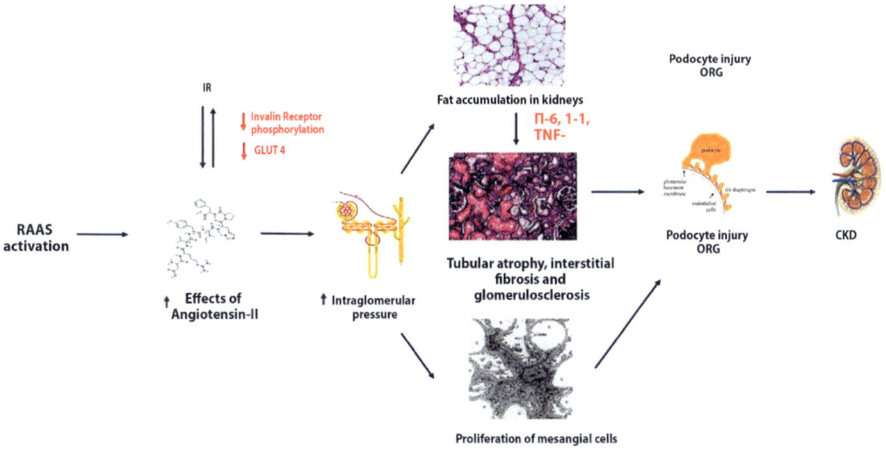

Figure 13.6. A history of obesity poses a substantial risk, with studies showing strong correlations between body weight and kidney health.

Source: Forcina G, Luciano M, Frattolillo V, Mori S, Monaco N, Guarino S, Marzuillo P, Miraglia del Giudice E, Di Sessa A. Kidney Damage in Pediatric Obesity: Insights from an Emerging Perspective. *Journal of Clinical Medicine*. 2024; 13(23):7025. https://doi.org/10.3390/jcm13237025

Another important risk factor found in recent studies is hyperuricemia. Having high uric acid levels can harm the body's metabolism and also contribute to the development of diabetic nephropathy. Experts have found that women, especially in some areas, are at greater risk of nephropathy, which results in differences in the occurrence of the disease among populations. Not being active enough has also been related to a greater chance of getting advanced nephropathy, which shows the link between lifestyle and health outcomes. The cumulative impact of these risk factors necessitates that patients and healthcare providers engage in proactive management, particularly monitoring blood sugar levels and encouraging regular physical activity as effective approaches to mitigate the adverse effects associated with diabetic nephropathy risk (Adi et al., 2019). Besides these common risk factors, what a person does and has done medically can make it much more likely for a diabetic person to develop nephropathy. In fact, having a history of obesity is a major risk, since many studies have found a strong link between weight and kidney health. In addition, taking oral contraceptives may increase the risk of diabetes, especially for women, showing how reproductive health and diabetes are related. They show that thorough patient evaluations should consider both the patient's diet and metabolic health to prevent diabetic nephropathy. Collectively, these insights suggest that a multifactorial approach is essential, focusing not only on glycemic control but also on broader health indicators such as uric acid levels, physical activity, and weight management to reduce the burden of nephropathy in diabetic patients (Buja et al., 2010) (Figure 13.6).

13.2.1. Genetic Predisposition to Diabetic Nephropathy

The likelihood of developing diabetic nephropathy is greatly affected by a person's genetic factors if they have diabetes. As previously noted, diabetic nephropathy is a leading cause of kidney disease, affecting approximately 40% of patients with type 1 and type 2 diabetes, with its manifestation typically characterized by increased urinary albumin excretion (UAE) in the absence of other renal diseases (Umarovna KN, 2023). Genetics is an important reason why some people develop this condition, not only hyperglycemia and hypertension from the environment. Research shows that some alleles may increase the risk, pointing out the connection between genes and the environment. Identifying these genetic markers may help develop interventions that focus on those who have a greater chance of getting diabetic nephropathy. New studies highlight that advanced genomic and bioinformatics methods are very useful in finding out the genetic factors behind diabetic nephropathy. With the prevalence of diabetes continuously increasing globally, a significant proportion of affected individuals will ultimately develop nephropathy, making it imperative to identify risk factors associated with this condition (Maxwell et al., 2013). Meta-analyses and the use of integrated pathways are now helping us learn more about diseases that people are predisposed to. Genetic, epigenetic, and transcriptomic studies are used together to improve our knowledge of the biological factors that lead to diabetic nephropathy. If these findings are used in healthcare, it may help doctors identify Omics profiles that aid in early diagnosis and improve patient outcomes as well as the use of healthcare resources. Also, finding out which genes affect diabetic nephropathy can greatly help in managing the disease. If doctors can identify genetic risks, they can choose more suitable ways to prevent diseases for each patient. For example, those considered at high risk might gain from regular check-ups and changes in their lifestyle to lower the risk of nephropathy. Moreover, understanding the genetic factors involved in diabetic nephropathy may help find new treatment options. Taking care of the genetic factors that lead to diabetic nephropathy improves our knowledge of the disease and could help develop new ways to treat and manage diabetes-related problems (Figure 13.7).

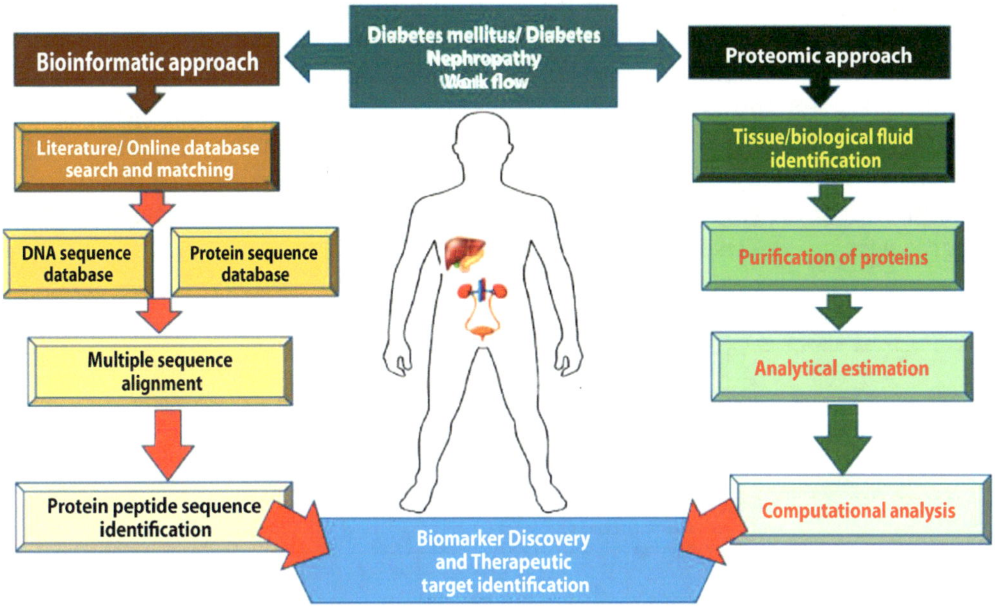

Figure 13.7. Emerging research underscores the utility of advanced genomic and bioinformatic techniques in deciphering the genetic contributors to diabetic nephropathy.

Source: Oh J-W, Muthu M, Haga SW, Anthonydhason V, Paul P, Chun S. Reckoning the Dearth of Bioinformatics in the Arena of Diabetic Nephropathy (DN)—Need to Improvise. *Processes*. 2020; 8(7):808. https://doi.org/10.3390/pr8070808

13.2.2. Lifestyle Factors Contributing to Kidney Damage

How lifestyle choices affect kidney health is best seen by looking at the diet of those who are likely to develop diabetic nephropathy. Diets high in protein have been questioned for a long time because they may influence the rate at which the kidneys filter blood and function. Taking in the right amounts of carbohydrates, fats, and protein may help prevent the worsening of diabetic nephropathy. It is suggested that paying attention to the source of your proteins and reducing glycotoxins can help slow the decline of kidney function. By aligning with recommendations for restricted caloric intake and improved dietary habits, individuals can significantly mitigate their risk of developing complications associated with diabetic nephropathy, ultimately enhancing their overall health outcomes (Iacobini et al., 2017). Being active physically is important for kidney health, mainly because it helps control high blood pressure and blood sugar levels. Being active regularly may ease the effects of obesity and metabolic syndrome, which are both important causes of diabetic nephropathy. If you exercise for at least 150 minutes each week at a moderate intensity, you can improve your heart and help your body manage blood sugar. Besides, resistance training helps build muscle, makes insulin function better, and supports healthy blood pressure. Because of these effects, the chances of chronic kidney disease are reduced, which helps maintain the kidneys' function. Consequently, encouraging physical activity as part of an integrated lifestyle approach is essential for individuals with diabetes to safeguard their kidneys from damage and prolong their well-being (Ekström et al., 2017). Smoking and drinking alcohol increase the chances of kidney damage in people who have diabetes. Cigarette smoke has many harmful substances that can damage the kidneys and speed up the progress of kidney disease through different types of inflammation. Besides, too much alcohol can cause hypertension and make diabetes harder to control, which increases the chance of kidney problems. Actions aimed at stopping smoking and cutting back on alcohol have been shown to help people at risk of chronic kidney disease, proving that it is important to adopt many healthy habits. Dealing with these bad habits is very important for managing diabetic nephropathy, since it can result in better kidney health and fewer complications from kidney failure. Encouraging patients to adopt tobacco-free and moderate drinking lifestyles forms an integral part of effective kidney health strategies (Iacobini et al., 2017) (Figure 13.8).

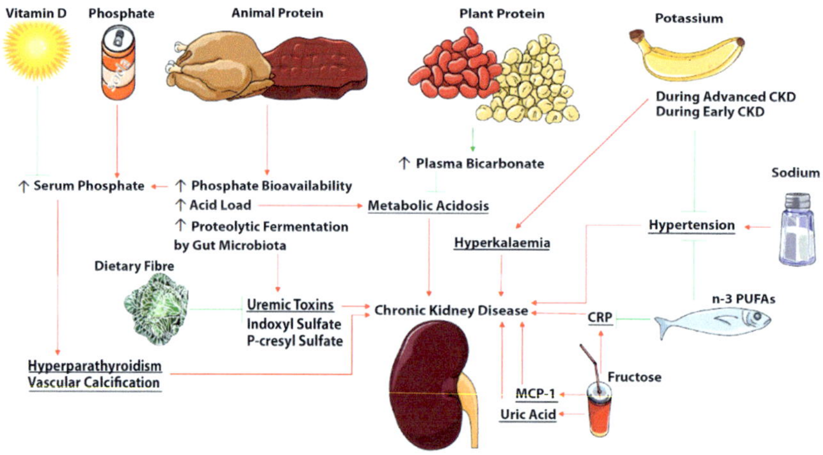

Figure 13.8. The interplay between lifestyle factors and kidney health is illuminated by examining dietary choices, particularly in individuals at risk for diabetic nephropathy.

Source: Snelson M, Clarke RE, Coughlan MT. Stirring the Pot: Can Dietary Modification Alleviate the Burden of CKD? *Nutrients*. 2017; 9(3):265. https://doi.org/10.3390/nu9030265

13.2.3. Duration and Control of Diabetes as Risk Factors

It is well known that the longer a person has diabetes, the greater the risk of diabetic nephropathy, which is an important concern for diabetes management. With time, diabetes becomes more likely to cause complications, and one of these is chronic kidney disease. If hyperglycemia goes on for a long period, it can cause changes in the structure of the kidneys, which may result in nephropathy. In a study involving patients with diabetes, it was shown that a significant proportion, approximately 47.25%, had prolonged diabetes duration correlating with their nephropathy risk, underscoring the importance of early diagnosis and intervention (Haque et al., 2023). Therefore, the length of time a person has had diabetes is a strong sign of nephropathy, which requires quick and effective actions to limit the damage caused by diabetes. Keeping blood sugar under control is an important factor that can lead to diabetic nephropathy. High blood glucose levels, which show poor glycemic control, increase the chance of renal complications because constant high glucose can harm the nephrons. The same study highlighted that a majority of patients, around 72%, developed nephropathy primarily due to high glucose levels, indicating that effective management of blood sugar can significantly alter the trajectory of kidney health in diabetic patients (Haque et al., 2023). In addition, studies keep showing that sticking to a proper HbA1c level helps prevent both the occurrence and the seriousness of diabetic nephropathy. So, managing blood sugar well is important for care because it can reduce the chances of getting diabetic nephropathy. Besides, hypertension and lipid disorders can also make diabetes more dangerous if it is not well controlled for a long period. It is clear from research that how long a person has had diabetes, how well blood pressure is controlled, and the severity of nephropathy are all related. For instance, elevated blood pressure was identified as a significant risk factor, with 53.33% of nephropathy patients also having hypertension (Haque et al., 2023). The appearance of retinopathy and neuropathy in people with diabetes shows how these conditions are closely linked, and this can make the risks of diabetes even greater. That is why taking care of blood sugar, blood pressure, and lipids is important for preventing diabetic nephropathy and protecting kidney function in people at risk (Figure 13.9).

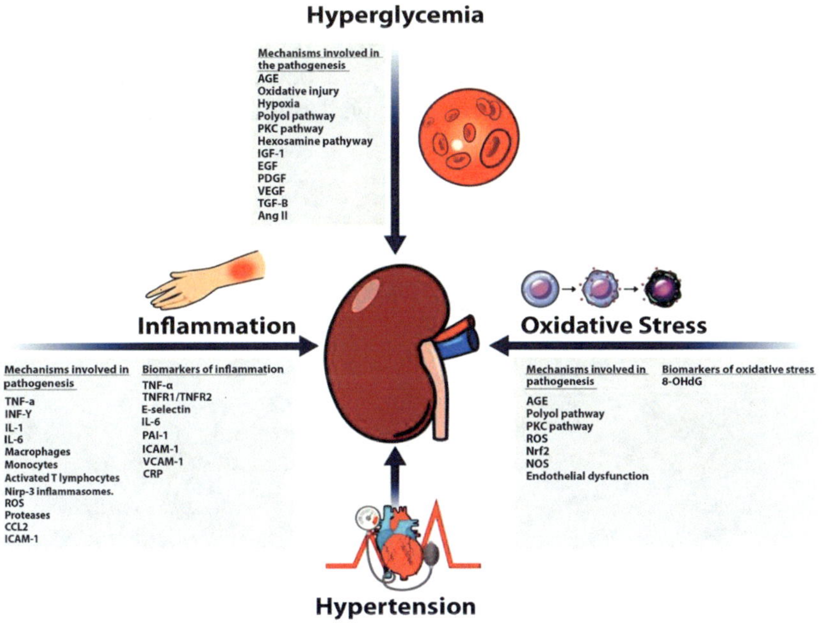

Figure 13.9. Factors such as longer exposure to hyperglycemia can lead to structural changes in renal tissue, ultimately precipitating nephropathy.

Source: https://www.e-dmj.org/upload/thumbnails/dmj-2021-0329f1.jpg

13.3. Symptoms and Diagnosis

At first, diabetic nephropathy appears in a mild way, and the early signs are often ignored until the kidneys have suffered serious damage. Some of the main symptoms are persistent proteinuria, which means too much protein in the urine and can be found during a routine urinalysis. This symptom means that the kidneys' filtration barrier is not working properly. Edema and hypertension may appear in patients as a result of fluid retention. Being aware of these early symptoms is very important for healthcare providers, as they can show the need for additional tests and treatment. It is very important to diagnose diabetes and its complications as soon as possible to prevent the disease from getting worse. Doctors usually depend on both clinical observations and laboratory tests to correctly diagnose diabetic nephropathy. At first, the test usually checks the amount of albumin in the urine and labels it as microalbuminuria or macroalbuminuria depending on the quantity. Additionally, serum creatinine tests and glomerular filtration rate (GFR) calculations are instrumental in evaluating kidney function. Because of new technological developments, urinary proteomics is now becoming an important tool for better diagnoses than the usual methods. Recent studies underscore the potential of urinary biomarkers, such as collagen fragments and uromodulin, to provide deeper insights into disease mechanisms and progression (Magalhães et al., 2016). Such biomarkers make it easier for doctors to decide on the best treatment plan for their patients. Also, the link between diabetes and mental health is important in determining the symptoms and diagnosis of diabetic nephropathy. Research highlights the higher prevalence of depressive symptoms among individuals with type 2 diabetes, which can complicate both the management and progression of nephropathy (Cardona et al., 2019). Because of these two problems, it is important to combine mental health screenings with regular diabetes care. If practitioners take into account both the mental and physical aspects of a patient, they can better understand their health. To sum up, managing diabetic nephropathy well requires acknowledging its psychological aspects as well as other factors (Figure 13.10).

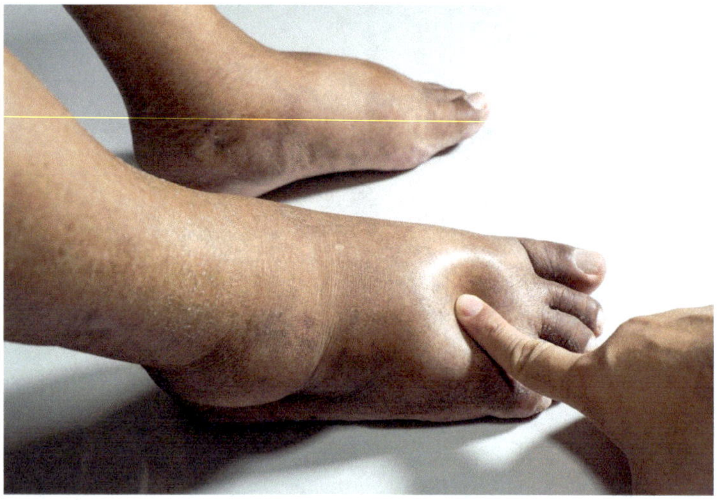

Figure 13.10. Patients may also experience signs of fluid retention, resulting in edema or hypertension.

Source: https://vohrawoundcare.com/wp-content/uploads/2023/02/What-is-Edema-min.jpg

13.3.1. Early Signs of Diabetic Nephropathy

Since the early symptoms of diabetic nephropathy are usually mild and can be missed, it is very important to detect the condition early to stop it from getting worse. Microalbuminuria is one of the early signs, as it shows a moderate rise in albumin in the urine, not enough to be called proteinuria. Having microalbuminuria signals that kidney damage might be developing; it indicates that glomerular permeability is higher, which is a main symptom of nephropathy. In addition, people with diabetes usually have renal hemodynamic changes, including glomerular hyperfiltration, which means the kidneys filter blood more rapidly. If these early changes are monitored, healthcare providers can find out what to do to stop the condition from worsening and help patients achieve better long-term results. In addition to microalbuminuria, declining glomerular filtration rates (GFR) are another observable sign of early diabetic nephropathy. If the kidneys are not working properly, routine blood tests will show a drop in renal function. New research has shown that there are several types of diabetic kidney disease, which means some patients can have kidney problems without albuminuria. These nonalbuminuric renal impairments suggest a more complex pathology at play among diabetic patients, with alterations in glomerular structure and function that require comprehensive evaluations (Magalhães et al., 2016). Early signs should be recognized since not every patient shows increased albumin, so kidney health in diabetes should be managed using several approaches. With new advances in urinary proteomics, it may be possible to find early signs of diabetic nephropathy. Using urinary biomarkers such as collagen fragments, serum albumin, and uromodulin, researchers are finding better ways to monitor kidney function than the traditional methods. Several studies on kidney diseases have proven that these biomarkers are more sensitive and specific, which suggests they could be useful in clinical settings. Identifying these proteins early on not only aids in the diagnosis of diabetic nephropathy but also enables better prognostic assessments, thereby facilitating a more proactive management of diabetes-related kidney complications (Magalhães et al., 2016). As doctors learn more about these first signs, they can choose treatments that may greatly influence the progress of nephropathy in diabetic patients (Figure 13.11).

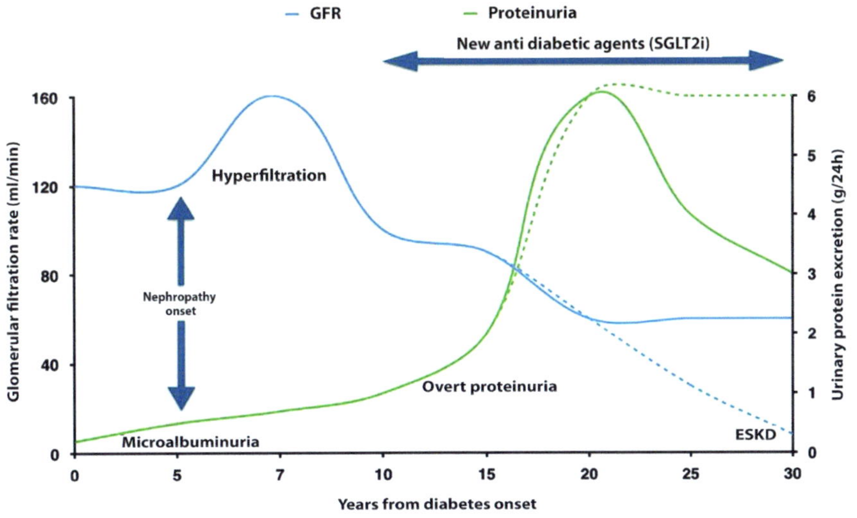

Figure 13.11. Declining glomerular filtration rates (GFR) are another observable sign of early diabetic nephropathy.

Source: Santoro D, Torreggiani M, Pellicanò V, Cernaro V, Messina RM, Longhitano E, Siligato R, Gembillo G, Esposito C, Piccoli GB. Kidney Biopsy in Type 2 Diabetic Patients: Critical Reflections on Present Indications and Diagnostic Alternatives. *International Journal of Molecular Sciences.* 2021; 22(11):5425. https://doi.org/10.3390/ijms22115425

13.3.2. Diagnostic Tests for Kidney Function

It is very important to diagnose diabetic nephropathy in the early stages of kidney disease for diabetic patients. A fundamental component of diagnosing kidney function involves evaluating markers such as serum creatinine and blood urea nitrogen (BUN). Biomarkers give the first indication of kidney function, helping doctors find cases of impaired renal filtration. Additionally, the estimation of glomerular filtration rate (GFR) is essential for determining the severity of kidney dysfunction. GFR can be calculated using creatinine levels, along with a person's age, sex, and race, so the assessment can be more specific. GFR calculations are very important for diabetic patients, since a drop in GFR usually means the disease is getting worse and requires regular screening and proper care. In the process of diagnosing kidney health, urine tests are very important, especially in diabetic nephropathy. Urine albumin excretion rates are important because they show kidney damage before the serum creatinine or GFR levels are affected. The presence of microalbuminuria, defined as 30-300 mg of albumin per gram of creatinine, serves as an early warning sign that kidney injury may be developing due to diabetes (Magalhães et al., 2016). Moreover, new findings in urinary proteomics, including the identification of collagen fragments and uromodulin, have increased the ability to diagnose diseases.

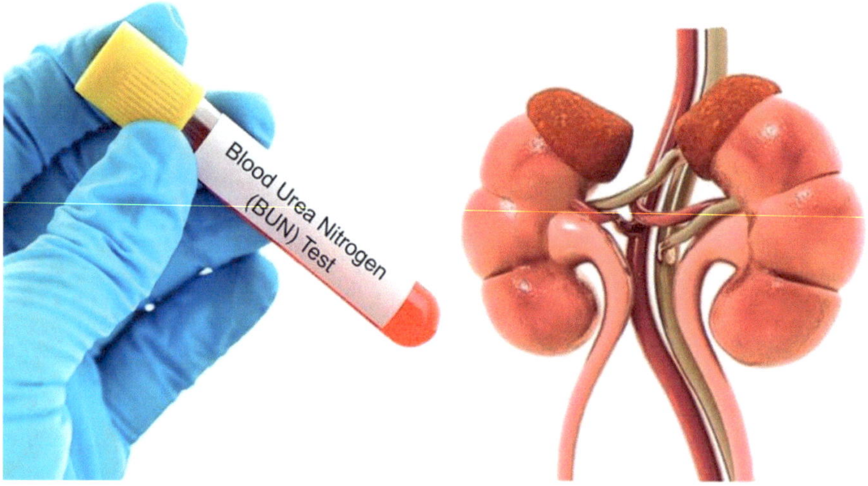

Figure 13.12. Blood urea nitrogen (BUN).

Source: https://requestatest.com/includes/uploads/blog/BUN.jpg

They enabled doctors to detect kidney damage more accurately and reliably than the previous methods. As a result, urinary proteomics presents a potential shift in diagnostic methods that could significantly enhance clinical decision-making for diabetic nephropathy patients (Magalhães et al., 2016). Along with regular biochemical tests, ultrasound imaging can give more information about the kidneys and how they are functioning in people with diabetic nephropathy. With the help of imaging, doctors can find structural problems such as renal hypertrophy or obstructions that can make diabetes control more difficult. Still, ultrasound is commonly used when simpler methods do not provide enough information about the kidneys. While imaging alone doesn't provide a comprehensive evaluation of kidney function, it complements other diagnostic tests by offering a broader perspective on renal health (Magalhães et al., 2016). Together, these tests and imaging studies help clinicians create a stronger way to diagnose patients. This way of managing diabetes helps detect nephropathy early and provides treatment to enhance patient results (Figure 13.12).

13.3.3. Importance of Regular Screening in Diabetic Patients

Screening should be done regularly by diabetic patients to help avoid problems such as diabetic nephropathy. As diabetes continues, the chance of kidney damage rises a lot. Identifying changes in the kidneys, for example, microalbuminuria, at an early stage can prevent the disease from worsening. The American Diabetes Association (ADA) emphasizes that routine screening for kidney function, alongside other important health assessments, can help in the timely management of diabetic complications. For instance, implementing best practice alerts (BPA) within electronic medical records has resulted in improved adherence to recommended screening guidelines, achieving adherence rates exceeding 90% for key assessments (DeSalvo et al., 2019). Taking such steps is important for making sure diabetic patients get proper care and better results. In addition, screening regularly is important not only for finding nephropathy but also for managing diabetes as a whole. Patients with diabetes, particularly those on treatments like highly active antiretroviral therapy (HAART), may experience increased risk for conditions such as insulin resistance and glucose intolerance (Wiwanitkit, 2007).

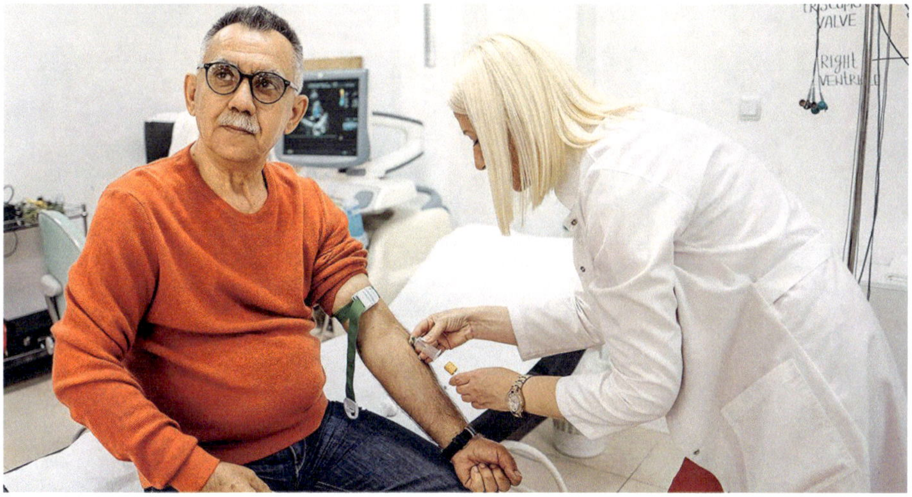

Figure 13.13. Regular screening is crucial for diabetic patients, particularly in the context of preventing complications such as diabetic nephropathy.

Source: https://media.post.rvohealth.io/wp-content/uploads/2023/02/blood-draw-senior-male-1200-628-facebook-1200x628.jpg.

Monitoring a patient's condition all the time helps healthcare professionals adjust treatment and manage the effects of diabetes on different organs, for example, the kidneys. Healthcare providers can address all aspects of a patient's health and lower the risk of long-term diabetes complications by checking blood pressure, lipids, and kidney function at regular intervals. Regular screening encourages preventative care that is necessary for dealing with diabetic nephropathy. Regular assessments by healthcare providers allow them to spot patients at risk and treat them before any serious harm happens. In this way, early detection of microalbuminuria helps doctors combine lifestyle changes and prescribe medicines to help protect the kidneys. Therefore, since the number of people with diabetes is rising, public health should focus on regular screenings to help reduce the effects of diabetes on healthcare systems. By doing so, not only are we safeguarding individual health, but we are also enhancing the sustainability of healthcare services dedicated to managing diabetes and its myriad complications (DeSalvo et al., 2019). In the end, sticking to regular screening is very important in managing diabetes, so patients can stay healthy and enjoy a good quality of life (Figure 13.13).

13.4. Stages of Diabetic Nephropathy

Diabetic nephropathy is usually described in five stages, and each stage is marked by certain biochemical and clinical features that show changes in the kidneys. Initially, the disease begins with hyperfiltration, where glomerular filtration rate (GFR) increases as a compensatory mechanism due to elevated blood glucose levels. At this stage, patients usually do not show any symptoms, but their kidney blood flow may change. When the disease progresses, it is possible to detect mild albuminuria, which means the glomeruli are starting to be damaged. Since this condition may predict worsening of the kidneys, it is necessary to screen and monitor those who are at risk as soon as possible.

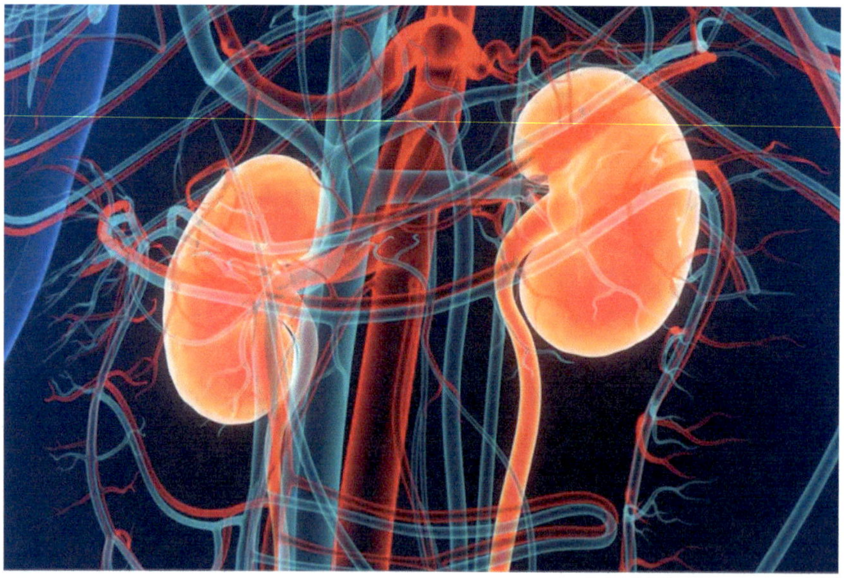

Figure 13.14. The early signs of renal impairment become more pronounced during this stage, with hypertensive complications contributing further to renal damage.

Source: https://img.lb.wbmdstatic.com/vim/live/webmd/consumer_assets/site_images/article_thumbnails/miniBEADs/high_blood_pressure_and_kidney_disease_minibead/1800x1200_getty_rf_high_blood_pressure_and_kidney_disease_minibead.jpg?resize=750px:*&output-quality=75

In the next phase of diabetic nephropathy, patients experience moderate albuminuria as well as high blood pressure. Due to kidney failure, the body is not able to keep proteins, so albumin appears in the urine, a condition known as microalbuminuria. Hypertension-related complications happen more often in this stage, which leads to even greater damage to the kidneys. When hyperglycemia and hypertension occur together, they can make kidney problems develop and progress faster. Although patients do not show obvious symptoms yet, research indicates that taking care of blood glucose levels can greatly slow the disease's progression during this important stage, so it is important to use careful management in healthcare settings. In the advanced stages of diabetic nephropathy, patients experience macroalbuminuria and a significant decline in GFR, culminating in end-stage renal disease (ESRD) if left untreated. When renal function decreases a lot, it becomes necessary to use dialysis or transplant a new kidney. New research in epidemiology has revealed different forms of kidney disease, where albuminuria is not always present, so doctors may need to change their approach to treatment. The introduction of sodium-glucose cotransporter 2 (SGLT2) inhibitors has emerged as a promising strategy to mitigate these changes, as these agents have shown nephroprotective effects beyond mere glycemic control (Busetto et al., 2016; Barutta et al., 2019). This new insight into diabetic nephropathy makes it clear that we should keep looking for better ways to help patients (Figure 13.14).

13.4.1. Classification of Nephropathy Stages

Understanding the stages of nephropathy is important for handling diabetic nephropathy because it describes how kidney disease develops in diabetic patients. The progression of diabetic nephropathy begins by showing microalbuminuria, which means the kidneys are damaged to some extent. Because this stage is often overlooked, it is important since it lets clinicians act early and possibly slow down the disease. If the condition gets worse, patients might develop macroalbuminuria, which means their urine contains much more protein. Moving from one stage to another may cause both changes in patient outcomes and the way kidney disease is treated, so it is important for the classification system to cover albuminuria, changes in renal function, and changes in kidney tissue. Analyzing miRNA and urinary proteins may help improve the way nephropathy is classified. It has been found in recent studies that urinary microRNA levels change during different stages of diabetic nephropathy, so these molecules might be used as biomarkers to monitor the disease. In particular, renal fibrosis and growth factor signaling, important factors in diabetic nephropathy, are connected to certain microRNAs. They can help reveal the reasons behind kidney injury and add to our understanding of nephropathy stages, apart from blood pressure and blood sugar levels. This integration of advanced biomarker analysis can contribute to improved individualized treatment and monitoring strategies tailored to each patient's unique progression of diabetic nephropathy (Argyropoulos et al., 2013). Apart from microRNAs, profiling the proteins found in urine is now widely used to identify the stages of nephropathy in people with type 2 diabetes. Using high-resolution capillary electrophoresis together with mass spectrometry, researchers have been able to distinguish between people with and without diabetic nephropathy, proving the method's strong accuracy. Studies done recently have shown that proteomics can detect unique biomarkers in urine, helping to spot and predict further kidney damage. Urinary proteome analysis may find collagen fragments that can indicate the early stages of diabetes-related kidney damage, which could help with early treatment and a better outcome. As the understanding of diabetic nephropathy evolves, these advanced classification methods may reshape clinical paradigms, emphasizing proactive management of renal health (Kottgen et al., 2010) (Figure 13.15).

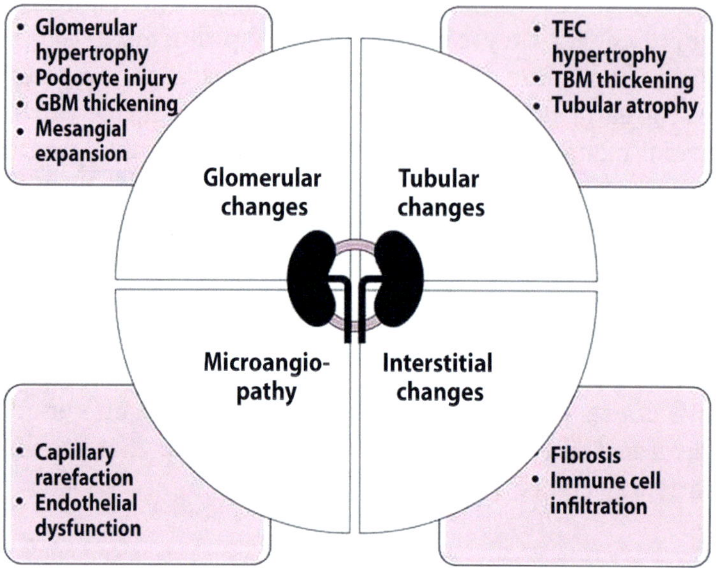

Figure 13.15. The classification of nephropathy stages is critical in understanding and managing diabetic nephropathy, as it outlines the progression of kidney disease in patients with diabetes.

Source: Młynarska E, Buławska D, Czarnik W, Hajdys J, Majchrowicz G, Prusinowski F, Stabrawa M, Rysz J, Franczyk B. Novel Insights into Diabetic Kidney Disease. *International Journal of Molecular Sciences*. 2024; 25(18):10222. https://doi.org/10.3390/ijms251810222

13.4.2. Progression from Microalbuminuria to End-stage Renal Disease

The progression from microalbuminuria to end-stage renal disease (ESRD) represents a critical concern in the management of diabetic nephropathy. Small amounts of albumin found in the urine due to microalbuminuria usually show up before the kidneys are seriously affected. With the progression of diabetic nephropathy, it can result in macroalbuminuria, releasing more albumin, which hurts the kidneys and lowers their function. The advancement of the disease is linked to glycemic control, high blood pressure, and other metabolic factors that make kidney damage worse. It is important to detect microalbuminuria in diabetic patients as it greatly increases the risk of ESRD, showing why early management is essential to avoid severe kidney damage. Taking care of diabetes is important to prevent microalbuminuria from becoming ESRD. It has been found that controlling blood sugar effectively reduces the risk of renal disease and other complications. Research suggests that higher HbA1c variability is associated with a significant increase in the risk of both micro- and macrovascular complications, including renal impairments (Gorst et al., 2015). Hence, using therapies that help control blood glucose can prevent diabetic nephropathy from getting worse. In addition, making changes to diet and exercise is important for a complete approach, since it helps control blood sugar and also boosts heart health, which is linked to kidney function in people with diabetes. Furthermore, new research points out that changing the diet can help stop diabetic nephropathy by controlling the amount of macronutrients and glycotoxins. Adjustments in protein intake, particularly focusing on the source of protein and incorporation of protective micronutrients, have gained traction as viable strategies in the prevention of nephropathy progression (Iacobini et al., 2017). When patients get nutritional education, they can choose healthy meals, which may help them avoid or delay the progression to ESRD. With more research being done on the effects of certain diets, healthcare providers should make sure to include these interventions in their management plans for diabetic nephropathy, so they can be more active in fighting kidney disease (Figure 13.16).

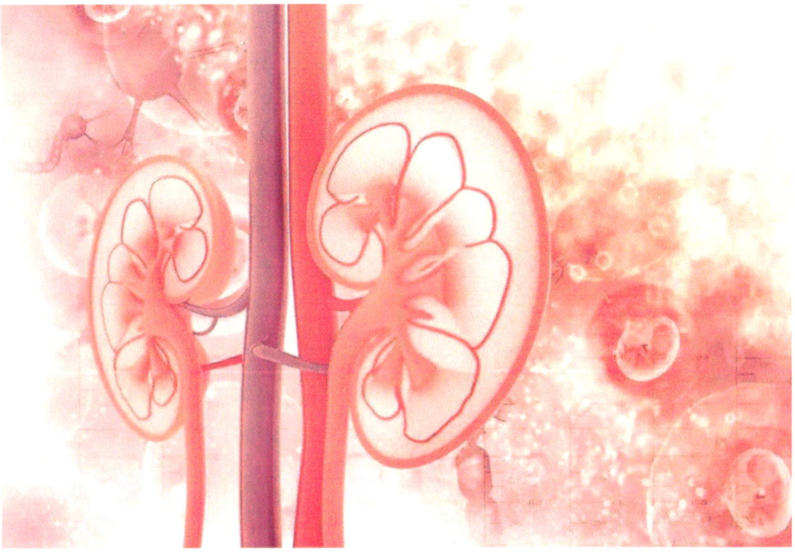

Figure 13.16. Microalbuminuria, characterized by the presence of small amounts of albumin in the urine, serves as an early indicator of kidney dysfunction, often preceding more severe complications.

Source: https://diabetesmantra.com/wp-content/uploads/2024/02/kidney_G_894952686_11zon-1024x682.jpg.webp

13.4.3. Implications of Each Stage for Patient Management

It is very important to understand the effects of each stage of the disease to give the patient the best possible care. At the beginning, diabetic nephropathy with only mild proteinuria needs to be watched and treated through lifestyle changes. Patients are advised to regulate their blood sugar, eat healthier meals, and exercise on a regular basis. Taking this approach helps to slow down kidney damage and reduces the chances of heart problems in people with diabetes. For this reason, healthcare providers should focus on teaching patients how to manage their health by themselves. Because of these early interventions, it is important to create a treatment plan that matches each patient's diabetes and other health conditions. As the disease progresses to the moderate stage, patients should start taking medicines as part of their treatment. This stage is often marked by increased albuminuria and a decline in glomerular filtration rate (GFR). It is at this point that the implementation of stricter blood pressure control, typically through the use of angiotensin-converting enzyme (ACE) inhibitors, becomes essential. Also, it is very important for patients to take their prescribed medicines, since evidence shows that individualized treatment plans for hyperglycemia should be adjusted according to each patient's kidney health. Recent studies highlight notable heterogeneities in diabetic kidney disease phenotypes, necessitating tailored strategies that address not only albuminuric traits but also those with progressive renal decline independent of albuminuria (Barutta et al., 2019). For this reason, regular evaluations are necessary since they impact the care provided. When diabetic nephropathy reaches its final stages and kidney function is seriously impaired, managing the patient's care becomes even more important. It is now important to include nephrologists, dietitians, and diabetes educators in the patient's care. Sometimes, patients need treatments such as dialysis or a kidney transplant, which can make treatment more challenging. Knowing the natural course of diabetic nephropathy allows providers to plan for possible problems and help patients get ready for different treatments. In addition, explaining the disease and what treatments are available to patients can help them be more ready for future care. Continuous evaluation of patient outcomes, alongside the economic implications of various treatment modalities, remains vital to optimize care in this complex stage of diabetic nephropathy (Martin et al., 2025) (Figure 13.17).

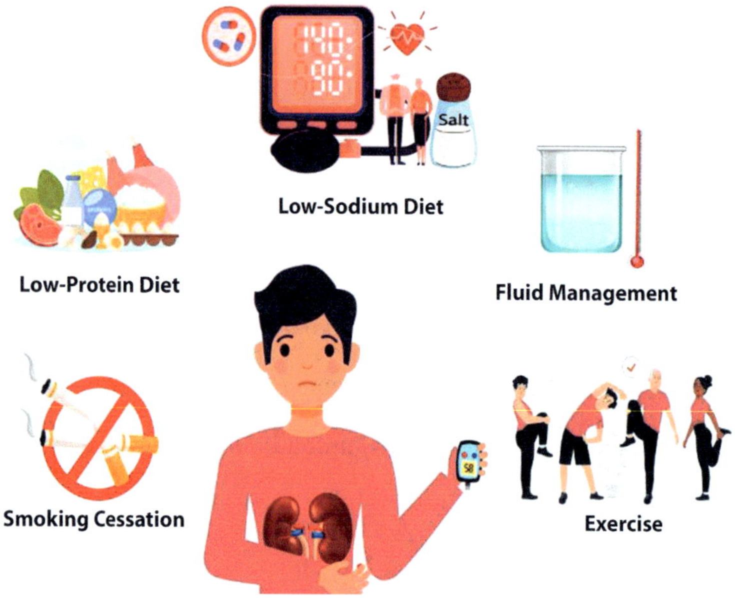

Figure 13.17. Early-stage diabetic nephropathy, characterized by mild proteinuria, often requires regular monitoring and lifestyle adjustments.

Source: https://www.ckbhospital.com/wp-content/uploads/2024/07/Diet-and-Lifestyle-Changes-1-01-1-scaled.webp

13.5. Treatment and Management

To manage diabetic nephropathy, it is important to use a variety of approaches that help slow its progress and avoid complications. The main part of this strategy is to keep blood glucose levels as steady as possible. The American Diabetes Association usually advises patients to set personal goals, with an HbA1c level below 7% as the main aim. It is very important since controlling glucose within a safe range can greatly reduce the chances of developing kidney problems known as nephropathy. Additionally, pharmacological agents such as angiotensin-converting enzyme (ACE) inhibitors or angiotensin II receptor blockers (ARBs) are instrumental in managing blood pressure, thereby providing nephroprotective effects. They do not just slow the development of kidney disease, but also help the heart, which is very important for diabetics because they have a higher risk of heart problems. Changing diet is becoming an important part of managing and treating diabetic nephropathy. Recently, focusing on diet changes has demonstrated that lessening protein intake may help stop kidney disease from getting worse. New studies have started to focus on the proteins people eat and the glycotoxins found in their foods. Researchers have found that a proper diet full of protective nutrients can help the kidneys work more efficiently while reducing the pressure on them. Also, adding nutritional education to patient management plans encourages people to make healthier food choices, which improves their health in general. Such dietary adaptations, coupled with an individualized treatment plan, contribute significantly to prolonging renal function in diabetic patients, marking a transition towards a more holistic management approach (Iacobini et al., 2017). In addition, it is important to use screening methods to find diabetic nephropathy early. By following the screening guidelines from the American Diabetes Association, it becomes clear that checking urine microalbumin-to-creatinine ratios is very important. They are used to find early signs of nephropathy as well as to help choose the best treatment options. Recently, Texas Children's Hospital showed that using electronic alerts in medical records helped doctors follow the screening guidelines, showing how technology can be useful in healthcare management. If healthcare providers keep their screening compliance rate above 90%, they can quickly notice any change in kidney function and alter the patient's treatment plan. Such methods exemplify the significant role of structured clinical frameworks in optimizing both early detection and ongoing management of diabetic nephropathy (DeSalvo et al., 2019) (Figure 13.18).

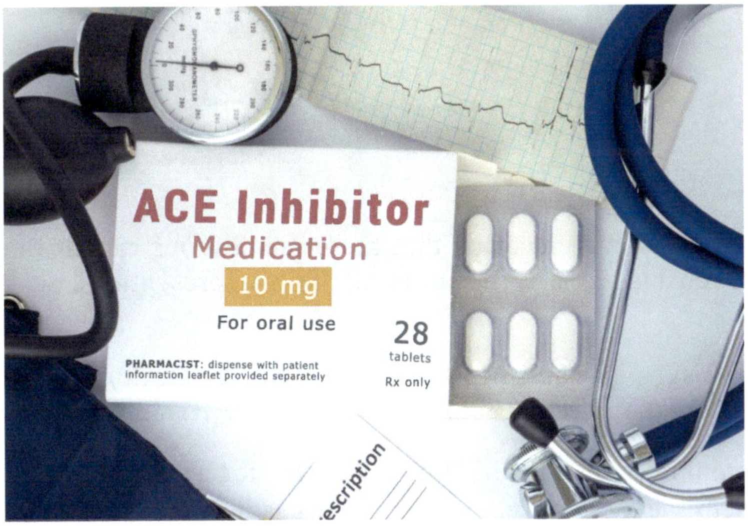

Figure 13.18. Pharmacological agents such as angiotensin-converting enzyme (ACE) inhibitors or angiotensin II receptor blockers (ARBs) are instrumental in managing blood pressure, thereby providing nephroprotective effects.

Source: https://medshadow.org/wp-content/uploads/2020/03/ACE-inhibitors-scaled.jpeg

13.5.1. Pharmacological Interventions for Diabetic Nephropathy

Treatments for diabetic nephropathy have advanced a lot, mainly because of new medicines that help slow its progression and benefit patients. Central to this approach is the utilization of angiotensin-converting enzyme (ACE) inhibitors, which have been shown to lower proteinuria and slow renal decline in diabetic patients. They achieve this by blocking the renin-angiotensin-aldosterone system, which causes the afferent arteriole to widen and lessen the pressure inside the kidney's filtering area. Studies involving patients with diabetes have proven that these drugs lower the risk of end-stage renal disease. Consequently, ACE inhibitors have become a cornerstone in the treatment protocols for diabetic nephropathy, underscoring the importance of early intervention to preserve kidney function and enhance overall health outcomes for individuals suffering from diabetes and its complications (Prabhakar, 2024).

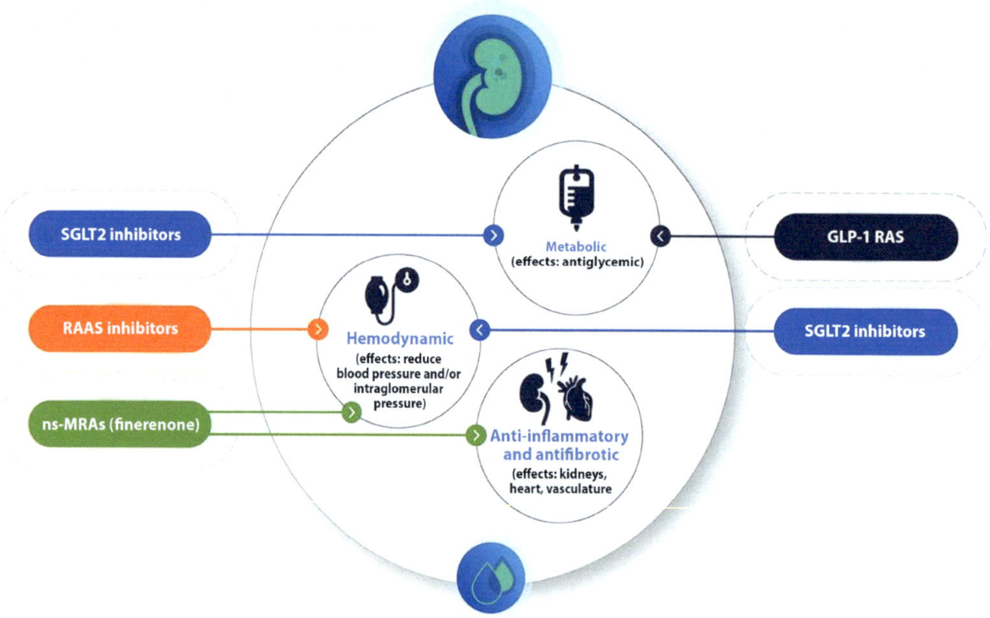

Figure 13.19. Clinical trials have revealed that these medications can significantly decrease the risk of progression to renal failure and cardiovascular events, presenting a dual benefit for patients with diabetes.

Source: https://media.springernature.com/lw1200/springer-static/image/art%3A10.1186%2Fs12882-024-03652-5/MediaObjects/12882_2024_3652_Fig1_HTML.png

Along with ACE inhibitors, SGLT2 inhibitors have attracted a lot of attention in treating diabetic nephropathy. They help the kidneys remove extra glucose, which benefits blood sugar levels and has a protective effect on the kidneys. It is shown by research that SGLT2 inhibitors help keep blood sugar levels under control and also protect the kidneys by reducing both high filtration and inflammation in the renal tubules. It has been found through clinical trials that these drugs reduce the chance of renal failure and cardiovascular events in diabetes patients. Their incorporation into treatment regimens represents a shift towards more comprehensive pharmacological strategies that address both glycemic control and the prevention of renal complications in diabetic patients (Huwiler et al., 2013).

Moreover, discovering new medicines has made it possible to treat diabetic nephropathy with a wider range of drugs. In recent times, researchers have examined how S1P receptor modulators work in the renal system because they have strong bioactive effects. Sphingosine 1-phosphate (S1P) has been implicated in various kidney functions and is believed to play a role in the pathophysiology of diabetic nephropathy. Studies suggest that controlling S1P signaling may help treat kidney problems linked to diabetes, which suggests new treatments could be developed for this pathway. The continuing evolution of pharmacological strategies underscores the importance of innovative therapies that not only address hyperglycemia but also focus on the multifactorial nature of diabetic nephropathy, aiming for a holistic approach to treatment (Prabhakar, 2024) (Figure 13.19).

13.5.2. Role of Lifestyle Modifications in Treatment

Proper management of diabetic nephropathy depends on making major lifestyle changes that can slow the disease. Since diabetes can cause chronic kidney disease, it is necessary to include diet, regular activity, and weight management in the treatment plan. If you eat a diet that is rich in nutrients and low in sodium, saturated fats, and sugars, you can help control blood glucose and lower your blood pressure, which are important for preventing diabetic nephropathy. Besides, regular exercise improves the way insulin works and helps people lose weight, which reduces the risks of diabetes complications.

It has been shown that following a planned diet and exercise program can help patients control their metabolism, which reduces the risks of renal impairment. Besides changing what they eat and how much they exercise, patients need to be educated to help manage diabetes and lower the risk of diabetic nephropathy. When people are informed about their illness, they are more likely to handle it well and this can have a big impact on their health. Educational interventions aimed at increasing awareness can lead to significant improvements in lifestyle choices, as evidenced by studies indicating that such strategies are associated with reductions in HbA1c levels and cholesterol management (Rao et al., 2015). Besides giving information, these programs help patients create habits that involve regular health check-ups, taking their medications, and checking their blood pressure and blood glucose.

Making sure care plans are specific to each patient can motivate them to change their lifestyles and manage both the physical and mental aspects of diabetes. In addition, using behavioral strategies in combination with medical care helps people stick to changes in their lifestyle. Taking into account both mental and behavioral aspects can lead to better results in people with diabetic nephropathy. Evidence suggests that lifestyle changes, when supported by behavioral modification techniques such as goal-setting and self-monitoring, lead to better management of diabetes and consequently, a lower risk of developing nephropathy (Busetto et al., 2015). If healthcare providers are part of setting goals, patients can understand their treatment plans and feel motivated to stick to them. In the end, making lasting changes to one's lifestyle works to stabilize kidney function and also improve the quality of life for people with diabetic nephropathy, proving how helpful these changes can be for the long term (Figure 13.20).

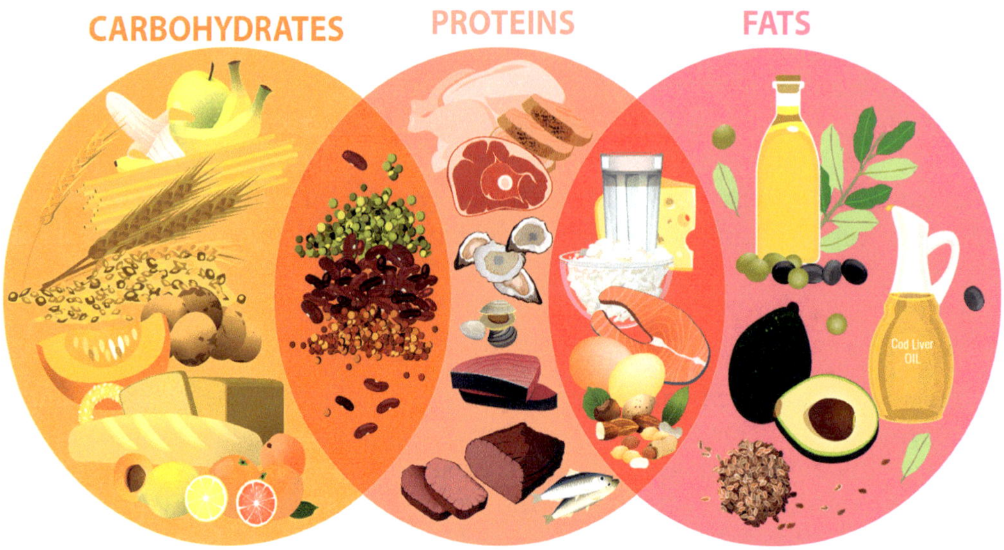

Figure 13.20. A well-balanced diet that emphasizes nutrient-rich food while limiting sodium, saturated fats, and sugars can significantly help in regulating blood glucose levels and reducing hypertension, both of which are contributing factors to diabetic nephropathy.

Source: https://i0.wp.com/blog.rsfh.com/wp-content/uploads/2023/01/4629b-shutterstock_1131777815_converted.png?resize=1271%2C675&ssl=1

13.5.3. Importance of Multidisciplinary Care in Management

Since diabetic nephropathy can be complicated and diabetes causes many different problems, it needs to be managed thoroughly. Using the approach of multidisciplinary care, patients are cared for by endocrinologists, nephrologists, dietitians, and diabetes educators. Using this model, patients are educated better and decisions are made together, always keeping the patient's needs in mind. When specialists communicate, patients are given treatment plans that focus on their kidney health and their general health. When team members cooperate well, the disease can be influenced in a positive way, as seen by better blood sugar and kidney results in patients receiving this type of care. Moreover, since many patients with diabetic nephropathy have other related health problems, multidisciplinary care is very important. People like John, who have foot ulcers, show that it is important for different specialists to work together. A diabetic foot ulcer should be treated by caring for the wound, checking glucose levels, changing medications, and making changes to lifestyle. If specialists from different fields join forces, they can tackle the main issues that cause complications and avoid them in the future. This care model stresses the use of preventive measures and helps patients become more involved, which leads to better health for everyone. If the management plan is followed, as in John's case, the rate of hospitalization can be reduced and patients' lives can improve. Having interprofessional care frameworks in place has been proven to lead to major improvements in quality and how satisfied patient are. It has been found that having quality indicators helps manage chronic kidney disease and track the results of patient care. In one study, a suite of thirteen clinical and process indicators was developed, which revealed remarkable improvements across several critical areas, including blood pressure control and engagement in advanced care planning (Awdishu et al., 2019). Working together as a team makes it easier to monitor patients and also encourages everyone on the team to be responsible. Regularly checking these metrics makes it possible to improve treatment plans and encourages everyone to keep improving. By using this approach, it is proven that multidisciplinary care is valuable for diabetic nephropathy since it results in improved health and higher satisfaction among patients (Figure 13.31).

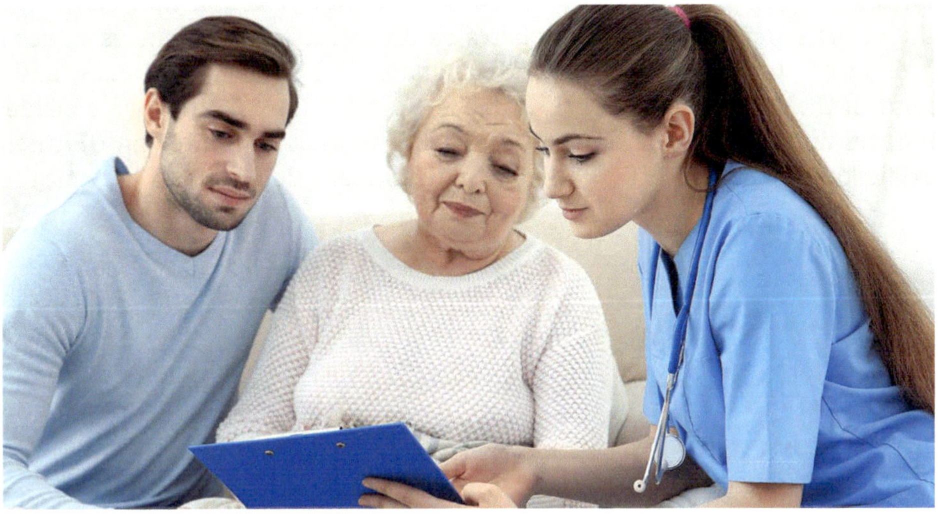

Figure 13.21. By fostering communication among various specialists, patients receive tailored treatment plans that address not only their kidney health but also their overall well-being.

Source: https://patientbetter.com/wp-content/uploads/2023/10/Treatment-options-health-advocacy.jpg

A CLOSER LOOK

Glomerular Filtration Rate (GFR)

Glomerular Filtration Rate (GFR) is a key measure of kidney function that estimates how much blood the kidneys filter per minute. It demonstrates the ability of the kidneys to get rid of waste and extra water in the blood. Factors used to calculate GFR are age, sex, race, and the level of creatinine found in the blood. Values of GFR above 90 mL/min/1.73 m^2 are considered normal, but lower numbers mean the kidneys are not working properly. Monitoring GFR helps diagnose and stage chronic kidney disease (CKD) and guides treatment decisions to prevent further kidney damage.

Summary

In summing up, we should understand that several molecular processes are involved in the development of diabetic nephropathy. A number of studies have found that problems with proteolytic systems are key in the development of diabetic nephropathy, suggesting possible early detection tools. The discovery of urinary peptides that change in nephropathy patients opens up the chance to use peptidomics to learn about the disease. Scientists study proteases such as MMP-2 and MMP-9 to see how they are related to urine tests and changes in the kidneys, which helps them improve the detection of diabetic nephropathy. Such research deals with current clinical problems and also helps create medicines to prevent further kidney damage. In addition, looking into epigenetic changes, especially DNA methylation, is helping to reveal a new aspect of diabetic nephropathy. Studies conducted recently have found a connection between certain CpG sites and the start of nephropathy in people with type 1 diabetes. Applying the Illumina Infinium HumanMethylation27 BeadChip, researchers have found important places in the genome that could signal the risk of nephropathy. Since DNA methylation changes with patient age and the length of diabetes, this suggests that personalized medicine could be useful. Repeating these findings in bigger patient groups could bring about new discoveries in the care and treatment of diabetic nephropathy. To summarize, since diabetic nephropathy is complex, it calls for an approach that combines information from proteomic and epigenetic studies. Looking at the molecular details can explain how diseases occur, which may guide clinical decisions. Besides, discovering urinary biomarkers and epigenetic risk factors could help find cancer early and provide better treatment, leading to better patient outcomes. As time goes on, it will be important for basic science and clinical research to work together to turn these findings into helpful therapies. To summarize, the results highlight the need to keep researching diabetic nephropathy, as it may lead to better ways to control and prevent this serious condition.

The progression of diabetic nephropathy (DN) is a multifaceted issue that warrants thorough investigation to enhance patient outcomes. Key factors influencing the advancement of renal complications in individuals with Type 1 Diabetes (T1D) include the presence of specific microRNAs that exhibit differential expression at various stages of nephropathy. According to a study, the microRNA levels in urine were found to be very different between patients who had overt nephropathy and those who did not develop kidney problems throughout their diabetes. These findings emphasize the potential of microRNAs as biomarkers for early detection and risk stratification of DN, suggesting that monitoring these molecular indicators could inform therapeutic interventions to halt or slow disease progression (Argyropoulos et al., 2013). Also, knowing how renal fibrosis and growth factors work may help find new ways to treat kidney diseases. Apart from microRNAs, oxidative stress plays a major part in the development of diabetic nephropathy. As a result of this mechanism, the kidney can suffer serious damage that ends up causing kidney dysfunction. Research utilizing a novel hyperpolarized (13)C dehydroascorbate (DHA) sensor has demonstrated that diabetic conditions lead to a marked decline in renal redox capacity, long before overt histological changes are observed. The early identification of oxidative stress in renal tissues, as indicated by diminished antioxidant levels and heightened expression of NADPH oxidase, underscores the relevance of targeting oxidative stress in therapeutic strategies (Kautzky-Willer et al., 2013). With the help of advanced imaging, researchers can check the kidneys and take action to reduce the harm caused by oxidative damage. Using information from microRNA profiling and oxidative stress tests gives a complete picture of diabetic nephropathy. All of these studies together give important knowledge that may help doctors change the way they detect and treat this serious condition. If healthcare providers use urinary microRNAs and advanced imaging, they may improve the early detection and monitoring of DN. As such, future research should continue to explore the interplay between molecular markers and oxidative stress, ultimately informing the creation of evidence-based strategies aimed at improving the prognosis for individuals affected by diabetes-related kidney disease (Argyropoulos et al., 2013; Bok et al., 2014).

References

1. Abdolrahim, M., Jazayeri, H. E., Rabiee, M., Rajab, A., et al. (2017). Evaluation of glycated albumin (GA) and GA/HbA1c ratio for diagnosis of diabetes and glycemic control: A comprehensive review. https://core.ac.uk/download/213086982.pdf (accessed on 11th June 2025).
2. Adi, M. S., Hadisaputro, S., Nugroho, H., Suhartono, S., et al. (2019). Faktor risiko kejadian nefropati diabetika pada wanita. https://core.ac.uk/download/234033539.pdf (accessed on 11th June 2025).
3. Agabiti-Rosei, E., Cruickshank, J. K., Dominiczak, A., Erdine, S., et al. (2016). 2016 European Society of Hypertension guidelines for the management of high blood pressure in children and adolescents. https://core.ac.uk/download/46165193.pdf (accessed on 11th June 2025).
4. Alpers, C. E., Hudkins, K. L., Kirk, E., LeBoeuf, R. C., et al. (2004). Hyperglycemia and hyperlipidemia act synergistically to induce renal disease in LDL receptor-deficient BALB mice. https://core.ac.uk/download/16432946.pdf (accessed on 11th June 2025).
5. Awdishu, L., Moore, T., Morrison, M., Trzebinska, E., et al. (2019). A primer on quality assurance and performance improvement for interprofessional chronic kidney disease care: A path to Joint Commission certification. https://core.ac.uk/download/323064308.pdf (accessed on 11th June 2025).
6. Bahamonde, J., Ezquer, F., Ezquer, M., Giraud Billoud, M., et al. (2017). Tubulointerstitial injury and proximal tubule albumin transport in early diabetic nephropathy induced by type 1 diabetes mellitus. https://core.ac.uk/download/159301014.pdf (accessed on 11th June 2025).
7. DeSalvo, D., Bartz, S. K., Mockler, B., & Sonabend, R. Y. (2019). Use of Best Practice Alerts to Improve Adherence to Evidence-Based Screening in Pediatric Diabetes Care. *Journal of Nursing & Interprofessional Leadership in Quality & Safety, 2* (1). Retrieved from https://digitalcommons.library.tmc.edu/uthoustonjqualsafe/vol2/iss1/7(accessed on 11th June 2025).
8. Barutta, F., De Nicola, L., Di Paolo, S., Gesualdo, L., et al. (2019). Diabetic kidney disease: New clinical and therapeutic issues. Joint position statement of the Italian Diabetes Society and the Italian Society of Nephrology on "the natural history of diabetic kidney disease and treatment of hyperglycemia in patients with type 2 diabetes and impaired renal function." https://core.ac.uk/download/231749247.pdf (accessed on 11th June 2025).
9. Bascands, J. L., Delles, C., Denis, C., Husi, H., et al. (2017). Urinary peptidomes analysis reveals proteases involved in diabetic nephropathy. https://core.ac.uk/download/132585012.pdf (accessed on 11th June 2025).
10. Bland, R., Hills, C. E., & Squires, P. E. (2009). SGK1 in the kidney: Disrupted sodium transport in diabetes and beyond. https://core.ac.uk/download/20442635.pdf (accessed on 11th June 2025).
11. Bok, R., Jen, K. Y., Keshari, K. R., Kurhanewicz, J., et al. (2014). Noninvasive *in vivo* imaging of diabetes-induced renal oxidative stress and response to therapy using hyperpolarized 13C dehydroascorbate magnetic resonance. https://core.ac.uk/download/323074740.pdf (accessed on 11th June 2025).
12. Buja, A., Helgadottir, A., Subramanian, A., Teschendorff, A. E., Maxwell, A. P., Teschendorff, A. E., O'Connor, A. S., et al. (2010). Genome-wide DNA methylation analysis for diabetic

nephropathy in type 1 diabetes mellitus. https://core.ac.uk/download/1688838.pdf (accessed on 11th June 2025).

13. Busetto, L. (2015). Timing of bariatric surgery in people with obesity and diabetes. https://core.ac.uk/download/53528626.pdf (accessed on 11th June 2025).
14. Cardona, T., & Pullicino, G. (2019). Depression in patients with type 2 diabetes in Maltese primary care. https://core.ac.uk/download/288638616.pdf (accessed on 11th June 2025).
15. De Gabriele, R. (2008). Assessment and management of diabetic ulcers in the primary health care setting. https://core.ac.uk/download/46602206.pdf (accessed on 11th June 2025).
16. Defeudis, G., Di Emidio, C., Gianfrilli, D., Lenzi, A., et al. (2015). Erectile dysfunction and its management in patients with diabetes mellitus. https://core.ac.uk/download/54528262.pdf (accessed on 11th June 2025).
17. Derakhshanpour, F., Farsinia, M., Mirkarimi, K., Vakili, M., et al. (2015). Depression and quality of life in patients with type 2 diabetes. https://core.ac.uk/download/52205715.pdf (accessed on 11th June 2025).
18. Dragoş, C., Mociran, M., & Hâncu, N. (2009). Risk factors and severity of diabetic retinopathy in Maramureş. https://core.ac.uk/download/pdf/26977706.pdf (accessed on 11th June 2025).
19. Ekström, T. J., Nordfors, L., Shiels, P. G., Stenvinkel, P., et al. (2017). Current epigenetic aspects the clinical kidney researcher should embrace. https://core.ac.uk/download/84340482.pdf (accessed on 11th June 2025).
20. Gorst, C., Cavalot, C. S. K., Kontopantelis, E., Foo, G., Heatlie, G., Hermann, M., et al. (2015). Long-term glycemic variability and risk of adverse outcomes: A systematic review and meta-analysis. https://core.ac.uk/download/41991337.pdf (accessed on 11th June 2025).
21. Guzik, T. J., Petrie, J. R., & Touyz, R. M. (2018). Diabetes, hypertension, and cardiovascular disease: Clinical insights and vascular mechanisms. https://core.ac.uk/download/153444565.pdf (accessed on 11th June 2025).
22. Haque, A., Mohammad Saifuddin, M. D., Kadir, M. R., Mithila, S. T., Saha, S. K., Moni, T. T., et al. (2023). Diabetic nephropathy and its risk factors among patients with diabetes mellitus—An observational study. https://core.ac.uk/download/570905622.pdf (accessed on 11th June 2025).
23. Heerspink, H. J. L., Mischak, H., & Pena, M. J. (2016). Proteomics for prediction of disease progression and response to therapy in diabetic kidney disease. https://core.ac.uk/download/84148392.pdf (accessed on 11th June 2025).
24. Kautzky-Willer, A., Stich, K., Hintersteiner, J., Kautzky, A., Kamyar, M. R., Saukel, J., Johnson, J., & Lemmens-Gruber, R. (2013). Sex-specific-differences in cardiometabolic risk in type 1 diabetes: a cross-sectional study. *Cardiovascular diabetology*, *12*, 78. https://doi.org/10.1186/1475-2840-12-78(accessed on 11th June 2025).
25. Huwiler, A., Koch, A., & Pfeilschifter, J. M. (2013). Sphingosine 1-phosphate in renal diseases. https://core.ac.uk/download/16515935.pdf (accessed on 11th June 2025).
26. Iacobini, C., Menini, S., Pesce, C., Pugliese, G., et al. (2017). Dietary interventions to contrast the onset and progression of diabetic nephropathy: A critical survey of new data. https://core.ac.uk/download/80314820.pdf (accessed on 11th June 2025).

27. Kapke, D. R. (2015). Childhood type II diabetes: The risks and complications. https://core.ac.uk/download/58826199.pdf (accessed on 11th June 2025).

28. Kottgen, A., Alkhalaf, A., Levey, A. S., Julian, B. A., Janssen, B., Tiran, B., et al. (2010). Multicentric validation of proteomic biomarkers in urine specific for diabetic nephropathy. https://core.ac.uk/download/110262.pdf (accessed on 11th June 2025).

29. Argyropoulos, C., Wang, K., McClarty, S., Huang, D., Bernardo, J., Ellis, D., Orchard, T., Galas, D., & Johnson, J. (2013). Urinary microRNA profiling in the nephropathy of type 1 diabetes. *PloS one*, *8*(1), e54662. https://doi.org/10.1371/journal.pone.0054662(accessed on 11th June 2025).

30. Magalhães, P., Mischak, H., & Zürbig, P. (2016). Urinary proteomics using capillary electrophoresis coupled to mass spectrometry for diagnosis and prognosis in kidney diseases. *Current opinion in nephrology and hypertension*, *25*(6), 494–501. https://doi.org/10.1097/MNH.0000000000000278(accessed on 11th June 2025).

31. Martin, D., Ting, J., & Haas, M. (2025). A Markov model of diabetic retinopathy progression for the economic evaluation of a novel DR prognostic device, *CHERE Working Paper 2007/14*. https://core.ac.uk/download/pdf/7070858.pdf (accessed on 11th June 2025).

32. Maxwell, A. P., & McKnight, A. J. (2013). Bioinformatic resources for diabetic nephropathy. https://core.ac.uk/download/16500310.pdf (accessed on 11th June 2025).

33. P. K. Prabhakar. Glucose to Complications: Understanding Secondary Effects in Diabetes Mellitus. Sumat. Med. J. [Internet]. 2024May1 [cited 2025Jul.23];7(2):87-95. Available from: https://talenta.usu.ac.id/smj/article/view/15998(accessed on 11th June 2025).

34. Rao, L. S. (2015). Redesigning treatment strategies in type 2 diabetes by treatment intensification and patient education. https://core.ac.uk/download/33562651.pdf (accessed on 11th June 2025).

35. Wiwanitkit, V. (2007). Primary care for diabetes in HIV-infected patients. https://core.ac.uk/download/pdf/86947.pdf (accessed on 11th June 2025).

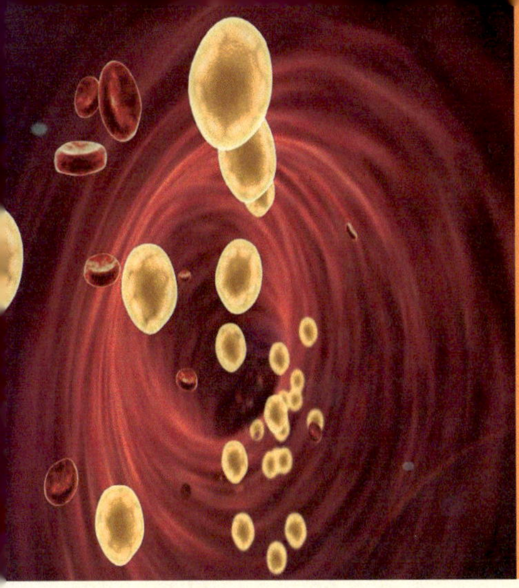

Chapter 14

BLOOD LIPID ABNORMALITIES

Contents

Introduction

Lately, the study of blood lipid abnormalities has become more important because of its strong effect on public health. When lipids like cholesterol and triglycerides are present in high amounts, the risk of heart diseases increases, so it is important to study the reasons behind this. These abnormalities may be caused by genetic factors or by the way a person lives, making it difficult to understand what affects cardiovascular health. Because metabolic syndromes are increasing among adolescents and people worldwide, the risks of abnormal lipid levels are very significant. It is important to educate people about lipid issues to help design strategies that reduce the number of heart-related illnesses. Gaining knowledge about lipids in the human body helps us see how abnormalities can happen. Lipids are active parts of cells and are involved in many metabolic processes that affect energy storage, hormone production, and cellular communication. The composition and functionality of erythrocytes, or red blood cells, are indicative of metabolic health, as recent studies highlight their intricate involvement in sustaining homeostasis and responding to systemic metabolic changes (de Oliveira & Saldanha, 2010). Because of this, we should examine both blood lipids and erythrocyte behavior, because problems in either area may point to bigger health problems. For this reason, research should focus on how lipids affect cells and how this relates to various diseases. In addition, it is becoming more obvious that lifestyle plays a role in lipid abnormalities, especially among younger people. Metabolic syndrome, a group of risk factors, points to the role of behavior in affecting a person's lipid levels. Sedentary behaviors, poor dietary habits, and substance use are pivotal contributors that warrant attention (Bekel et al., 2020). New data about high rates of lipid abnormalities in adolescents underlines the importance of teaching about these issues and taking action in the community. Learning about the effects of these choices on blood lipids will help plan future public health actions to lower the rate of related health issues. If we focus on these environmental and behavioral factors and create suitable solutions, the population can become healthier and enjoy better cardiovascular health in the future (Figure 14.1).

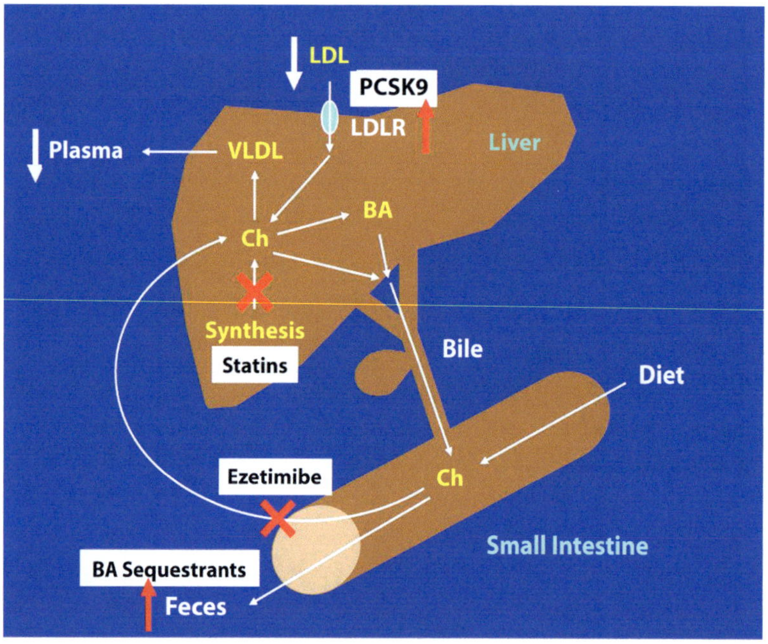

Figure 14.1. Elevated lipid levels, including cholesterol and triglycerides, are linked to increased risk factors for cardiovascular diseases, necessitating a deeper understanding of their underlying mechanisms.

Source: https://static.elsevier.es/multimedia/16652681/0000001600000OS1/v1_201906111104/S1665268119310415/v1_201906111104/en/main.assets/gr7.jpeg

14.1. Types of Blood Lipids

Learning about the different blood lipids is necessary to explain their effects on metabolic health, mainly in cases of lipid abnormalities. Some of the main types of blood lipids are triglycerides, cholesterol, and phospholipids. Triglycerides are the main type of fat and provide most of the body's energy; they are kept in adipose tissue and used when we are fasting or exercising. Triglycerides are usually higher in people with obesity and metabolic syndrome, which points to their importance for the heart. In contrast, cholesterol exists in two principal forms, low-density lipoprotein (LDL) and high-density lipoprotein (HDL), each possessing distinct physiological roles that can impact disease risk. LDL cholesterol is called bad cholesterol as it has a connection to atherosclerosis, whereas HDL cholesterol is referred to as good cholesterol because it helps remove cholesterol from the arteries and protects against heart disease. Phospholipids are another major type of lipid in blood, and they help create cell membranes and take part in lipid signaling. Phospholipids, having both hydrophilic and hydrophobic parts, assemble into lipid bilayers that play a key role in how cells are built. The flexibility and strength of the cell membrane are important for its functions, and this is made possible by their dynamic nature. Some phospholipids are transformed into bioactive lipid mediators that have an effect on inflammation and the health of the heart. Problems in the metabolism of phospholipids can result in diseases, mainly when looking at how increased levels of certain phospholipids are connected to inflammation. By knowing what lipids do, we can see their significance in both healthy and unhealthy conditions, especially in examining heart diseases. Besides, how different lipids interact can make blood lipid abnormalities more complicated. Recent studies have unveiled the role of proteins like proprotein convertase subtilisin kexin 9 (PCSK9) in lipid metabolism, as evidenced by various cohorts examining individuals with concurrent health challenges such as HIV/HCV coinfection. Studies reveal that HIV/HCV patients tend to have less LDL cholesterol but higher PCSK9 levels, which raises questions about what causes dyslipidemia in these people. For example, such results can cover blood lipids as well as cardiovascular risks, so it's necessary to understand how different blood lipids relate to health. For this reason, each type of blood lipid has its own purpose and also interacts with the others, which is important for understanding metabolic health and blood lipid problems (Figure 14.2).

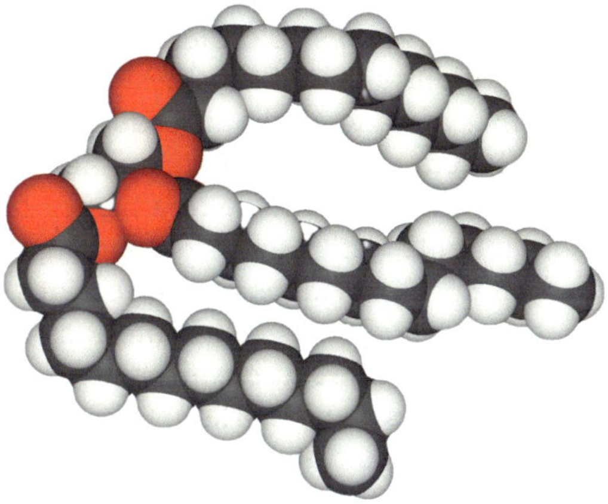

Figure 14.2. Triglycerides, the most abundant type of fat in the body, serve as a primary energy source; they are stored in adipose tissue and released during fasting or physical activity.

Source: https://upload.wikimedia.org/wikipedia/commons/6/64/Trimyristin-3D-vdW.png

14.1.1. Cholesterol

Cholesterol, which is a lipid molecule, is important for cells and hormones. The liver is the main place where it is made, although some can come from certain foods. Cholesterol is usually examined in the context of blood lipid abnormalities because it is linked to heart health. High-density lipoprotein (HDL) cholesterol is deemed good cholesterol as it facilitates the removal of excess cholesterol from the bloodstream, while low-density lipoprotein (LDL) cholesterol is often classified as bad cholesterol, as elevated levels are associated with an increased risk of atherosclerosis and other cardiovascular diseases. The levels of these lipoproteins in the blood can give a clue about a person's risk of heart disease, so it is important to maintain healthy cholesterol levels. Researchers have paid a lot of attention to the link between cholesterol levels and metabolic syndrome. Metabolic syndrome is a combination of obesity, hypertension, and dyslipidemia, and all these factors increase the risk of heart disease. It has been found that overweight or at-risk adolescents are increasingly developing metabolic syndrome, which is related to abnormal cholesterol levels. According to studies, 35.2% of overweight adolescents may have metabolic syndrome, which resembles the situation in the United States, where similar problems have been noted. This surge in cholesterol-related issues among the youth underscores the urgency of addressing dietary habits and lifestyle choices to mitigate long-term health risks associated with dyslipidemia and metabolic disorders (Kok et al., 2008). In addition, chronic conditions greatly affect lipid metabolism, as shown by the changes seen in people with cancer and chronic infections. Studies have found that some treatments, for example, rIFN-gamma, can lead to higher triglyceride levels in patients, which adds to the complications of their lipid profile. Although total cholesterol levels do not vary, changes in triglycerides and the related processes, such as poor lipid removal, imply that the body's overall conditions have a strong impact on cholesterol. Such interactions point out the strong relationship between health disorders and lipid metabolism, which explains why cholesterol is a key marker for spotting unusual blood lipid levels. This underscores the need for comprehensive strategies to monitor and manage cholesterol levels, especially in vulnerable populations impacted by comorbidities (Bradley et al., 1986) (Figure 14.3).

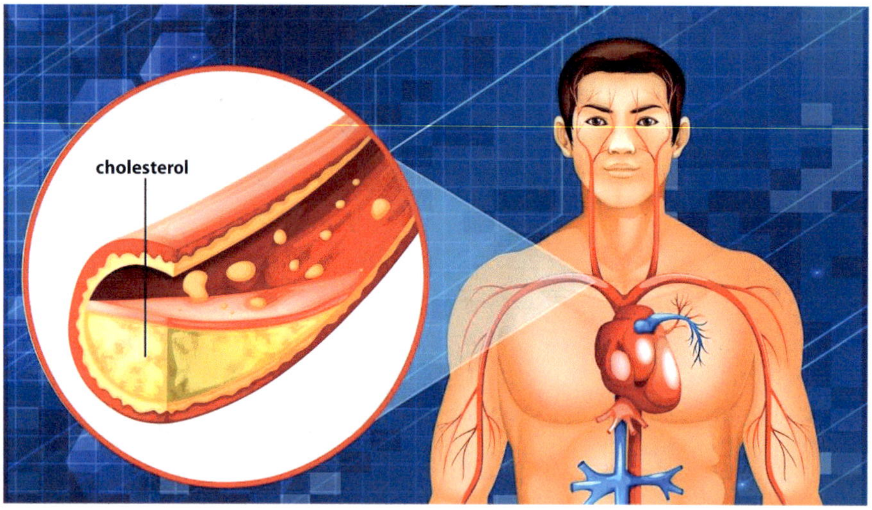

Figure 14.3. Cholesterol, a lipid molecule essential for various physiological functions, plays a critical role in cellular structure and hormone production.

Source: https://www.drvaidyaslab.com/wp-content/uploads/2023/08/high-cholestrol-1.jpg

14.1.2. Triglycerides

Triglycerides play an important part in blood lipid abnormalities since they are linked to cardiovascular disease and metabolic syndromes. Having high levels of triglycerides, often caused by poor eating and not enough exercise, is now known to increase the risk of heart problems. Research indicates that high triglyceride levels can instigate a cascade of metabolic alterations, influencing other lipid profiles, including low-density lipoprotein (LDL) cholesterol and high-density lipoprotein (HDL) cholesterol. Also, the link between triglycerides and insulin resistance has been established, as people with insulin resistance often have high triglycerides, adding to their chances of getting metabolic syndrome. For this reason, healthcare providers need to carefully check triglyceride levels in people who are at risk of lipid problems and heart disease. More studies explain the ways in which triglycerides cause problems in metabolism. It has been found that having central obesity is a major sign that triglyceride levels will be high, increasing the chances of developing high blood pressure and impaired glucose tolerance. Longitudinal studies have revealed that when people's waistlines get larger, their triglyceride levels go up, showing a link between obesity and lipid problems. In particular, research shows that a person's waist size at the start can help predict how triglyceride levels will change in the future. As a result, dietary changes and exercise habits may help reduce triglycerides and also stop other heart-related problems from getting worse. The genetic aspects of triglyceride metabolism should be considered, especially when it comes to obesity-related changes in lipid levels. Looking into a specific genetic variant called ANGPTL4-E40K has uncovered links between our genes and how lipids are controlled in the body. As a result of this mutation, lipoprotein lipase is blocked, which makes triglyceride levels fall and HDL cholesterol rise in people who are obese. Studies on populations have found that having this mutation leads to better lipid profiles, unlike non-carriers who usually suffer from high triglycerides and related issues. For this reason, it is important to use personalized methods to address blood lipid problems, especially in people who are obese, since ANGPTL4-E40K is a genetic factor. Studying how genes affect triglycerides may help create better ways to treat and control the condition in both hospitals and the community (Figure 14.4).

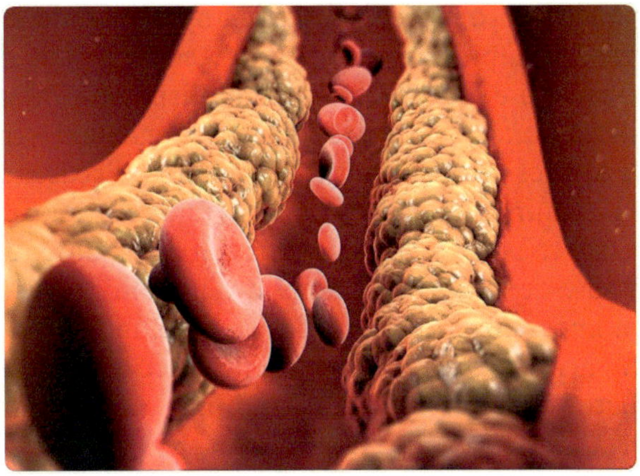

Figure 14.4. The role of triglycerides in the context of blood lipid abnormalities is critical due to their association with cardiovascular disease and metabolic syndromes.

Source: https://www.news-medical.net/image-handler/picture/2021/5/shutterstock_1848796216.jpg

14.1.3. Phospholipids

Phospholipids are necessary for cellular membranes because they ensure the membrane stays fluid and intact. As a result of having glycerol, two fatty acids, and a phosphate group, these lipids can arrange themselves in bilayers because they are amphipathic. Phospholipids' fatty acid structure affects the membranes and is strongly linked to numerous health outcomes, mainly those related to lipid metabolism and the formation of abnormal blood lipids. Recent studies underline the importance of long-chain polyunsaturated fatty acids (LC-PUFAs) in phospholipids, suggesting that dietary intake and genetic factors, such as single nucleotide polymorphisms (SNPs) in desaturase enzymes, significantly affect LC-PUFA concentrations in the body, ultimately influencing metabolic health and disease susceptibility (Heinrich et al., 2009). Disorders in phospholipid metabolism are related to many health conditions, and psoriasis is one of them, as it is linked to changes in blood lipids. According to research, people with psoriasis are more likely to get dyslipidemia, which can increase their chances of developing heart disease. Lipid molecules in serum and skin from psoriatic patients have different patterns that show the effects of lipid metabolism and inflammation. The interplay between phospholipids and inflammatory processes suggests that targeting lipid metabolism could offer novel therapeutic strategies for managing inflammatory diseases such as psoriasis, which is increasingly understood as an immunometabolic disorder (Chodorowska et al., 2010). In addition, knowing how phospholipids relate to blood lipid problems can affect other chronic diseases besides psoriasis. Besides high levels of low-density lipoproteins, dyslipidemia is also a sign of phospholipid metabolism imbalance. Such an imbalance may harm the cell membrane and cell signals, eventually leading to the development of various metabolic disorders. Since phospholipids, genes, and diet play a complex role in health, further studies are needed to find out how these lipids impact disease and what can be done to reduce their effects. Hence, phospholipids play a key role in blood lipid problems, so more attention should be given to their influence and regulation in the treatment of chronic diseases (Figure 14.5).

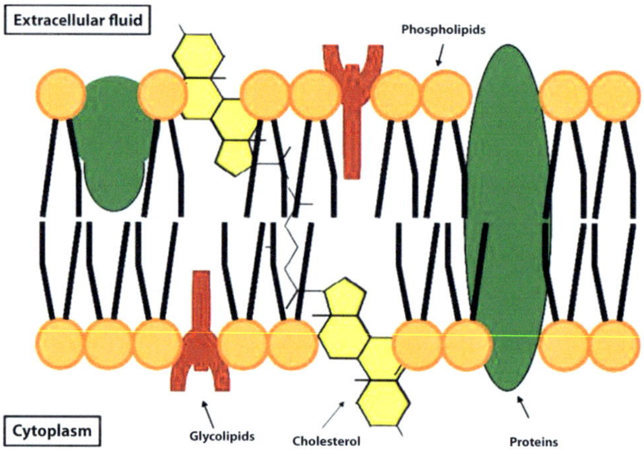

Figure 14.5. Phospholipids serve as fundamental components of cellular membranes, playing a pivotal role in maintaining membrane fluidity and structural integrity.

Source: https://www.bocsci.com/upload/image/classification-and-function-of-phospholipids-1.jpg

14.2. Causes of Blood Lipid Abnormalities

There are many genetic, lifestyle, and environmental reasons behind blood lipid abnormalities. Genetic predispositions, particularly mutations in cholesterol metabolism genes, can lead to disorders such as familial hypercholesterolemia, where individuals exhibit markedly elevated levels of low-density lipoprotein (LDL) cholesterol. Therefore, early steps are often required to manage lipid levels well. Besides genetics, the way people eat and exercise greatly affects their lipid levels. Having a diet rich in saturated fats and sugars may boost triglyceride and cholesterol levels, while being physically active frequently usually helps reduce them. It is very important to understand these different causes to design effective prevention and treatment plans for people with lipid abnormalities and related heart diseases. In addition, blood lipid abnormalities can be caused by insulin resistance and long-term inflammation in the body. Insulin resistance, commonly seen in conditions such as type 2 diabetes, leads to altered lipid metabolism, contributing to elevated triglycerides and reduced high-density lipoprotein (HDL) levels. Moreover, persistent inflammation may interfere with lipid balance and affect the way lipoproteins work. Research also suggests that complications during pregnancy, as indicated by the work of Sattar and Greer (2002), may predispose women to later vascular and metabolic diseases, underscoring a potential link between maternal health and offspring lipid profiles. To manage lipid abnormalities well, it is necessary to look at these physiological factors. Lifestyle changes and medical treatments can give us valuable information about managing high or low blood lipid levels. Taking statins is now the usual approach to lowering LDL cholesterol and decreasing the risk of heart problems. Still, the basic part of any successful intervention are dietary adjustments and physical activity. Eating a balanced diet that is high in omega-3 fatty acids, fiber, and antioxidants can greatly affect cholesterol levels and heart health. Additionally, the advancement of research methodologies, such as proteomic analysis, has opened new avenues for understanding the molecular mechanisms involving erythrocyte membranes and their role in lipid transport, potentially unveiling further targets for therapeutic intervention (de Oliveira & Saldanha, 2010). So, it is necessary to combine changes in lifestyle with medical care to effectively manage blood lipid abnormalities (Figure 14.6).

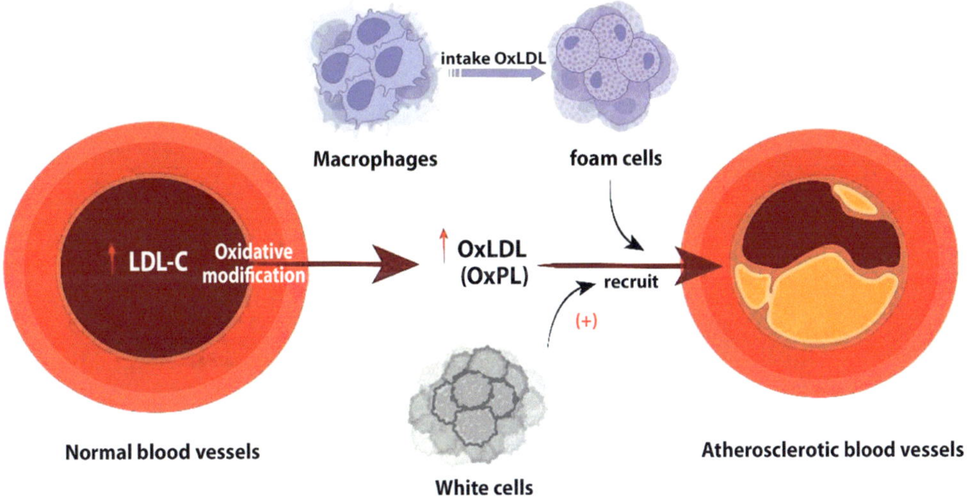

Figure 14.6. Chronic inflammation can disrupt lipid homeostasis, influencing the function and composition of lipoproteins.

Source: Xu L, Yang Q, Zhou J. Mechanisms of Abnormal Lipid Metabolism in the Pathogenesis of Disease. *International Journal of Molecular Sciences*. 2024; 25(15):8465. https://doi.org/10.3390/ijms25158465

14.2.1. Genetic Factors

More and more, people are realizing that genetic factors play a major role in causing blood lipid abnormalities and in heart health. Having certain genes can change a person's lipid levels, which may raise the risk of atherosclerosis and coronary artery disease. New studies have pointed out that certain genetic changes play a big role in how lipids are handled in the body. As an illustration, alterations in genes responsible for lipid transport and metabolism can lead to changes in lipid levels in people, proving that genetics and the environment are closely related. It indicates that screening the genes of people at risk for lipid problems is necessary, as it can guide the right treatments. One significant area of research involves the investigation of quantitative trait loci (QTL) associated with triglyceride levels in humans.

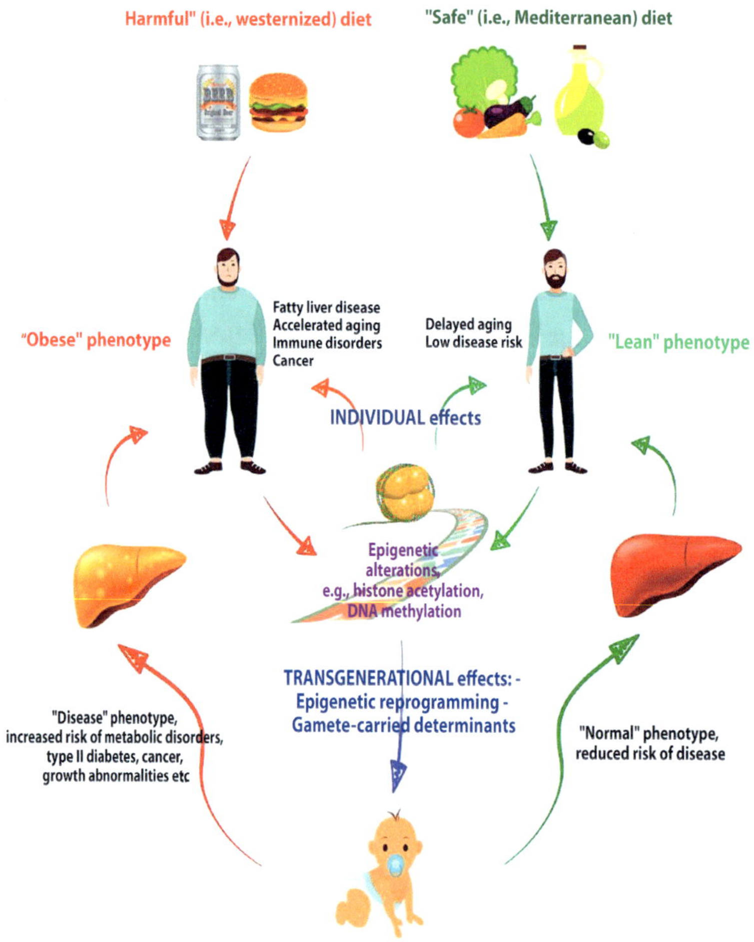

Figure 14.7. Genetic factors can intersect with environmental influences, such as lifestyle and dietary habits, leading to variations in lipid profiles among individuals.

Source: Tiffon C. The Impact of Nutrition and Environmental Epigenetics on Human Health and Disease. *International Journal of Molecular Sciences*. 2018; 19(11):3425. https://doi.org/10.3390/ijms19113425

As an example, a study found that a QTL on chromosome 7q36 points to the INSIG1 gene as a possible factor in triglyceride regulation. The promoter variant rs2721 was found to correlate with elevated triglyceride levels among individuals, suggesting a direct link between genetic variation and lipid metabolism (Kissebah et al., 2010). In particular, people with two copies of the T allele had higher triglyceride levels and lower INSIG1 expression. The fact that this gene acts as a feedback regulator in cholesterol and fatty acid synthesis shows that genes can directly affect lipid problems, stressing the need for more genetic research in handling dyslipidemia. Along with particular gene changes, the way a person's genes are organized matters a lot for lipid metabolism. Having different lifestyles and diets can cause genetic factors to influence lipid levels in people differently. For instance, some people have a genetic reason for high cholesterol, but others can keep their cholesterol in check by changing their lifestyle. The combination of genes and the environment is very important when it comes to personalized medicine in blood lipid abnormalities. Understanding these interactions not only informs risk assessment but also aids in devising tailored therapeutic strategies for individuals based on their unique genetic backgrounds and lifestyle factors (Ware et al., 2014) (Figure 14.7).

14.2.2. Dietary Influences

What people eat has a big impact on blood lipid abnormalities, and certain foods are very important for controlling cholesterol and triglycerides. Diets rich in saturated fats and trans fats have been identified as significant contributors to elevated LDL (low-density lipoprotein) cholesterol, often termed "bad" cholesterol. These fats can be found in most processed foods. Alternatively, taking in polyunsaturated and monounsaturated fats, mostly from fish, nuts, and olive oil, has been linked to good lipid levels.

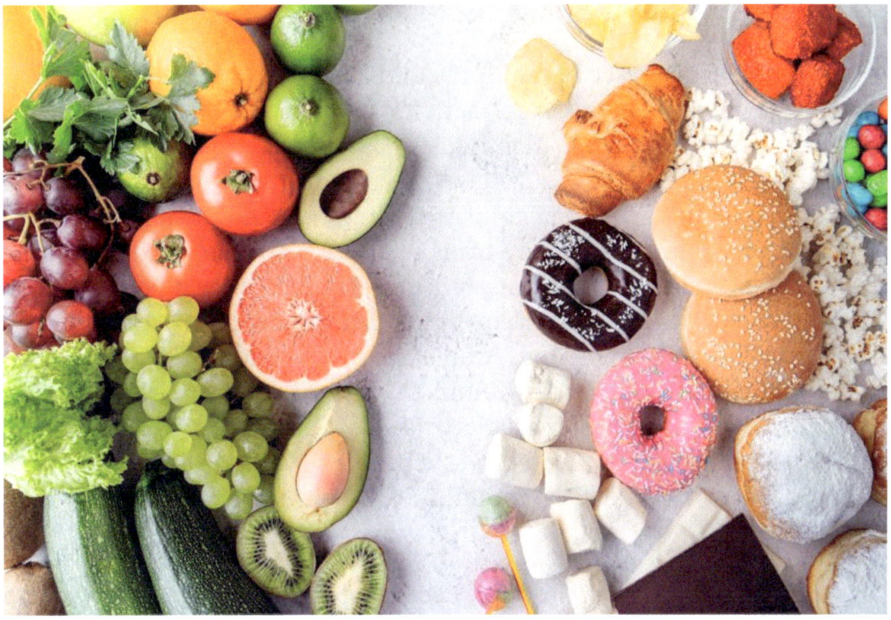

Figure 14.8. Diets rich in saturated fats and trans fats have been identified as significant contributors to elevated LDL (low-density lipoprotein) cholesterol, often termed "bad" cholesterol.

Source: https://sa1s3optim.patientpop.com/assets/images/provider/photos/2659779.jpg

This dietary shift not only reduces LDL cholesterol but also enhances HDL (high-density lipoprotein) cholesterol levels, which serve a protective role against cardiovascular disease. For this reason, fat selection is important for handling blood lipid problems and lowering heart disease risks.

Taking enough dietary fiber is also important for managing blood lipid levels. Soluble fiber, present in oats, legumes, and some fruits, has been proven to help reduce LDL cholesterol by combining with bile acids in the intestine and eliminating them from the body. A decrease in LDL cholesterol is necessary to reduce the danger of atherosclerosis and other heart problems. Also, eating lots of fiber is good for health, as it helps control blood sugar, improves appetite, and may help weight loss. Eating whole grains, fruits, and vegetables every day is a useful way to support metabolism and deal with lipid problems. Therefore, increasing fiber in the diet should be a main part of any strategy meant to improve lipid levels. In addition, the importance of phytochemicals and omega-3 fatty acids cannot be ignored when talking about blood lipid problems. It has been found that omega-3 fatty acids in fatty fish and flaxseeds can greatly lower triglycerides and improve the heart. For instance, (Hasani-Ranjbar et al., 2012) highlights how certain natural substances can influence metabolic variables linked to lipid disorders, suggesting a potential therapeutic avenue through nutritional intervention. Furthermore, (Bradley et al., 1986) emphasizes the impact of immune-mediated processes on triglyceride metabolism, illustrating the delicate interplay between dietary influences and underlying biological mechanisms. So, it is important to eat foods that are rich in phytochemicals, omega-3 fatty acids, and low in processed fats to manage lipid abnormalities. This way of thinking points out that diet should be included in overall health strategies for controlling blood lipids (Figure 14.8).

14.2.3. Lifestyle Choices

The way people live can greatly affect blood lipids and reduce the risk of cardiovascular diseases. Individuals who engage in regular physical activity tend to maintain healthier lipid profiles, as exercise has been shown to elevate high-density lipoprotein (HDL) cholesterol levels while simultaneously lowering low-density lipoprotein (LDL) cholesterol and triglycerides. In addition, diet can change blood lipid levels; for example, including fish and nuts in can help improve lipid abnormalities. Alternatively, eating too many trans fats and saturated fats can worsen lipid levels, which may result in long-term health problems. It is important to inform people about these factors, so they can be treated promptly and maintain better health, especially if they are at higher risk due to their health conditions or medicines. Some diets, for example, vegan diets, seem to help with blood lipid abnormalities. It has been found that these diets are related to a lower risk of chronic diseases, such as obesity, cardiovascular disease, and type two diabetes, mainly because they contain a lot of fiber and less saturated fat. Vegan diets shoud be carefully planned to avoid nutrient deficiencies such as vitamin B12, vitamin D and omega-3 fatty acids.

Certain medications may lead to metabolic syndrome. For example, second-generation antipsychotics are associated with weight gain, becoming diabetic, or getting high cholesterol, so they require routine monitoring according to the guidelines.

Improving quality in healthcare, including education for staff, has made it more likely that screening rules are followed. They help providers learn more and also encourage them to be more involved in caring for patients. When healthcare providers add lifestyle changes to treatment, patients with blood lipid issues can enjoy a much better quality of life and achieve better health in the future (Figure 14.9).

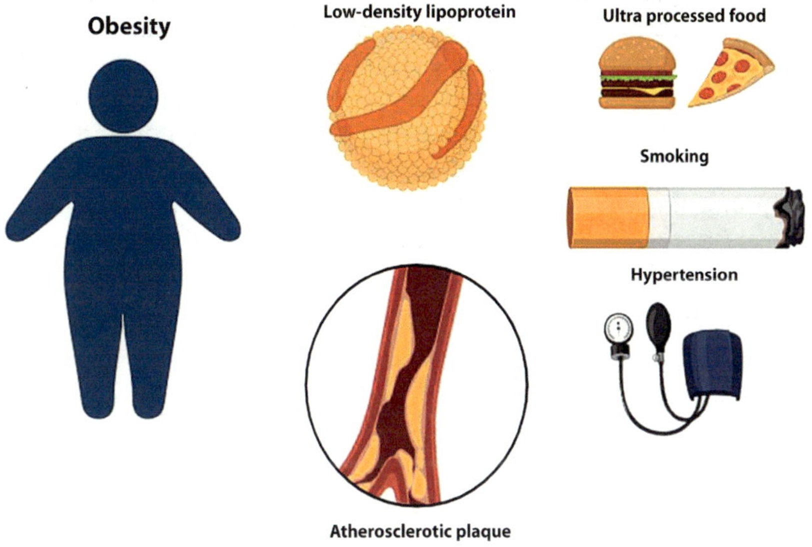

Figure 14.9. Lifestyle choices play a pivotal role in the management and prevention of blood lipid abnormalities, which are increasingly recognized as critical risk factors for cardiovascular diseases.

Source: Almohtasib Y, Fancher A J, Sawalha K (March 21, 2024) Emerging Trends in Atherosclerosis: Time to Address Atherosclerosis From a Younger Age. Cureus 16(3): e56635. doi:10.7759/cureus.56635

14.3. Health Implications of Abnormal Lipid Levels

Having abnormal lipid levels can harm many parts of the body and raise the chances of chronic health problems. Dyslipidemia, characterized by elevated levels of triglycerides and low-density lipoprotein (LDL) cholesterol, is closely associated with cardiovascular diseases, including coronary artery disease and stroke. High levels of LDL cholesterol in the arteries cause atherosclerosis, which reduces the size of blood vessels and restricts blood flow. In addition, when lipids are not within normal range, it can cause insulin resistance, which is a first step toward type 2 diabetes. As a result, the connection between lipid problems and these metabolic conditions shows that it is important to have effective ways to monitor and treat them. If these abnormalities in lipids are not managed, they may cause serious long-term problems, showing why it is important to educate and treat dyslipidemia. In addition to cardiovascular risks, abnormal lipid levels are implicated in the development of nonalcoholic fatty liver disease (NAFLD), a condition now recognized as the most common liver disease linked to metabolic disorders. When people's lifestyles get worse, the number of NAFLD cases in the world keeps rising, as it is currently at around 25%. Abnormal lipid metabolism, marked by increased fatty acids and triglycerides, overwhelms the liver's capacity for fat processing and export, thereby promoting the transition from simple steatosis to more severe forms such as nonalcoholic steatohepatitis (NASH) and cirrhosis. It is especially worrying that hepatocellular carcinoma can result from advanced liver disease. Thus, understanding the mechanisms of lipid metabolism can inform targeted interventions and facilitate the development of precise treatments to combat NAFLD and its systemic repercussions (Alonso et al., 2019). In addition, having abnormal lipid levels can affect more than metabolic and heart health; it may also raise the risk of premature death. Increased lipid levels might cause inflammation in the whole body, which is now seen as an important factor in the development of many chronic diseases, including some cancers and disorders affecting the brain. Noticing the warning signs of dyslipidemia allows healthcare professionals to determine if a condition is serious or not and helps them diagnose and treat patients earlier. Making changes to one's diet and exercising more can greatly affect how diseases develop and improve the health of the population. The multifaceted consequences of abnormal lipid levels necessitate a comprehensive approach to prevention and management, emphasizing the importance of early identification and intervention strategies in enhancing patient quality of life (Basavarajaiah et al., 2010) (Figure 14.10).

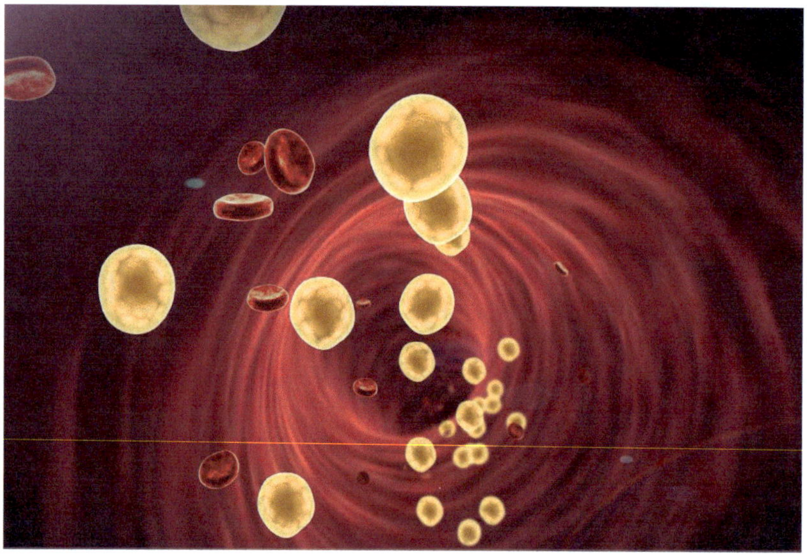

Figure 14.10. Dyslipidemia, characterized by elevated levels of triglycerides and low-density lipoprotein (LDL) cholesterol, is closely associated with cardiovascular diseases, including coronary artery disease and stroke.

Source: https://cdn-prod.medicalnewstoday.com/content/images/articles/321/321844/blood-cells-and-lipid-particles-in-artery-to-represent-dyslipidemia.jpg

14.3.1. Cardiovascular Diseases

The intricate relationship between blood lipid abnormalities and cardiovascular diseases (CVD) underscores a critical area of study within cardiovascular health. Elevated levels of low-density lipoprotein (LDL) cholesterol and triglycerides are well-documented risk factors for atherogenesis, leading to the development of atherosclerosis and subsequent cardiovascular events. The inflammatory reactions in these diseases prove that dyslipidemia leads to damage to blood vessels. Having many small, dense LDL particles is a main concern since they are more likely to cause heart problems than the larger, less dense particles. As a result, these lipid problems worsen the tendency for cholesterol plaque to form in blood vessels and also cause inflammation that leads to heart and brain problems. Even though cholesterol is still the main marker for dyslipidemia, recent findings suggest that the health of the gut microbiota affects both lipid metabolism and inflammation linked to CVD. Short-chain fatty acids (SCFAs), produced during the fermentation of dietary fibers by gut bacteria, have been linked to the regulation of cholesterol levels and immune responses that impact cardiovascular health. It has been found that SCFAs reduce inflammation and affect several metabolic pathways that are often out of balance in people with cardiovascular diseases, especially those with diabetes as well. Because of this connection, strategies that help produce more SCFAs through diet may improve lipid profiles and reduce the risk of heart disease. Therefore, knowing about the gut-lipid-heart axis might help find new ways to prevent or control CVD. Also, the link between obesity, inflammation, and heart disease is becoming easier to see. Problems like obesity can cause major changes in metabolism, resulting in abnormal lipid levels and increasing the risk of heart disease. For example, research indicates that chronic infection, such as that stemming from parasitic diseases, can exacerbate lipid and glucose metabolism in obese individuals, leading to an increased risk of diabetes and atherosclerosis (Andrada et al., 2016). Therefore, the findings suggest that managing cardiovascular disease should focus on lipid problems as well as the metabolic and inflammatory processes that are common in chronic diseases. Healthcare providers can use this knowledge to develop treatments that help people from many groups maintain healthy hearts (Figure 14.11).

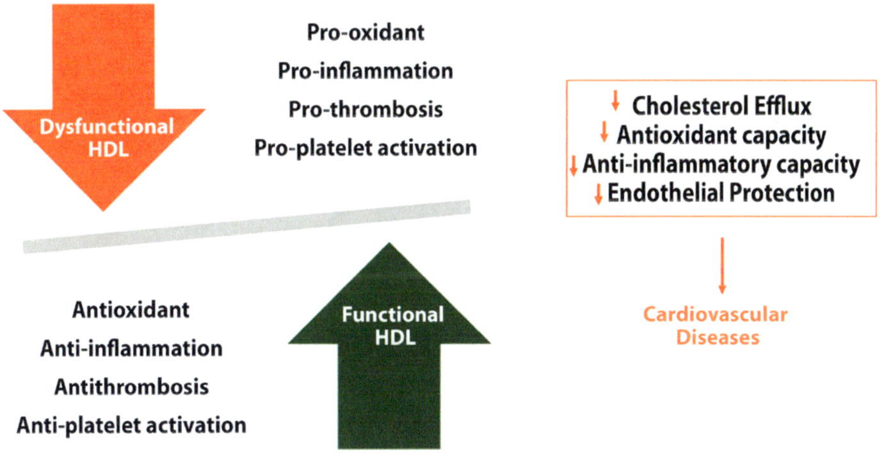

Figure 14.11. Elevated levels of low-density lipoprotein (LDL) cholesterol and triglycerides are well-documented risk factors for atherogenesis, leading to the development of atherosclerosis and subsequent cardiovascular events.

Source: Madaudo C, Bono G, Ortello A, Astuti G, Mingoia G, Galassi AR, Sucato V. Dysfunctional High-Density Lipoprotein Cholesterol and Coronary Artery Disease: A Narrative Review. *Journal of Personalized Medicine.* 2024; 14(9):996. https://doi.org/10.3390/jpm14090996

14.3.2. Metabolic Syndrome

Metabolic syndrome greatly increases a person's chances of developing cardiovascular disease and other severe health problems. The main features of this syndrome are central obesity, problems with lipids, high blood pressure, and insulin resistance. All these factors lead to an environment that causes endothelial dysfunction, and the development of atherosclerosis. According to Slee (2012), chronic kidney disease (CKD) often exacerbates these metabolic disturbances, leading to a vicious cycle where each component accelerates the others. Due to an overactive renin-angiotensin-aldosterone system, blood pressure and insulin resistance progress.

The lipid abnormalities associated with metabolic syndrome, such as elevated triglycerides and reduced high-density lipoprotein (HDL) cholesterol, reflect critical perturbations in lipid metabolism. Although there can be a genetic cause, dyslipidemia often stems from a poor diet and a lack of exercise, which are typical in those with metabolic syndrome. Lipid problems seen in people with metabolic syndrome may associated with a rise in inflammatory markers and adipocytokines. These lipid abnormalities are accompanied by atherosclerosis, and heart disease and death. As identified in Joseph et al. (2017), the gut microbiota plays a role in metabolic pathways and inflammation, suggesting that dietary interventions aimed at enhancing short-chain fatty acid production could positively influence lipid profiles and overall metabolic health. A good approach to metabolic syndrome involves changes in diet, medications, and lifestyle habits. Diets rich in fiber and healthy fats, such as the Mediterranean diet, can improve lipid levels and reduce insulin resistance. Such dietary patterns may enrich gut microbiota diversity, thereby producing short-chain fatty acids that help regulate immune and metabolic pathways, as noted in Joseph et al., (2017). Medications used to manage lipids, blood pressure, and insulin sensitivity along with lifestyle changes help patients reach better results. Awareness of metabolic syndrome and early action can result in improved blood lipids and cardiovascular health for those at risk (Figure 14.12).

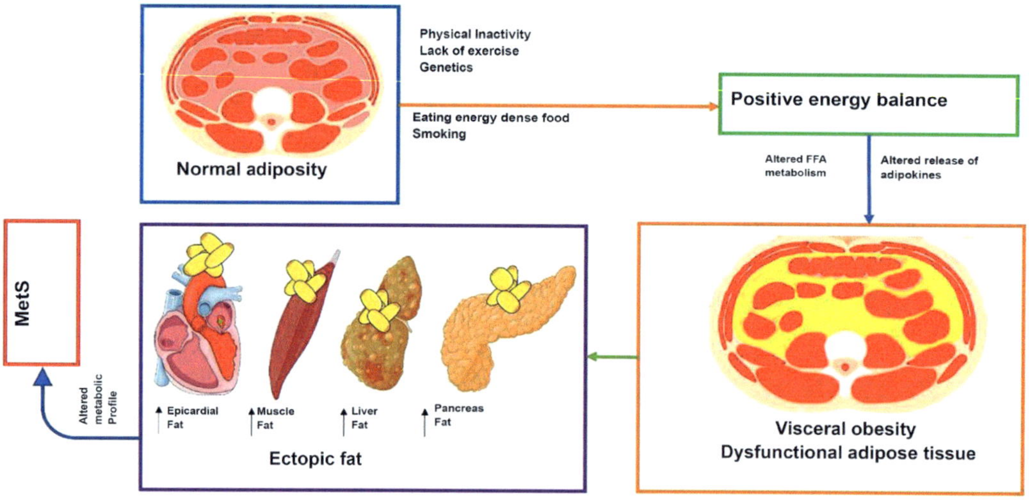

Figure 14.12. Metabolic syndrome is a multifaceted disorder that significantly contributes to the risk of cardiovascular disease and other serious health conditions.

Source: https://media.springernature.com/lw1200/springer-static/image/art%3A10.1186%2Fs10020-024-01019-y/MediaObjects/10020_2024_1019_Fig2_HTML.png

14.3.3. Pancreatitis

In pancreatitis, an abnormal activation of pancreatic enzymes results in the digestion of the pancreas and surrounding tissues. It is leads to edema, necrosis and inflammation of the pancrease.

Elevated triglycerides, which are frequently seen in patients with metabolic syndrome, in addition to excessive alcohol consumption, certain medications, and genetic predispositions are frequent causes of pancreatitis. Triglyceride levels over 1000 mg/dL greatly raise the risk of pancreatitis. If lipid abnormalities are corrected, and lifestyles changes to manage metabolic syndrome and limiting alcohol consumption are implemented, the risk of pancreatitis can be reduced. (Figure 14.13).

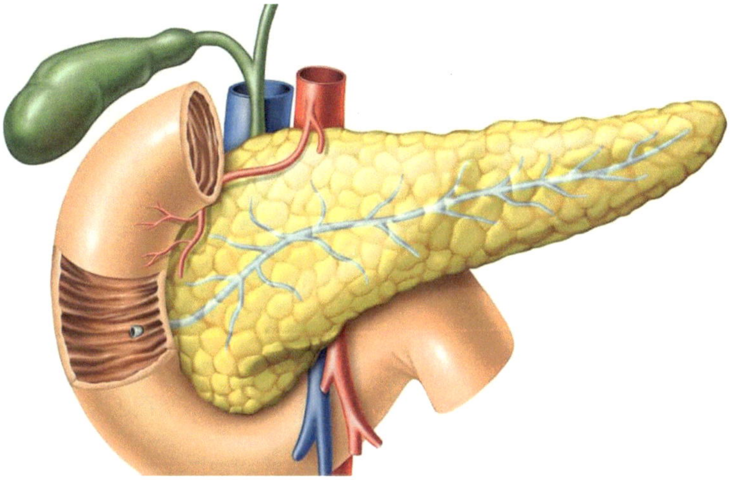

Figure 14.13. Pancreatitis.

Source: https://www.carygastro.com/uploads/_1200x630_crop_center-center_82_none/Acute-Pancreatitis-FB.jpg?mtime=1591739831

14.4. Diagnosis of Blood Lipid Abnormalities

To assess cardiovascular health and assess the risk of atherosclerosis, it is vital to diagnose blood lipid abnormalities. The diagnostic process typically begins with a comprehensive lipid panel, which measures total cholesterol, low-density lipoprotein (LDL) cholesterol, high-density lipoprotein (HDL) cholesterol, and triglycerides. People with high LDL and triglycerides and low HDL are more likely to suffer from cardiovascular problems. Lipid profiles are best interpreted considering a patient's general health, habits, and their family's medical background. Lipids should be monitored regularly, especially in patients who have obesity, diabetes or lead a sedentary life. More investigation may focus on finding secondary reasons for dyslipidemia, which can be linked to problems such as a low thyroid, liver disease, or some drugs. It is very important to find these secondary causes because fixing the main problem may solve the lipid abnormalities. Genetic factors may lead to familial hyperlipidemia or similar inherited problems with lipid metabolism. Along with changing their lifestyle, some patients with high lipid levels may need to take medications as well. With these methods, clinicians are able to design a plan that helps patients reduce their cardiovascular risk and maintain good health. Dietary modifications have a significant impact of lipid levels. These include lowering the consumption of carbohydrate intake, saturated fats and increasing the consumption of foods high in omega-3 fatty acids can have a major effect on their lipid levels. Taking care of blood lipid abnormalities can help prevent heart disease and reduce its health complications (Figure 14.14).

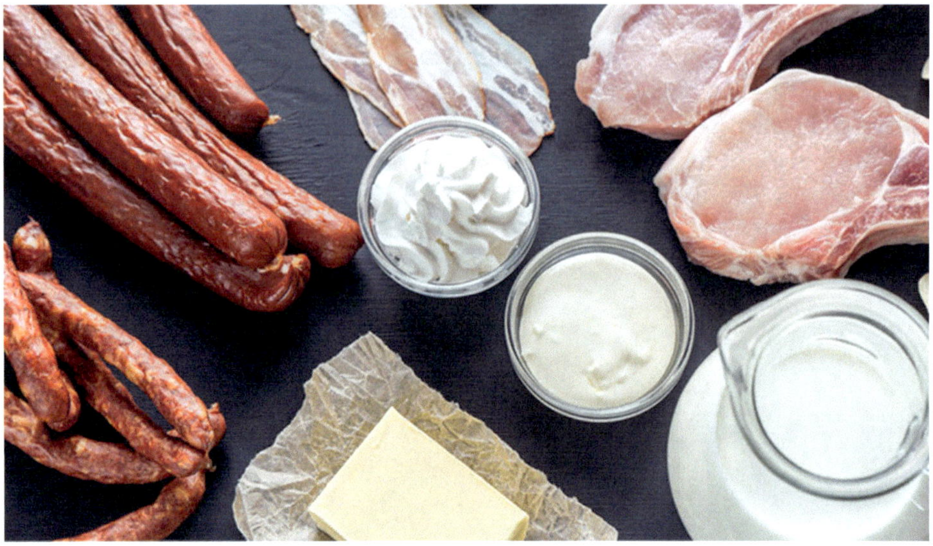

Figure 14.14. Education concerning dietary choices, such as reducing saturated fat intake and increasing omega-3 fatty acids, can significantly impact lipid profiles.

Source: https://www.heart.org/-/media/AHA/H4GM/Article-Images/saturated-fat.jpg?sc_lang=en

14.4.1. Blood Tests and Lipid Panels

Blood tests and lipid panels are very important for assessing the heart and for finding problems with blood lipids. A lipid panel checks the amounts of cholesterol and triglycerides in the blood to determine a person's likelihood of heart disease and similar conditions. The standard components of a lipid panel include low-density lipoprotein (LDL), high-density lipoprotein (HDL), total cholesterol, and triglycerides. The amount of these lipids in a person's blood can be used by healthcare providers to identify dyslipidemia, which is usually a warning sign for serious health complications. Spotting high levels of LDL or triglycerides in blood tests is important, since it enables early action to be taken. As a result, it is advised that regular lipid tests be done, mainly for those who are obese or have a family history of high cholesterol. The implications of lipid profiles extend beyond mere measurements, as they can indicate broader metabolic disturbances, such as those seen in nonalcoholic fatty liver disease (NAFLD). Studies have found that a large number of children with NAFLD have dyslipidemia that should be managed by a doctor, and the first step is to check their lipid levels. It was found in a cohort study that 14% of children had high LDL cholesterol levels at the start, showing how useful blood tests are for spotting people at risk. After applying dietary changes, many of these children reached the recommended levels for lipids, proving that lifestyle changes play a key role. This information proves that lipid screening should be done early in children to help detect and prevent health problems. In addition, lipid panels give both doctors and patients important information that helps them decide on changes in diet and daily habits. If someone's triglyceride levels are high, as shown by lipid testing, they may be eligible for special dietary advice or drug therapy. The study found that more than half of the children diagnosed with NAFLD had dyslipidemia, proving that checking lipid levels is important in clinical practice. With this information, healthcare providers and patients can have active talks about lowering cardiovascular risks. They can support patients in following their treatment plans, making the outcomes better. To summarize, blood tests and lipid panels are necessary for finding, measuring, and managing problems with blood lipids, which can help people stay healthy and well in the long run (Figure 14.15).

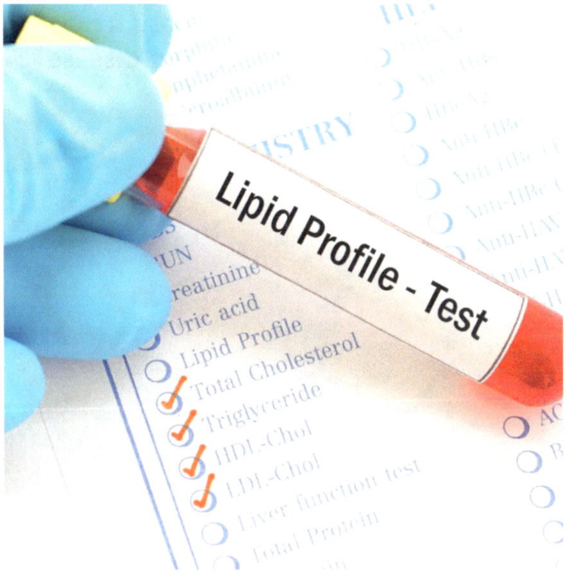

Figure 14.15. Blood tests and lipid panels serve as critical diagnostic tools in the assessment of cardiovascular health, particularly in relation to blood lipid abnormalities.

Source: https://walkin-clinic.co.uk/wp-content/uploads/2024/05/Lipid-Profile-1.webp

14.4.2. Interpretation of Results

The interpretation of blood lipid test results is very important for both doctors and public health officials. High levels of low-density lipoprotein (LDL) cholesterol and triglycerides, coupled with low high-density lipoprotein (HDL) levels, are key indicators of metabolic dysfunction. To understand these lipid profiles, all the results from blood tests must be carefully examined. The results need to be understood in light of the patient's general health, including what they eat, how much they exercise, and their genetic background, as these can have a strong effect on lipid metabolism. Moreover, the intricacies of lipid interactions and their implications on cardiovascular health underscore the importance of not merely focusing on threshold values but also considering the broader metabolic context in which these abnormalities exist, as highlighted by recent findings on erythrocyte function and adhesion molecule expression (de Oliveira & Saldanha, 2010). The results of lipid profiles are most important when trying to identify people at risk for metabolic syndrome. New research points out that a strict methodology should be used to assess interventions for correcting lipid levels. For instance, while the effects of herbal treatments like Anethum graveolens (dill) have shown some promise in reducing triglyceride levels in patients with metabolic syndrome, the overall impact on lipid profiles requires careful scrutiny (Hasani-Ranjbar et al., 2012). Because of these findings, healthcare professionals should be careful when suggesting dietary supplements, since changes in laboratory tests may not always matter in the patient's condition. Because of this complexity, it is important to understand how each lipid marker affects the whole body's metabolism. It is also necessary to keep in mind that blood lipid levels vary from one population to another. Results should be interpreted considering the patient's age, sex, and ethnicity, since these factors are key in lipid metabolism and heart disease. Genetic polymorphisms can affect the way some populations react to diet and medicine meant to improve their lipid levels. So, taking these factors into account allows for better management of blood lipid problems. By knowing these details, doctors can read lipid results more accurately, choose treatments that fit each patient, and thus achieve better health results and lower risks for heart disease (Figure 14.16).

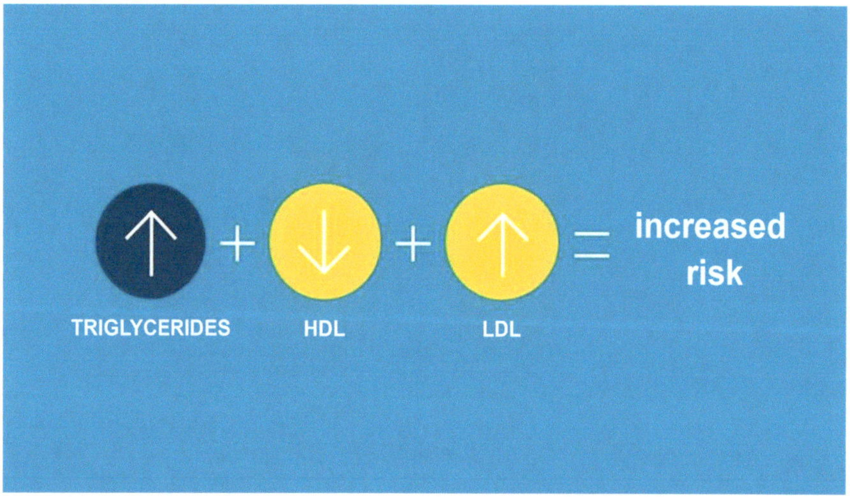

Figure 14.16. High levels of low-density lipoprotein (LDL) cholesterol and triglycerides, coupled with low high-density lipoprotein (HDL) levels, are key indicators of metabolic dysfunction.

Source: https://www.heart.org/-/media/Images/Health-Topics/Video-Thumbnails/Cholesterol-What-is-video.jpg?h=720&w=1280&sc_lang=en&hash=F8D2ECB14D2EBAE8E346EE18D9DC91A6

14.4.3. Risk Assessment

Assessing the risk of blood lipid abnormalities is key in finding people who are more likely to develop heart diseases. By examining parameters such as total cholesterol, low-density lipoprotein (LDL) cholesterol, and high-density lipoprotein (HDL) cholesterol, healthcare providers can stratify patients according to their potential for adverse health outcomes. People who have higher LDL cholesterol and lower HDL cholesterol levels have a high risk of getting atherosclerosis, which may result in heart attacks and strokes. Moreover, blood lipid assessments are particularly poignant in populations with conditions such as polycystic ovary syndrome (PCOS), where dyslipidemia is a common finding. Women with PCOS not only exhibit unfavorable lipid profiles but also display additional cardiovascular risks, highlighting the necessity for comprehensive risk assessment to manage and mitigate these conditions effectively (Cascella et al., 2004). Blood lipid abnormalities should be assessed by considering a patient's lifestyle as well. Factors such as diet, physical activity, and body mass index (BMI) can significantly influence lipid levels and metabolic health. In such cases, those with little exercise and unhealthy diets tend to have unusual lipid levels, which increases their chance of heart problems. Regular cardiovascular tests that check blood lipid levels can help people change their lifestyle when necessary. Sometimes, using medications is necessary when the lipid levels are very high. Thiazolidinediones (TZDs), such as rosiglitazone and pioglitazone, can notably enhance lipid profiles while also targeting the underlying insulin resistance commonly found in type 2 diabetes. This multifaceted approach emphasizes that understanding risk through lipid assessment is crucial for appropriate intervention and disease prevention (Honisett et al., 2007). It is important to move from assessing the risks of individuals to planning strategies for the whole population when dealing with blood lipid problems. If people improve their diets and increase physical activity, public health can help lower the number of dyslipidemias and heart problems. Such programs usually concentrate on people who are at risk, such as those with serious health problems or financial issues that make it hard for them to choose healthy ways of living. When healthcare practitioners organize community programs, they can stress the role of regular lipid screening for keeping people healthy. Therefore, assessing risk helps patients and also supports strategies that reduce the number of cardiovascular disease cases in the public. Therefore, using blood lipid tests in risk assessment helps achieve better health and saves money on cardiovascular disease treatment (Figure 14.17).

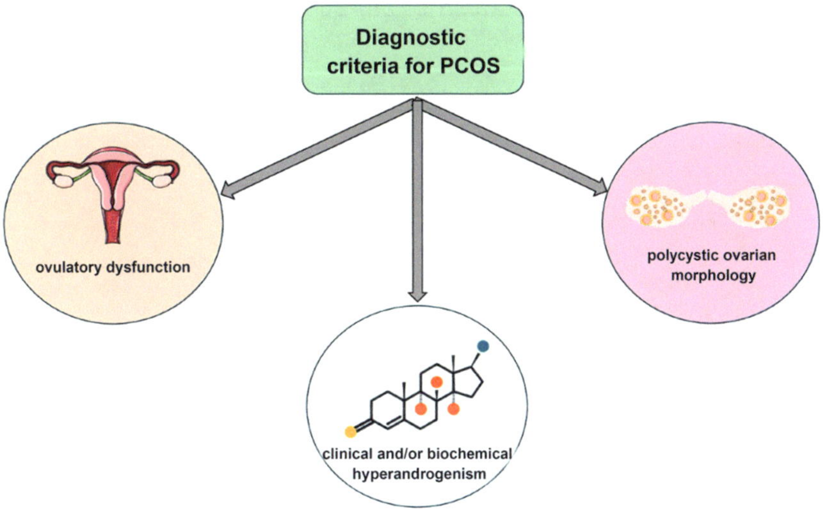

Figure 14.17. Women with PCOS not only exhibit unfavorable lipid profiles but also display additional cardiovascular risks, highlighting the necessity for comprehensive risk assessment to manage and mitigate these conditions effectively

Source: Pililis S, Lampsas S, Kountouri A, Pliouta L, Korakas E, Livadas S, Thymis J, Peppa M, Kalantaridou S, Oikonomou E, et al. The Cardiometabolic Risk in Women with Polycystic Ovarian Syndrome (PCOS): From Pathophysiology to Diagnosis and Treatment. *Medicina*. 2024; 60(10):1656. https://doi.org/10.3390/medicina60101656

14.5. Treatment Options

Taking care of blood lipid problems can prevent heart diseases and improve a person's overall health. Most people are recommended to change their lifestyle, take medicines, and get advanced care when it is required. A healthy diet, frequent exercise and smoking cessation can improve the lipid panel. If needed, statins and fibrates are medications given to people with dyslipidemia. Statins are especially recognized for reducing LDL cholesterol and lowering the risk of heart-related issues.

Statins are considered the first-line medication due to their proven benefits in reducing low-density lipoprotein (LDL) cholesterol levels and decreasing the risk of heart attacks and strokes. If statins are not effective, ezetimibe or PCSK9 inhibitors can be added. Ezetimibe blocks the intestines from absorbing cholesterol, while PCSK9 inhibitors raise the liver's ability to remove LDL cholesterol from the blood. It is necessary to select treatment plans that are tailored to every patient's lipid problems. With advances in therapy and technology, lipid disorders are being targeted with gene therapy and monoclonal antibodies. For instance, studies done recently with gene editing have indicated that controlling genes responsible for lipid control can help lower cholesterol. Medicines being tested for how they affect lipid transport and metabolism seem promising for managing severe dyslipidemia that does not respond to usual treatments. Since science is always progressing, the options for treating blood lipid abnormalities must change, so personalized medicine is necessary. Monitoring patient response to treatments and incorporating novel therapies into management strategies ensures a comprehensive approach to prevent cardiovascular complications and promote long-term health outcomes (Ambale-Venkatesh et al., 2017; Couce et al., 2020) (Figure 14.18).

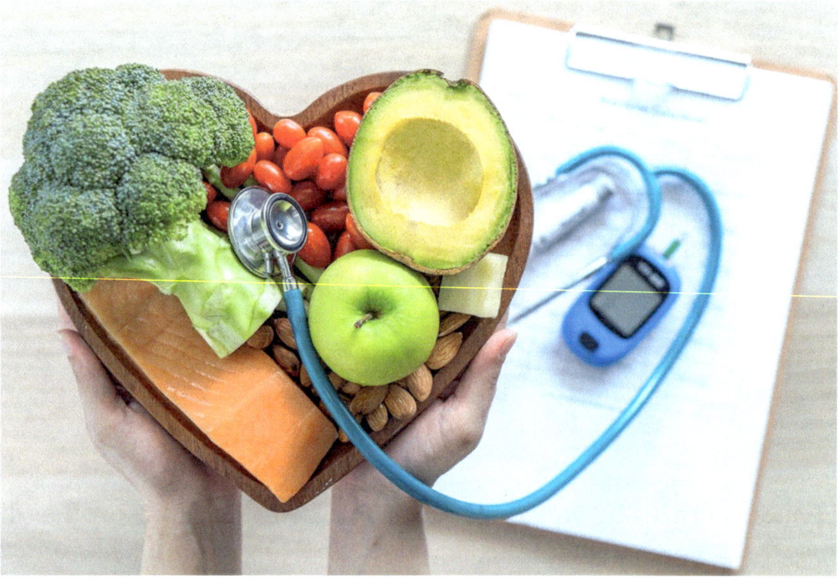

Figure 14.18. Lifestyle changes such as adopting a heart-healthy diet, increasing physical activity, and quitting smoking can significantly lower cholesterol levels and improve lipid profiles.

Source: https://www.bestdoctorsinsurance.com/wp-content/uploads/2023/08/shutterstock_1926525272.webp

14.5.1. Lifestyle Modifications

Making certain lifestyle changes is very important for managing and preventing blood lipid abnormalities.. Diets high in fruits, vegetables, whole grains, and healthy fats, can correct dyslipidemias , lower inflammation and improve the function of the immune system. The connection between dietary choices and cardiovascular health is underscored by recent findings that link short-chain fatty acids (SCFAs) derived from the fermentation of dietary fibers to beneficial metabolic pathways, crucial for combating disorders like cardiovascular disease and type II diabetes, as noted in the research surrounding gut microbiota (Joseph et al., 2017). In addition to diet, engaging in moderate to vigorous exercise enhances lipid metabolism, facilitating the reduction of triglycerides and the elevation of high-density lipoprotein (HDL) cholesterol. For children, particularly those with conditions like nonalcoholic fatty liver disease (NAFLD), implementing structured physical activity alongside dietary adjustments can lead to significant improvements in lipid profiles. A longitudinal study demonstrated that after one year of standardized dietary recommendations and increased physical activity, a remarkable percentage of participants achieved their lipid goals (Alazraki et al., 2018). As a result, it is important to use both diet and exercise together, since this can bring lasting improvements in lipid levels and result in better health. In addition, the mental side of making lifestyle changes is very important. While the primary focus of research has often been on the implications of dietary quality and quantity, there is a compelling case for examining how lifestyle changes can simultaneously target both mental and physical health interventions (Joseph et al., 2017). When lifestyle changes are made, they address blood lipid problems and also help people live a better life in many areas of well-being (Figure 14.19)

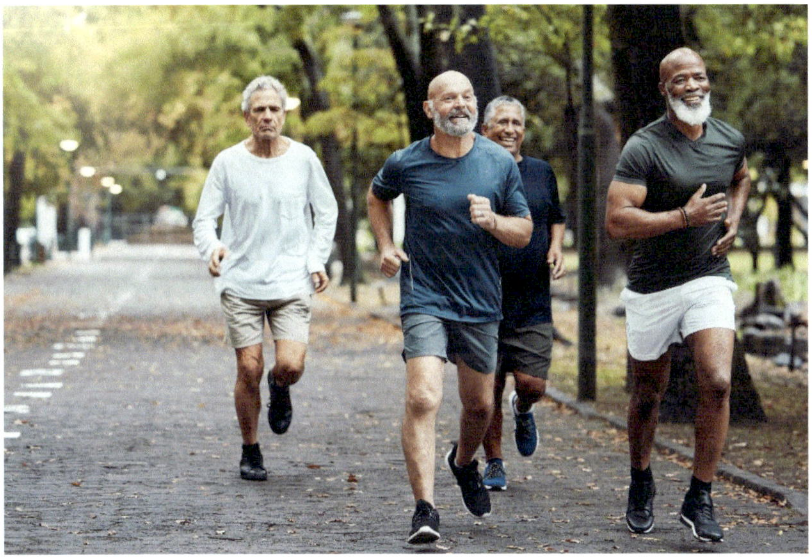

Figure 14.19. Engaging in moderate to vigorous exercise enhances the body's lipid metabolism, facilitating the reduction of triglycerides and the elevation of high-density lipoprotein (HDL) cholesterol, often referred to as the good cholesterol.

Source: https://www.news-medical.net/images/news/ImageForNews_768543_17047719291831057.jpg

14.5.2. Pharmacological Interventions

When it comes to blood lipid problems, medicines are essential in handling dyslipidemias that may result in serious heart-related risks. A broad spectrum of medications targets lipid profiles, particularly by lowering low-density lipoprotein (LDL) cholesterol and triglycerides while potentially elevating high-density lipoprotein (HDL) cholesterol. Among the most commonly prescribed drugs, statins stop HMG-CoA reductase and lower the amount of cholesterol produced inside the liver. Also, new treatments like PCSK9 inhibitors and ezetimibe have become available for patients who either have side effects from statins or do not get the desired results from taking them alone. It is important to look at a patient's risk factors, the way they react to treatment, and their general health to design the best drug regimen for lipid management. Besides statins and PCSK9 inhibitors, fibrates and niacin can be used to treat high blood lipids. Fibrates are mainly helpful for patients with high triglycerides because they increase lipolysis and reduce the liver's production of triglycerides. Although niacin is helpful in raising HDL cholesterol, it may cause side effects like flushing and discomfort in the stomach. New therapies, such as novel drugs and gene therapy, are being studied. Understanding the genetic factors influencing lipid metabolism could tailor treatment to a person's genes. Moreover, using changes in diet and lifestyle along with drugs is more effective in treating blood lipid issues, as it provides a variety of treatments that help patients the most (Figure 14.20).

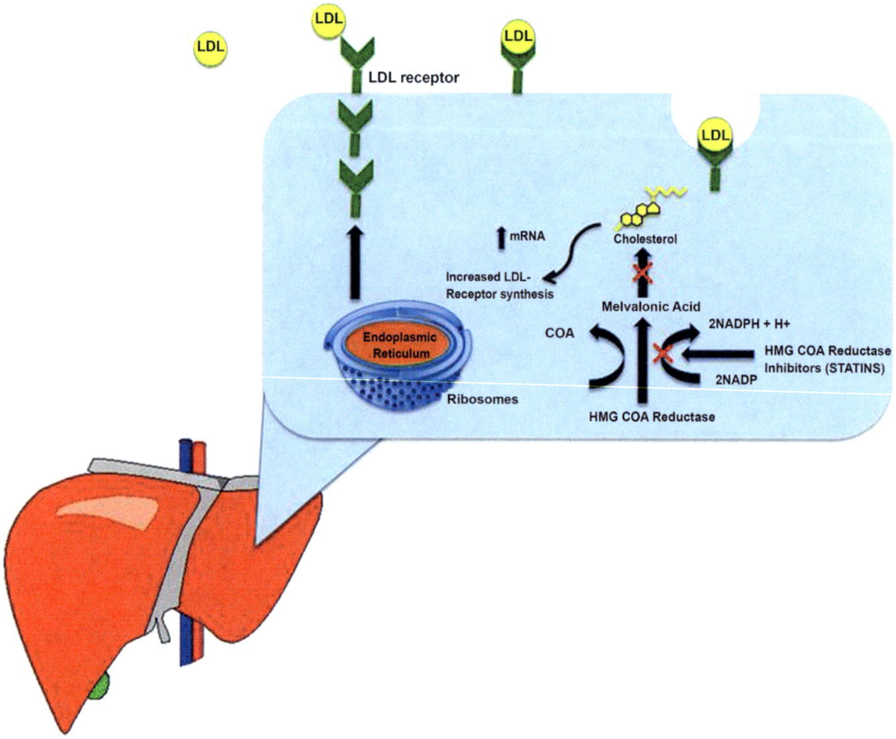

Figure 14.20. Statins, among the most extensively prescribed agents, function by inhibiting HMG-CoA reductase, thus reducing endogenous cholesterol production.

Source: https://www.researchgate.net/publication/325252975/figure/fig1/AS:962674242383883@1606530833367/Statins-inhibit-HMG-CoA-reductase-thereby-decreasing-intracellular-synthesis-of.gif

14.5.3. Monitoring and Follow-up

Following up and monitoring patients is essential for managing blood lipid problems, since it strongly affects patient results and the success of treatment. By checking lipid levels regularly, healthcare professionals can review the success of treatments, find out if there are risks for heart diseases, and make sure the treatment is effective. It is recommended to have a lipid profile test every six months to a year, mainly for patients who have a family history of dyslipidemia or any heart problems. Setting follow-up schedules according to each person's risk factors helps deal with changes in lipid levels quickly and encourages them to stick to their treatment and lifestyle changes. Lifestyle modifications usually involve dietary changes, frequent exercise, and weight management. Drug intervention is usually delayed until lifestyle changes have been implemented for an adequate time (Ware et al. (2014)). Concentrating on lifestyle improves overall care for patients and motivates them to take part in managing their health, which leads to better outcomes. Moreover, using technology and telemedicine has made it much easier to manage blood lipid problems. Digital health tools help people keep track of their lipid levels and follow the prescribed medicines, and they also make it easier for patients to communicate with their doctors. Because the information is updated in real time, doctors can quickly change the patient's treatment plan according to their needs. Technology can also help patients with personalized tools and reminders, encouraging them to follow recommendations. (Figure 14.21).

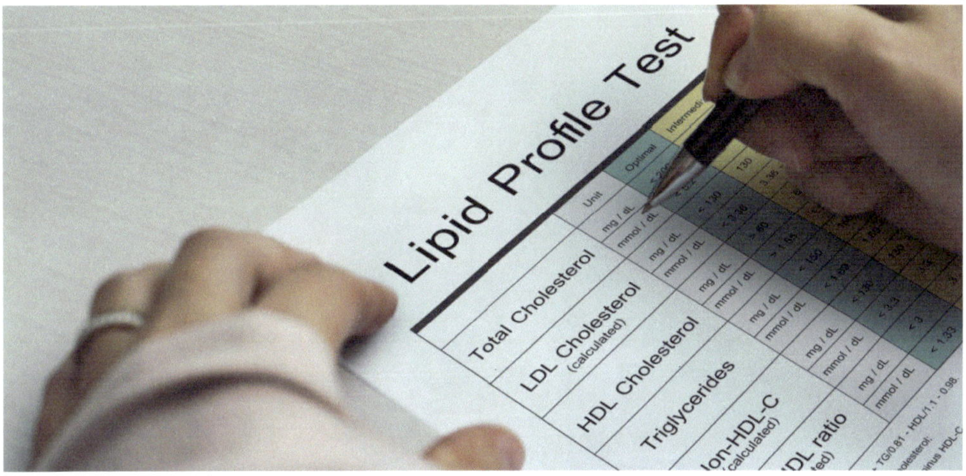

Figure 14.21. Monitoring and follow-up are critical components in the management of blood lipid abnormalities, significantly influencing patient outcomes and treatment efficacy.

Source: https://images.apollo247.in/pd-cms/cms/2023-07/Shutterstock_561584608.jpg

A CLOSER LOOK

HIGH-DENSITY LIPOPROTEIN (HDL) CHOLESTEROL

High-Density Lipoprotein (HDL) cholesterol is often called the "good" cholesterol because it helps remove excess cholesterol from the bloodstream and transport it to the liver for disposal. A higher level of HDL cholesterol is linked to a lower chance of heart disease and stroke, as it stops the growth of fatty plaques in the arteries. Making sure to exercise often, eat a good diet, and not smoke can boost HDL levels. A high HDL level, above 60 mg/dL, is usually seen as protective from cardiovascular disease.

Summary

When blood lipids are not normal, it becomes a health concern, mainly because of changes in triglycerides, cholesterol, and different lipoproteins. There are many reasons for these abnormalities, including diet, metabolic syndromes, genetics, and certain medications. Even certain cancer treatments such as RIFN-gamma treatment can cause significant increase in triglycerides. Chronic conditions such as cancer or infections are also associated with hypertriglyceridemia. Such findings highlight the complexity of lipid metabolism regulation, which can be influenced by biochemical mediators released from immune cells under certain conditions, thus linking inflammation and lipid profiles in significant ways (Bradley et al., 1986). Another challenge in this area is that mothers' health is now understood to play a big role in shaping their children's future health. It has been found that not getting enough nutrition as a mother during pregnancy can affect the child's development and increase the risk of vascular diseases in the future. As Naveed Sattar and Ian Greer (2002) note, issues that arise during pregnancy may not only affect the immediate well-being of the mother and child but can also set the stage for metabolic disorders, linking maternal health to long-term vascular risks. The fact that maternal and fetal health are both considered means that lipids affect health in many ways, not only in the present but also in the future. The connection between nutrition, metabolism, and blood lipids underlines the importance of using all-around approaches. As scientists discover the links between lipid metabolism, chronic diseases, and maternal health, it is clear that there should be more public health efforts to change people's diets and improve their metabolism. Educating people who are pregnant and those with chronic diseases could help avoid the complications of blood lipid abnormalities. Also, further studies on what affects lipid metabolism can lead to better treatments. Knowing more about these topics helps with current health problems and encourages actions that can prevent diseases in the future.

References

1. Abumrad, N. A., Allum, F., Arnett, D. K., Aslibekyan, S., et al. (2016). *Higher Chylomicron Remnants and LDL Particle Numbers Associate with CD36 SNPs and DNA Methylation Sites that Reduce CD36.* https://core.ac.uk/download/74479156.pdf (accessed on 11th June 2025).
2. Aguilar-Salinas, C. A., American Diabetes Association, Aryal, M., Boyle, J. P., Davies, M. J., Dewey, F. E., Eckel, R. H., et al. (2019). *ANGPTL4 Gene E40K Variation Protects Against Obesity-Associated Dyslipidemia in Participants with Obesity.* https://core.ac.uk/download/195777348.pdf (accessed on 11th June 2025).
3. Aguirre-Betolaza, A., Martínez, I., Corres, P., Francisco-Terreros, S., et al. (2020). *A Metabolically Healthy Profile Is a Transient Stage When Exercise and Diet Are Not Supervised: Long-Term Effects in the EXERDIET-HTA Study.* https://core.ac.uk/download/322929946.pdf (accessed on 11th June 2025).
4. Alazraki, A., Jain, A. K., Wells, A., Hernandez, A., Towbin, A., Mencin, A., Sternberg, A., et al. (2018). *Clinically Actionable Hypercholesterolemia and Hypertriglyceridemia in Children with Nonalcoholic Fatty Liver Disease.* https://core.ac.uk/download/228066177.pdf (accessed on 11th June 2025).
5. Alonso, C., Lu, S. C., Mato, J. M., Noureddin, M., et al. (2019). *Biomarkers and Subtypes of Deranged Lipid Metabolism in Non-Alcoholic Fatty Liver Disease.* https://core.ac.uk/download/323078743.pdf (accessed on 11th June 2025).
6. Ambale-Venkatesh, B., Bluemke, D. A., Butt, A. A., Chew, M., et al. (2017). *Subclinical Myocardial Disease by Cardiac Magnetic Resonance Imaging and Spectroscopy in Healthy HIV/Hepatitis C Virus-Coinfected Persons.* https://core.ac.uk/download/323078609.pdf (accessed on 11th June 2025).
7. Andrada, M. C., Aoki, M. P., Cabalén, M. E., Cabral, M. A., et al. (2016). *Chronic Trypanosoma cruzi Infection Potentiates Adipose Tissue Macrophage Polarization Toward an Anti-Inflammatory M2 Phenotype and Contributes to Diabetes Progression in a Diet-Induced Obesity Model.* https://core.ac.uk/download/159288522.pdf (accessed on 11th June 2025).
8. Azar, R., Jonnalagadda, S., Kerr, T. A., Prakash, R., et al. (2007). *Pancreatitis Following Olanzapine Therapy: A Report of Three Cases.* https://core.ac.uk/download/83101025.pdf (accessed on 11th June 2025).
9. Azran, C., Batterham, R. L., Busetto, L., Dicker, D., et al. (2017). *Practical Recommendations of the Obesity Management Task Force of the European Association for the Study of Obesity for the Post-Bariatric Surgery Medical Management.* https://core.ac.uk/download/141699962.pdf (accessed on 11th June 2025).
10. Basavarajaiah, S., Giese, E. A., International Olympic Committee Medical Commission, & Ingle, L. (2010). *Pre-Participation Cardiac Screening in Young Athletes: Models and Criteria.* https://core.ac.uk/download/29019018.pdf (accessed on 11th June 2025).
11. Becque, M. D., Boreham, C., Corigliano, G., Lee, S., McMahan, C. A., Shea, S., & Thompson, P. D. (2007). *Special Article: Physical Activity, Physical Fitness, And Cardiovascular Risk Factors in Childhood.* https://core.ac.uk/download/83049283.pdf (accessed on 11th June 2025).
12. Bekel, G. E., & Thupayagale-Tshweneagae, G. (2020). *Prevalence and Associated Factors of Metabolic Syndrome and Its Individual Components Among Adolescents.* https://media.neliti.

com/media/publications/300772-prevalence-and-associated-factors-of-met-7bc6a11e.pdf (accessed on 11th June 2025).

13. Bowman, S. J., Giles, I. P., Ioannou, Y., Rahman, A., et al. (2005). *Review of Presentations at the 6th European Lupus Meeting 3–5 March 2005.* https://core.ac.uk/download/1669257.pdf (accessed on 11th June 2025).

14. Bradley, W. A., Gianturco, S. H., Gutterman, J. U., Kurzrock, R., et al. (1986). *Recombinant Gamma Interferon Induces Hypertriglyceridemia and Inhibits Post-Heparin Lipase Activity in Cancer Patients.* https://core.ac.uk/download/323066542.pdf (accessed on 11th June 2025).

15. Joseph, J., Depp, C., Shih, P. B., Cadenhead, K. S., & Schmid-Schönbein, G. (2017). Modified Mediterranean Diet for Enrichment of Short Chain Fatty Acids: Potential Adjunctive Therapeutic to Target Immune and Metabolic Dysfunction in Schizophrenia?. *Frontiers in neuroscience, 11,* 155. https://doi.org/10.3389/fnins.2017.00155(accessed on 11th June 2025).

16. Cameron, A. J., Alberti, K. G. M. M., Alessi, M. C., Barr, E. L. M., Boyko, E. J., Cameron, A. J., Carr, M. C., et al. (2008). *Central Obesity as A Precursor to The Metabolic Syndrome in the AusDiab Study and Mauritius.* http://hdl.handle.net/10536/DRO/DU:30021308 (accessed on 11th June 2025).

17. Cascella, T., Colao, A., Zullo, F., Tauchmanovà, L., Lombardi, G., et al. (2004). *The Cardiovascular Risk of Young Women with Polycystic Ovary Syndrome: An Observational, Analytical, Prospective Case-Control Study.* https://core.ac.uk/download/55016624.pdf (accessed on 11th June 2025).

18. Chodorowska, G., Michalak-Stoma, A., Pietrzak, A., Szepietowski, J., et al. (2010). *Lipid Disturbances in Psoriasis: An Update.* https://core.ac.uk/download/pdf/8437406.pdf (accessed on 11th June 2025).

19. Ware, Lisa & Rennie, Kirsten & Gafane-Matemane, Lebo & Collard, Jade & Nell, Tarryn & Schutte, Aletta. (2014). Physical activity and hypertension in South African adults. Conference: Society for Endocrinology, Metabolism and Diabetes South Africa 2014 Annual Scientific MeetingAt: Durban, South Africa(accessed on 11th June 2025).

20. Couce, M. L., Otero, F. J., Piechnik, M., Sawamoto, K., et al. (2020). *Mucopolysaccharidosis IVA: Diagnosis, Treatment, And Management.* https://core.ac.uk/download/299811588.pdf (accessed on 11th June 2025).

21. Deeks, S., Ganz, P., Grunfeld, C., Hsue, P., et al. (2016). *HIV and Hepatitis C-Coinfected Patients Have Lower Low-Density Lipoprotein Cholesterol Despite Higher Proprotein Convertase Subtilisin Kexin 9 (PCSK9): An Apparent "PCSK9-lipid paradox."* https://core.ac.uk/download/323063369.pdf (accessed on 11th June 2025).

22. Denno, D. M., Musser, C. A., Nelson, Z. C., Tarr, P. I., et al. (2016). *Chapter Five. Systematic Review Results by Biomarker Classifications.* https://core.ac.uk/download/70385873.pdf (accessed on 11th June 2025).

23. Fiehn, O., Ismail, I. T., & Showalter, M. R. (2019). *Inborn Errors of Metabolism in The Era of Untargeted Metabolomics and Lipidomic.* https://core.ac.uk/download/323068986.pdf (accessed on 11th June 2025).

24. Sattar, N., & Greer, I. A. (2002). Pregnancy complications and maternal cardiovascular risk: opportunities for intervention and screening?. *BMJ (Clinical research ed.), 325*(7356), 157–160. https://doi.org/10.1136/bmj.325.7356.157(accessed on 11th June 2025).

25. Grimes, L. R., Webster, G. F., & Webster, T. G. (2017). *Laboratory Tests in Patients Treated with Isotretinoin: Occurrence of Liver and Muscle Abnormalities and Failure of AST and ALT to predict liver abnormality*. https://core.ac.uk/download/129191066.pdf (accessed on 11th June 2025).
26. Hasani-Ranjbar, S., Keshtkar, A., Larijani, B., Mansouri, A., et al. (2012). *The Effect of 12 Weeks Anethum graveolens (dill) on Metabolic Markers in Patients with Metabolic Syndrome: A Randomized Double Blind Controlled Trial*. https://core.ac.uk/download/52204793.pdf (accessed on 11th June 2025).
27. Heinrich, J., Illig, T., Koletzko, B., Lattka, E., et al. (2009). *FADS Gene Cluster Polymorphisms: Important Modulators of Fatty Acid Levels and Their Impact on Atopic Diseases*. https://core.ac.uk/download/16432559.pdf (accessed on 11th June 2025).
28. Hester, E. R. (2017). *The Benefits and Concerns of Veganism in Women's Health*. https://core.ac.uk/download/58824999.pdf (accessed on 11th June 2025).
29. Honisett, S., Komesaroff, P. A., & Stojanovska, L. (2007). *The Anti-Atherogenic Effects of Thiazolidinediones*. https://core.ac.uk/download/10826553.pdf (accessed on 11th June 2025).
30. Kissebah, A. H., Almasy, A., Austin, M., Barrett, C., Brown, M., Connelly, M., Cox, N., et al. (2010). *INSIG1 Influences Obesity-Related Hypertriglyceridemia in Humans*. https://core.ac.uk/download/45950.pdf (accessed on 11th June 2025).
31. Kitsiou, A., Caforio, A. L. P., Porta-Sanchez, A., Vahanian, A., Iung, B., Carrera, C., Szymanski, C., et al. (2013). *ESC Core Curriculum for The General Cardiologist (2013)*. https://core.ac.uk/download/55756305.pdf (accessed on 11th June 2025).
32. Kok, F. J., Li, Y., Ma, G., Piao, J., et al. (2008). *Prevalence of the Metabolic Syndrome in Chinese Adolescents*. https://core.ac.uk/download/pdf/29257767.pdf (accessed on 11th June 2025).
33. de Oliveira, S., & Saldanha, C. (2010). An overview about erythrocyte membrane. *Clinical hemorheology and microcirculation*, *44*(1), 63–74. https://doi.org/10.3233/CH-2010-1253(accessed on 11th June 2025).
34. Oswald, L. A. S. (2015). *Feline Hyperthyroidism: A Longitudinal Comparative Study of Patients in The Presence or Absence of Concurrent Chronic Kidney Disease*. https://core.ac.uk/download/61483975.pdf (accessed on 11th June 2025).
35. Slee, A. D. (2012). *Exploring Metabolic Dysfunction in Chronic Kidney Disease*. https://core.ac.uk/download/17352998.pdf (accessed on 11th June 2025).

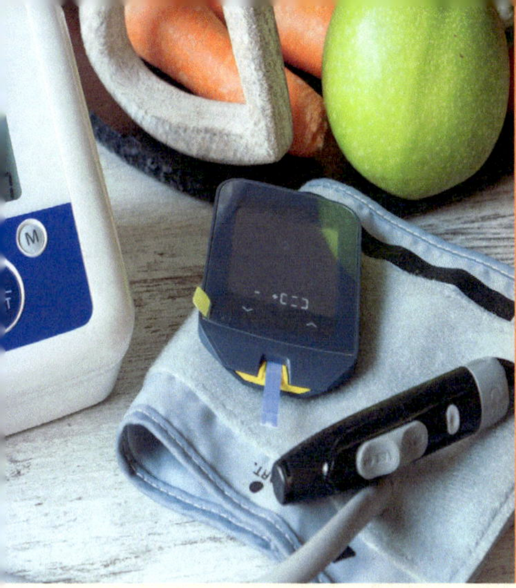

Chapter 15

HYPERTENSION IN DIABETES

Contents

Introduction

The strong relationship between hypertension and diabetes causes a major public health issue because these two conditions work together to increase heart disease and death. Often, diabetes and hypertension, a disease with high blood pressure, occur together in patients. Studies in the last few years have found that people with diabetes are more likely to develop hypertension, and it is thought that about half of these patients have high blood pressure. As a result of these conditions being linked, the risk of serious problems such as stroke, heart attack, and other heart diseases increases. Therefore, it is important to learn about hypertension in diabetics to create effective ways to lower the risks it causes. If we look at the demographics of those affected by hypertension, we can see that the disease and its results differ greatly among people with diabetes. For instance, a population-based study noted that individuals of African origin exhibited a lower 10-year risk estimate for coronary heart disease (CHD) compared to their white and South Asian counterparts. In particular, South Asians were found to have the highest total risk of cardiovascular diseases. This proves that diabetes patients should be treated for hypertension differently, as ethnicity has a major effect on their cardiovascular risk. To deal with these differences, primary care doctors should use culturally appropriate and proven guidelines that fit the needs of patients from different backgrounds, leading to improved healthcare results. It is very important to handle hypertension in diabetic people, given that it is closely linked to a higher risk of stroke. It has been found that poor blood pressure control is linked to a large number of strokes. Keeping blood pressure levels below 150/90 mm Hg every day is vital in clinical practice, since it greatly reduces the risk of stroke. This shows that healthcare providers should pay close attention to and treat hypertensive patients with diabetes. If blood pressure control is emphasized in healthcare, the risk of severe neurological problems can be lowered, which benefits the lives and health of those affected by these conditions (Figure 15.1).

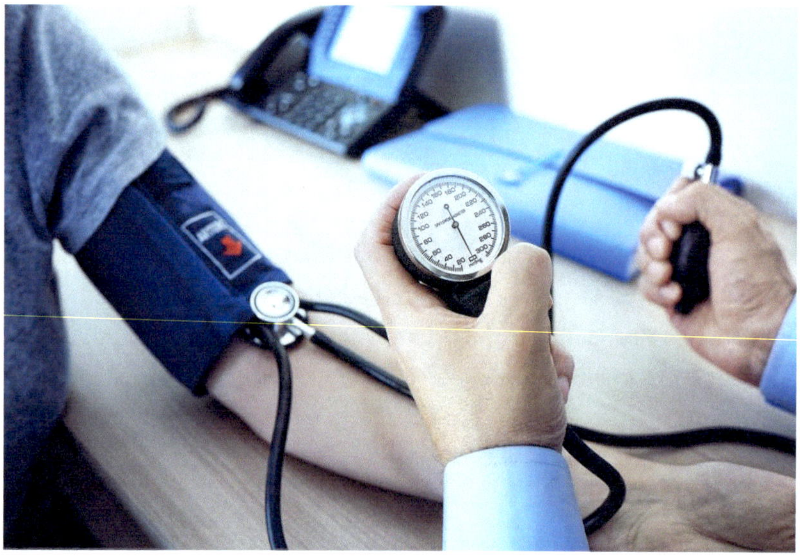

Figure 15.1. Hypertension.

Source: https://gumlet.assettype.com/down-to-earth%2Fimport%2Flibrary%2Flarge%2F2023-09-19%2F0.12714200_1695102088_istock-873891794.jpg?format=auto

15.1. Pathophysiology of Hypertension in Diabetes

Many metabolic problems in diabetes interact to cause damage to blood vessels in hypertension. When someone has type 2 diabetes, insulin resistance causes nitric oxide to be produced differently and leads to more activity in the sympathetic nervous system, which results in blood vessels constricting. The sympathetic nervous system's overactivity causes hypertension to get worse by raising the heart rate and making the blood vessels narrower. Glycation of proteins is another problem caused by high blood glucose in diabetic patients, and it makes blood vessels lose their elasticity. As a result of this, the arteries become stiffer, so the heart finds it harder to handle more blood, which increases blood pressure. To summarize, these mechanisms show that problems with glucose metabolism and high blood pressure are closely related and can seriously affect the heart health of people with diabetes.

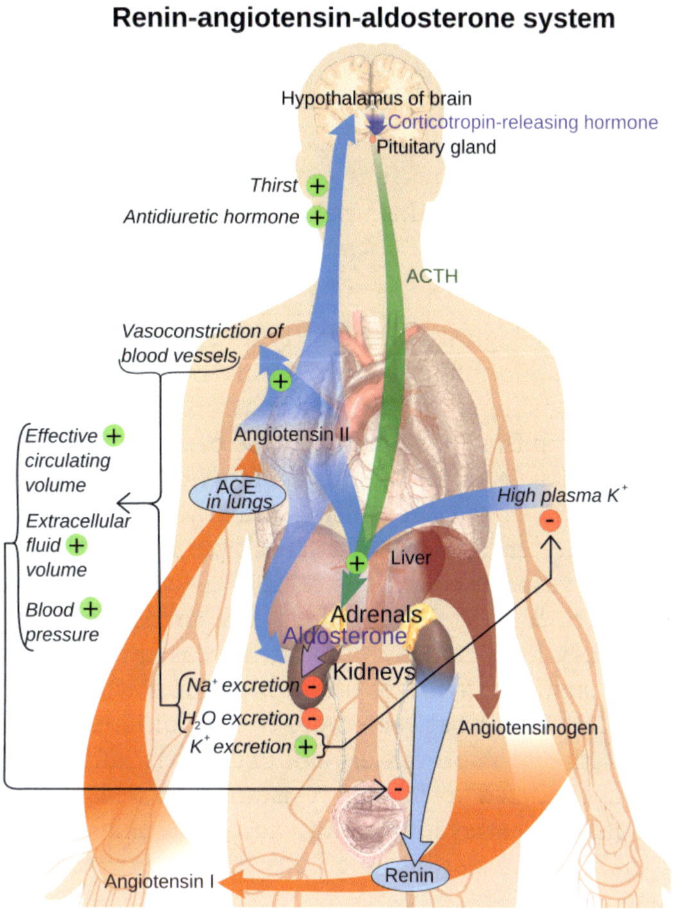

Figure 15.2. The renin-angiotensin-aldosterone system (RAAS) also becomes activated in the context of obesity and insulin resistance, promoting sodium retention and vascular tone, thereby elevating blood pressure.

Source: By Mikael Häggström - All used images are in public domain., Public Domain, https://commons.wikimedia.org/w/index.php?curid=8458370

In addition, the connection between diabetes and hypertension is made more complicated by the fact that obesity and metabolic syndrome are common among people with diabetes. Cytokines and free fatty acids are among the many bioactive substances secreted by adipose tissue, and they help cause inflammation and abnormal lipid levels. This situation can bring about inflammation and reorganization of blood vessels, which may result in hypertension. The renin-angiotensin-aldosterone system (RAAS) also becomes activated in the context of obesity and insulin resistance, promoting sodium retention and vascular tone, thereby elevating blood pressure. Since these factors are linked, it is necessary to handle hypertension in diabetes by looking at many aspects and using a comprehensive approach. Taking care of these linked pathways is very important for lowering the heart disease risks of people with diabetes. To treat high blood pressure in diabetic patients well, it is important to know what causes it. ACE inhibitors and angiotensin receptor blockers are commonly used first-line medicines for high blood pressure, and they also safeguard the kidneys, which is especially helpful for people with diabetes. They help to control the negative effects of high blood sugar on the kidneys and stop diabetic nephropathy from getting worse. Even so, diuretics are often prescribed, but should be used with care since they can bring about electrolyte imbalances, which is a big concern for diabetics. Also, making healthy changes in eating, exercise, and weight management is important for the treatment plan. Recognizing the unique way hypertension affects diabetes patients makes it possible to use more suitable treatments, which in turn helps these patients and reduces their risk of heart issues (Figure 15.2).

15.1.1. Insulin Resistance and Its Effects

Insulin resistance is a core pathological feature of type 2 diabetes mellitus (DM2), significantly influencing various metabolic abnormalities and chronic conditions, including hypertension. As the body becomes resistant to insulin, it has trouble controlling blood sugar, which results in high blood sugar levels. In people with DM2, insulin resistance eventually reduces the pancreas's ability to secrete enough insulin, which leads to various metabolic problems. Besides impairing blood glucose, insulin resistance also leads to hypertension and other heart problems, so it is a key factor in treating diabetes-related hypertension. As noted in multiple studies, the interrelationship between insulin resistance and various vascular conditions reveals the complexities that complicate the care of patients with DM2 (Stafford & Elasy, 2007). There is a connection between hypertension and insulin resistance because they both contribute to an increased risk of heart problems. Elevated blood pressure is observed significantly more often in patients with diabetes compared to those without, suggesting a clear connection between these two conditions (Guzik et al., 2018). The main reasons are the problems with the blood vessels and body-wide inflammation, which can develop due to the metabolic changes linked to insulin resistance. In addition, when insulin resistance occurs, lipid metabolism changes a negatively and causes inflammation in the blood vessels. All these changes together make arteries stiffer and help atherosclerosis develop. As a result of this relationship, hypertension makes insulin resistance worse, which increases the chances of heart-related health problems. Consequently, understanding these connections is crucial for effective interventions and therapeutic strategies designed to mitigate hypertension in diabetic patients (Guzik et al., 2018). To treat hypertension in patients with insulin resistance, both blood sugar and heart health should be managed. Pharmacological options, such as thiazolidinediones, may offer dual benefits by enhancing insulin sensitivity while concurrently impacting blood pressure regulation (Stafford & Elasy, 2007). In addition, dietary changes and being more active are important ways to reverse insulin resistance and the effects it has on hypertension. They can ease chronic inflammation and improve the function of blood vessels, which leads to better heart health. As ongoing research continues to elucidate the mechanisms linking diabetes, insulin resistance, and hypertension, clinicians are empowered to develop targeted strategies that not only focus on glycemic management but also holistically address cardiovascular risks, ultimately improving patient outcomes in this growing population (Stafford & Elasy, 2007) (Figure 15.3).

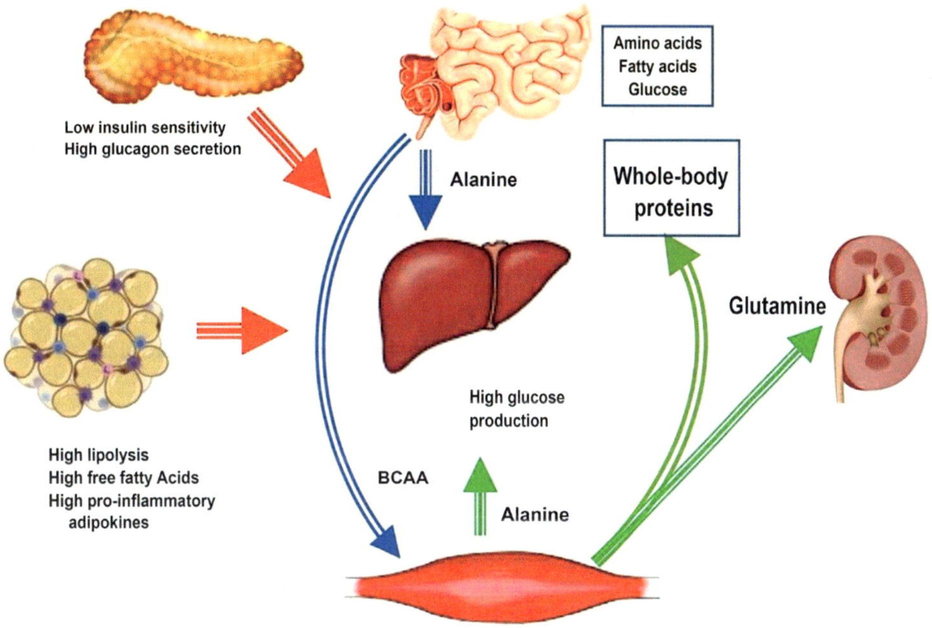

Figure 15.3. Insulin resistance is a core pathological feature of type 2 diabetes mellitus (DM2), significantly influencing various metabolic abnormalities and chronic conditions, including hypertension.

Source: Petroni ML, Brodosi L, Marchignoli F, Sasdelli AS, Caraceni P, Marchesini G, Ravaioli F. Nutrition in Patients with Type 2 Diabetes: Present Knowledge and Remaining Challenges. *Nutrients.* 2021; 13(8):2748. https://doi.org/10.3390/nu13082748

15.1.2. Role of the Renin-Angiotensin System

The renin-angiotensin system (RAS) serves a pivotal role in regulating blood pressure and fluid balance, thus significantly contributing to the pathophysiology of hypertension, particularly in diabetic patients. The RAS is started when renin from the kidneys turns angiotensinogen from the liver into angiotensin I. Subsequently, angiotensin I is converted into the potent vasoconstrictor angiotensin II by angiotensin-converting enzyme (ACE) primarily in the lungs. Angiotensin II makes blood vessels narrower and also causes the adrenal glands to release aldosterone, which results in the body holding onto sodium and water. Hyperactivity in this system in diabetic people can worsen hypertension and its problems. Because the RAS is often overactive in these patients, it leads to higher rates of heart disease, so it is important to focus on RAS management in treating hypertension in diabetes. Studies have found that the RAS is greatly affected when a person has insulin resistance and obesity, which are common in type 2 diabetes. The enzyme 11β-hydroxysteroid dehydrogenase type 1 (11β-HSD1) has been implicated in promoting local glucocorticoid regeneration, enhancing insulin resistance, and increasing blood pressure. There are significant increases in angiotensinogen, angiotensin II, and aldosterone in the blood of genetically modified mice that overexpress this enzyme, as well as higher blood pressure. This indicates that having too much RAS activity might be linked to hypertension as well as to the metabolic problems that are often found in people with diabetes. As a result, it is important to understand how RAS activation affects metabolism when managing hypertension in diabetic patients, since this could help improve the outcomes of treatment. Angiotensin-converting enzyme inhibitors (ACE-I) and angiotensin II receptor blockers (ARBs) represent cornerstone therapies in the treatment of hypertension, specifically catering to individuals with diabetes. It is recommended to use ACE inhibitors by clinical guidelines because they help lower blood pressure and also protect the kidneys, especially for people with diabetic nephropathy. It is worth noting that ACE-I users might have a constant cough, which can make some practitioners suggest using ARBs instead. They are able to target the RAS more precisely, which could reduce negative effects and still control blood pressure well. Doctors are still studying how these medications affect hypertensive patients with diabetes in the long run, which is why it's important to keep an eye on their kidney function and electrolytes during treatment. By learning about the RAS in diabetes, healthcare providers can improve their methods of handling hypertension in this group (Figure 15.4).

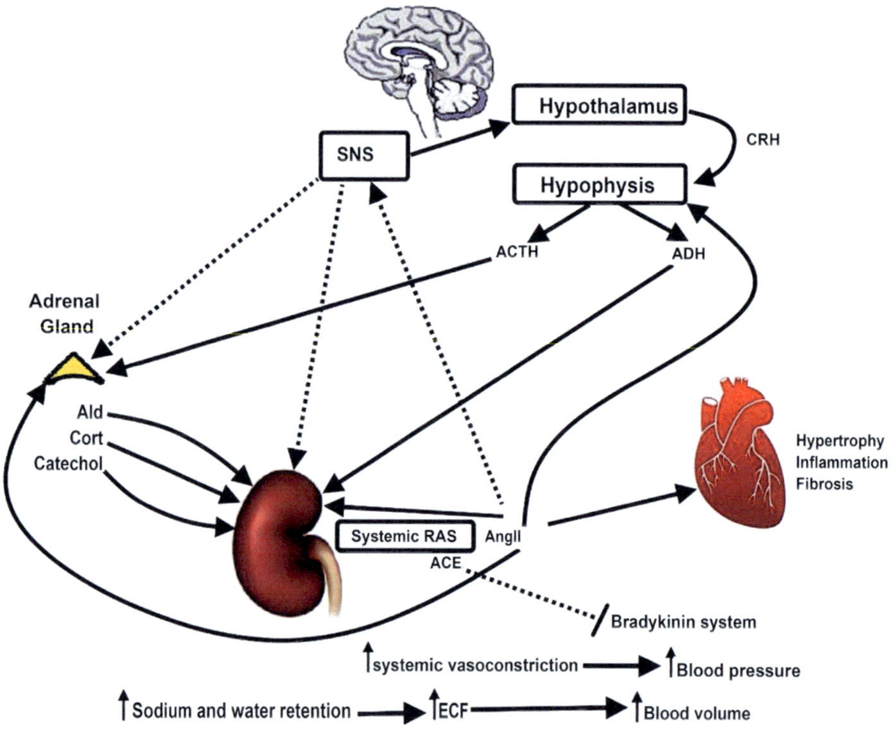

Figure 15.4. The renin-angiotensin system (RAS) serves a pivotal role in regulating blood pressure and fluid balance, thus significantly contributing to the pathophysiology of hypertension, particularly in diabetic patients.

Source: https://static.elsevier.es/multimedia/25300180/0000006900000001/v1_202202280604/S2530018022000099/v1_202202280604/en/main.assets/gr2.jpeg

15.1.3. Impact of Inflammation on Blood Pressure

People with diabetes are more likely to show the relationship between inflammation and blood pressure, since diabetes is commonly linked to hypertension. Blood pressure can rise when someone has chronic inflammation caused by obesity and insulin resistance. In adipose tissues, the release of pro-inflammatory cytokines results in problems with blood vessels and higher activity of the sympathetic nervous system. According to studies, high levels of serum angiotensin II are related to hypertension, especially in diabetic people who are obese. If angiotensin II rises, it can cause more inflammatory markers to be released, which in turn makes hypertension worse. This relationship indicates that targeting inflammation might offer therapeutic avenues for managing hypertension in diabetic populations, thereby underscoring the necessity of comprehensive interventions that address both inflammation and blood pressure regulation (Al-Daghri et al., 2012). In addition, the link between oral health and inflammation is becoming more important in hypertension, mainly for diabetic patients. Periodontitis and similar conditions can result in systemic inflammation that might interfere with the functioning of the blood vessels. Inflammatory factors produced by oral infections may increase the problems with the endothelium, which can lead to more vascular complications. Patients with stomatitis caused by dentures were found to have reduced flow-mediated dilation, which points to poor vascular health.

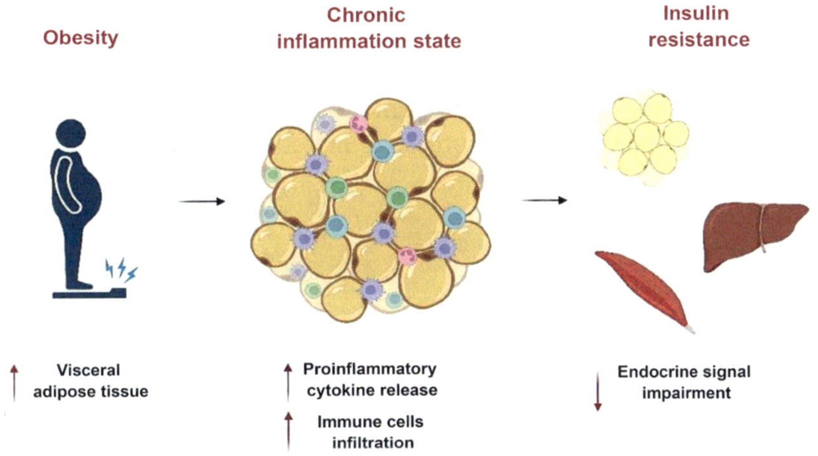

Figure 15.5. Chronic inflammatory states, induced by factors such as obesity and insulin resistance, contribute significantly to elevated blood pressure levels.

Source: Secchiero P, Rimondi E, Marcuzzi A, Longo G, Papi C, Manfredini M, Fields M, Caruso L, Di Caprio R, Balato A. Metabolic Syndrome and Psoriasis: Pivotal Roles of Chronic Inflammation and Gut Microbiota. *International Journal of Molecular Sciences*. 2024; 25(15):8098. https://doi.org/10.3390/ijms25158098

These results indicate that ongoing oral inflammatory diseases might lead to hypertension, which makes it more difficult to control diabetes. Consequently, addressing oral health proactively could serve as an integral component in mitigating hypertension risks in diabetics by reducing systemic inflammation (Cześnikiewicz-Guzik et al., 2014). Besides, when inflammation, obesity, and diabetes are present, it becomes more difficult to control blood pressure. When people have more body fat, their pro-inflammatory adipokines rise, which may result in insulin resistance and high blood pressure. TNF-α and leptin levels found in the bloodstream are strongly linked to systolic blood pressure in people with hypertension and diabetes. In this situation, weight management, healthy food choices and exercise become key approaches to reduce inflammation and, therefore, blood pressure. These types of strategies can help prevent hypertension and also boost the general health of the body. As research continues to elucidate the pathways linking inflammation, obesity, and hypertension, developing therapies that simultaneously target these factors will likely yield the most effective outcomes for diabetic patients facing hypertension (Al-Daghri et al., 2012; Cześnikiewicz-Guzik et al., 2014) (Figure 15.5).

15.2. Prevalence of Hypertension in Diabetic Patients

Both diabetes and hypertension are common in the same individuals, making it a major problem for public health since they tend to worsen each other's symptoms. It is very common for diabetes patients to also have hypertension, as experts say that about 60% of those with diabetes also have high blood pressure. The connection is mainly because of diabetes-related vascular issues, which may cause the arteries to stiffen and make the body's circulation harder. For this reason, having hypertension along with diabetes makes it more difficult to treat and also greatly increases the risk of heart attacks and strokes, so it is important to treat both conditions at the same time. It is more complicated for patients when diabetes has lasted a long time, their blood sugar is not well controlled, and they have hypertension.

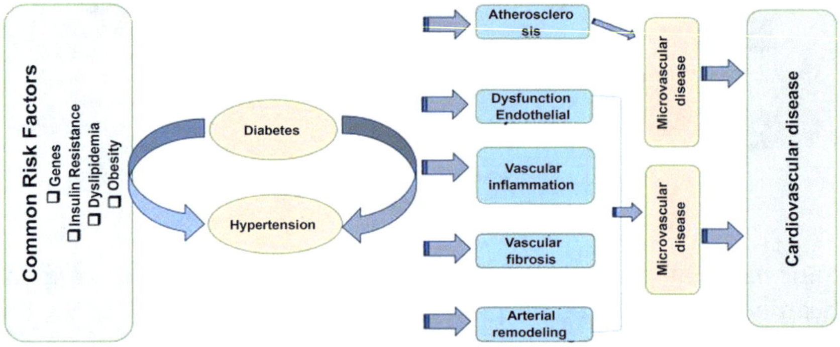

Figure 15.6. The relationship between diabetes duration, glycemic control, and the prevalence of hypertension further complicates patient management.

Source: https://media.springernature.com/lw685/springer-static/image/art%3A10.1007%2Fs13410-022-01143-7/MediaObjects/13410_2022_1143_Fig3_HTML.png

It has been proven that diabetes lasting for a longer period often causes hypertension, since long-term high blood sugar weakens the blood vessels. In addition, the degree of blood sugar control, shown by HbA1c, is a sign that someone may develop hypertension. If HbA1c levels are high, it can result in diastolic dysfunction in diabetic people, which may eventually cause hypertension. Addressing the dual challenges of controlling blood glucose levels and managing blood pressure is vital for minimizing the risk of complications associated with hypertension in diabetic patients, reinforcing the urgency for proactive monitoring and intervention strategies (Jain et al., 2018).

Because hypertension in diabetics is caused by several factors, it is important to know about the risk factors that can be changed. Among the factors, physical inactivity, poor diet, and not managing weight properly are very important in causing hypertension. Also, recent studies suggest that systemic hypertension may appear in patients with diabetes and no visible microvascular damage, which means diabetic retinopathy and hypertension can happen separately. For this reason, it is important to use careful monitoring, even if microalbuminuria or other diabetes problems are not present. Ultimately, early identification and management of hypertension within the diabetic population are essential steps for reducing the burden of cardiovascular diseases and preserving overall health (Irsath, 2015) (Figure 15.6).

15.2.1. Statistical Data on Co-Occurrence

There is strong evidence in the statistics that hypertension and diabetes often appear together. According to recent studies, diabetes increases a person's risk of hypertension, and the two conditions are found together in up to 10.8% of some populations. The connection between these two diseases is mainly because of common risk factors such as being overweight, leading a sedentary lifestyle, and genetic background. It is important for healthcare providers to recognize these similarities because they need to use a complete approach when diagnosing diabetes patients. Furthermore, the information from statistics supports the use of specific strategies that help patients handle both hypertension and diabetes at the same time, leading to better results and less pressure on the healthcare system. Knowing these relationships allows medical professionals to create better prevention and treatment measures. The importance of co-occurrence is also shown in studies that focus on the grouping of cardiovascular risk factors. Researchers who use hierarchical clustering analysis have found that there are different profiles in populations that have both hypertension and diabetes. It is found in the study that overweight or obese individuals are more likely to have these conditions together with other risks, such as having high levels of lipids in the blood. With these clusters, healthcare professionals can spot high-risk people and plan interventions that fit their needs. Using statistics on how these health conditions interact, practitioners can help find and manage patients with several cardiovascular risks, which benefits the population's health and lowers costs.

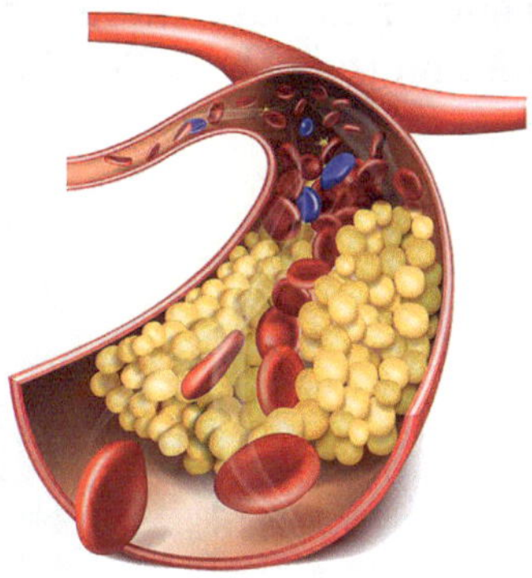

Figure 15.7. Hyperlipidemia.

Source: https://www.heartbeats.org.nz/wp-content/uploads/2023/02/hyperlipidemia.jpg

Furthermore, these conditions have effects that go beyond a single person's health, also changing the healthcare system. Studies that include the whole population show that having hypertension and diabetes often leads to significant disability. It has been proven through statistical analysis that when hypertension occurs alongside ischemic heart disease, the chance of disability rises greatly. Recognizing these connections is necessary for making public health policies and dividing resources, because it proves that care should be integrated to manage different health issues. Since the number of senior citizens is rising, it is important to notice the links between chronic diseases such as hypertension and diabetes to help with public health planning and providing healthcare where it is most needed (Figure 15.7).

15.2.2. Demographic Variations

Different racial and ethnic groups have different ways in which hypertension and diabetes are related. It has been found that African American and Hispanic populations have a higher chance of having both conditions than Caucasian populations. The difference in obesity and lifestyle-related diseases is mainly because of genetic, socio-economic, and environmental factors. Moreover, the way a culture views health care can shape how these health problems are managed and the chance of people seeking help from a doctor. It is important to recognize these demographic differences, since they guide public health efforts to reduce health gaps. These interventions can help solve these problems and improve health, proving that cultural awareness is important for handling hypertension in people with diabetes from different groups. Also, the age, gender, and economic status of a person can strongly influence the occurrence and control of hypertension in diabetics. Older people often have more insulin resistance and different reactions in their hearts, which makes them more likely to develop hypertension.

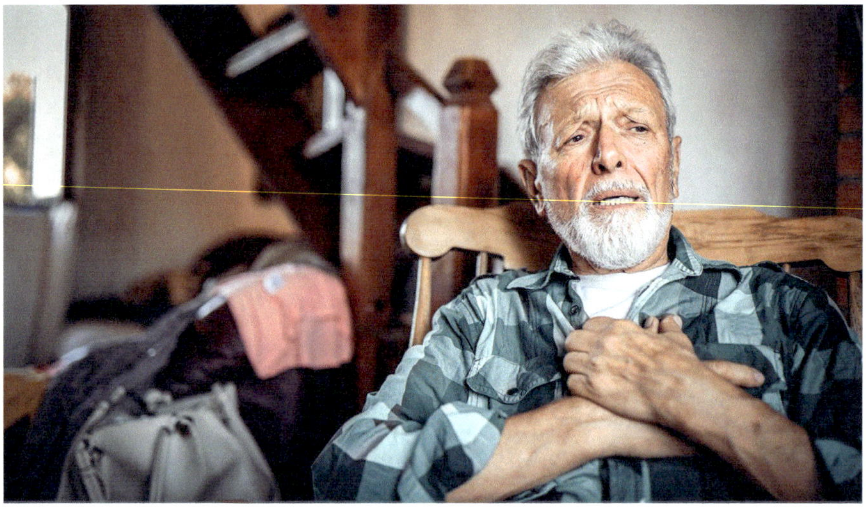

Figure 15.8. Older adults often experience increased insulin resistance and altered cardiovascular responses, making them more susceptible to hypertension.

Source: https://media.post.rvohealth.io/wp-content/uploads/2023/09/senior-male-with-chest-pain-1296-728-header.jpg

After menopause, women often experience hypertension because the hormonal changes that happen then affect the health of their blood vessels. A person's social and financial situation can make it harder or easier to get health care, learn, and choose a healthy lifestyle, which all play a big role in diabetes and hypertension management. For instance, those with low incomes may not be able to get enough healthy food or regular medical treatment, which makes their health problems worse. So, it is necessary for medical practice to consider these demographic differences to ensure that all populations receive the care they need. Therefore, the connections between lifestyle and demographic factors mean that hypertension in diabetes needs to be managed carefully. It seems that tobacco use and dietary habits are different among various groups and play a major role in metabolic health. For example, a study found that smokeless tobacco use is associated with lower adiponectin levels, which are crucial for metabolic regulation, highlighting a significant health disparity affecting specific populations, particularly among young men (Ahmad et al., 2015). Similarly, barriers in health care access, particularly among American Indian and Alaska Native communities, inhibit effective management of both conditions, leading to heightened health disparities (Jones et al., 2015). Noticing these relationships gives us important knowledge to help develop public health programs that reduce the risks of hypertension in diabetic patients from various backgrounds. When health practitioners understand the many aspects of these relationships, they can provide interventions that help all individuals with chronic conditions (Figure 15.8).

15.2.3. Risk Factors Contributing to Hypertension

Obesity, not being active, and poor diet are some of the factors that link hypertension and diabetes. It is well known that obesity is a major cause of hypertension, since the extra fat leads to higher vascular resistance and affects the hormones insulin and leptin. In the past several decades, obesity has become much more common among people with diabetes, which has caused hypertension rates to increase.

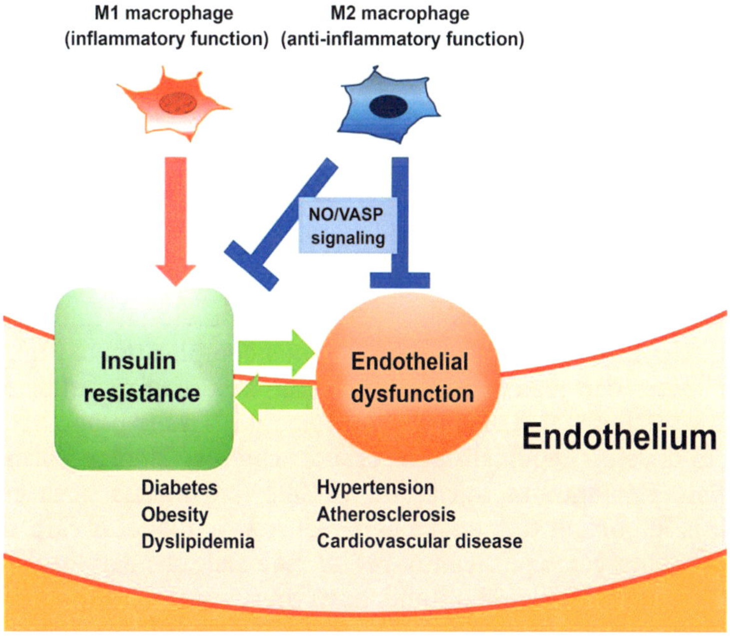

Figure 15.9. Endothelial dysfunction plays a crucial role in the pathogenesis of both hypertension and diabetes, indicating a shared pathway for these conditions.

Source: Takeda Y, Matoba K, Sekiguchi K, Nagai Y, Yokota T, Utsunomiya K, Nishimura R. Endothelial Dysfunction in Diabetes. *Biomedicines.* 2020; 8(7):182. https://doi.org/10.3390/biomedicines8070182

Also, not moving enough adds to the problem; regular exercise helps keep body weight healthy and benefits the heart. A diet high in sodium and low in potassium can lead to high blood pressure.

These factors cause one problem to worsen the other. For this reason, people with hypertension and diabetesare instructed to lower their intake of processed foods, which are often high is sodium. Both hypertension and diabetes are linked by endothelial dysfunction, showing that they may have a similar pathway. Because the endothelium cannot dilate as it should, there is an increase in vascular resistance and high blood pressure. In people with diabetes, high blood sugar can result in oxidative stress and encourage inflammation and changes in the blood vessels. Biochemical factors such as advanced glycation end products play a role in causing endothelial dysfunction, which brings the two conditions together. Besides, when the renin-angiotensin-aldosterone system is overactive, it can increase blood pressure and make the body resistant to insulin. These common mechanisms reinforce the understanding that managing endothelial health, through lifestyle changes or pharmacological interventions, is essential for reducing both hypertensive and diabetic complications, as each condition perpetuates the severity of the other (Guzik et al., 2018). In addition, factors like a person's age, gender, and ethnicity can strongly affect the chances of developing hypertension and diabetes. Experts have found that older people are more likely to have high blood pressure because of stiff arteries and reduced kidney function. It is also important to note that men have hypertension at a younger age than women, but after menopause, the difference between the two groups narrows. Certain ethnic groups, for example, African Americans, are more likely to deal with hypertension and diabetes, which may be related to their financial situation, the foods they eat, and genetics. It is essential for healthcare professionals to know these demographic variables, as this allows them to customize care for people from different backgrounds. By focusing on these demographic factors, public health initiatives can more effectively combat the growing prevalence of hypertension within the context of diabetes (Budoff et al., 2017) (Figure 15.9).

15.3. Complications Associated with Hypertension and Diabetes

The presence of both hypertension and diabetes in an individual causes major public health concerns because the two conditions can lead to serious complications. High blood pressure that often accompanies diabetes can make it more likely for a person to suffer from stroke or heart failure. Those who have diabetes usually have problems with their blood vessels, which makes it more likely for them to develop hypertension. Diabetes can also change hormone and metabolism levels, which increases resistance in the blood vessels and makes both conditions get worse together. Therefore, it is important to manage hypertension in diabetes care since studies indicate that lowering blood pressure can significantly reduce the risk of heart problems in these people. Because of this, it is important to understand how these two conditions are related to create better treatment plans for reducing the number of deaths and serious illnesses in affected people. In addition, the occurrence of microvascular problems in diabetes underlines how important it is to control hypertension. High blood pressure often makes conditions such as diabetic retinopathy, nephropathy, and neuropathy worse, which can seriously affect a person's long-term health. For instance, nephropathy, which may cause end-stage renal disease, is more common in patients who have both diabetes and hypertension. Research shows that people with high blood pressure are more likely to damage their kidneys, which means that diabetic patients should have their blood pressure managed and checked often. Moreover, if hypertension is not well managed, it can result in more retinopathy since the increased pressure in the blood vessels can cause leakage and harm the vision. Taking care of these microvascular issues by closely managing hypertension can help improve the overall care of diabetes patients. The different effects of hypertension and diabetes on men and women are important to notice, since they may affect the way these conditions are treated. Studies reveal that women with type 1 diabetes usually have higher total cholesterol, which may put them at a different risk for heart problems than men. Hyperlipidemia is frequently observed with hypertension in diabetic patients, which makes it more difficult to treat them. It has also been noticed that women tend to follow their hypertension treatment less often than men. As a result of this gap, women with diabetes may develop more complications, so it is important to give them individualized care. If healthcare providers notice and deal with these gender differences, they can improve the results of treatment and ensure patients follow instructions, which lowers the risk of complications linked to hypertension and diabetes (Figure 15.10).

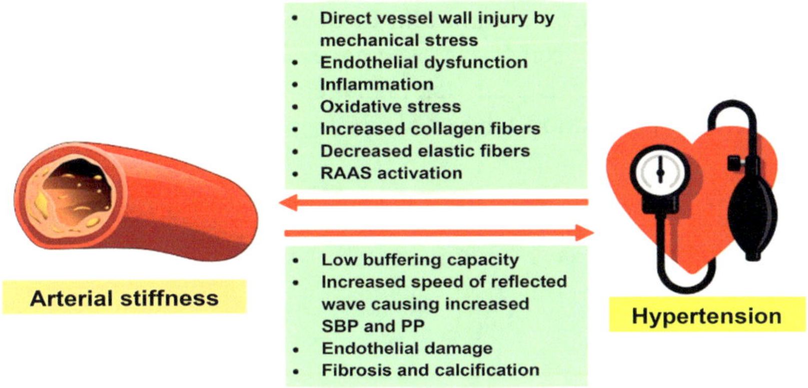

Figure 15.10. Patients with diabetes often experience endothelial dysfunction and increased arterial stiffness, which heightens hypertension prevalence.

Source: https://media.springernature.com/lw685/springer-static/image/art%3A10.1186%2Fs40885-023-00258-1/MediaObjects/40885_2023_258_Fig1_HTML.png

15.3.1. Cardiovascular Disease Risks

The interrelationship between diabetes and hypertension significantly amplifies the risks associated with cardiovascular diseases (CVD), a leading cause of mortality among affected individuals. When diabetes mellitus affects metabolism, it results in obesity and insulin resistance, which are the main risk factors for hypertension. Although insulin therapy is key for controlling blood sugar, it can cause weight gain and raise the risk of heart problems due to more fat and water in the body. Recently, studies have explained how weight gain caused by insulin can increase the risk of heart disease, mainly through problems with the endothelium and increased oxidative stress. As these physiological changes occur, they contribute to a cascading effect that worsens hypertension and dyslipidemia, thus fortifying the connection between diabetes management and cardiovascular health outcomes, underscoring the importance of vigilant monitoring and intervention strategies in this population (Jha et al., 2024). It is also found through research that variations in demographic factors can lead to different risks of CVD for people with hypertension and diabetes, so special approaches are needed. A study assessing coronary heart disease (CHD) risk across different ethnic groups revealed significant disparities, suggesting that South Asian individuals are at particularly elevated risk due to combined cardiovascular disease (CVD) factors. The 10-year risk of combined CVD for South Asian people is much higher than for white and African origin groups, so doctors should pay more attention to screening and managing these populations. Especially, setting lower standards for identifying and managing hypertension in high-risk groups could help find the condition early and prevent future heart problems. Thus, recognizing these demographic distinctions allows for more targeted interventions, ultimately aiming to reduce the burden of cardiovascular complications linked to diabetes-induced hypertension (Cappuccio et al., 2002). To manage hypertension in diabetic patients, a strategy that covers both weight loss and heart health should be used. Dietary changes and exercise improve cardiovascular health.. In addition, healthcare providers should make sure patients understand that not managing weight gain from insulin therapy may result in heart-related issues. Tailored treatment plans and proper changes to medications are important for lowering the impact of hypertension on CVD in people with diabetes. Additionally, ongoing clinical research should aim to develop innovative therapeutic options that address these challenges, ultimately reinforcing the necessity for a comprehensive framework that integrates diabetes care with cardiovascular risk management, thereby promoting improved health outcomes in this vulnerable population (Jha et al., 2024) (Figure 15.11).

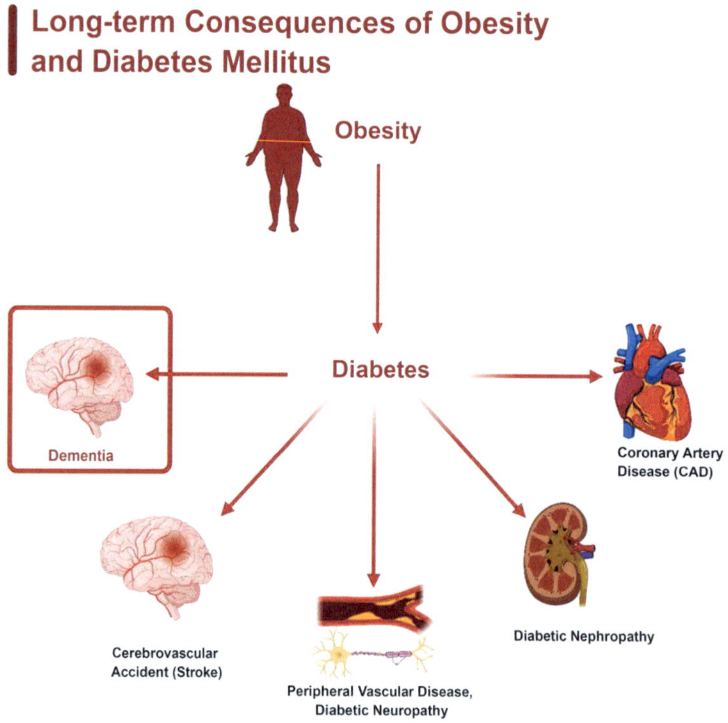

Figure 15.11. Diabetes mellitus fundamentally alters metabolic processes, leading to complications such as obesity and insulin resistance, which are crucial risk factors for hypertension.

Source: Selman A, Burns S, Reddy AP, Culberson J, Reddy PH. The Role of Obesity and Diabetes in Dementia. *International Journal of Molecular Sciences*. 2022; 23(16):9267. https://doi.org/10.3390/ijms23169267

15.3.2. Kidney Damage and Nephropathy

The relationship between hypertension and kidney damage in diabetic people is an important issue since it helps cause nephropathy. Diabetic nephropathy, characterized by persistent albuminuria and a gradual decline in glomerular filtration rate (GFR), is often exacerbated by the presence of hypertension. Increased blood pressure results in higher pressure inside the kidney's filtering units, which causes scarring and more damage to the kidneys. Even though the relationship is not simple, it is mainly highlighted by the fact that both types of diabetes cause high blood sugar and increase oxidative stress and inflammation in the body. Such factors lead to the early stages of kidney damage and also make it harder to control blood pressure, so diabetics with hypertension need comprehensive care.

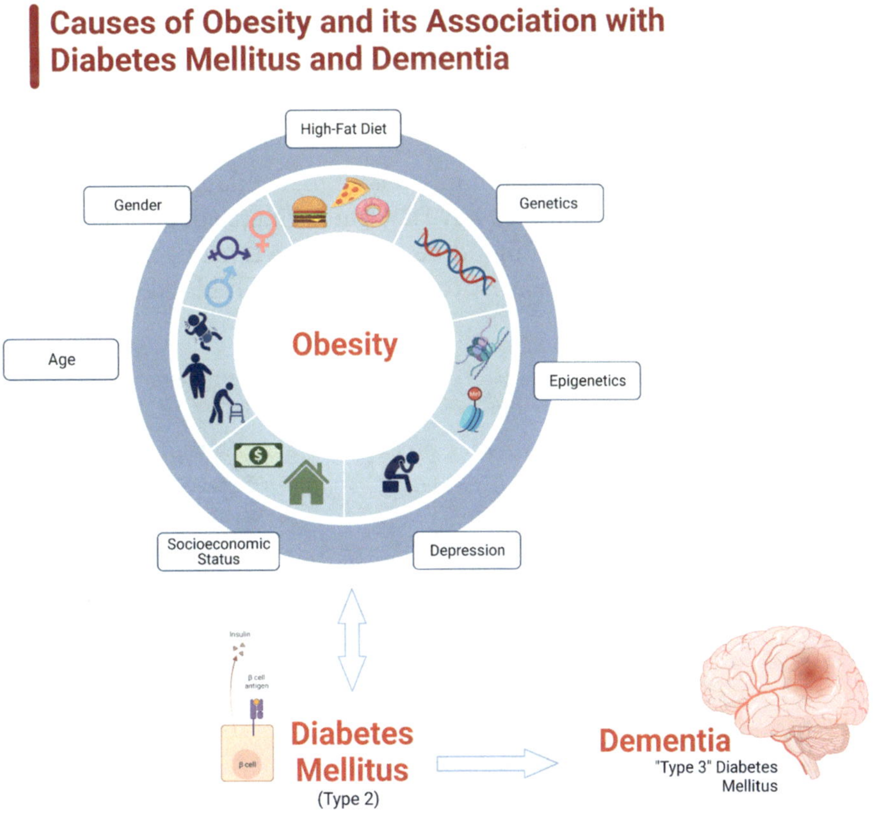

Figure 15.12. Obesity has multiple causes and is associated with diabetes and dementia

Source: Selman A, Burns S, Reddy AP, Culberson J, Reddy PH. The Role of Obesity and Diabetes in Dementia. *International Journal of Molecular Sciences.* 2022; 23(16):9267. https://doi.org/10.3390/ijms23169267

Using diet to manage hypertension and diabetic nephropathy is important, as it gives a natural method for treatment. Evidence shows that dietary changes can slow down the progression of kidney disease by tackling metabolic problems in the body. Traditionally, dietitians have suggested lowering calories and changing the amount of protein in a person's diet to help protect kidney function. New studies are exploring how particular substances in foods, for example, glycotoxins, can make nephropathy worse. As professionals strive to expand dietary recommendations, the emphasis has now shifted toward identifying functional foods that can provide protective effects against diabetic nephropathy, thereby integrating nutrition into a comprehensive plan for patients managing hypertension and diabetes (Iacobini et al., 2017). Cellular mechanisms in diabetic nephropathy indicate that it is important to understand specific risk factors, for example, genetic background and hormones. Emerging research points to the involvement of serum and glucocorticoid-induced kinase-1 (SGK1) as a critical regulator in the pathological processes leading to kidney damage. SGK1's action on several sodium transport pathways in the kidney epithelia affects sodium reabsorption, which plays a role in regulating both fluids and blood pressure. If SGK1 is not working properly, it can cause sodium to be retained, which may result in hypertension for diabetic patients. Thus, the intersection of SGK1 function, sodium transport, and nephropathy illustrates the multifaceted nature of kidney damage in the context of diabetes, reinforcing the need for targeted interventions that address both hypertension and nephropathy simultaneously (Bland et al., 2009) (Figure 15.12).

15.3.3. Vision Problems and Retinopathy

There are many health effects of the connection between hypertension and diabetes, mainly related to vision and retinopathy. Those with diabetes have a greater chance of getting diabetic retinopathy, which is a problem that affects the retinal blood vessels. Hypertension makes the situation worse by putting more pressure on the blood vessels; together with high blood sugar, it creates a setting that can harm the retina.

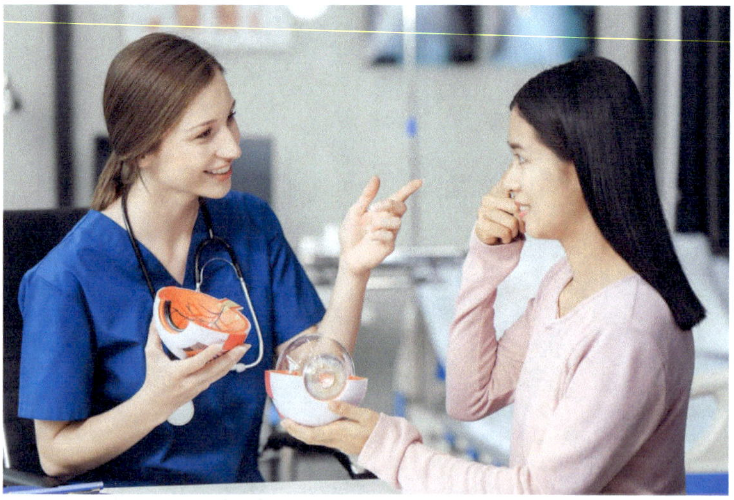

Figure 15.13. Individuals with diabetes are at an elevated risk for developing diabetic retinopathy, a condition characterized by damage to the retina's blood vessels.

Source: https://cdn.prod.website-files.com/64eec5ed1ea74a7194cd16a3/673b7dcc50ce0645aca1071b_1.%20Retinopathy%20-%20Header.jpg

It is especially common in adolescents and young adults with type II diabetes, who are more at risk because of the growing problem of obesity and little exercise. As emphasized in recent studies, understanding the relationship between these two chronic conditions is critical for preventing long-term vision impairment and associated co-morbidities (Kapke et al., 2015). Often, diabetic retinopathy advances silently until serious harm has been done, which is why diabetic patients, and those with hypertension in particular, should have regular eye check-ups. At first, these diseases may only show as mild retinopathy, but if not watched properly, they can get worse. In children, the long-term effects of hypertension and diabetes may result in a high number of vision problems at an early age. It has been found that early diagnosis and treatment can greatly improve the outcomes for these people and possibly stop damage to their retina. Comprehensive management strategies addressing both blood sugar control and blood pressure regulation are essential to mitigate the risks associated with these interconnected health issues (Foering, 2018). Moreover, the consequences of retinopathy include changes in people's social and emotional well-being, not only vision. Having a vision impairment often makes it harder for a person to learn, earn an income, and do basic tasks. In addition, it may slow down a child's development, adding to the difficulties faced by young people with diabetes and hypertension. In the long run, people with dementia may need more medical help and rely on support services more often. So, teaching at-risk people about healthy habits and regularly checking their vision is very important. This multifaceted strategy highlights the urgent need for awareness and proactive measures to combat the dual challenges presented by hypertension and diabetes, particularly concerning visual health (Kapke et al., 2015) (Figure 15.13).

15.4. Diagnostic Criteria for Hypertension in Diabetic Patients

Because diabetes and heart problems are linked, it is very important to diagnose hypertension in diabetic patients. The usual guidelines state that hypertension is diagnosed when a person's blood pressure is regularly above 130/80 mmHg. This limit is especially important for diabetic patients since they are more likely to suffer from heart-related health problems and death. The American Diabetes Association points out that regularly checking blood pressure is important for people with diabetes. Because of the relationship between diabetes and hypertension, it is important to find and treat diabetes early to avoid possible problems. In addition, knowing the special changes in the body of diabetic patients, such as increased resistance in their blood vessels and different endothelial function, is necessary to manage their hypertension in the best way. Besides the numbers used for hypertension, monitoring blood sugar levels is important in making the diagnosis. It has been found that high HbA1c levels in diabetic patients make them more likely to develop hypertension. In particular, having poor control over blood sugar increases the risk of high blood pressure, so managing blood sugar levels may play a key role in preventing hypertension. Since diabetes may result in cardiovascular disease, it is important to handle hypertension by including glycemic management in the patient's overall care plan. This approach can help manage hypertension well and also boost the health of patients with diabetes, which shows why an integrated model of care is important. Also, making positive lifestyle changes is very important for diabetic people with hypertension, according to different health organizations. An active lifestyle and weight control are useful ways to manage mild hypertension without using drugs. These suggestions are in line with the South African Hypertension Society, which suggests starting with lifestyle changes and using medicine only when necessary in people with low risk. Applying these lifestyle changes has helped some people keep their blood pressure and blood sugar within safe levels, which reduces the stress on healthcare services. As diabetes management continues to evolve, the incorporation of diagnostic criteria for hypertension focused on both pharmacological and lifestyle approaches will remain vital for optimizing patient outcomes in this increasingly prevalent population (Alsaad et al., 2015; Ware et al., 2014) (Figure 15.14).

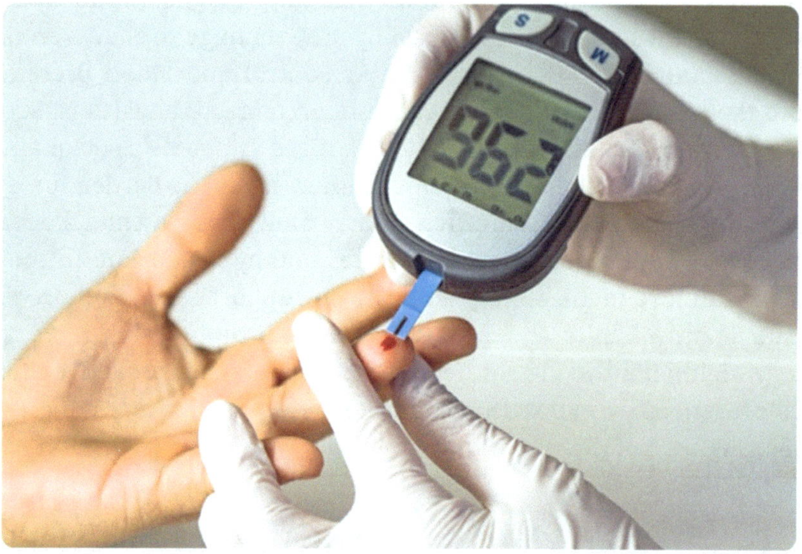

Figure 15.14. Poor glycemic control, indicated by elevated HbA1c levels, can exacerbate the incidence of hypertension among diabetic patients.

Source: https://www.news-medical.net/image-handler/picture/2018/10/shutterstock_271701911.jpg

15.4.1. Blood Pressure Measurement Guidelines

Effective management of hypertension in diabetic patients hinges not only on accurate diagnosis but also on standardized blood pressure (BP) measurement guidelines. The way BP is measured can cause differences in readings, which may lead to improper care of hypertension. It has been found through studies that the first BP reading may be different from the average of several readings taken over time. As these results show, it is crucial to have clear blood pressure measurement guidelines, mainly for people with diabetes who require precise results. The clinical consequences of these discrepancies can adversely affect treatment regimens, making it essential for healthcare providers to adhere to established guidelines that promote consistency and accuracy in BP assessments (Bilo et al., 2006). The integration of electronic health records (EHRs) in managing hypertension presents both advantages and challenges in establishing effective BP measurement practices. EHR data can be used by healthcare providers to design electronic indicators that help track patients with hypertension and diabetes. Still, since these guidelines are interpreted differently, they can result in the same type of differences as traditional methods. It is important to use a careful method to link the EHR indicators with recommended ways to manage blood pressure, so that patients get the right care from dependable data. The experiences of numerous provider organizations in refining these electronic indicators reveal both the potential for improvement and the obstacles that must be addressed in order to standardize care (Brian L Hazlehurst et al., 2008). In the end, using the same blood pressure measurement guidelines helps improve how hypertension is managed in people with diabetes. With more research, it is expected that researchers will pay more attention to strict protocols, which will help unify different methods. Proper training on these guidelines is needed by clinicians to reduce the variation in BP readings and achieve better health results. Furthermore, when healthcare professionals join forces to improve these measurement methods, the strategies used will stay effective and able to change along with changes in diabetes care. Such collective efforts are essential in addressing the complexities associated with hypertension management in diabetic patients, ultimately leading to enhanced patient safety and better clinical outcomes (Bilo et al., 2006) (Figure 15.15).

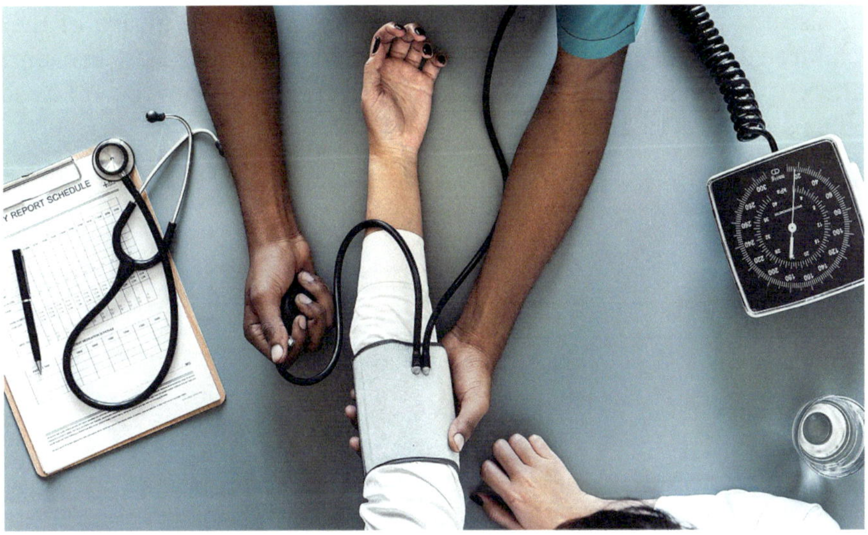

Figure 15.15. Clinicians must be equipped with comprehensive training on these guidelines to minimize variability in BP readings and improve health outcomes.

Source: https://upload.wikimedia.org/wikipedia/commons/thumb/c/c6/Blood_pressure_monitoring.jpg/1200px-Blood_pressure_monitoring.jpg

15.4.2. Importance of Regular Monitoring

It is important to check for hypertension regularly in people with diabetes to prevent serious health problems in the future. Hypertension is a common condition for diabetic patients, and it often makes the risks from both diseases worse. Regular checks on blood pressure help doctors see any changes and act fast, which can prevent serious heart problems like heart attacks and strokes. Because of this ongoing attention, doctors can create treatment plans that fit the patient's needs and help them live better. If hypertension is found early, patients can quickly change their habits and take the necessary medicines, following a proactive approach. For this reason, it is crucial to add complete monitoring steps to diabetes care to lower the risks of high blood pressure in this group. The framework for managing chronic non-communicable diseases (NCDs) emphasizes the necessity of regular monitoring in addressing hypertension effectively. According to (Harries et al., 2009), a standardized approach to healthcare can significantly improve patient outcomes when managing conditions like diabetes and hypertension. Identifying risk factors that can be changed during routine checks allows healthcare providers to address diabetes and hypertension at the same time. Because there is a link between the two, it is important to address both conditions at the same time. Regularly checking the results of interventions helps clinicians collect useful data for wider efforts to reduce the impact of NCDs. For this reason, a reliable system for monitoring is necessary to help both patients and the public. According to studies, it has become more important to monitor children and adolescents regularly because hypertension cases in this population are increasing. The guidelines synthesized from extensive research highlight the critical need for regular blood pressure assessments in younger demographics, as they are often overlooked in routine check-ups (Agabiti-Rosei et al., 2016). If tracking is done from an early stage, it can help prevent the development of serious health problems in the future, mainly for those who are at risk due to family or lifestyle factors. This points out that doctors and nurses are responsible for patient care and also for making sure parents and communities are aware of the importance of checking their children's blood pressure, especially if they have diabetes. Preventive actions can help ensure healthier people in the future and greatly decrease the number of hypertension cases and related problems (Figure 15.16).

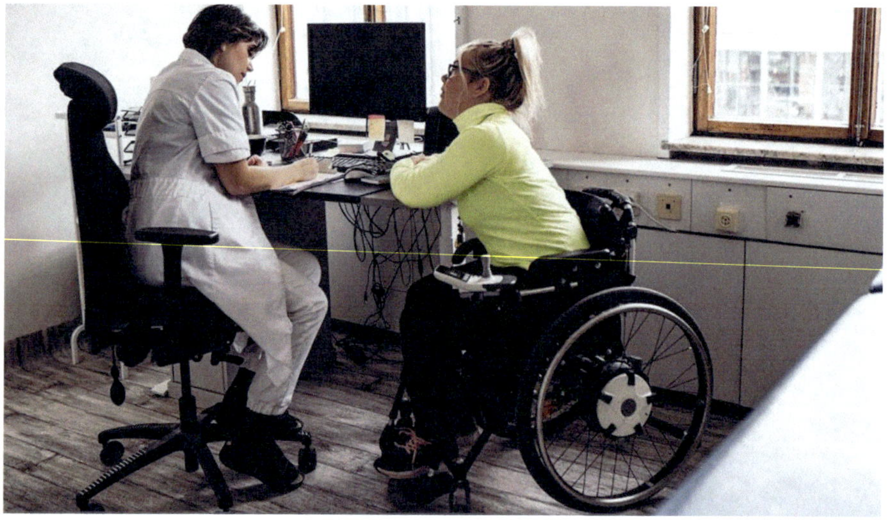

Figure 15.16. Regular monitoring of hypertension among individuals with diabetes is essential for effective management and prevention of long-term complications.

Source: https://i0.wp.com/post.medicalnewstoday.com/wp-content/uploads/sites/3/2022/03/diabetes_hypertension_GettyImages1321467313_Header-1024x575.jpg?w=1155&h=1528

15.4.3. Differentiating Between Types of Hypertension

The causes of hypertension are many and therefore require careful study of its various types. The most common type of hypertension is called primary or essential hypertension, and it is present in about 90-95% of cases. Most of the time, its reason is not clear and it is affected by genes, personal habits, and the environment. Secondary hypertension, on the other hand, is caused by specific conditions, for example, endocrine issues or kidney problems, and should be managed and diagnosed in a specific way. A clear differentiation between these types is imperative, especially within diabetic populations, where the risk of kidney disease elevates the chances of secondary hypertension (Marjina et al., 2020). With this knowledge, healthcare providers can design suitable treatments, leading to better patient results. Besides primary and secondary hypertension, there are other types of hypertension that matter in diabetes management. For instance, isolated systolic hypertension (ISH), characterized by elevated systolic pressure with a normal diastolic reading, is prevalent among older adults and often linked with increased cardiovascular risk. In addition, white-coat hypertension can make it challenging to determine if a person is truly hypertensive, especially for diabetics whose stress and anxiety may raise their blood pressure levels at the doctor's office. Identifying these variations ensures that healthcare practitioners deliver appropriate pharmacological and non-pharmacological interventions (Kautzky-Willer et al., 2013), thus enhancing the management of hypertension amid the complexities of diabetes. The condition also becomes more complicated when cases like malignant hypertension need to be treated quickly. Since this type of acute disease may damage vital organs, it is necessary to diagnose and treat it quickly. Moreover, when antihypertensive drugs do not lower blood pressure in people with diabetes, it becomes a serious issue. Because diabetes and hypertension often make each other worse, it is important to use strong management methods that include changing habits and sticking to medications. When healthcare professionals use evidence to identify the type of hypertension, they can give timely and suitable care to diabetic patients, which reduces the risk of heart problems and helps them stay healthier (Figure 15.17).

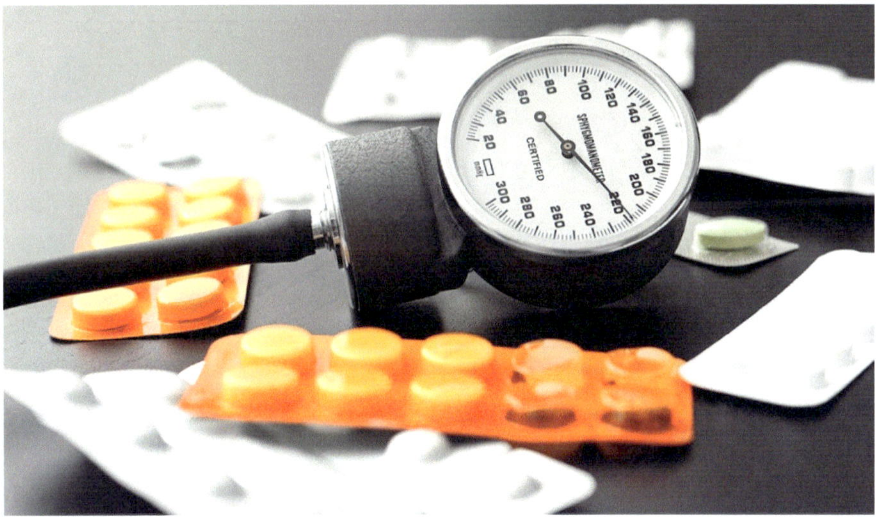

Figure 15.17. Resistant hypertension.

Source: https://d14d5nk8lue86f.cloudfront.net/s3fs-public/2022-11/Endothelin%20Receptor%20 Antagonist%20Effective%20in%20Resistant%20Hypertension%20PRECISION.jpg

A CLOSER LOOK

CORONARY HEART DISEASE (CHD)

Coronary Heart Disease (CHD) is a condition characterized by the narrowing or blockage of the coronary arteries, which supply blood and oxygen to the heart muscle. Most of the time, this happens because fatty deposits called plaques develop, which is known as atherosclerosis. CHD can lead to chest pain (angina), heart attacks, and other serious heart problems. Some of the risks are high blood pressure, high cholesterol, smoking, diabetes, obesity, and a lack of exercise. Managing heart health means changing habits, using medicines, and occasionally undergoing surgery to boost blood flow and prevent heart problems.

Summary

The relationship between hypertension and diabetes makes it hard to manage patients and can greatly affect their outcomes. Hypertension is common among people with diabetes, as it affects about 70% of them. It is probably because of shared processes in the body, such as insulin resistance, abnormal lipid levels, and inflammation. Besides, people with hypertension have a higher risk of heart disease, kidney disease, and eye disease, which leads to greater illness and death. It has been found that good blood pressure control greatly lessens these risks, making it important for diabetic patients to be regularly monitored. The relationship between body mass index (BMI) and health care utilization in individuals with diabetes is particularly relevant when considering hypertension management. It has been found that normal-weight diabetic patients use more health care resources than do overweight and obese diabetic patients. Because of this, people with normal weight diabetes may need more care and have worse health outcomes, leading to more difficulties in hypertension management. It appears from the evidence that, in spite of the need for more care, normal weight patients may encounter obstacles that prevent them from controlling their blood pressure well. Such insights emphasize the need for tailored intervention strategies that address the unique challenges of hypertension within this demographic (Bertakis et al., 2015). Creating and using effective risk models and scores for type 2 diabetes is very important for improving patient outcomes, especially in cases of hypertension. A review of current models has pointed out several statistical aspects, but many are not widely used in clinical settings because they are complicated or do not have clear goals. It has been found that assessing diabetes risk helps improve outcomes, so early screening and treatment could lessen the burden of hypertension in these patients. While new tools such as risk scores are promising, the problem is still how to make sure they are used by doctors and patients. Strategies aimed at increasing awareness and facilitating risk assessment could potentially foster better management of hypertension in diabetic individuals (Dent et al., 2011).

References

1. Agabiti-Rosei, E., Cruickshank, J. K., Dominiczak, A., Erdine, S., et al. (2016). *2016 European Society of Hypertension Guidelines for The Management of High Blood Pressure in Children and Adolescents*. https://core.ac.uk/download/46165193.pdf (accessed on 11th June 2025).
2. Ahmad, S., Ahmed, J., Ali, A., Hussain, M., et al. (2015). Association of hypoadiponectemia with smokeless/dipping tobacco use in young men. https://core.ac.uk/download/42366369.pdf (accessed on 11th June 2025).
3. Ahmed, N., Ford, G. A., Kaste, M., Lees, K. R., et al. (2009). *Relationship of Blood Pressure, Antihypertensive Therapy, And Outcome in Ischemic Stroke Treated with Intravenous Thrombolysis: Retrospective Analysis from Safe Implementation of Thrombolysis in Stroke-International Stroke Thrombolysis Register (SITS-ISTR)*. https://core.ac.uk/download/110121.pdf (accessed on 11th June 2025).
4. Akrom, A., Dania, H., O. M., S., Saputri, Y., et al. (2019). Validation of diabetes mellitus patient behavior questionnaire in primary health care service. https://core.ac.uk/download/480550032.pdf (accessed on 11th June 2025).
5. Alsaad, S., Binmoammar, T., Hassounah, S. O. A., Majeed, F. A., et al. (2015). The impact of poor glycemic control on the prevalence of erectile dysfunction in men with type 2 diabetes mellitus: A systematic review. https://core.ac.uk/download/77006748.pdf (accessed on 11th June 2025).
6. Alsweiler, J., Brown, J., Crowther, C. A., Downie, A. B., et al. (2018). Treatments for women with gestational diabetes mellitus: An overview of Cochrane systematic reviews. https://core.ac.uk/download/187724799.pdf (accessed on 11th June 2025).
7. Angleman, S., Fratiglioni, L., & Marengoni, A. (2011). Prevalence of disability according to multimorbidity and disease clustering: A population-based study. https://core.ac.uk/download/pdf/29572301.pdf (accessed on 11th June 2025).
8. Aristimuño, G., Benetos, A., Blacher, J., Chaturvedi, N., Chobanian, A., Conroy, R. M., Drukteinis, A., et al. (2008). Risk factors and target organ damage: Is there a special case for prehypertension? https://core.ac.uk/download/1395617.pdf (accessed on 11th June 2025).
9. Awdishu, L., Singh, R. F., Saunders, I., Yam, F. K., Hirsch, J. D., Lorentz, S., Atayee, R. S., Ma, J. D., Tsunoda, S. M., Namba, J., Mnatzaganian, C. L., Painter, N. A., Watanabe, J. H., Lee, K. C., Daniels, C. D., & Morello, C. M. (2019). Advancing Pharmacist Collaborative Care within Academic Health Systems. *Pharmacy (Basel, Switzerland)*, *7*(4), 142. https://doi.org/10.3390/pharmacy7040142(accessed on 11th June 2025).
10. Aubert, G., Busetto, L., Butz, S., Kenyon, C. J., Contreras, R., Cowley, M. A., De la Sieera, C., et al. (2003). Transgenic amplification of glucocorticoid action in adipose tissue causes high blood pressure in mice. https://core.ac.uk/download/20448745.pdf (accessed on 11th June 2025).
11. Auerbach, A. D., Bachman, D. J., Baer, D. M., Benaroia, M., Bowling, C. B., Bruce, B., Bulpitt, C. J., et al. (2017). Computer-assisted versus oral-and-written history taking for the prevention and management of cardiovascular disease: A systematic review of the literature. https://core.ac.uk/download/151170821.pdf (accessed on 11th June 2025).
12. Awdishu, L., Moore, T., Morrison, M., Trzebinska, A., et al. (2019). A primer on quality assurance

and performance improvement for interprofessional chronic kidney disease care: A path to Joint Commission certification. https://core.ac.uk/download/323064308.pdf (accessed on 11th June 2025).

13. Bae, S., Kurian, A. K., Lykens, K., Singh, A., et al. (2012). Racial and ethnic differences in cardiovascular disease risk factors in U.S. older women: Findings from Behavioral Risk Factor Surveillance Survey, 2003 & 2004. https://digitalscholarship.unlv.edu/cgi/viewcontent.cgi?article=1086&context=jhdrp (accessed on 11th June 2025).
14. Barbot, M., Ceccato, F., & Scaroni, C. (2019). The pathophysiology and treatment of hypertension in patients with Cushing's syndrome. https://core.ac.uk/download/211056096.pdf (accessed on 11th June 2025).
15. Al-Daghri NM, Bindahman LS, Al-Attas OS, Saleem TH, Alokail MS, Alkharfy KM, et al. (2012) Increased Circulating ANG II and TNF-α Represents Important Risk Factors in Obese Saudi Adults with Hypertension Irrespective of Diabetic Status and BMI. PLoS ONE 7(12): e51255. https://doi.org/10.1371/journal.pone.0051255(accessed on 11th June 2025).
16. Bertakis, K. D., Franks, P., & Jerant, A. (2015). Body mass index and health care utilization in diabetic and nondiabetic individuals. https://core.ac.uk/download/323069407.pdf (accessed on 11th June 2025).
17. Biller, B. M. K., Colao, A., De Martino, M. C., Isidori, A., et al. (2016). *Complications of Cushing's Syndrome: State of the Art.* https://core.ac.uk/download/54532161.pdf (accessed on 11th June 2025).
18. Bilo, H. J. G., Groenier, K. H., Houweling, S. T., Kleefstra, N., et al. (2006). Pitfalls in blood pressure measurement in daily practice. https://core.ac.uk/download/pdf/12919819.pdf (accessed on 11th June 2025).
19. Bland, R., Hills, C. E., & Squires, P. E. (2009). SGK1 in the kidney: Disrupted sodium transport in diabetes and beyond. https://core.ac.uk/download/20442635.pdf (accessed on 11th June 2025).
20. Borghi, C., Grassi, G., Rosei, E. A., Savoia, C., et al. (2017). Personalized medicine—A modern approach for the diagnosis and management of hypertension. https://core.ac.uk/download/96884785.pdf (accessed on 11th June 2025).
21. Bosworth, H. B., Heisler, M. M., Hofer, T. P., Hogan, M. M., et al. (2010). Study protocol: The Adherence and Intensification of Medications (AIM) study–A cluster randomized controlled effectiveness study. https://core.ac.uk/download/pdf/8472048.pdf (accessed on 11th June 2025).
22. Budoff, M., Cademartiri, F., Diederichsen, A., Gueret, P., et al. (2017). Diabetes and male sex are key risk factor correlates of the extent of coronary artery calcification: A Euro-CCAD study. https://core.ac.uk/download/287622217.pdf (accessed on 11th June 2025).
23. Helleputte, S., De Backer, T., Lapauw, B., Shadid, S., Celie, B., Van Eetvelde, B., Vanden Wyngaert, K., & Calders, P. (2020). The relationship between glycaemic variability and cardiovascular autonomic dysfunction in patients with type 1 diabetes: A systematic review. *Diabetes/metabolism research and reviews*, *36*(5), e3301. https://doi.org/10.1002/dmrr.3301(accessed on 11th June 2025).
24. Cappuccio, F., Kerry, S. M., Oakeshott, P., Strazzullo, P., et al. (2002). Application of Framingham

risk estimates to ethnic minorities in United Kingdom and implications for primary prevention of heart disease in general practice: Cross sectional population-based study. https://core.ac.uk/download/44322.pdf (accessed on 11th June 2025).

25. Cheung, B. M. Y. (2002). Blockade of the renin-angiotensin system. https://core.ac.uk/download/37883952.pdf (accessed on 11th June 2025).

26. Ciccarese, P., Kumar, A., Piazza, M., Smith, B., et al. (2004). Context-based task ontologies for clinical guidelines. https://core.ac.uk/download/131212561.pdf (accessed on 11th June 2025).

27. Ware, Lisa & Rennie, Kirsten & Gafane-Matemane, Lebo & Collard, Jade & Nell, Tarryn & Schutte, Aletta. (2014). Physical activity and hypertension in South African adults. Conference: Society for Endocrinology, Metabolism and Diabetes South Africa 2014 Annual Scientific MeetingAt: Durban, South Africa(accessed on 11th June 2025).

28. Cosentino, F., & Guzik, T. J. (2018). Epigenetics and immunometabolism in diabetes and aging. https://core.ac.uk/download/153371255.pdf (accessed on 11th June 2025).

29. Cruickshank, K., Du, X., Holmes, S., McNamee, R., et al. (1997). Case-control study of stroke and the quality of hypertension control in north west England. https://core.ac.uk/download/1667396.pdf (accessed on 11th June 2025).

30. Cześnikiewicz-Guzik, M., Dróżdż, M., Filip, M., Guzik, T., et al. (2014). Denture-related stomatitis is associated with endothelial dysfunction. https://core.ac.uk/download/42353840.pdf (accessed on 11th June 2025).

31. Dent, T., Greenhalgh, T., Mathur, R., Meads, C., et al. (2011). Risk models and scores for type 2 diabetes: Systematic review. https://core.ac.uk/download/20271037.pdf (accessed on 11th June 2025).

32. Stafford, J. M., & Elasy, T. (2007). Treatment update: thiazolidinediones in combination with metformin for the treatment of type 2 diabetes. *Vascular health and risk management, 3*(4), 503–510.(accessed on 11th June 2025).

33. Foering, A. (2018). Pediatric type II diabetes mellitus: Examining the upward trend. https://core.ac.uk/download/158970346.pdf (accessed on 11th June 2025).

34. Gailey, A., Goldman, D., Lakdawalla, D., Michaud, P. C., & Zheng, Y. (2025). International differences in longevity and health and their economic consequences. https://core.ac.uk/download/pdf/6354917.pdf (accessed on 11th June 2025).

35. Guzik, T. J., Petrie, J. R., & Touyz, R. M. (2018). Diabetes, hypertension, and cardiovascular disease: Clinical insights and vascular mechanisms. https://core.ac.uk/download/153444565.pdf (accessed on 11th June 2025).

36. Harries, A. D., Harries, A. D., Harries, A. D., Daar, A. S., Janssens, B., Maher, D., Maher, D., et al. (2009). A global framework for action to improve the primary care response to chronic non-communicable diseases: A solution to a neglected problem. https://core.ac.uk/download/pdf/9417460.pdf (accessed on 11th June 2025).

37. Hazlehurst, B. L., Sittig, D. F., Kind, E. A., Krizak, J. T., Fowles, J. B., Weiner, J. P., Chan, K. S., et al. (2008). Performance measures using electronic health records: Five case studies. https://core.ac.uk/download/71353765.pdf (accessed on 11th June 2025).

38. Heier, M., Karl, F. M., Laxy, M., Mess, F., et al. (2019). Change in physical activity after diagnosis

of diabetes or hypertension: Results from an observational population-based cohort study. https://core.ac.uk/download/343309156.pdf (accessed on 11th June 2025).

39. Hidayah, A. N., Pauzi, R. Y., Setyanto, M. R., Wahyudin, A., et al. (2025). The relationship between blood pressure and blood sugar levels: The moderating role of age and gender. https://core.ac.uk/download/641608741.pdf (accessed on 11th June 2025).

40. Kautzky-Willer, A., Stich, K., Hintersteiner, J., Kautzky, A., Kamyar, M. R., Saukel, J., Johnson, J., & Lemmens-Gruber, R. (2013). Sex-specific-differences in cardiometabolic risk in type 1 diabetes: a cross-sectional study. *Cardiovascular diabetology, 12*, 78. https://doi.org/10.1186/1475-2840-12-78 (accessed on 11th June 2025).

41. Iacobini, C., Menini, S., Pesce, C., Pugliese, G., et al. (2017). Dietary interventions to contrast the onset and progression of diabetic nephropathy: A critical survey of new data. https://core.ac.uk/download/80314820.pdf (accessed on 11th June 2025).

42. Irsath, S. (2015). Predictors of diabetic retinopathy in patients with type 2 diabetes mellitus with normoalbuminuria. https://core.ac.uk/download/235667486.pdf (accessed on 11th June 2025).

43. Jain, M., Kiyawat, P., & Sarkar, U. K. (2018). Echocardiographic evaluation of diastolic dysfunction in type 2 diabetes mellitus with normal systolic function and correlation with duration of diabetes mellitus and HbA1C. https://core.ac.uk/download/539911997.pdf (accessed on 11th June 2025).

44. Jeanne, A. (2024). Obesity, hypertension, and type 2 diabetes: Assessment and pathophysiological interconnections. *Research Invention Journal of Scientific and Experimental Sciences*. https://www.semanticscholar.org/paper/7ef0da51b013f74e39da1e2e05ba58bcfc5ab84b (accessed on 11th June 2025).

45. Jha, M. (2024). Insulin-induced weight gain as a potential risk factor for cardiovascular disease: A narrative review. https://core.ac.uk/download/618348877.pdf (accessed on 11th June 2025).

46. Jones, K. M., Lannon, S. M., Raglan, G. B., Schulkin, J., et al. (2015). Obstetrician-gynecologists' knowledge of health disparities and barriers among American Indian/Alaska Native women in Washington State. https://digitalscholarship.unlv.edu/cgi/viewcontent.cgi?article=1352&context=jhdrp (accessed on 11th June 2025).

47. Kapke, D. R. (2015). Childhood type II diabetes: The risks and complications. https://core.ac.uk/download/58826199.pdf (accessed on 11th June 2025).

48. Kitsiou, A., Caforio, A. L. P., Porta-Sanchez, A., Vahanian, A., Iung, B., Carrera, C., Szymanski, C., et al. (2013). *ESC Core Curriculum for The General Cardiologist (2013)*. https://core.ac.uk/download/55756305.pdf (accessed on 11th June 2025).

49. Koval, A. M., Nakamura, M., Newman, J. D., Schwartz, J., et al. (2013). Cost-effectiveness of secondary screening modalities for hypertension. https://core.ac.uk/download/161454698.pdf (accessed on 11th June 2025).

50. Kupzyk, K. A., Tran, D. M., & Zimmerman, L. M. (2018). Using cluster analysis to identify subgroups of college students at increased risk for cardiovascular disease. https://digitalscholarship.unlv.edu/cgi/viewcontent.cgi?article=1260&context=nursing_fac_articles (accessed on 11th June 2025).

51. Marjina., Narang, R. K., Sharma, A., et al. (2020). Management of hypertension with conventional and herbals drugs. https://core.ac.uk/download/328146104.pdf (accessed on 11th June 2025).

52. Motala, A. A., Swai, A. B., Perry, A. C., Muhihi, A., Walker, A. R., Filmer, D., Hu, D., et al. (2009). Gender-related differences in the prevalence of cardiovascular disease risk factors and their correlates in urban Tanzania. https://core.ac.uk/download/pdf/11307378.pdf (accessed on 11th June 2025).

53. Pop, C., Petriş, A., Pop, L., & David, L. (2025). Pillars of blood pressure management in patients with type 2 diabetes mellitus: Insights from recent trials and emerging perspectives. *Journal of Clinical Medicine, 14*. https://www.semanticscholar.org/paper/779821cafb6671ada656000621cda7d628b88e61 (accessed on 11th June 2025).

54. Savoy, J., Thorpe, R. J. Jr. (2019). Examining race differences in blood pressure control among people with chronic kidney disease. https://digitalscholarship.unlv.edu/cgi/viewcontent.cgi?article=1932&context=jhdrp (accessed on 11th June 2025).

55. Silverstein, J. M. (2016). Hyperglycemia induced by pareptide in patients with Cushing's disease or acromegaly. https://core.ac.uk/download/83100992.pdf (accessed on 11th June 2025).

56. Vaismoradi, M. (2022). Effectiveness of community pharmacy diabetes and hypertension care program: An unexplored opportunity for community pharmacists in Pakistan. https://core.ac.uk/download/519702227.pdf (accessed on 11th June 2025).

INDEX

D

E

F

G

S

T

U

V

W